BROCA'S REGION

BROCA'S REGION

EDITED BY

Yosef Grodzinsky

Katrin Amunts

OXFORD

UNIVERSITY PRESS

2006

Oxford University Press

Oxford University Press, Inc., publishes works that further
Oxford University's objective of excellence
in research, scholarship, and education.

Oxford   New York
Auckland   Cape Town   Dar es Salaam   Hong Kong   Karachi
Kuala Lumpur   Madrid   Melbourne   Mexico City   Nairobi
New Delhi   Shanghai   Taipei   Toronto

With offices in
Argentina   Austria   Brazil   Chile   Czech Republic   France   Greece
Guatemala   Hungary   Italy   Japan   Poland   Portugal   Singapore
South Korea   Switzerland   Thailand   Turkey   Ukraine   Vietnam

Published by Oxford University Press, Inc.
198 Madison Avenue, New York, New York 10016
www.oup.com

Oxford is a registered trademark of Oxford University Press

Library of Congress Cataloging-in-Publication Data

Broca's region / edited by Yosef Grodzinsky, Katrin Amunts.
p. cm.
Includes bibliographical references and index.
ISBN-13 978-0-19-517764-0
ISBN 0-19-517764-9
1. Broca, Paul, 1824–1880. 2. Neurolinguistics. 3. Psycholinguistics. 4. Frontal
lobes. 5. Sign language. 6. Aphasia. I. Grodzinsky, Yosef. II. Amunts, Katrin.
QP399.B76 2005
612.8'2336—dc22   2004023816

1 3 5 7 9 8 6 4 2

Printed in the United States of America
on acid-free paper

Contents

Contributors

FRANCISCO ABOITIZ
Departamento de Psiquiatría
Escuela de Medicina
Pontificia Universidad Católica de Chile
Santiago
Chile
faboitiz@puc.cl

KATRIN AMUNTS
Brain Mapping
Institut für Medizin
Forschungszentrum Jülich
Jülich
Germany
k.amunts@fz-juelich.de

MICHAEL ARBIB
Computer Science Department
Neuroscience Program and USC Brain Project
University of Southern California
Los Angeles, CA
arbib@pollux.usc.edu

SERGEY AVRUTIN
UiL OTS
Utrecht University
Utrecht
The Netherlands
Sergey.Avrutin@let.uu.nl

CONRADO BOSMAN
Departamento de Psiquiatría
Escuela de Medicina
Pontificia Universidad Católica de Chile
Santiago
Chile
cabosman@puc.cl

ENZO BRUNETTI
Departamento de Psiquiatría
Escuela de Medicina
Pontificia Universidad Católica de Chile
Santiago
Chile
ebrunnet@canela.med.uchile.cl

STEFANO F. CAPPA
Università Vita Salute and Istituto Scientifico
  San Raffaele
Milano
Italy
stefano.cappa@hsr.it

LAILA CRAIGHERO
Department of Biomedical Sciences
Section of Human Physiology
University of Ferrara
Ferrara
Italy
laila.craighero@unife.it

DAN DRAI
Weizmann Institute of Science
Rehovot
Israel
DanDrai@gmail.com

KAREN EMMOREY
Director
Laboratory for Language and Cognitive
  Neuroscience
San Diego State University
San Diego, CA
kemmory@mail.sdsu.edu

LUCIANO FADIGA
Department of Biomedical Sciences
Section of Human Physiology
University of Ferrara
Ferrara
Italy
luciano.fadiga@unife.it

GEREON R. FINK
Kognitive Neurologie
Institut für Medizin
Forschungzentrum Jülich
Jülich
Germany
g.fink@fz-juelich.de

ANGELA D. FRIEDERICI
Max Planck Institute for Human Cognitive and
  Brain Sciences
Leipzig
Germany
angelafr@cbs.mpg.de

NAAMA FRIEDMANN
School of Education
Tel Aviv University
Tel Aviv
Israel
naamafr@post.tau.ac.il

RICARDO GARCÍA
Departamento de Psiquiatría
Escuela de Medicina
Pontificia Universidad Católica de Chile
Santiago
Chile
rgarcia@med.puc.cl

YOSEF GRODZINSKY
Department of Linguistics
McGill University
Montreal, Quebec
Canada
Yosef.grodzinsky@mcgill.ca

JENNIFER M. GURD
Department of Psychology
University of Hertfordshire
Hatfield
United Kingdom
and
Neuropsychology Unit
University Department of Clinical Neurology
Radcliffe Infirmary
Oxford
United Kingdom
jennifer.gurd@clinical-neurology.ox.ac.uk

PETER HAGOORT
F.C. Donders Centre for Cognitive Neuroimaging
Nijmegen
The Netherlands
peter.hagoort@fcdonders.ru.nl

LUTZ JÄNCKE
Department of Neuropsychology
Institute for Psychology
University of Zürich
Zürich
Switzerland
ljaencke@psychologie.unizh.ch

KYLE JOHNSON
Department of Linguistics
University of Massachusetts
Amherst, MA
kbj@linguist.vmass.edu

ZINA M. MANJALY
Kognitive Neurologie
Institut für Medizin
Forschungzentrum Jülich
Jülich
Germany
z.manjaly@fz-juelich.de

JOHN C. MARSHALL
Neuropsychology Unit
University Department of Clinical Neurology
Radcliffe Infirmary
Oxford
UK
john.marshall@clinical-neurology.ox.ac.uk

MARTIN E. MEYER
Department of Neuropsychology
Institute for Psychology
University of Zürich
Zürich
Switzerland
mmeyer@access.unizh.ch

DANIELA PERANI
Università Vita Salute and Istituto Scientifico
    San Raffaele
Milano
Italy
daniela.perani@hsr.it

MICHAEL PETRIDES
Montreal Neurological Institute
McGill University
Montreal, Quebec
Canada
michael.petrides@mcgill.ca

ALICE ROY
Department of Biomedical Sciences
Section of Human Physiology
University of Ferrara
Ferrara
Italy
alice.roy@unife.it

LEWIS P. SHAPIRO
San Diego State University
School of Speech, Language, and Hearing
    Sciences
San Diego, CA
shapiro@mail.sdsu.edu

KLAAS E. STEPHAN, MD
Wellcome Department of Imaging Neuroscience
Institute of Neurology
University College London
London
UK
kstephan@fil.ion.ucl.ac.uk

CYNTHIA K. THOMPSON
Northwestern University
Communication Sciences and Disorders
Evanston, IL
ckthom@northwestern.edu

KARL ZILLES
Institut für Medizin
Forschungzentrum Jülich
Jülich
Germany
and
C. and O.Vogt für Hirnforschungs Institut
Heinrich-Heine-Universität
Düsseldorf, Germany
k.zilles@fz-juelich.de

Introduction

Broca's region has been in the news ever since scientists first hit upon the idea that particular cognitive functions can be localized to parts of the cerebral cortex. Its discoverer, Paul Broca, was one of the first scientists to argue that there is a direct connection between a concrete piece of behavior—in this case, the use of language, or what Broca called "articulated speech"—and a specific cortical region. Today, Broca's region is probably the most famous part of the human brain: it is featured in virtually every introductory psychology course and textbook and in many, if not all, introductory anatomy and linguistics courses, and for over a century, it has persisted as the focus of intense research and much debate. The name has even penetrated popular culture, serving as the title for a best-selling popular science book by Carl Sagan.

This region is not famous for nothing: as language is one of the most distinctive human traits, it would seem to follow that the cognitive mechanisms that support it are quite complex, and the tissues in which these mechanisms are housed have interesting characteristics and important implications for how brain function relates to behavior. Thus, Broca's region features prominently in the study of brain–behavior relations.

The first studies of Broca's region focused on language pathologies caused by brain lesions. The results of this early work by Broca, Wernicke, and their contemporaries captivated the public's imagination. Among the language pathologies, Broca's aphasia attracted attention as no other disorder ever had. It even made it to Broadway, through the protagonist of Arthur Kopit's play *Wings*—stroke victim Emily Stilson, an aphasic patient whose compelling plight, as described in the play's synopsis, is that she is "an ex-aviatrix who loses speech . . . and slowly regains power of language and life."

Broca's discoveries were also an important, driving force behind the more general effort to relate complex behavior to particular parts of the cerebral cortex, which, significantly, produced the first brain maps. Incorrect paths such as phrenology notwithstanding, during the heyday of Broca's work, research aimed at identifying the cerebral localization of cognitive function was flourishing and the study of aphasic syndromes was the flagship of neuropsychology. During these early years, the investigation into brain and behavior was based almost solely upon lesion studies. Although researchers were able to analyze lesions at the level of brain macroscopy and functional deficit, this is, unfortunately, where their analyses ended. On an anatomical level, researchers were not aware of the underlying principles of cellular dysfunction and disconnectivity, and of the huge amount of variability among different subjects. On a behavioral level, their distinctions were crude because they were not aware of the structural properties of language and cross-linguistic variation.

Although much has been discovered since Broca claimed that the region contains "the faculty of articulated language," even today, these problems have not been completely solved. Technological advancements have made more detailed studies possible, but there is still no general agreement among anatomists on what constitutes the underlying microstructure of Broca's region or even on the name of the region itself. In the early twentieth century, anatomists distinguished a strict sense of Broca's region from the more general sense of it. Just to make matters perfectly confusing, later researchers also referred to this particular piece of neural tissue as Broca's area and Broca's complex. The term "Broca's area" seems to be misleading because it suggests that it is a single entity, characterized by a certain homogeneity in structure, connectivity, and function (almost as if it were a Brodmann area), whereas it has become increasingly clear that it actually includes cortical areas with different functional specializations and connectivity.

In an analogous situation, there is also no general agreement on how the cognitive functions related to Broca's region should be characterized. It is, however, quite clear that modality-based divisions of the type found in standard neurology texts—speaking, understanding, repeating, naming, and so on—are not good enough units of measure and that creating divisions based on either psychological mechanisms or linguistically motivated concepts also fails to tell the whole story.

If it is so difficult to come to an understanding of each of these things alone, then how can we so easily claim that the anatomy and functional role of this part of the brain are related to each other? Initially established as the exclusive domain of clinical neurologists, the study of brain/language relations increasingly required deeper expertise in specialized domains. The field was transformed when psychologists entered with experimental methods and linguists entered with analytic categories and theoretical conceptions. Later, when new methods has been developed, neuroscientists, biomedical engineers, and computer scientists became interested. Today, particularly as a result of important advances made in neuroimaging during the past two decades, Broca's region and, for that matter, all language areas are being investigated from every angle from which we can manage to approach them.

The careers of the editors of this volume illustrate the phenomenon: Our long-term research program has always focused on Broca's region, and we currently use fMRI as a method of investigation. However, while one of us studies the structure of this region primarily by looking at cells, cellular architecture, cortical layers, and borders, the other editor is primarily concerned with words, phrases, sentences, and grammatical rules and the way in which they are instantiated in neural tissue.

Indeed, as the volume of research into the relations between brain and language has created several communities, each importing its own concepts, methods, and considerations, we thought that it was time to stop and reflect together, and that is the purpose of this book. In it, we tried to do what is generally considered to be nearly impossible: to mix intellectual traditions and cultures and to juxtapose rather disparate bodies of knowledge, styles of reasoning, and forms of argumentation. At the same time, we made every effort to produce a book that is both relevant and accessible to a broad audience.

To this end, we invited scientists with diverse backgrounds to contribute their particular take at the Broca's Region Workshop, hoping that a coherent and perhaps even a novel picture would emerge. Although the participants share a special interest in Broca's region, their backgrounds and approaches—neuroanatomy, physiology, evolutionary biology, cognitive psychology, clinical neurology, functional imaging, speech and language research, computational biology, and psychological, neurological, and theoretical linguistics—represent all the myriad angles from which we currently approach Broca's region.

We met at the Forschungszentrum in Juelich, Germany, on June 4 through 6, 2004. As one would expect, the meeting was unusual. At times it became tense, but it was never dull. We are happy to report that it reflected a genuine effort on everyone's part to listen, accommodate, and, most of all, understand.

We offer the readers of this volume the product of our Broca's Region Workshop—contributions made by the participants and their research teams, amended after they were presented to the workshop's diverse audience. To underscore the richness of viewpoints contained herein and to give readers an idea of the level of interaction that took place, we have included parts of the discussion that we recorded during the workshop. Because Broca's region is such an historically significant concept and rich area, we added a collection of classic and recent-yet-classic papers. Along with cutting-edge science, we wish to remind readers of the celebrated past from which much may be learned. These historical chapters include the first two papers written by Paul Broca, as well as some work by two of the most important neurologists of the nineteenth century, Carl Wernicke and John Hughlings-Jackson. We also included parts of twentieth-century papers by Korbinian Brodmann, Norman Geschwind, Harold Goodglass, Roman Jakobson, Jay Mohr, and Arnold Pick.

The resulting volume, we believe, reflects the state of the art. We hope that it will stimulate more interdisciplinary work, as the project called "Broca's region," which encompasses the study of brain/language relations, is far from being finished.

We are grateful to the speakers/contributors, who helped bring the workshop and book to life. We were supported by Oxford University Press, with Catharine Carlin at the wheel; by the Forschungszentrum Juelich GmbH, the chairman of its board of directors, Joachim Treusch, and the director of its Institute of Medicine, Karl Zilles; and by the Centre for Research on Language, Brain, and Mind at McGill University, and its director, Shari Baum. We would also like to thank Katie Clark and Andrea Santi for their help. Without these individuals and organizations, neither the workshop nor the book would ever have happened. Their help and generosity were invaluable in creating and carrying out this project.

Katrin Amunts
Yosef Grodzinsky

I

MATTERS ANATOMICAL

1

The Origin of Broca's Area and Its Connections from an Ancestral Working Memory Network

Francisco Aboitiz

Ricardo García

Enzo Brunetti

Conrado Bosman

Language has been historically considered the hallmark of human uniqueness. Darwin (1871) proposed a species-specific, instinctive tendency to acquire language (Pinker, 1995, p. 20) but never ventured to propose a detailed account of evolutionary language origins. Not long before Darwin's publication, Paul Broca (1861) had presented the brain of his patient Tan to the *Société d' Anthropologie* in Paris, which firmly established the role of the left inferior frontal lobe in language production. Relatively soon after Broca, Carl Wernicke (1874) proposed the first anatomical model for language perception and production, which despite many posterior modifications remains roughly valid today. Thus, even if the concepts of human evolution by natural selection and of the localization of the language faculty were quite contemporaries, very little was proposed in the way to understand the evolutionary bases of language origins.

A significant attempt to explain the evolutionary origins of language occurred a century later, when Norman Geschwind (1964) proposed that the ability to give names to objects relied on the capacity to establish cross-modal, corticocortical associations, something that nonhuman primates were apparently unable to do. Subsequent studies showed that apes are able to name objects and actions if trained in sign language (Premack, 1983). Furthermore, recent evidence indicates that word learning—even after single exposure—can occur in the domestic dog (Kaminski et al., 2004). However, the fact remains that apes (and probably dogs) are much slower than humans in learning cross-modal associations and in the ability to learn sign words (Aggleton, 1993; Nahm et al., 1993). Thus, it may seem that the ability to give names, although greatly facilitated in the human species, is based on a neural substrate whose precursor exists in other animals. This is entirely compatible with a gradualistic darwinian interpretation of language origins.

Nevertheless, apes trained in sign language were never able to go beyond a two- or three-word organization in their utterances and definitely lacked any hint of grammatical organization. This evidence strengthened the contemporary theory of universal grammar, prescribing that all languages share common combinatorial principles that are genetically determined and unique with regard to other cognitive processes found in humans and other animals (Chomsky, 1978). One important observation regarding the innateness of language is that while learning language, children may produce complex grammatical utterances that they apparently never heard before. This supports a genetic tendency to learn language in our species. Furthermore, Chomsky has argued that because no hints of syntax precursors are found in nonhuman animals, syntax most likely arose in evolution as the result of a single biological macromutation. Nevertheless, gradualistic interpretations for the origins of syntactic rules have been proposed in the latest years (Dennett, 1995; Pinker, 1995; Pinker and Bloom, 1990), partly based on observations on how children acquire grammatical rules.

Many authors have located syntactical processing in Broca's area (corresponding to Brodmann's areas 44 and 45) (Embick et al., 2000). However, studies indicate that Broca's area participates in several other neurocognitive processes, including working memory, gesture recognition, mirror drawing, and aspects of musical analysis (Bookheimer 2002; Dronkers et al., 1992; Gruber, 2002; Maess et al., 2001; Patel, 2003; Rizzolatti et al., 1992). Of particular interest is the finding of "mirror neurons" in the inferior frontal lobe, which participate in the recognition of one's own actions and of actions performed by others in the human and monkey ventral premotor cortex (Gallese et al., 1996; Iacoboni et al., 1999; Rizzolatti et al., 1996, 2002); these have been proposed to be the phylogenetic precursors of Broca's language area (Arbib and Bota, 2003; Rizzolatti and Arbib, 1998). An additional issue is that damage to Broca's area alone usually does not produce long-lasting severe aphasia; the surrounding areas and underlying white matter must be damaged as well (Dronkers et al., 1992; Pinker, 1995). In this context, we (Aboitiz, 1995; Aboitiz and García, 1997) originally proposed that the neural device involved in language comprehension and production is not isolated from the rest of the brain. Rather, this system belongs to a large-scale corticocortical network reciprocally connecting higher-order areas in the temporoparietal lobes with prefrontal areas (other components such as the basal ganglia and certain thalamic nuclei may also participate). Among the functions of this overall network are several processes that require sustained neural activity for intervals of a few seconds or longer, such as attention, language, imitation, and especially working memory.

In this chapter, we provide an updated version of this theory. Since our original proposal, much neuroanatomical, neuroimaging, and neurolinguistic evidence has accumulated that calls for a revision of some of the issues presented in those times. In particular, neuroanatomical findings on animals and imaging studies in humans, especially on linguistic working memory, have revealed a much finer-grained picture of the anatomy and connectivity of the language areas and its nonhuman homologues and of their function in the human brain. We begin with a brief overview of our original proposals and then discuss new evidence from comparative neuroanatomy, brain imaging, and cognitive neuroscience, to end with a discussion on the possible role of neuropsychological processes like working memory in semantic and syntactic processing.

OVERVIEW OF THE ORIGINAL HYPOTHESIS

In our original articles (Aboitiz, 1995; Aboitiz and García, 1997a, b), we placed special emphasis on working memory, a specific form of short-term memory that maintains perceptual information and long-term memory online while executing a certain cognitive task (Baddeley, 1992; Baddeley and Hitch, 1974). Like the language network, the neural system for working memory relies on extensive temporoparietal–prefrontal connections. Working memory has been proposed to be subdivided into a general, all-purpose executive system and "slave" systems involved in sensorimotor rehearsal: one of such systems is the visuospatial sketchpad, which maintains online visuospatial information, and the other is the phonological loop, allowing internal rehearsal of phonological utterances. However, sensorimotor working memory networks may be more complex than just a visuospatial sketchpad and a phonological loop; there are probably subdivisions in these components, as well as additional components involving other perceptual and processing domains (Levy and Goldman-Rakic, 2000; Romanski et al., 1999a). We suggested that the phonological loop in particular may have been essential to early language origins, in the sense that it participated in learning complex utterances that were acquired by imitation. A circuit involving inferior parietal, intraparietal, and inferior frontal areas (including Broca's area) differentiated into a working memory device involved in the imitation and internal rehearsal of complex vocalizations. This is not to exclude gestural communication, which may have co-occurred with these early vocalizations. However, in early hominids, there were limits to the complexity of utterances that could be learned. The increase in brain size was related to the development of more complex neuronal networks, allowing the generation of elaborate vocal utterances with primitive syntactic rules (Aboitiz, 1988, 1996). Initially, the language areas were able to coordinate phonemes and morphemes into primitive words, and eventually some sequences of words. Shortly, our claim is that the language areas originated from a primitive working memory device involved in the imitation of complex utterances, which eventually served as a template from which brain organization for modern language evolved. Language processing requires a very efficient working memory system, in terms of phonology, syntax, and meaning. In this sense, additional working memory circuits were subsequently recruited in the evolution of human communication, producing the structural and semantic complexities of modern language.

CONNECTIVITY AND HOMOLOGY ISSUES

As mentioned earlier, a major issue in our proposal concerns the structural similarity of language-related networks and the networks involved in working memory. Because connectivity studies cannot be performed in humans, neuroscientists have had to rely in nonhuman primates to study these neural projections. However, cortical areas in the monkey and human are not easily comparable, and a major problem has been to establish specific nonhuman homologies for the language areas. In our original article (Aboitiz and García, 1997a), we tentatively proposed a framework for homology between the human language areas and their primate counterparts based on the available evidence at that time (Barbas and Pandya, 1989; Preuss and Goldman-Rakic, 1991a). Shortly, we followed Preuss and Golman-Rakic (1991a) in their suggestion of an area 45 inside the macaque's inferior arcuate sulcus, between subareas 6V and 8Ar, and proposed that Broca's region could be conceived as a differentiation of the ventral premotor region (ventral

area 6 of the monkey). In the human, we suggested the existence of a network connecting Broca's area (areas 44 and 45) and frontal granular cortex (areas 9 and 46) with regions in the superior temporal lobe (specifically, area Tpt in the posterior superior temporal gyrus and, to a lesser extent, area TE), and we emphasized connections between the supramarginal gyrus (more specifically, area 40) and Broca's area. The latter proposal was mainly based on previous findings in the monkey, indicating connections from intraparietal (7ip) and inferior parietal (7b) areas to the anterior and the posterior banks of the inferior arcuate sulcus, respectively (Cavada and Goldman-Rakic, 1989; Petrides and Pandya, 1984; Preuss and Goldman-Rakic, 1991a, b, c). Although area Tpt was found to project strongly to the dorsal moiety of the arcuate sulcus (Petrides and Pandya, 1988), it was also observed sending projections to the inferior arcuate sulcus (Deacon, 1992).

In the past years, much evidence has appeared regarding the cytoarchitecture and connectivity of these areas, which, although implying modifications to our proposed scheme, confirms its main points of a Broca's area homolog in the inferior bank of the arcuate sulcus with strong connections with the superior temporal, intraparietal, and inferior parietal regions (see Fig. 3 in Aboitiz and García, 1997a). Connections of intraparietal and inferoparietal regions with area 45 and the inferior arcuate sulcus have been confirmed (Lewis and Van Essen, 2000; Preuss and Goldman-Rakic, 1991a). Nevertheless, a reconsideration of this scheme, claiming a parallel segregation of the prefrontal–temporoparietal projections to Broca's area, has come from additional data associated with physiological and anatomical refinements of the primate auditory cortical system (Kaas and Hackett, 2000; Romanski and Goldman-Rakic, 2001; Romanski et al, 1999a, b). This evidence is reviewed later.

The current understanding of the anatomical organization of the auditory cortex specifies a concentric organization, with a core region containing the primary auditory area and other rostral areas, a belt region surrounding the core region, and a more lateral, parabelt region (Hackett et al., 1998). Very interestingly, and in analogy with the visual system, two different processing streams have been identified in the primate auditory cortex, one projecting caudally and more involved with spatial auditory information (the "where" stream), and the other projecting rostrally and processing the intrinsic features of auditory stimuli including speech (the "what" stream) (Kaas and Hackett, 1999; Tian et al., 2001). Supporting this evidence, the injection of retrograde and anterograde tracers into several areas of prefrontal cortex has shown a rostrocaudal gradient of reciprocal cortical connectivity between prefrontal regions and belt and parabelt auditory association areas (Romanski et al., 1999a). Thus, rostral and orbital regions of prefrontal cortex are connected with rostral belt and parabelt areas, whereas caudal regions in the sulcus principalis and the inferior convexity of the prefrontal cortex are reciprocally connected with caudal belt and parabelt auditory association areas. More specifically, the "where" pathway projects mainly to prearcuate areas 8a and 46, and the "what" pathway projects to the frontal pole (area 10), the rostral principal sulcus (area 46), and the ventral prefrontal cortex (areas 12 and 45) (Hackett et al., 1999; Rauschecker and Tian, 2000; Romanski et al., 1999a, 1999b). Furthermore, Romanski and Goldman-Rakic (2002) identified an auditory domain in the monkey prefrontal cortex, located in areas 12lat, 12orb, and 45 (which receive projections from the "what" pathway), in which most neurons preferred vocalizations than other acoustic stimuli, whereas some neurons were also responsive to visual stimuli. In general, the caudal parabelt ("where") provides auditory projections to the region related to directing eye movements and to the dorsal prefrontal cortex, and the rostral parabelt ("what") projects to the ventral/orbital prefrontal cortex and the granular frontal cortex, perhaps more related to the human Broca's area.

Area Tpt, located in the posterior superior temporal gyrus, deserves some special consideration. This area was originally described by Pandya and Sanides (1973) and by Galaburda and Sanides (1980) in the macaque and the human, respectively. Considering its relation to the human planum temporale, this area was considered to be an integral element of Wernicke's posterior language area (Galaburda et al., 1978). On the other hand, according to the concentric belt–parabelt array proposed by Hackett et al. (1998), area Tpt is located near the posterolateral parabelt region and topographically close to the "where" stream. We see later that although this area projects to dorsal and ventral aspects of the prefrontal cortex, its emphasis is to more dorsal areas, consistent with the projections of the caudal parabelt. Furthermore,

recent analyses indicate that more than being a language-specific area, the planum temporale (and perhaps, consequently, area Tpt) is related to the analysis of many types of spectrally complex sounds, working as a node (a "hub") that distributes projections to several higher-order areas (Binder et al., 1996; Griffiths and Warren, 2002).

Another topographic and connectional scheme is that provided by Petrides and Pandya (1994, 1999, 2001). These authors considered that the macaque area 45 (comparable to the human area 45 because it displays large pyramidal neurons in layer IIIc, a well-defined layer IV, and medium-size neurons in layer V) could be subdivided into areas 45A and 45B, which are different from the more dorsally located frontal eye fields. Importantly, they describe a dysgranular area 44 in the caudal bank of the lower limb of the arcuate sulcus, adjacent to area 45B. In addition, areas 47 and 12 were considered to correspond to human area 47, sharing with area 45 a complex, multimodal input. Nevertheless, area 47/12 receives more heavy projections from rostral inferotemporal visual areas and temporal limbic areas, whereas area 45 receives input from the superior temporal gyrus (including area Tpt) and the upper bank of the superior temporal sulcus. It will be important to determine to what extent Petrides and Pandya's (2001) areas 45 and 47/12 relate to Romanski and Goldman-Rakic's (2002) areas 45 and 12lat/12orb, respectively. Area Tpt and other caudal stream auditory areas have an important projection to the more dorsal area 8Ad, which is linked to the parieto-occipital region but is also connected to area 45. Finally, area 46 was found to be smaller than previously thought, being restricted to an anterior part and to the cortex inside the sulcus principalis. The posterior part of area 46 corresponded instead to a part of area 9 and was called area 9/46 (ventral and dorsal).

In our view, this new cumulus of neuroanatomical evidence allows us to refine our early connectional model subserving human language origins (Aboitiz and García, 1997a, b) (Fig. 1–1, see color insert). In fact, the recent data regarding the architecture and prefrontal–temporoparietal connectivity confirm our previous proposal suggesting several pathways running in parallel from inferoparietal and inferotemporal regions to the inferior frontal cortex: first, (1) the inferoparietal and intraparietal zones corresponding to areas 7ip and 7b of the monkey (perhaps partly related

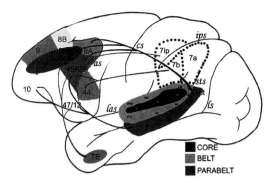

FIGURE 1–1. Diagram indicating some connections between the parietotemporal and the inferior prefrontal areas in the monkey. The auditory region in the superior temporal lobe is subdivided into core, belt, and parabelt regions, and has two main processing streams: the rostral belt and parabelt (the "what" pathway, RTL and RP), which projects to the inferior convexity of the prefrontal lobe; and the caudal belt and parabelt (the "where" pathway, CM, CL, and CP), which projects to more dorsolateral areas. The intraparietal and inferior parietal regions (7ip, 7b) project to the inferior convexity. Numbers indicate Brodmann's areas. Data from Hackett et al. (1998), Romanski et al. (1999a, 1999b), and Petrides and Pandya (2001, 1999). as, arcuate sulcus; cs, central sulcus; ips, intraparietal sulcus; las, lateral sulcus; ls, lunate sulcus; ps, principal sulcus; sts, superior temporal sulcus.

to the gyrus supramarginalis in humans, especially area 7b) connect with the inferior periarcuate region, including area 45. As we have mentioned before, in humans, the inferior parietal region could be connected to the caudal belt region configuring a temporoparietal–prefrontal pathway subserving a phonological–rehearsal loop. However, this connection has not been demonstrated in the monkey. In addition, a dual stream of auditory projections targets distinct prefrontal domains: (2) a spatial "where" pathway connects the caudal belt regions with the caudal dorsolateral prefrontal cortex (areas 8 and 46) including a posterior parietal relay through areas 7ip and 7a, and (3) a "what" stream connects the rostral belt and parabelt regions to the inferior periarcuate convexity where area 45 is located. Finally, there is an inferotemporal projection connecting area TE with area 45 whose function is probably to transmit object relevant information to Broca's area. Note that Petrides

and Pandya (1988, 1994, 1999, 2001) describe a projection from area Tpt, the superior temporal gyrus and the superior temporal sulcus to dorsal frontal areas (related to eye movements) but also to area 45, which receives projections from the "what" pathway (Hackett et al., 1999; Rauschecker and Tian, 2000; Romanski et al., 1999a, b). In this sense, the inferior arcuate sulcus (including area 45) may partly serve as an interface between both the "where" and the "what" streams in the inferior frontal lobe.

A quite recent proposal for macaque homologies with the human language areas was outlined by Arbib and Bota (2003) and was based on Rizzolatti and Arbib's (1998) concept of a mirror system for grasping as the neuronal precursor of Broca's area. These authors propose that a network involving the anterior intraparietal sulcus and ventral premotor area F5 of the macaque anchors a cortical circuit for hand movements and grasping. F5 contains so-called mirror neurons whose activity matches the execution and observation of hand movements. Furthermore, F5 can be subdivided into F5ab, containing "canonical" motor neurons, and F5c, which contains mirror neurons. According to Arbib and Bota, F5 may be compared with human areas 44 and 45, and F5c corresponds to at least part of area 44. Area 45 may contain two subareas: a dorsal one related to the frontal eye fields and a ventral one distinct from the frontal eye fields. Further studies are needed to determine exactly and to what extent areas F5ab and F5c correspond to Petrides and Pandya's (1994) areas 45A, 45B, and 44 and with Romanski and Goldman-Rakic's (2002) areas 45 and 12lat/12orb, respectively. Although it may be premature to propose detailed homologies in these as yet ill-defined regions, this view is in general terms consistent with our proposals. In general, we agree that a region in or surrounding the inferior arcuate sulcus, receiving projections from superior temporal, inferior parietal, and intraparietal areas, may be the best candidate for homology with Broca's area. Because in the human frontal lobe the language-related region extends beyond the boundaries of areas 44 and 45 (Dronkers et al., 1992), it is perhaps advisable to consider the connections of a relatively wide region surrounding the primate inferior arcuate sulcus instead of focusing on the strict homologues of areas 44 and 45. In this chapter, we emphasized these two areas mainly because at this point they are the best known in terms of language processing.

WORKING MEMORY

Phonological working memory has been shown to be important for language learning. Patients with working memory deficits show impairments in long-term phonological learning, and a link has been observed between performance in the phonological loop and vocabulary level in children (Baddeley et al., 1988; Gathercole and Baddeley, 1990). According to Baddeley (2000), this suggests that the loop might have evolved to enhance language acquisition. In our original proposal (Aboitiz and García, 1997a) and following earlier evidence (Awh et al., 1995; Frackowiak, 1994; Habib, 1996; Paulesu et al., 1993; Salmon et al., 1996), we proposed that the "slave" component of verbal working memory contained a storage component, or phonological buffer, which included the left hemispheric postero parietal cortex (the supramarginal gyrus, Brodmann's area 40), and a rehearsal component including the left hemisphere frontal speech areas. We proposed that phonological representations were initially processed in the posterior language areas, stored transiently in inferior parietal areas, and then transferred to Broca's area for rehearsal. On the other hand, we suggested that granular frontal areas (areas 9 and 46) might participate in more complex working memory functions related to higher-level syntactic and semantic processing and in discourse planning (Aboitiz and García, 1997a, b).

Shortly after our publication, Smith and Jonides (1998) reviewed much of the neuroimaging studies for human working memory, providing an essentially similar picture in which verbal working memory was dissociable into a transient storage component in the left posterior parietal cortex and a rehearsal component in Broca's area and its vicinities. In this context, Kirchhoff et al. (2000) showed that a left prefrontal–temporal circuit including Broca's area and lateral temporal cortex mediates novel verbal episodic encoding and that the magnitude of activity in that region predicted whether an event (word) would be subsequently remembered. In addition, in articulatory suppression experiments that interfere with the phonological rehearsal mechanism, Gruber (2001, 2002) observed a specific activation pattern involving inferior parietal areas and anterior prefrontal cortex, while in conditions of subvocal rehearsal there was activation of intraparietal areas and Broca's area. Note that the pattern of activation in conditions of articulatory suppression resembles the "mirror system" circuit for movements and grasping proposed by Arbib and Bota (2003). Thus, the "slave" verbal working memory circuit may involve two main circuits, one involving rehearsal and perhaps overlapping with a mirror system circuit, and the other, related to transient phonological storage (Gruber, 2001, 2002).

In our view, one paradigmatic example of the role of working memory in language processing is the case of conduction aphasia. Usually, this type of aphasia results from lesions in the supramarginal gyrus, and even lesions of the insula that perhaps impair fibers in the underlying white matter (Greenfield, 1992). Like in Wernicke's aphasia, there are paraphasias and relatively fluent speech production, and like Broca's aphasia, there is preserved comprehension (Damasio, 1992). A diagnostic characteristic of conduction aphasia is the inability to repeat sentences presented to the patient. We proposed that because the capacity to repeat sentences requires a functional short-term memory (Trortais, 1974), the deficit in conduction aphasia may result from interruption of a verbal working memory circuit, either by damage to the subcortical white matter or, more likely, by direct damage to inferior parietal (intraparietal?) areas that transiently store phonological information (Aboitiz and García, 1997a). Smith and Jonides (1998) also called attention to a possible deficit in the storage component of verbal working memory in conduction aphasia. Along this line, it has been proposed that subjects with conduction aphasia comprehend and are able to access lexical–semantic information about words but demonstrate a deficit in retrieving the stored phonological representations of these items (Anderson et al., 1999). A related interpretation is that the supramarginal gyrus (area 40) and Broca's area are involved in speech perception only indirectly through their role in phonological working memory: the left supramarginal gyrus alone might represent an interface between speech-related auditory representations and frontal, motor systems, whereas the left supramarginal gyrus together with Broca's area mediates explicit access to speech segments (Hickok, 2000a; Hickok and Poeppel, 2000).

Summarizing, there is substantial evidence indicating that temporoparietal–prefrontal working memory systems are strongly implicated in language acquisition and in language processing, which suppports our main proposal that a specialization of working memory–related networks may have been at the basis of language origins. Perhaps the phonological rehearsal system including an incipient Broca's area and intraparietal and inferior parietal regions was especially relevant in the very early stages of language evolution. This may have been fundamental for learning complex utterances by imitation. In later stages, a transient phonological store located in the inferior parietal lobe evolved together with working memory systems for complex syntax, lexicon, and semantics (Aboitiz, 1995; Aboitiz and García, 1997a).

As mentioned previously (page 7), Arbib and Bota (2003) proposed a sequence of events for language origins starting from a complex imitation system for grasping, followed by a manual-based communication system in which imitation of others is an important element; this "mirror system" eventually participates in the generation of protospeech, which gives the vocal apparatus sufficient flexibility, and eventually language originates. In other words, the hand-based parietoprefrontal imitation system provided the behavioral flexibility necessary to generate a diversity of vocalizations that could evolve into language. (Note that this series of steps, if they occurred, might have taken place prior to the establishment of a phonological loop, which in our view served as the basis for primitive language networks.) We agree that the hand-based and orofacial mirror neuron system probably had a role in gestural communication and that imitation was possibly an important element in early prelinguistic evolution. However, we are not so sure yet about the stronger claim that gestural language was ancestral to vocal communication. Phylogenetic evidence indicates that external meaning is transmitted mostly by vocal communication in nonhuman primates (Acardi, 2003; Seyfarth and Cheney, 2003). In addition, in wild chimpanzees gestural communication is more limited than vocal communication (Acardi, 2003). Perhaps a more parsimonious hypothesis is that gestural and vocal communication coevolved to a large extent. Furthermore, we have suggested that the frontal auditory domain described by Romanski and Goldman-Rakic (2002) may belong to, or be the precursor of, a vocalization mirror system similar to the mirror system for grasping described by Rizzolatti and Arbib (1998). This system may have participated in vocal imitative behavior, permitting to compare heard vocalizations with own productions, and therefore may have been fundamental in early

language evolution (Bosman et al., 2004; see also Jürgens, 2003).

The discovery of a family with members bearing a mutation in gene *FOXP2* and showing severe language disorders (Lai et al., 2001) has prompted an intensive search for the functions of this gene. Imaging analyses indicate underactivation of Broca's area in subjects carrying the mutation (Liégeois et al., 2003). *FOXP2* has been hypothesized to be linked to the mirror system for grasping (Liégeois et al., 2003; Corballis, 2004), while there is evidence indicating that the deficit in *FOXP2* function produces an impairment in nonword repetition, a condition related to a deficit in the storage of phonological information in working memory (Watkins et al., 2002). Recently, we proposed an integrative approach to the study of this gene, including its participation in mirror system circuits and in working memory networks (Bosman et al., 2004).

SEMANTICS AND SYNTAX

Two main characteristics of language are semantics and syntax. *Semantics* concerns meaning, or the reference to the external world or the internal state of the individual, while *syntax* has to do with rules specifying an internal order of utterances. Concerning semantics, Geschwind (1964) already proposed that it was based on associative interactions between the language areas and sensory or limbic areas, a line that Pulvermuller (1999) has pursued with a more modern associative approach. In our view, which is similar to those just presented, semantics was achieved by integration of the language/working memory networks with other (working memory) networks related to online maintenance of sensory and mnemonic percepts. This integration was perhaps initially with limbic areas, to signal emotional state, and to motor areas, to signal specific behaviors. For example, associations between mirror neurons and auditory neurons in the frontal cortex may have provided the basis for the first utterances signaling specific behaviors (Hauk et al., 2004). In subsequent stages, integration with other, more widespread brain systems possibly allowed the generation of content words (Pulvermuller, 1999). Next, we discuss the possibility that higher levels of syntax involve the integration of Broca's area with neighboring cognitive systems of the frontal lobe and other cortical areas (this may include processing of abstract words, which serve a grammatical function; Pulvermuller, 1999).

Many researchers now consider that syntactic processing takes place in Broca's area and neighboring regions (operculum, insula, and subjacent white matter in which connections with other brain regions occur). Beside the well-known lesion studies, some electroencephalographic and imaging reports have confirmed this view. Electrophysiologically, two kinds of evoked potentials, the P600 (Osterhout and Holcomb, 1992) and the left anterior negativity (Friederici et al., 1993; Münte et al., 1993), have been related to errors in syntactic processing. Although both the source and the syntactic specificity of the P600 have been challenged (Patel et al., 1998), the left anterior negativity has been found to be more specific and its topographic arrangement suggests a source related to Broca's area (Patel, 2003). Interestingly, it was also found that harmonic musical processing may be processed in Broca's area; an anterior negativity component (ERAN [early right anterior negativity]) was elicited by harmonically inappropriate chords, localized in Broca's area and its right hemisphere homologue (Maess et al., 2001), suggesting similar mechanisms in syntactic and harmonic processing (Patel, 2003).

Several imaging reports have shown activation of Broca's area and surrounding regions related to syntactic processing (Caplan et al., 1998; Dapretto and Bookheimer, 1999; Friederici et al., 2000; Indefrey et al., 2001; Meyer et al., 2000; Moro et al., 2001; Ni et al., 2000; Stromswold et al., 1996; Tettamanti et al., 2001). For example, a study detected that Broca's area is specifically activated with ungrammatical sentences (Embick et al., 2000), and another study detected an increase in signal in the left infero frontal gyrus (especially area 45) with online performance of sentences with "real" syntactic rules compared with sentences with "unreal" rules (Musso et al., 2003). The interpretation of the latter result was that Broca's area disengages with the learning of unreal grammars, which possibly are learned with the participation of other, nonlinguistic systems.

It has been argued that the inferior frontal gyrus activity associated with syntactic processing may partly reflect working memory demands rather than syntactic processing per se (Bookheimer, 2002). Nevertheless, the two possibilities may not be exclusive. Besides its involvement in phonological processing, working memory seems to participate in syntactic pro-

cessing (see also Chapter 13). Caplan and Waters (1999) claim that syntax processing requires a specialized working memory system that is separated from the working memory system underlying sentence meaning and other functions. They propose a system for "interpretive processing" that deals with complex syntax and is more related to Broca's area and a system for "postinterpretive processing" that analyzes complex meaning, which may be more widely distributed. Furthermore, Martin and Saffran (1997) emphasize that there are several parallel but interacting working memory circuits in language: the semantic, the lexical, and the phonological systems. In addition, Fiebach et al. (2001) argue that there exists a separate cognitive or neural resource that supports syntactic working memory processes necessary for the temporary maintenance of syntactic information for the parser, whereas in an fMRI study, Cooke et al. (2002) report that the left inferior frontal cortex is recruited to support the cognitive resources required to maintain long-distance syntactic dependencies during the comprehension of complex grammatical sentences. Although there may still be some disagreement on the details of how many working memory levels operate in language processing, it is fair to say that working memory participates at the phonological, the lexical, the syntactic, and the semantic levels. However, these components may be relatively independent of each other: impairment to one particular working memory domain (say, phonological) may leave relatively undamaged other working memory components (lexical, syntactic, semantic) and vice versa. This is consistent with the neurobiological concept of several parallel working memory networks subserving distinct cognitive domains (Levy and Goldman-Rakic, 2000; Romanski et al., 1999a). Also along this line, it is important to recall Fuster's assertion that rather than one memory system in the cerebral cortex, each processing system has its own memory device (Fuster, 1995).

In a comprehensive study of the linguistic characteristics of Broca's aphasics, Grodzinsky (2000) claimed that Broca's area and neighboring regions do not participate in all syntax but only in some syntactic rules: in language comprehension, Broca's area keeps track of the transformationally moved phrasal constituents. For example, when transforming a canonical sentence into a passive form ("the boy kissed the girl" → "the girl was kissed by the boy"), the components are moved in order in relation to the verb. In verbal transformations, moved constituents leave a "trace" that is normally tracked by the listener in order to appropiately understand it. According to Grodzinsky, Broca's aphasics have special problems with verbal transformations because for some reason, traces are "deleted" and therefore roles are impossible or more difficult to track (the trace deletion hypothesis [TDH]). Interestingly, the more complex the transformation, or the longer the distance between a trace and its antecedent, the more difficult it is to track the moved constituents for Broca's aphasics. A relatively common interpretation of Grodzinsky's proposal is that trace deletion reflects a deficit in working memory (for example, Hickok, 2000b; Müller, 2000, Stowe, 2000, Szelag and Pöppel, 2000). Similarly, Pinker (1995) had already proposed a role of short-term memory for tracing constituents in phrasal transformations. Grodzinsky argues that it remains to be shown that there is a direct connection between working memory resources and formal elements of syntactic processing. Another point is that when phrasal constituents are moved, there must exist neuronal mechanisms involved in the detection of traces and their extraction sites. This may be detected at the lexical level, there being key words that permit the connection with other elements located distantly in the phrase. Finally, Grodzinsky (2000) also claims that in speech production, Broca's aphasics have problems in constructing appropriate syntactic trees in a manner similar to children's grammar. Specifically, they cannot construct trees below the tense node.

What is so special about syntax? A fundamental characteristic of syntax is that it does not merely consist of linear order within a sequence of words; rather, it relies on the hierarchical or recursive relations between words in such a way that not just any order is possible and that there are constraints with regard to the types of grammar that can be learned (Chomsky, 1978; Marcus et al., 2003). How is this performed in the brain? At least Pinker (1995) claimed that short-term memory plays an important role in syntactic processing. More recently, Patel (2003) compared two different theories of syntactic and harmonic processing: the dependency locality theory (DLT) (Gibson, 1998, 2000) and the tonal pitch space theory (TPS) (Lerdhal, 2001), respectively. In DLT, distances between related words are computed and stored as the sentence is perceived in time, whereas in TPS, distances between chords and some predefined "anchor" chords are being computed in a similar way. When explaining the similarity between syntactic and harmonic processing, Patel explicitly claims not to be invoking a special memory system or a symbol-manipulating system but rather considers the cognitive theories of processing in the two domains. However, Patel finally claims that "in DLT, integration can be understood as activating the representation of an incoming word while also reactivating a prior dependent word whose activation has decayed in proportion to the distance between words. In TPS, integration can be understood as activating an incoming chord while maintaining activation of another chord which provides the context for the incoming chord's interpretation" (Patel, 2003, p. 678). This interpretation is strongly reminiscent of managing online information during working memory tasks.

It may be argued that most syntactical processing is performed implicitly, without conscious involvement, whereas working memory operates largely in explicit form. We consider that the short-term memory networks required for syntactic processing may be quite similar in organization (although not necessarily in location) to the working memory networks described for other linguistic tasks. The implicit/explicit distinction perhaps has to do with other parameters that are not fundamental for the implementation of these networks.

Summarizing, our main claim has been that the language circuit arose as a specialization of a circuit involved in phonological working memory, which eventually incorporated other working memory systems involved in syntax, the lexicon, and semantics. This is reminiscent of Martin and Saffran's (1997) proposal of different but interacting working memory domains involved in language processing: the semantic, the lexical, and the phonological systems, and Caplan and Waters' (1999) two working memory systems, an "interpretive" component analyzing syntax and a "postinterpretive" component analyzing the semantic contents.

Anatomically, these networks may correspond to a relatively restricted system involving the language areas and neighboring regions for phonological and syntactic processing and, more widespread, bilateral networks related to meaning and semantics. In order to be efficient, working memory must create a frame in which all the online items are ordered and have some definite relations between them. In this sense, there is some sort of "syntax" intrinsic to all working memory systems. We consider that a primordium of the formal elements that appear in modern syntax may have occurred in the organization of the primitive linguistic working memory systems but, perhaps more important, as rules that permitted the "traduction" from one working memory system to another. For example, a "presyntax" may have emerged as a strategy to superpose the temporal (phonological and syntactical) working memory frames in which the different components of an utterance are retained, with a visuospatial/episodic frame that generates a mental "image" of an action or an event (this need not be purely visual) associated with that utterance. Thus, the hierarchical organization of a syntactically ordered sentence may be partly related to the requirements to transform this temporally ordered online information (in which Broca's area may play a special role, in both phonological and syntactic processing) into a perhaps more distributed, visuospatial sketchpad describing the meaning of a given sentence, and vice versa. In this sense, perhaps one main innovation in language origins and in human neural evolution was the ability to "translate" complex working memory codes from one functional domain (i.e., sequential) into another (i.e., visuospatial working memory and episodic memory) and vice versa. Modern language, then, may be generated by an imbricated and coordinated macroscopic working memory system, which involves several reciprocally interacting subsystems (lexical, semantic, syntactic, phonological). The uniqueness of syntax, and of the human brain, is perhaps partly related to the translating mechanisms required for the reciprocal interaction between these different subsystems. This view is consistent with recent fMRI research identifying three separate regions of functional specialization in the inferior frontal gyrus: phonology, syntax, and semantics (Bookheimer, 2002).

FINAL COMMENTS

We have proposed a revised version of our original hypothesis that language networks emerged as a specialization of temporoparietal–prefrontal networks involved in cognitive processes that require sustained activity, like working memory, attention, and movement imitation. In this context, Arbib and Bota (2003) made a contrast between our theory being "retrospective" (looking at what is in the human brain—working memory—and tracking it back to the monkey brain) and theirs being "prospective" (finding what is in the monkey—hand coordination—which may have served as a substrate for human language), which we believe may be misleading. We have followed standard phylogenetic methodology: first, identified in the monkey the networks that can be homologous to the language-related neural networks, and second, asked for the functions of these networks in the monkey, one of which is working memory. Because working memory is seen to operate at many levels of language processing (phonological, lexical, syntactic, and semantic), we conclude that corticocortical language networks originated from preexisting working memory networks in the primate brain (of course, this is far from saying that working memory mechanisms explain all aspects of language processing). A good analogy for our strategy comes from the evolution of the eye: although image formation is a highly derived characteristic, there are other, more basic functions, like photoreception, which are central to vision but insufficient for producing an image, that are shared by other species whose visual organs lack image-forming properties; these functions permit us to track the phylogenetic ancestry of the eyes. Simply put, our hypothesis points to a function (working memory) that is present in the monkey and participates in language processing. On the other hand, although in humans and monkeys the inferior frontal region participates in hand movements and other functions, at this point there is no evidence that manual coordination is involved in language processing. Nevertheless, a "mirror system" initially involved in decoding orofacial gestures and body posture may have also participated in communication. We are not sure which came first, oral or gestural communication, but we believe that these two may have relied on related, interacting temporoparietal–prefrontal networks in the cerebral cortex. Furthermore, a mirror system for vocalizations may have been fundamental for early learning of complex vocalizations and vocal communication (Bosman et al., 2004; Jürgens, 2003). We consider that a crucial element that allowed the processing of increasingly complex utterances was an expanded phonological working memory capacity, possibly based on supratemporal/inferoparietal–inferior prefrontal networks. Utterances begun to acquire relatively complex meanings by virtue of associative interactions of the language regions with other brain regions; this required a notable expansion of the working memory capacity and of the neural networks underlying it. Finally, we propose that syntax emerged as a neuronal strategy to efficiently "translate" a phonological, sequential working memory code into an episodic, visuospatial memory code that represents the meaning of the respective utterances. In a way, the rules for syntax may perhaps be partly understood as a strategy that permits the transmission of information between the different working memory codes that make up the elements of language; that is, it relates to a binding mechanism that permits the different networks to interact during human communication.

ACKNOWLEDGMENTS   Juan Montiel prepared Figure 1–1. Part of the work presented here was financed by the Millenium Center for Integrative Neuroscience.

References

Aboitiz, F. (1988). Epigenesis and the evolution of the human brain. *Medical Hypotheses, 25,* 55–59.

Aboitiz, F. (1995). Working memory networks and the origin of language areas in the human brain. *Medical Hypotheses, 44,* 504–506.

Aboitiz, F. (1996). Does bigger mean better? Evolutionary determinants of brain size and structure. *Brain, Behavior and Evolution, 47,* 225–245.

Aboitiz, F., & García, R. (1997a). The evolutionary origin of the language areas in the human brain. A neuroanatomical perspective. *Brain Research. Brain Research Reviews, 25,* 381–396.

Aboitiz, F., & García, R. (1997b). The anatomy of language revisited. *Biol. Research, 30,* 171–183.

Acardi, A.C. (2003). Is gestural communication more sophisticated than vocal communication in wild chimpanzees? *The Behavioral and Brain Sciences, 26,* 210–211.

Aggleton, P. (1993). The contribution of the amygdala to normal and abnormal emotional states. *Trends in Neuroscience, 16,* 328–334.

Anderson, J.M., Gilmore, R., Roper, S., Crosson, B., Bauer, R.M., Nadeau, S., Beversdorf, D.Q., et al. (1999). Conduction aphasia and the arcuate fasciculus: A reexamination of the Wernicke-Geschwind model. *Brain and Language, 70,* 1–12.

Arbib, M., & Bota, M. (2003). Language evolution: Neural homologies and neuroinformatics. *Neural Networks: The Official Journal of the International Neural Network Society, 16,* 1237–1260.

Awh, E., Smith, E.E., & Jonides, J. (1995). Human rehearsal processes and the frontal lobes: PET evidence. *Annals of New York Academy of Science, 769,* 97–118.

Baddeley, A. (2000). The episodic buffer: A new component of working memory? *Trends in Cognitive Sciences, 4,* 417–423.

Baddeley, A. (1992). Working memory. *Science, 255,* 556–559.

Baddeley, A.D., & Hitch, G.J. (1974). Working memory. In G.A. Bower (Ed.), *The psychology of learning and motivation* (pp. 47–89). New York: Academic Press.

Baddeley, A.D., Papagno, C., & Vallar, G. (1988). When long-term learning depends on short-term memory. *Journal of Memory and Language, 27,* 586–595.

Barbas, H., & Pandya, D.N. (1989). Architecture and intrinsic connections of the prefrontal cortex in the rhesus monkey. *The Journal of Comparative Neurology, 286,* 353–375.

Binder, J.R., Frost, J.A., Hammeke, T.A., Rao, S.M., & Cox, R.W. (1996). Function of the left planum temporale in auditory and linguistic processing. *Brain, 119,* 1239–1247.

Bookheimer, S. (2002). Functional fMRI of language: New approaches to understanding the cortical organization of semantic processing. *Annual Review of Neuroscience, 25,* 151–188.

Bosman, C., García, R., & Aboitiz, F. (2004). FOXP2 and the language working memory system. *Trends in Cognitive Sciences, 6,* 251–252.

Broca, P. (1861). Remarques sur le siege de la faculté du langage articulé, suivies d'une observation d'aphémie (perte de la parole). *Bulletin of Society of Anatomy, 36,* 330–357.

Cavada, C., & Goldman-Rakic, P. (1989). Posterior parietal cortex in rhesus monkey: II. Evidence for segregated cortico–cortical networks linking sensory and limbic areas with the frontal lobe. *The Journal of Comparative Neurology, 287,* 422–445.

Caplan, D., & Waters, G.S. (1999). Verbal working memory and sentence comprehension. *Behavioral and Brain Sciences, 22,* 77–126.

Caplan, D., Alpert, N., & Waters, G. (1998). Effects of syntactic structure and propositional number on patterns of regional cerebral blood flow. *Journal of Cognitive Neurosciences, 10,* 541–552.

Chomsky, N. (1978). *Rules and representations.* New York: Columbia University Press.

Cooke, A., Zurif, E.B., DeVita, C., Alsop, D., Koenig, P., Detre, J., et al. (2002). Neural basis for sentence comprehension: grammatical and short-term memory components. *Human Brain Mapping, 15,* 80–94.

Corballis, M.C. (2004). FOXP2 and the mirror system. *Trends in Cognitive Science, 8,* 95–96.

Damasio, A.R. (1992). Aphasia. *New England Journal of Medicine, 326,* 531–539.

Dapretto, M., & Bookheimer, S.Y. (1999). Form and content: Dissociating syntax and semantics in sentence comprehension. *Neuron, 24,* 427–432.

Darwin, C. (1871). *The descent of man and selections in relation to sex.* London: John Murray.

Deacon, T.W. (1992). Cortical connections of the inferior arcuate sulcus cortex in the macaque brain. *Brain Research, 573,* 8–26.

Dennett, D.C. (1995). *Darwin's dangerous idea. Evolution and the meanings of life.* New York: Simon and Schuster.

Dronkers, N.F., Shapiro, J.K., Redfern, B., & Knight, R.T. (1992). The role of Broca's area in Broca's aphasia. *Journal of Clinical and Experimental Neuropsychology, 14,* 52–53.

Embick, D., Marantz, A., Miyashita, Y., O'Neil, W., & Sakai, K.L. (2000). A syntactic specialization for Broca's area. *Proceedings of National Academy of Science USA, 97,* 6150–6154.

Fiebach, C.J., Schlesewsky, M., & Friederici, A.D. (2001). Syntactic working memory and the establishment of filler-gap dependencies: Insights from ERPs and fMRI. *Journal of Psycholinguistic Research, 30,* 321–338.

Frackowiak, R.S. (1994). Functional mapping of verbal memory and language. *Trends in Neuroscience, 17,* 109–115.

Friederici, A.D., Opitz, B., & Von Cramon, D.Y. (2000). Segregating semantic and syntactic aspects of processing in the human brain: An fMRI investigation of different word types. *Cerebral Cortex, 10,* 698–705.

Friederici, A.D., Pfeifer, E., & Hahne, A. (1993). Event-related brain potentials during natural speech processing: Effects of semantic, morphological and syntactic violations. *Cognitive Brain Research, 1,* 183–192.

Fuster, J. (1995). *Memory in the cerebral cortex.* Cambridge, MA: MIT Press.

Galaburda, A.M., & Sanides, F. (1980). Cytoarchitectonic organization of the human auditory cortex. *Journal of Comparative Neurology, 190,* 597–610.

Galaburda, A.M., & Pandya, D.N. (1983). The intrinsic architectonic and connectional organization of the superior temporal region of the rhesus monkey. *Journal of Comparative Neurology, 221,* 169–184.

Galaburda, A.M., Sanides, F., & Geschwind, N. (1978). Human brain: Cytoarchitectonic left-right asymmetries in the temporal speech region. *Archives of Neurology, 35,* 812–817.

Gallese, V., Fadiga, L., Fogassi, L., & Rizzolatti, G. (1996). Action recognition in the premotor cortex. *Brain, 119,* 593–609.

Gathercole, S.E., & Baddeley, A.D. (1990). The role of phonological memory in vocabulary acquisition: A study of young children learning new names *British Journal of Psychology, 81,* 439–454.

Geschwind, N. (1964). The development of the brain and the evolution of language. *Mon. Ser. Lang. Ling., 1,* 155–169.

Gibson, E. (1998). Linguistic complexity: Locality of syntactic dependencies. *Cognition, 68,* 1–76.

Gibson, E. (2000). The dependency locality theory: A distance-based theory of linguistic complexity. In Y. Miyashita, A. Marantaz, & W. O'Neill (Eds.), *Image, language, brain* (pp. 95–126), Cambridge, MA: MIT Press.

Greenfield, P.M. (1992). Language, tools and brain: The ontogeny and phylogeny of hierarchically organized sequential behavior. *Behavioral and Brain Sciences, 14,* 531–595.

Griffiths, T.D., & Warren, J.D. (2002). The planum temporale as a computational hub. *Trends in Neuroscience, 25,* 348–353.

Grodzinsky, Y. (2000). The neurology of syntax: Language use without Broca's area. *Behavioral and Brain Science, 23,* 1–71.

Gruber, O. (2001). Effects of domain-specific interference on brain activation associated with verbal working memory task performance. *Cerebral Cortex, 11,* 1047–1055.

Gruber, O. (2002). The coevolution of language and working memory capacity in the human brain. In V. Gallese and M. Stamenov (Eds.), *Mirror neurons and the evolution of brain and language* (pp. 77–86). Advances in Consciousness Research Series. Amsterdam: John Benjamins.

Habib, M., Demonet, J.F., & Frackowiak, R. (1996). Cognitive neuroanatomy of language: Contribution of functional cerebral imaging. *Review of Neurology, (Paris), 152,* 249–260.

Hackett, T.A., Stepniewsk, I., & Kaas, J.H. (1999). Prefrontal connections of the parabelt auditory cortex in macaque monkeys. *Brain Research, 817,* 45–58.

Hackett, T.A., Stepniewska, I., & Kaas, J.H. (1998). Subdivisions of auditory cortex and ipsilateral cortical connections of the parabelt auditory cortex in macaque monkeys. *Journal of Comparative Neurology, 394,* 475–495.

Hauk, O., Johnsrude, I., & Pulvermuller, F. (2004). Somatotopic representation of action words in human motor and premotor cortex. *Neuron, 41,* 301–307.

Hickok, G. (2000a). Speech perception, conduction aphasia and the functional neuroanatomy of language. In J. Grodzinsky, L. Shapiro, & D. Swinney (Eds.), *Language and the brain* (pp. 87–104). New York: Academic Press.

Hickok, G. (2000b). The left frontal convolution plays no special role in syntactic comprehension. *Behavioral and Brain Sciences, 23,* 35–36.

Hickock, G., & Poeppel, D. (2000). Towards a functional neuroanatomy of speech perception *Trends in Cognitive Science, 4*, 131–138.

Iacoboni, M., Woods, R.P., Brass, M., Bekkering, H., Mazziota, J.C., & Rizzolatti, G. (1999). Cortical mechanisms of human imitation. *Science, 286*, 2526–2528.

Jürgens, U. (2003). From mouth to mouth and hand to hand: on language evolution. *Behavioral and Brain Sciences, 26*, 229–230.

Kaas, J.H., & Hackett, T.A. (2000). Subdivisions of auditory cortex and processing streams in primates. *Proceedings of the National Academy of Sciences USA, 97*, 11793–11799.

Kaas, J.H., & Hackett, T.A. (1999). What' and 'where' processing in auditory cortex. *Nature Neuroscience, 2*, 1045–1047.

Kaminski, J., Call, J., & Fischer, J. (2004). Word learning in a domestic dog: Evidence for "fast mapping." *Science, 304*, 1682–1683.

Indefrey, P., Hagoort, P., Herzog, H., Seitz, R., & Brown, C. (2001). Syntactic processing in left prefrontal cortex is independent of lexical meaning. *Neuroimage, 14*, 546–555.

Kirchhoff, B.A., Wagner, A.D., Maril, A., & Stern, C.E. (2000). Prefrontal-temporal circuitry for episodic encoding and subsequent memory. *Journal of Neuroscience, 20*, 6173–6180.

Lai, C.S., Fisher, S.E., Hurst, J.A., Vargha-Khadem, F., & Monaco, A.P. (2001). A forkhead-domain gene is mutated in a severe speech and language disorder. *Nature, 413*, 519–523.

Lerdhal, F. (2001). *Tonal pitch space*. Oxford: Oxford University Press.

Levy, R., & Goldman-Rakic, P.S. (2000). Segregation of working memory functions within the dorsolateral prefrontal cortex. *Experimental Brain Research, 133*, 23–32.

Lewis, J.W., & Van Essen, D.C. (2000). Corticocortical connections of visual, sensorimotor, and multimodal processing areas in the parietal lobe of the macaque monkey. *Journal of Comparative Neurology, 428*, 112–137.

Liegeois, F., Baldeweg, T., Connelly, A., Gadian, D.G., Mishkin, M., & Vargha-Khadem, F. (2003). Language fMRI abnormalities associated with FOXP2 gene mutation. *Nature and Neuroscience, 6*, 1230–1237.

Maess, B., Koelsch, S., Gunter, T.C., & Friederici, A.D. (2001). Musical syntax is processed in Broca's area: An MEG study. *Nature and Neuroscience, 4*, 540–545.

Marcus, G.F., Vouloumanos, A., & Sag, I.A. (2003). Does Broca's area play by the rules? *Nature and Neuroscience, 6*, 651–652.

Martin, N., & Saffran, E.M. (1997). Language and auditory-verbal short-term memory impairments: Evidence for common underlying processes. *Cognitive Neuropsychology, 14*, 641–682.

Meyer, M., Friederici, A., & Von Cramon, D. (2000). Neurocognition of auditory sentence comprehension: Event related fMRI reveals sensitivity to syntactic violations and task demands. *Cognitive Brain Research, 9*, 19–33.

Moro, A., Tettamanti, M., Perani, D., Donati, C., Cappa, S., & Fazio, F. (2001). Syntax and the brain: Disentangling grammar by selective anomalies. *Neuroimage, 13*, 100–118.

Müller, R.A. (2000). A big "housing" problem and a trace of neuroimaging: Broca's area is more than a transformation center. *Behavioral Brain Sciences, 23*, 42.

Munte, T.F., Heinze, H.J., & Mangun, G.R. (1993). Dissociation of brain activity related to syntactic and semantic aspects of language. *Journal of Cognitive Neuroscience, 5*, 335–344.

Musso, M., Moro, A., Glauche, V., Rijntjes, M., Reichenbach, J., Büchel, C., et al. (2003). Broca's area and the language instinct. *Nature and Neuroscience, 6*, 774–781.

Nahm, F.K.D., Tranel, D., Damasio, H., & Damasio, A.R. (1993). Cross-modal associations and the human amygdala. *Neuropsychologia, 31*, 727–744.

Ni, W., Constable, R., Mencl, W., Pugh, K., Fulbright, R., Shaywitz, S., Shaywitz, B., et al. (2000). An event-related neuroimaging study distinguishing form and content in sentence processing. *Journal of Cognitive Neuroscience, 12*, 120–133.

Osterhout, L., & Holcomb, P.J. (1992). Event-related brain potentials elicited by syntactic anomaly. *Journal of Memory and Language, 31*, 785–806.

Pandya, D.N., & Sanides, F. (1973). Architectonic parcellation of the temporal operculum in rhesus monkey and its projection pattern. *Z. Nature Entwickl. Gesch, 139*, 127–161.

Patel, A.D. (2003). Language, music, syntax and the brain. *Nature and Neuroscience, 7*, 674–681.

Patel, A.D., Gibson, E., Ratner, J., Besson, M., & Holcomb, P.J. (1998). Processing syntactic relations in language and music: An event-related potential study. *Journal of Cognitive Neuroscience, 10*, 717–733.

Paulesu, E., Frith, C.D., & Frackowiak, R.S. (1993). The neural correlates of the verbal component of working memory. *Nature, 362*, 342–345.

Petrides, M., & Pandya, D.N. (2001). Comparative cytoarchitectonic analysis of the human and the macaque ventrolateral prefrontal cortex and corticocortical connection patterns in the monkey. *European Journal of Neuroscience, 16*, 291–310.

Petrides, M., & Pandya, D.N. (1999). Dorsolateral prefrontal cortex: Comparative cytoarchitectonic analysis in the human and the macaque brain and corticocortical connection patterns. *European Journal of Neuroscience, 11*, 1011–1036.

Petrides, M., & Pandya, D. (1994). Comparative architectonic analysis of the human and the macaque frontal cortex. In F. Boller & J. Grafman (Eds.), *Handbook of neuropsychology* (pp. 17–58). Amsterdam: Elsevier.

Petrides, M., & Pandya, D.N. (1988). Association fiber pathways to the frontal cortex from the superior temporal region in the rhesus monkey. *Journal of Comparative Neurology, 273*, 52–66.

Petrides, M., & Pandya, D.N. (1984). Projections to the frontal cortex from the posterior parietal region in the rhesus monkey. *Journal of Comparative Neurology, 228*, 105–116.

Pinker, S. (1995). *The language instinct: How the mind creates language.* New York: Harper Perennial.

Pinker, S., & Bloom, P. (1990). Natural language and natural selection. *Behavioral and Brain Sciences, 13*, 707–784.

Premack, D. (1983). The codes of man and beasts. *Behavioral and Brain Sciences, 6*, 125–167.

Preuss, T., & Goldman-Rakic, P.S. (1991a). Myelo- and cytoarchitecture of the granular frontal cortex and surrounding regions in the strepsirhine primate Galago and the anthropoid primate Macaca. *Journal of Comparative Neurology, 310*, 429–474.

Preuss, T., & Goldman-Rakic, P.S. (1991b). Architectonics of the parietal and temporal association cortex in the strepsirhine primate Galago compared to the anthropoid primate Macaca. *Journal of Comparative Neurology, 310*, 475–506.

Preuss, T., & Goldman-Rakic, P.S. (1991c). Ipsilateral cortical connections of granular frontal cortex in the strepsirhine primate Galago, with comparative comments on anthropoid primates. *Journal of Comparative Neurology, 310*, 507–549.

Pulvermüller, F. (1999). Words in the brain's language. *Behavioral and Brain Sciences, 22*, 253–336

Rauschecker, J.P., & Tian, B. (2000). Mechanisms and streams for processing of "what" and "where" in auditory cortex. *Proceedings of the National Academy of Science USA, 97*, 11800.

Rizzolatti, G., & Arbib, M.A. (1998). Language within our grasp. *Trends in Neuroscience, 21*, 188–194.

Rizzolatti, G., Fogassi, L., & Gallese, V. (2002). Motor and cognitive functions of the ventral premotor cortex. *Current Opinions in Neurobiology, 12*, 149–154.

Rizzolatti, G., Fadiga, L., Gallese, V., & Fogassi, L. (1996). Premotor cortex and the recognition of motor actions. *Cognitive Brain Research, 3*, 131–141.

Romanski, L.M., & Goldman-Rakic, P.S. (2002). An auditory domain in primate prefrontal cortex. *Nature and Neuroscience, 5*, 15–16.

Romanski, R.L., Tian, B., Mishkin, M., Goldman-Rakic, P.S., & Raushecker, J.P. (1999a). Dual streams of auditory afferents target multiple domains in the primate prefrontal cortex. *Nature and Neuroscience, 2*, 1131–1136.

Romanski, R.L., Bates, J.F., & Goldman-Rakic, P.S. (1999b). Auditory belt and parabelt projections to the prefrontal cortex in the rhesus monkey. *Journal of Comparative Neurology, 403*, 141–157.

Salmon, E., Van der Linden, M., Collette, F., Delfiore, G., Maquet, P., Degueldre, C., et al. (1996). Regional brain activity during working memory tasks. *Brain, 119*, 1617–1625.

Seyfarth, R.M., & Cheney, D.L. (2003). Meaning and emotion in animal vocalizations. *Annals of New York Academy of Science, 1000*, 32–55.

Smith, E.E., & Jonides, J. (1998). Neuroimaging analyses of human working memory. *Proceedings of National Academy of Science USA, 95*, 12061–12068.

Stowe, L.A. (2000). Sentence comprehension and the left inferior frontal gyrus: Storage, not comprehension. *Behavioral and Brain Sciences, 23*, 51.

Stromswold, K., Caplan, D., Alpert, N., & Rauch, S. (1996). Localization of syntactic comprehension by positron emission tomography. *Brain and Language, 52*, 452–473.

Szelag, E., & Pöppel, E. (2000). Temporal perception: A key to understand language. *Behavioral and Brain Sciences, 23*, 52.

Tettamanti, M., Alkadhi, H., Moro, A., Perani, D., Kollias, S., & Weniger, D. (2002). Neural correlates for the acquisition of natural language syntax. *NeuroImage, 17*, 700–709.

Tian, B., Reser, D., Durham, A., Kustov, A., & Rauschecker, J.P. (2001). Functional specialization in rhesus monkey auditory cortex. *Science, 292*, 290–293.

Trortais, A. (1974). Impairment of memory for sequences in conduction aphasia, *Neuropsychologia, 12*, 355–366.

Watkins, K.E., Vargha-Khadem, F., Ashburner, J., Passingham, R.E., Connelly, A., Friston, K.J., et al. (2002). Behavioural analysis of an inherited speech and language disorder: Comparison with acquired aphasia. *Brain, 125*, 452–464.

Wernicke, C. (1874). *Der aphasische Syntomemkomplex: Eine psychologische Studie auf anatomischer Basis.* Breslau: Cohn and Weigert.

2

A Multimodal Analysis of Structure and Function in Broca's Region

Katrin Amunts
Karl Zilles

A recent postmortem study of histological sections of a brain of a language genius, E.K., who spoke more than 60 languages, showed that the cytoarchitecture of cortical areas 44 and 45 as the putative correlates of Broca's region differed significantly from that of control brains (Amunts et al., 2004). The reported differences encompassed the cell architecture as well as interhemispheric cytoarchitectonic asymmetry. It was found that right area 45 differed with respect to the laminar pattern in supragranular and infragranular layers in the brain of E.K. compared with controls. Differences in left and right areas 44 were mainly associated with the heterogeneity of the volume fraction of cell bodies across cortical layers. Finally, the cytoarchitecture of areas 44 was more symmetrical in the brain of E.K. than in any control brain, whereas the architecture of area 45 was more asymmetrical. This combination was unique for the E.K. brain. It was concluded that the exceptional language competence of E.K. may be related to distinct cytoarchitectonic features in Broca's region (Amunts et al., 2004).

Only a few studies, however, correlated language with the underlying (micro)anatomy, although Broca's region was originally conceptualized as a speech center based on anatomical clinical observations performed by Pierre Paul Broca (1824–1880) in the middle of the nineteenth century (see the historical chapters in this volume). Broca and his colleague Aubertin examined a patient, Leborgne, who had lost articulated speech ("*aphemia*") after brain lesion in the third convolution of the frontal lobe of the left hemisphere (Broca, 1861a, b, 1863, 1865) (Fig. 2–1, see color insert). Leborgne could no longer pronounce more than a single syllable—"tan"—for that reason, he became famous as "Monsieur Tan." In addition to his inability to speak, he had paralysis of the right side. He seemed to be normal in all other aspects (Stookey, 1954).

"Broca's region" was the first brain region to which a circumscribed function, overt speech, had been related. A few years after Broca's first studies, Wernicke (1848–1904) proposed the first theory of language,

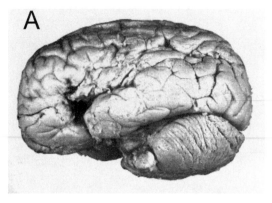 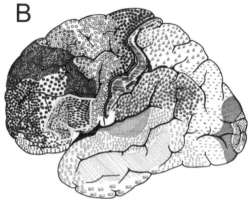

FIGURE 2–1. (A) Lateral view of the brain of Leborgne with lesion in the left frontal lobe. It was the first brain region to which a circumscribed function, overt speech, had been related. This speech region was called Broca's area (or region) and the syndrome that results from its damage was called Broca's aphasia. The lesion included the posterior portion of the left inferior frontal gyrus as seen on the photo- graph but also parts of subcortical white matter, temporal lobe, and inferior parietal lobe (Signoret et al., 1984). (B) Lateral view of Brodmann' map (1909). Areas 44 and 45 (marked by a bold line) occupy the posterior inferior frontal gyrus and, thus, have been assumed to constitute the microstructural correlates of Broca's region.

which postulated an anterior, motor speech center (Broca's region); a posterior, semantic language center (Wernicke's region); and a fiber tract, the arcuate fascicle, connecting the two regions (Lichtheim, 1885; Wernicke, 1874; see the historical part of this volume). These discoveries can be interpreted as the beginning of the scientific theory of the localization of cortical functions.

It has to be noticed, however, that the lesion of Leborgne's brain was huge (Fig. 2–1, see color insert). In addition to the involvement of the left inferior frontal lobe, the brain of Leborgne showed more posterior lesions. Broca interpreted these lesions as occurring after the onset of Leborgne's aphasia and as not being relevant for his speech disturbances (Kolb and Whishaw, 1996). As shown by recent magnetic resonance imaging (MRI) of Leborgne's brain, large parts of the subcortical white matter and parts of the middle frontal convolution, the insula, and the temporal pole of the left hemisphere were also lesioned. The lesion even reached the parietal lobe of the left hemisphere (Signoret et al., 1984).

Broca did not analyze the underlying microstructure of the lesion. Such an analysis was not feasible at this time, because Brodmann's famous map of the cytoarchitecture of cortical areas was published more than 40 years later (1909). According to Brodmann, the cytoarchitecture should be more or less constant within a cortical area (BA) but changes at its border. Although for the vast majority of cortical areas such an association was not rigorously tested, Brodmann was also convinced that every cytoarchitectonically defined cortical area subserves a certain function considering the existing electrophysiological and comparative anatomical data of that time, which came mainly from the analysis of movements and the motor system (Brodmann, 1912; Leyton and Sherrington, 1917; Vogt and Vogt, 1919a, 1926). He was careful enough, however, not to interpret his cytoarchitectonic map with respect to the Broca region as a center for articulated speech. This may be seen in the context that later lesion data of patients with aphasia were more difficult to interpret and that the question of the localization of function was still controversially discussed, such as by Hughling Jackson (see historical part of the book). The purely macroscopic description of Paul Broca and the huge extent of the lesion made it difficult to associate the lesion site in the following years with a Brodmann area (or a group of areas) as defined on a microstructural level.

Old (Vogt and Vogt, 1919b) and more recent electrophysiological studies in nonhuman primates have demonstrated that Brodmann's basic idea was true: neurons with similar receptive fields and response properties lie within the same cytoarchitectonic area. This has been shown by combined electrophysiological–neuroanatomical studies, such as of the motor system, in which monkey brains were sectioned and cell stained following electrophysiological stimulation and in which penetration sites were correlated with the cytoarchitectonic pattern. The experiments showed that response properties of neurons change across cytoarchitectonic borders (e.g., Luppino et al., 1991; Matelli et al., 1991; Tanji and Kurata, 1989).

Relationships between architecture, connectivity, and function have been less well analyzed for higher cognitive functions, such as, language, which are supported by neocortical association areas. The search for anatomical correlates of language requires alternative tools of analysis compared with, for example, the motor system, where many questions of structure–function relationship could be investigated in animals. It also requires a clear concept of what is language—not an easy task. Anatomoclinical observations of patients with brain lesion and aphasia represent such an alternative. However, "We are by no means justified to infer directly from a correlation between a localized defect and a defect in performance a relationship between the concerned area and

a definite performance. The facts allow only—*localization of defects*, but not a localization of performance. The latter remains a theoretical interpretation which can be tried only after a careful analysis of the functions corresponding to the performance and the defect" (Goldstein, 1946). An obvious but necessary prerequisite of anatomoclinical studies is a detailed analysis of the underlying "normal" anatomy and the microstructure, in particular (e.g., cyto-, receptor-, myeloarchitecture), as well as the connectivity of the relevant cortical areas.

The cortical areas corresponding to Broca's region (or Broca's area) comprise, according to many authors, BA 44 and 45 (Aboitiz and Garcia, 1997; Amunts et al., 1999; Kononova, 1949; Lieberman, 2002). Other authors used the term Broca's region either for Brodmann's area 45 (Hayes and Lewis, 1992) or for area 44 only (Galaburda, 1980), or they attributed BA 47 as well to Broca's region (Harasty et al., 1996). For an overview of the different meanings of the term "Broca's region," see Uylings et al. (1999). Finally, a Broca region in the "strict sense" was distinguished from a region in a "broader sense." The

A

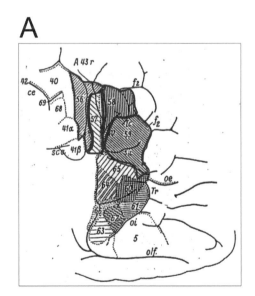

B

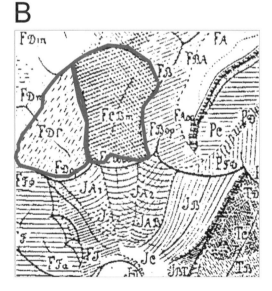

FIGURE 2–2. (A) Adopted cytoarchitectonic maps of an individual brain (right hemisphere) of Riegele (1931; see the historical part of this volume) and (B) von Economo and Koskinas (left hemisphere; 1925). Riegele defined a Broca region comprising areas 56 to 66 as well as 41 (nomenclature of Vogt), corresponding roughly to Brodmann's areas 44, 45, and 47 (1909). Areas 57, 58, and 59 constitute the Pars triangularis (area FDΓ of von Economo and Koskinas), whereas 56 constitutes the Pars opercularis (FCB$_m$ of von Economo and Koskinas). Note the different parcellation schemes of the different authors with respect to Broca's region.

latter also included orbitofrontal and deep opercular areas (Hervé, 1888; Riegele, 1931; Strasburger, 1938) (Fig. 2–2, see color insert).

Thus, the term "Broca region" is not used consistently in the literature with respect to the underlying microstructure. It is often applied as a clinical and/or historical concept of a center of language processing without keeping in mind a certain microstructurally defined cortical area. It seems to be not yet decided, whether the concept of "Broca region" is more than an historical one or an imprecise descriptor of a language center, that is, whether a functionally and/or anatomically defined unit is beyond the term. It seems to be reasonable, at least, to investigate this question using a *combination* of anatomical approaches (multimodal analysis of microstructure) with functional analysis of language (psycholinguistics) and, finally, clinical studies. Here we focus on the microstructure of the putative Broca region and how this anatomical information can be used for the interpretation of data from functional imaging studies (fMRI, positon-emission tomography [PET]) of language-related tasks.

THE ANATOMY OF BROCA'S REGION

Macrostructure

Two areas, Brodmann's areas 44 and 45, occupy the posterior portion of the inferior frontal gyrus (opercular and triangular parts, respectively), which makes them good candidates for microstructural correlates of Broca's region. It is not clear from brain macroscopic studies whether the most ventral part of BA 6 (inferior precentral gyrus) is also part of Broca's region, nor can it be excluded that parts of the cortex hidden in the depths of the Sylvian fissure or the orbital part of the inferior frontal gyrus (e.g., BA 47) also belong to Broca's region. The inferior posterior frontal cortex is a region, where many cytoarchitectonic areas are located in close neighborhood. As a possible consequence, the localization of the borders of these areas as well as their number differed between the maps of Brodmann (1909), von Economo and Koskinas (1925), the Russian school (Sarkisov et al., 1949), and Riegele (1931).

Furthermore, previous anatomical studies have demonstrated a considerable variability in the sulcal pattern of the infero frontal lobe (Amunts et al., 1999, 2004; Duvernoy, 1991; Ono et al., 1990; Tomaiuolo

et al., 1999). See also Petrides, this volume, Chapter 3. This concerns the shape of the sulci, the number of their segments, and their presence. Previous studies by our group have shown that the diagonal sulcus, which may subdivide the opercular part of the inferofrontal gyrus into an anterior and a posterior part, was present in only the half of the 20 observed hemispheres (Amunts et al., 1999). This sulcus has been interpreted as an indicator for a subdivision of BA 44 into an anterior and a posterior portion in the map of von Economo and Koskinas (1925).

Because of the considerable intersubject variability in the sulcal pattern, the question arises of how far this variability is also reflected on a microstructural level. To answer this question, we have applied quantitative tools of analysis of histological, cell body–stained sections of the human brain and have defined the borders of BA 44 and 45 in these sections using an algorithm-based approach (Schleicher et al., 1999).

Cytoarchitecture

In contrast to classic cytoarchitectonic studies, which were mainly based on purely visual inspection of histological sections and rather subjective cytoarchitectonic criteria such as the presence of large pyramidal cells and the distinctiveness of the laminar and columnar organization of the cortex, recent methodological progress enabled an observer-independent definition of the borders of BA 44 and 45 (Amunts et al., 1999; Schleicher et al., 1999; Zilles et al., 2002) based on the statistical evaluation of laminar changes in the grey level index (GLI), (Schleicher and Zilles, 1990). Even though these modern methods are observer independent, they search for borders along the same lines that Brodmann proposed, namely looking for abrupt changes in the cytoarchitecture. Observer-independent mapping includes (1) the measurement of the GLI as an estimate of the volume fraction of nerve cell bodies (Wree et al., 1982), (2) the calculation of profiles that quantified the laminar changes in the volume fraction from the cortical surface to the white matter, that is, the cytoarchitecture, and that covered in small equidistant intervals the putative border regions of the cytoarchitectonic areas, (3) the extraction of features from the profiles as numerical descriptors of the shape of the profiles, that is, cytoarchitecture, (4) the calculation of the Mahalanobis distances as measures of differences in shape

FIGURE 2–3. Algorithm-based definition of areal borders in the inferior frontal cortex of a left hemisphere. (A) Regions of interest are defined in cell body stained histological sections. (B) The GLI (Schleicher and Zilles, 1990) as a measure of the volume fraction of cell bodies is defined, and GLI (grey level index) images are obtained in which each pixel corresponds to a certain value grey value, that is, the *volume* fraction. The cortex is covered by consecutive traverses, reaching from the layer I–layer II border to the cortex–white matter border. Profiles are obtained along these traverses that quantify laminar changes in the GLI. (C) Multivariate statistical analysis is applied in order to define the positions of those profiles (here at positions 111 and 33) at which the shape of the profiles, that is, the cytoarchitecture, changes abruptly. (D) These positions indicate areal borders—in this section, the borders of BA 44. sprc/sfi, junction of the precentral and the inferior frontal sulcus; sd/sfi, junction of the diagonal and the inferior frontal sulcus.

———————————————→

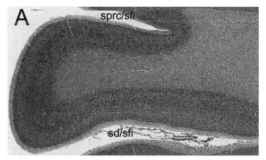

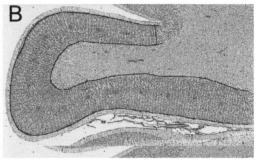

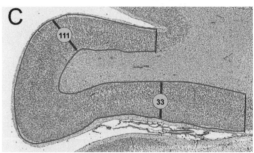

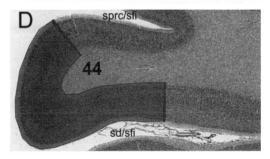

between profiles coming from different areas, and (5) the definition of areal borders at those locations at which the Mahalanobis distances showed significant values, thus indicating that the shape of the profile, that is, the cytoarchitecture, has changed abruptly (Fig. 2–3, see color insert). The Mahalanobis distance is a multivariate distance measure that quantifies shape differences between groups of profiles, that is, differences in the laminar pattern or cytoarchitecture. The larger the Mahalanobis distance, the larger are cytoarchitectonic differences, and vice versa—the smaller the distance, the more similar are the laminar patterns (Schleicher et al., 1999).

Locations of significant changes in the Mahalanobis distance function have been accepted as areal borders if they could be verified in serial histological sections. In contrast, if a border has been defined only on a single histological section, it was rejected.

Changes in the laminar patterns as detected by the observer-independent approach coincide well with changes in cytoarchitecture between BA 44 and 45 and the surrounding areas. For example, both BA 44 and 45 show conspicuous pyramidal cells in the deep part of layer III, whereas such cells are absent in neighboring BA 8, 9, and 46. In contrast to BA 6, which is interpreted as premotor cortex and is agranular (i.e., without an internal granular layer IV), BA 44 is dysgranular; that is, layer IV is visible, but pyramidal cells from the lower part of layer III and from the upper

part of layer V may intermingle with granular cells of layer IV. This blurs the appearance of layer IV as a separate layer containing granular cells exclusively.

When taking the layer IV criterion into account, dysgranular BA 44 seems to occupy an intermediate position between the more posterior agranular BA 6 and the more anterior granular BA 45. These transformations from the agranular (BA 6) via the dysgranular (BA 44) to the granular cortex (BA 45) may be interpreted as "gradations," or stepwise, architectonic differentiations of the frontal lobe in coronal directions that have been described by Sanides (1966) and Vogt and Vogt (1919b). In this context, it seems to be interesting to know to which of them (BA 45 or BA 6) BA 44 is more similar. Greater similarity of BA 44 to BA 6 would be an argument that BA 44 belongs to the "motor" family of cortical areas. If BA 44 is more similar to BA 45, this would be an argument of combining BA 44 and 45 into one family such as Broca's region.

Analyses of this kind, however, can be performed only on the basis of measurements and statistical analysis, not on pure visually guided descriptions. Dissimilarities of Brodmann's areas 44, 45, and 6 as well as the visual areas V1 and V2 (for internal comparison) therefore have been analyzed via GLI profiles as measures of cortical cytoarchitecture. Euclidean distances were calculated as multivariate measures of dissimilarity between profiles of different cortical areas (=interareal differences). Multidimensional scaling was applied for the visualization of interareal differences and for data reduction to a two-dimensional plane defined by dimension 1 and dimension 2 (Schleicher et al., 2000): the larger the dissimilarity in cytoarchitecture between two areas, the larger was the distance between them in the graph (Fig. 2–4, see color insert). The distances on the graph showed high similarities between Brodmann's areas 44 and 45. Both areas differed considerably from area 6 as well as from visual areas V1 and V2. Thus, BA 44 and 45 seem to belong to a

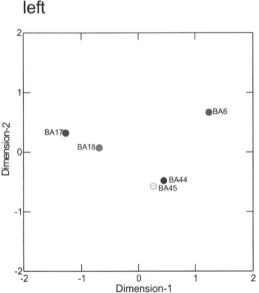

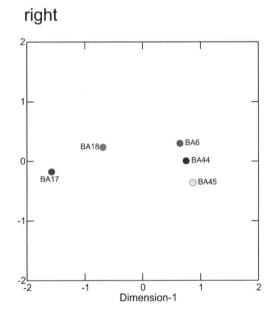

FIGURE 2–4. Cytoarchitectonic dissimilarities between Brodmann's areas (BA) 44, 45, and 6 and areas V1 and V2 for left and right hemispheres. Data are based on the analysis of 10 human postmortem brains. Euclidean distances were calculated as multivariate measures of dissimilarity between profiles of different cortical areas (=interareal differences). They are calculated using features that characterize the shape of the profiles of an area. Multidimensional scaling was applied for visualization of interareal differences and for data reduction to a two-dimensional plane defined by dimension 1 and dimension 2 (Schleicher et al., 2000). The greater the dissimilarity in cytoarchitecture between two areas, the larger

is the distance between them in the graph. Although left hemispheric areas 44 and 45 were found to be very similar in cytoarchitecture, both areas differed from area 6 and even more from visual areas V1 and V2. Differences in cytoarchitecture between areas 6 on the one hand and areas 44 and 45 on the other were less pronounced in the right hemisphere. Area 44 seems to take an intermediate position between areas 45 and 6 with respect to its cytoarchitecture, the location in rostrocaudal direction, and in receptorarchitecture (see Fig. 2–5). The two visual areas (V1 and V2) can clearly be distinguished on the basis of their cytoarchitecture from the three frontal ones (6, 44, and 45).

family of areas, and V1 and V2 belong to another family, whereas BA 6 does not belong to any of these two families but instead seems to belong to a third group. This would make sense with respect to the functional involvements as language—related, visual, and motor, respectively.

Receptorarchitecture

Further arguments come from the analysis of the distribution of different receptor binding sites of the classic neurotransmitters. Considering that receptor borders are even more likely to reflect functional distinctions than are cytoarchitectonic borders and that receptorarchitectonic borders coincide with cytoarchitectonic borders, as we show later, Brodmann's hypothesis regarding a correspondence between structure and function is further supported.

Unfixed frozen hemispheres (n = 4) were serially sectioned in the frontal plane by means of a cryostat microtome for large sections. Quantitative in vitro receptor autoradiography of various receptor subtypes of neurotransmitter systems was performed using tritiated ligands (Zilles et al., 2002). The laminar and regional distribution of glutamatergic (AMPA, kainate, NMDA), GABAergic (GABA$_A$, GABA$_B$), muscarinic cholinergic (M$_1$, M$_2$), noradrenergic (α_1, α_2), adenosinergic (A1), and serotonergic (5-HT$_{1A}$, 5-HT$_2$) receptors were examined in the inferofrontal lobe. Cell body staining was performed on adjacent sections for cytoarchitectonic analysis. The distribution of different receptor bindings sites revealed both interlaminar and regional differences. For example, the AMPA receptor binding site for glutamate shows a higher concentration in BA 6 than in BA 44 and in BA 45. There is a caudal-to-rostral gradient in the binding site concentrations from BA 4 over BA 6, BA 44 to BA 45 (Fig. 2–5, see color insert). [^{3}H]Prazosin labels the noradrenergic α_1 receptor and also shows a caudal-to-rostral gradient with higher concentrations of binding sites in BA 4 and BA 6 compared with BA 45.

In addition to differences in receptor densities between cortical areas, there are heterogeneities within a cortical area. For example, binding to the AMPA receptor subdivided BA 45 into a rostral part with higher concentrations in the supragranular layers and a caudal part with lower concentrations in these layers. The infragranular layers of both subdivisions show approximately similar values. The receptorarchitectonic findings agree with data from comparative cytoarchi-

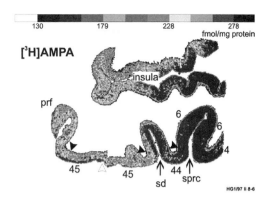

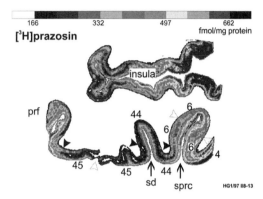

FIGURE 2–5. Regional distributions of glutamatergic AMPA and noradrenergic α_1 receptors (demonstrated with [^{3}H]AMPA and [^{3}H]prazosin) in horizontal sections through the human frontal lobe (Amunts, Palomero-Gallagher, and Zilles; unpublished observation). Grey value images were scaled, enhanced in contrast, and color coded (Zilles, 2003). The color scales indicate the total binding in fmol/mg protein. The receptors are heterogeneously distributed and, therefore, allow mapping of cortical areas including 4, 6, 44, and 45 (*arrowheads*). In addition to these cortical areas, subdivisions have been identified on the basis of receptorarchitectonic mapping (*open arrowheads*). Borders obtained by receptor architectonic mapping were compared with borders revealed by cytoarchitectonic mapping. Note the decrease in receptor density from caudal to rostral positions. The different architectonic techniques supplement each other and are the basis of multimodal architectonic mapping. sprc, precentral sulcus; sd, diagonal sulcus; prf, prefrontal cortex (*arrows*).

tectonic analysis of the human and macaque brain (Petrides and Pandya, 2001).

Another subdivision, in dorsoventral direction, can be found in coronal sections showing Brodmann's

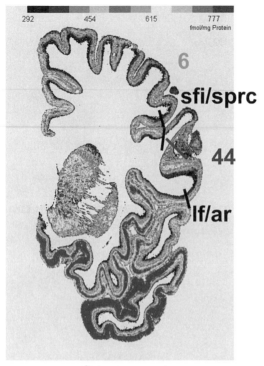

[³H] Ketanserin
Serotonin

FIGURE 2–6. Regional distributions of serotonergic 5-HT$_2$ receptors (demonstrated with [³H]ketanserin) in a coronal section through the human frontal lobe (Amunts, Palomero-Gallagher, and Zilles; unpublished observation). Designation of areas as in Figure 2–5. lf/ar, ascending branch of the lateral fissure. sfi, inferior frontal sulcus.

area 44. The 5-HT$_2$ receptor for serotonin subdivides a more dorsal part with lower binding site density from a more ventral part with higher density (Fig. 2–6, see color insert).

Evidence for a heterogeneity of BA 44 has been already provided in cytoarchitectonic studies, but the subdivision of BA 44 have not yet been mapped systematically (Amunts et al., 1999). Functional imaging studies revealed an activation pattern that seem to occupy only parts of BA 44, not the entire area. For example, the most ventral (and posterior) part of BA 44 had been activated in a syntactic task (Indefrey et al., 2001). Imagery of movement (a task that was not directly related to language) has shown to activate the most caudoventral part of BA 44 (Binkofski et al., 2000). On the other hand, phonological processing

seems to involve only the superior portion of the left pars opercularis of the inferofrontal gyrus, not the inferior one (Heim and Friederici, 2003). It has to be underlined, however, that these tasks have not specifically been conducted to evaluate the substructure of Broca's region. There is a considerable variability across studies (usually due to the use of different types of materials, different reference systems, statistical tools of analysis, smoothing, etc.), which makes it problematic to compare them directly (see, e.g., Poeppel et al., 1996).

The existing data on cytoarchitecture and receptorarchitecture as well as functional imaging data strongly suggest a further subdivision of both BA 44 and 45. As a consequence, the Brodmann's parcellation scheme seems to be not necessarily the adequate anatomical reference for functional activations obtained during fMRI and PET experiments. For other brain regions, such as the visual cortex, this discrepancy between Brodmann's map and functional, architectonic, and connectivity data has already been demonstrated (Zilles and Clarke, 1997). Retinotopic mapping (Sereno et al., 1995; Tootell et al., 1997) revealed a much more detailed map than the proposed tripartion of the visual cortex as proposed by Brodmann (1909).

Is it possible, as an alternative, to interpret functional imaging data with respect to gyri and sulci only, without relating them to cortical areas or subareas? There are, at least, two problems with this approach. The first concerns the intersubject variability in the shape, presence, and size of gyri and sulci (see earlier). The second is related to the variability in the localization of cortical borders with respect to the sulci.

Localization of BA 44 and 45 With Respect to Surrounding Sulci and Gyri

The definition of borders using an observer-independent approach has shown that the location of the borders does not coincide with sulcal markers, such as the crown of a gyrus or the depth of a sulcus. As an example, the dorsal border of BA 44 has been found in the ventral bank of the inferior frontal sulcus in some sections, but also in its dorsal bank in other sections. It never, however, reached the free surface of the middle frontal gyrus. The inferior frontal sulcus was sometimes interrupted and consisted of two, three, or even four independent segments. This was the case in 44% of the right hemispheres and 60% of the left hemispheres as reported by Ono et al. (1990). The dorsal border of BA 44 and 45 cannot continuously be approximated by the inferior frontal sulcus in half of the brains.

The same situation is true for the caudal border of BA 44 with respect to the inferior segment of the precentral sulcus and for the border between BA 44 and 45. The latter may be located either close to the ascending branch of the lateral fissure or in the region of the diagonal sulcus, or somewhere between these sulci. Thus, although it is true that BA 45 usually occupies the triangular part of the inferior frontal gyrus, and BA 44, the opercular part, the location of the *borders* of both areas to the surrounding sulci is less well defined by sulci. The more one moves from the free surfaces of the opercular and triangular parts into the depths of the surrounding sulci, the more uncertain is the localization of the borders of BA 44 and 45, respectively. This variability is additive to the variability of the opercular and triangular parts (Tomaiuolo et al., 1999).

Finally, two thirds of the cortex are hidden in the depths of the sulci, and not on the outer surface of the brain (Zilles et al., 1988). As a consequence, the size of the free surface of the opercular and triangular parts is not an indicator of the sizes, that is, the volumes, of BA 44 and 45. A relatively small extent of an area on the free surface may be associated with high volume values due to a large portion of the area that is hidden in the sulci, such as the precentral and the diagonal sulci (Fig. 2–7, see color insert).

Interhemispheric Differences

The volumes of both areas also varied considerably (by a factor of 10) between the postmortem brains. This variability was considerably larger than that in other brain regions, such as the hippocampus, where the volume varied by only a factor of 2 (Amunts et al., 2005). Volumes of left BA 44, however, were always larger than those of the right hemisphere (Amunts et al., 1999). This was in correspondence to data of Galaburda (1980). In contrast to BA 44, the volumes of BA 45 did not differ significantly between the hemispheres. Both areas, however, differed between the two hemispheres in cytoarchitecture as shown on quantitative cytoarchitectonic analysis (Amunts and Zilles, 2001). Thus, interhemispheric differences in the volume of BA 44 and cytoarchitectonic differences may be interpreted as anatomical correlates of language dominance and supplement

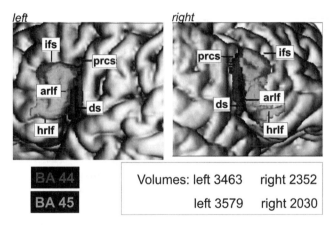

FIGURE 2–7. Surface rendering of Brodmann's area (BA) 44 (red) and BA 45 (yellow) in a postmortem brain of the left and the right hemispheres based on cell body stained histological sections and observer-independent definition of cytoarchitectonic borders in serial histological sections (Amunts et al., 1999). The volumes (in mm³) of the areas have been calculated using Cavalieri's principle. Note that the different extents of the areas on the free surface do not reflect their volumes. For example, BA 45 occupies a considerably larger portion of the free surface than BA 44, but the volumes show very similar values. In addition, BA 44 seems to be slightly larger on the right side as judged by its extent on the free surface, but the volume is greater on the left side by a factor of 1.5. arlf, ascending branch of the lateral fissure; ds, diagonal sulcus; hrlf, horizontal branch of the lateral fissure; ifs, inferior frontal sulcus; prcs, precentral sulcus.

earlier data on interhemispheric asymmetry on a cellular level (Hayes and Lewis, 1995, 1996; Jacobs et al., 1993).

Interestingly, interhemispheric differences in cytoarchitecture (i.e., interhemispheric asymmetry) as estimated by multivariate Euclidean distances were already found in 1-year-old infants (Amunts et al., 2003). Asymmetry tended to increase with age, which was significant in BA 45 but not in BA 44. An adult-like, left-larger-than-right asymmetry in the GLI was reached approximately at an age of 5 years in BA 45 and 11 years in BA 44. These time points indicate delayed development of the cytoarchitectonic asymmetry in Broca's region in comparison to that of the primary motor cortex (BA 4) (Amunts et al., 1997). It may be hypothesized that the delayed maturation is the microstructural basis of the development of language abilities and the influence of language practice on cytoarchitecture during childhood. Interhemispheric asymmetry in cytoarchitecture of BA 44 and 45 continues changing throughout life. We conclude that the cytoarchitectonic asymmetry of Brodmann's areas 44 and 45 is a result of microstructural plasticity that endures throughout almost the entire life span (Amunts et al., 1997). Considering functional imaging data suggesting that BA 44 is more involved in syntactic processes and BA 45 is more involved in semantic processes, the data on the developmental aspects of interhemispheric asymmetry fit nicely with behavioral findings that adult-like syntactic processes are observable only around the age of 10 years (Friederici and Kotz, 2003), whereas adult-like semantic processes are established much earlier (Friederici, 1983).

STRUCTURAL–FUNCTIONAL ANALYSIS OF BROCA'S REGION

BA 44 and 45 in Stereotaxic Space

Cytoarchitectonic borders of both areas on histological sections were reconstructed in three dimensions and warped to a common reference space, such as the T1-weighted MR single-subject brain of the Montreal Neurological Institute (MNI) (Collins et al., 1994; Evans et al., 1993; Holmes et al., 1998) and the reference brain of the ECHBD (Roland and Zilles, 1994). For warping, we have developed and applied

a combination of an affine preregistration and an elastic, nonlinear registration (Henn et al., 1997; Hömke et al., 2004; Mohlberg et al., 2003). The elastic transformation was computed by minimizing a nonlinear functional composed of the sum of squared differences between the two data sets and the elastic energy of the transformation field. This leads to a system of Navier-Lamé equations. The equations were solved with a full multigrid approach, that is, a multiscale approach with a multigrid as a solver at each scale. As a result of this step, the MR data of the original data sets of the brains coincided both in shape (sulcal pattern, external shape) and in size with the data set of the reference brain.

The superimposition of the 10 brain data sets in standard reference space enabled the calculation of probabilistic maps of each area. These maps show, for each voxel of the reference space, the frequency with witch a certain cortical areas was present in the sample of postmortem brains (Fig. 2–8, see color insert). The probabilistic maps of BA 44 and 45 and corresponding maps of other cortical areas and subcortical structures are available at http://www.fz-juelich.de/ime and http://www.bic.mni.mcgill.ca/cytoarchitectonics/. Both brains are applied as reference systems for functional imaging studies.

The application of a common reference brain for postmortem data of cytoarchitectonically defined areas (e.g., BA 44 and 45) and data obtained during paradigms testing for a certain component of language processing in an fMRI or a PET experiment enables the interpretation of functional activations with respect to the probabilistic maps. As an example, we show a combined fMRI and cytoarchitectonic study (Amunts et al., 2004), analyzing the involvement of BA 44 and 45 in a verbal fluency task. To do so, we combined data from a previous fMRI (Gurd et al., 2002) and from our cytoarchitectonic study (Amunts et al., 1999). In the fMRI experiment, verbal fluency was investigated in 11 healthy volunteers, who covertly produced words from predefined categories. A factorial design was used with factors verbal class (semantic versus overlearned fluency) and switching between categories (no versus yes). Cytoarchitectonic maps of BA 44 and 45 were derived from histological sections of 10 postmortem brains. Both the in vivo fMRI and postmortem MR data were warped to the common reference brain of the ECHBD (Roland and Zilles, 1994) using the above-mentioned elastic warp-

A

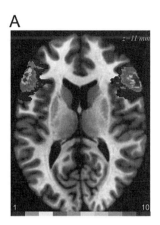

B

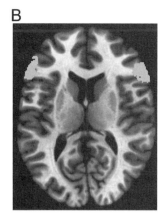

FIGURE 2–8. Probabilistic map of Brodmann's area 45 in standard stereotaxic space (T1-weighted single-subject brain of the MNI; Evans et al., 1993). (A) Complete probabilistic map showing the frequency with which Brodmann's area 45 was present in a particular voxel of the standard reference space. Fre-quencies are color-coded, whereby red means maxi-mal overlap of all 10 brains, dark orange corresponds to an overlap of 9 brains, etc. (B) 50% map of the area. All of the voxels are part of the 50% map that over-lapped in at least 5 of 10 brains.

ing tool. The cytoarchitectonic probability maps showed the involvement of left hemisphere areas with verbal fluency relative to the baseline. Semantic rel-ative to overlearned fluency showed greater involve-ment of left BA 45 than of 44. Thus, although both areas participate in verbal fluency, they do so differ-entially. Left BA 45 was more involved in semantic aspects of language processing, whereas BA 44 was probably involved in high-level aspects of program-ming speech production per se. The combination of functional data analysis with a new elastic warping tool and cytoarchitectonic maps opens new perspec-tives for analyzing the cortical networks involved in language (Horwitz et al., 1998; Stephan et al., 2003).

RESUME

The frontal cortex consists of numerous areas, each with a special architecture (cyto-, myelo-, receptor-, etc.), connectivity, and function. Quantitative tools of the analysis may assist in defining these cortical areas and their position in a hierarchy of cortical regions and subregions. They enable a reliable definition of areal borders and the consideration of intersubject variability.

In our particular case, receptorarchitecture sug-gests a further subdivision of BA 44 and 45. The com-bination of microstructurally defined maps and data obtained in fMRI studies investigating different as-pects of language may open further perspectives for analyzing language and underlying brain structure.

References

Aboitiz, F., & Garcia, G.L. (1997). The evolutionary ori-gin of language areas in the human brain. A neu-roanatomical perspective. *Brain Research Reviews*, 25, 381–396.

Amunts, K., Kedo, O., Kindler, M., Pieperhoff, P., Hömke, L., Schneider, F., Mohlberg, H., Shah, N.J., Habel, U., & Zilles, K. (2005). Cytoarchitec-tonic mapping of the human amygdala, hippocam-pal region, and entorhinal cortex. *Anatomy and Embryology*, in press.

Amunts, K., Schleicher, A., & Zilles, K. (2004). Out-standing language competence and cytoarchitec-ture in Broca's speech region. *Brain and Language*, 89, 346–353.

Amunts, K., Schleicher, A., Ditterich, A., & Zilles, K. (2003). Broca's region: Cytoarchitectonic asymme-try and developmental changes. *Journal of Com-parative Neurology*, 465, 72–89.

Amunts, K., Schleicher, A., Bürgel, U., Mohlberg, H., Uylings, H.B.M., & Zilles, K. (1999). Broca's region revisited: Cytoarchitecture and intersubject vari-ability. *Journal of Comparative Neurology*, 412, 319–341.

Amunts, K., Schmidt-Passos, F., Schleicher, A., & Zilles, K. (1997). Postnatal development of interhemispheric asymmetry in the cytoarchitecture of human area 4. *Anatomy and Embryology, 196,* 393–402.

Amunts, K., Weiss, P.H., Mohlberg, H., Pieperhoff, P., Gurd, J., Shah, J.N., et al. (2004). Analysis of the neural mechanisms underlying verbal fluency in cytoarchitectonically defined stereotaxic space—The role of Brodmann's areas 44 and 45. *Neuroimage, 22,* 42–56.

Amunts, K., & Zilles, K. (2001). Advances in cytoarchitectonic mapping of the human cerebral cortex. In T.P. Naidich, T.A. Yousry, & V.P. Mathews (Eds.), *Neuroimaging clinics of North America on functional MR imaging* (pp. 151–169). Philadelphia: Harcourt.

Binkofski, F., Amunts, K., Stephan, K.M., Posse, S., Schormann, T., Freund, H.-J., et al. (2000). Broca's region subserves imagery of motion: A combined cytoarchitectonic and fMRI study. *Human Brain Mapping, 11,* 273–285.

Broca, M.P. (1861a). Perte de la parole, ramollissement chronique et desstruction partielle du lob antérieur gauche de cerveau. *Bulletins de la Société d'Antrhopologie, 62,* 235–238.

Broca, M.P. (1861b). Remarques sur le siége de la faculté du langage articulé, suivies d'une observation d'aphemie (Perte de la Parole). *Bulletins et Memoires de la Societe Anatomique de Paris, 36,* 330–357.

Broca, M.P. (1863). Localisation des fonctions cérébrales. Siege du langage articulé. *Bulletins de la Société d'Anthropologie, Séance du 2 Avril,* 200–204.

Broca, M.P. (1865). Sur la siege de la faculté langage articulé. *Bulletin of the Society of Anthropology, 6,* 377–396.

Brodmann, K. (1912). Neue Ergebnisse über die vergleichende histologische Lokalisation der Großhirnrinde mit besonderer Berücksichtigung des Stirnhirns. *Anatomischer Anzeiger, Ergänzungsheft zum 41. Band,* 157–216.

Collins, D.L., Neelin, P., Peters, T.M., & Evans, A.C. (1994). Automatic 3D intersubject registration of MR volumetric data in standardized Talairach space. *Journal of Computer Assisted Tomography, 18,* 192–205.

Duvernoy H. (1991). *The human brain. Surface, three-dimensional sectional anatomy and MRI.* New York: Springer.

Evans, A.C., Collins, D.L., Mills, S.R., Brown, E.D., Kelly, R.L., and Peters, T.M. (1993). 3D statistical neuroanatomical models from 305 MRI volumes. 1813–1817. IEEE-NSS-MI Symposium.

Friederici, A.D. (1983). Children's sensitivity to function words during sentence comprehension. *Linguistics, 21,* 717–739.

Friederici, A.D., & Kotz, S.A. (2003). The brain basis of syntactic processes: functional imaging and lesions studies. *Neuroimage, 20,* S8–S17.

Galaburda, A.M. (1980). La region de Broca: Observations anatomiques faites un siecle apres la mort de son decoveur. *Revue Neurology (Paris), 136,* 609–616.

Goldstein, K. (1946). Remarks on localisation. *Confidia Neurologica, 7,* 25–34.

Gurd, J., Amunts, K., Weiss, P.H., Zafiris, O., Zilles, K., Marshall, J.C., et al. (2002). Posterior parietal cortex is implicated in continous switching between verbal fluency tasks: An fMRI study with clinical implications. *Brain, 125,* 1024–1038.

Harasty, J., Halliday, G.M., & Kril, J.J. (1996). Reproducible sampling regimen for specific cortical regions: Application to speech-related areas. *Journal of Neuroscience Methods, 67,* 43–51.

Hayes, T.L., & Lewis, D.A. (1992). Nonphosphorylated neurofilament protein and calbindin immunoreactivity in layer III pyramidal neurons of human neocortex. *Cerebral Cortex, 2,* 56–67.

Hayes, T.L., & Lewis, D.A. (1995). Anatomical specialization of the anterior motor speech area: Hemispheric differences in magnopyramidal neurons. *Brain and Language, 49,* 289–308.

Hayes, T.L., & Lewis, D.A. (1996). Magnopyramidal neurons in the anterior motor speech region. *Archives of Neurology, 53,* 1277–1283.

Heim, S., & Friederici, A.F. (2003). Phonological processing in language production. *Neuroreport, 14,* 2031–2033.

Henn, S., Schormann, T., Engler, K., Zilles, K., & Witsch, K. (1997). Elastische Anpassung in der digitalen Bildverarbeitung auf mehreren Auflösungsstufen mit Hilfe von Mehrgitterverfahren. In E. Paulus & F. M. Wahl (Eds.), *Mustererkennung* (pp. 392–399). Informatik aktuell. Berlin: Springer.

Hervé, G. (1888). *La circonvolution de Broca. Etude de morphologie cerebrale.* Paris: A. Davy.

Holmes, C.J., Hoge, R., Collins, L., Woods, R., Toga, A.W., & Evans, A.C. (1998). Enhancement of MR images using registration for signal averaging. *Journal of Computer Assisted Tomography, 22,* 324–333.

Hömke, L., Weder, B., Binkofski, F., & Amunts, K. (2004). Lesion mapping in MRI data—an application of cytoarchitectonic probabilistic maps. Second Vogt-Brodmann Symposium: The convergence of structure and function, P21. Jülich; Forschungszentrum Jülich GmbH.

Horwitz, B., Rumsey, J.M., & Donohue, B.C. (1998). Functional connectivity of the angular gyrus in normal reading and dyslexia. *Proceedings of the National Academy of Science USA*, 95, 8939–8944.

Indefrey, P., Brown, C.M., Hellwig, F., Amunts, K., Herzog, H., Seitz, R.J., et al. (2001). A neural correlate of syntactic encoding during speech production. *Proceedings of the National Academy of Science USA*, 98, 5933–5936.

Jacobs, B., Batal, H.A., Lynch, B., Ojemann, G., Ojemann, L.M., & Scheibel, A.B. (1993). Quantitative dendritic and spine analysis of speech cortices: A case study. *Brain and Language*, 44, 239–253.

Kolb, B., & Whishaw, I.Q. (1996). *Human neuropsychology*. New York: W.H. Freeman and Company.

Kononova, E.P. (1949). The frontal lobe (in Russian). In: S.A. Sarkisov, I.N. Filimonoff, & N.S. Preobrashenskaya (Eds.), *The cytoarchitecture of the human cortex cerebri* (pp. 309–343). Moscow: Medgiz.

Leyton, A.S.F., & Sherrington, C.S. (1917). Observations on the excitable cortex of the chimpanzee, orangutan, and gorilla. *Quarterly Journal of Experimental Physiology*, XI, 135–222.

Lichtheim, L. (1885). On aphasia. *Brain*, 7, 433–484.

Lieberman, P. (2002). On the nature and evolution of the neural bases of human language. *Yearbook of Physical Anthropology*, 45, 36–62.

Luppino, G., Matelli, M., Camarda, R.M., Gallese, V., & Rizzolatti, G. (1991). Multiple representations of body movements in mesial area 6 and the adjacent cingulate cortex: An intracortical microstimulation study in the macaque monkey. *Journal of Comparative Neurology*, 311, 463–482.

Matelli, M., Luppino, G., & Rizzolatti, G. (1991). Architecture of superior and mesial area 6 and the adjacent cingulate cortex in the macaque monkey. *Journal of Comparative Neurology*, 311, 445–462.

Mohlberg, H., Lerch, J., Amunts, K., Evans, A.C., & Zilles, K. (2003). Probabilistic cytoarchitectonic maps transformed into MNI space. Presented at the *9th International Conference on Functional Mapping of the Human Brain*, June 19–22, 2003, New York. Available on CD-Rom in *Neuroimage*, 19(2).

Ono, M., Kubik, S., & Abernathey, C.D. (1990). *Atlas of the cerebral sulci*. Stuttgart/New York: Thieme.

Petrides, M., & Pandya, D.N. (2001). Comparative cytoarchitectonic analysis of the human and the macaque ventrolateral prefrontal cortex and corticocortical connection patterns in the monkey. *European Journal of Neuroscience*, 16, 291–310.

Poeppel, D. (1996). A critical review of PET studies of phonological processing. *Brain and Language*, 55, 317–351.

Riegele, L. (1931). Die Cytoarchitektonik der Felder der Broca'schen Region. *Journal für Psychologie und Neurologie*, 42, 496–514.

Roland, P.E., & Zilles, K. (1994). Brain atlases—A new research tool. *Trends in Neuroscience*, 17, 458–467.

Sanides, F. (1966). The architecture of the human frontal lobe and the relation to its functional differentiation. *International Journal of Anatomy*, 5, 247–261.

Sarkisov, S.A., Filimonoff, I.N., & Preobrashenskaya, N.S. (1949). *Cytoarchitecture of the human cortex cerebri* (in Russian). Moscow: Medgiz.

Schleicher, A., Amunts, K., Geyer, S., Kowalski, T., Schormann, T., Palomero-Gallagher, N., et al. (2000). A stereological approach to human cortical architecture: Identification and delineation of cortical areas. *Journal of Chemcial Neuroanatomy*, 20, 31–47.

Schleicher, A., Amunts, K., Geyer, S., Morosan, P., & Zilles, K. (1999). Observer-independent method for microstructural parcellation of cerebral cortex: A quantitative approach to cytoarchitectonics. *Neuroimage*, 9, 165–177.

Schleicher, A., & Zilles, K. (1990). A quantitative approach to cytoarchitectonics: analysis of structural inhomogeneities in nervous tissue using an image analyser. *Journal of Microscopy*, 157, 367–381.

Sereno, M.I., Dale, A.M., Reppas, J.B., Kwong, K.K., Belliveau, J.W., Brady, T.I., et al. (1995). Borders of multiple visual areas in humans revealed by functional magnetic resonance imaging. *Science*, 268, 889–893.

Signoret, J.-L., Castaigne, P., Lhermitte, F., Abelanet, R., & Lavorel, P. (1984). Rediscovery of Leborgne's brain: Anatomical description wit CT scan. *Brain and Language*, 22, 303–319.

Stephan, K.E., Marshall, J.C., Friston, K.J., Rowe, J.B., Ritzl, A., Zilles, K., et al. (2003). Lateralized cognitive processes and lateralized task control in the human brain. *Science*, 301, 384–386.

Stookey, B. (1954). A note on the early history of cerebral localization. *Bulletin of the New York Academy of Medicine*, 30, 559–578.

Strasburger, E.H. (1938). Vergleichende myeloarchitektonische Studien an der erweiterten Brocaschen Region des Menschen. *Journal für Psychologie und Neurologie*, 48, 477–511.

Tanji, J., & Kurata, K. (1989). Changing concepts of motor areas of the cerebral cortex. *Brain Development*, 11, 374–377.

Tomaiuolo, F., MacDonald, B., Caramanos, Z., Posner, G., Chiavaras, M., Evans, A.C., et al. (1999). Morphology, morphometry and probability mapping of the pars opercularis of the inferior frontal gyrus: An in vivo MRI analysis. *European Journal of Neuroscience, 11,* 3033–3046.

Tootell, R.B.H., Mendola, J.D., Hadjikhani, N.K., Ledden, P.J., Liu, A.K., Reppas, J.B., et al. (1997). Functional analysis of V3A and related areas in human visual cortex. *The Journal of Neuroscience, 17,* 7060–7078.

Uylings, H.B.M., Malofeeva, L.I., Bogolepova, I.N., Amunts, K., & Zilles, K. (1999). Broca's language area from a neuroanatomical and developmental perspective. In P. Hagoort, & C. Brown (Eds.), *Neurocognition of language processing* (pp. 319–336). Oxford: Oxford University Press.

von Economo C., & Koskinas, G.N. (1925). *Die Cytoarchitektonik der Hirnrinde des erwachsenen Menschen.* Berlin: Springer.

Vogt, C., & Vogt, O. (1919a). Allgemeinere Ergebnisse unserer Hirnforschung. Vierte Mitteilung: Die physiologische Bedeutung unserer Rindenfelderung auf Grund neuer Rindenreizung. *Journal für Psychologie und Neurologie, 25,* 399–462.

Vogt, C., & Vogt, O. (1919b). Allgemeinere Ergebnisse unserer Hirnforschung. *Journal für Psychologie und Neurologie, 25,* 292–398.

Vogt, C., & Vogt, O. (1926). Die vergleichend-architektonische und die vergleichend-reizphysiologische Felderung der Großhirnrinde unter besonderer

Berücksichtigung der menschlichen. *Die Naturwissenschaften, 14,* 1192–1195.

Wernicke, C. (1874). *Der aphasische Symptomencomplex. Eine psychologische Studie auf anatomischer Basis.* Berlin: Springer Verlag.

Wree, A., Schleicher, A., & Zilles, K. (1982). Estimation of volume fractions in nervous tissue with an image analyzer. *Journal of Neuroscience Methods, 6,* 29–43.

Zilles, K. (2003). Architecture of the human cerebral cortex: Regional and laminar organization. In G. Paxinos, & J.K. Mai (Eds.), *Human nervous system* (pp. 997–1055). San Diego: Elsevier.

Zilles, K., Schleicher, A., Palomero-Gallagher, N., & Amunts, K. (2002). Quantitative analysis of cyto- and receptor architecture of the human brain. In J.C. Mazziotta and A. Toga (Eds.), *Brain mapping: The methods* (pp. 573–602). New York: Elsevier.

Zilles, K., Armstrong, E., Schleicher, A., & Kretschmann, H.J. (1988). The human pattern of gyrification in the cerebral cortex. *Anatomy and Embryology, 179,* 173–179.

Zilles, K., & Clarke, S. (1997). Architecture, connectivity and transmitter receptors of human extrastriate visual cortex. Comparison with non-human primates. In Rockland, et al. (Ed.), *Cerebral cortex. Vol. 12.* (pp. 673–742). New York: Plenum Press.

3

Broca's Area in the Human and the Nonhuman Primate Brain

Michael Petrides

The posterior part of the inferior frontal gyrus in the left hemisphere is traditionally considered to constitute the classic Broca's area (Dejerine, 1914), that is, the anterofrontal cortical area that is thought to play a critical role in certain aspects of language production (Geschwind, 1970; Grodzinsky, 2000). The posterior part of the inferior frontal gyrus exhibits two gross morphological subdivisions: the pars opercularis (Op) and the pars triangularis (Tr) (Fig. 3–1, see color insert). Although several attempts have been made to specify more precisely the critical zone for language within this general region on the basis of clinical–anatomical correlation studies (see, e.g., Alexander et al., 1989; Mohr et al., 1978), such endeavors have been of limited success because of the difficulty in obtaining lesions that are restricted to particular subdivisions of the inferior frontal region. The best evidence thus far has been obtained from electrical stimulation of the cerebral cortex carried out under local anesthesia during brain surgery to establish, in a particular patient, the precise part of the left hemisphere

that is critical for speech. This approach is motivated by the need to spare cortex critical for language. The critical region is considered to be the part of the cortex from which dysphasic speech arrest can be evoked by the application of electrical stimulation. Such studies have established that, in the lateral frontal lobe of the left hemisphere, dysphasic speech arrest occurs most reliably from stimulation of that part of the inferior frontal gyrus that lies immediately anterior to the lower end of the precentral gyrus, that is, the pars opercularis (Fig. 3–2, see color insert) (Duffau et al., 2003; Ojemann et al., 1989; Penfield and Roberts, 1959; Rasmussen and Milner, 1975). Stimulation of the ventral precentral region, which represents the orofacial motor region, also interferes with speech, but this interference is primarily due to dysarthria and evoked vocalization responses caused by disruption of normal activity in the motor circuits necessary for speech.

The term "Broca's area" is used inconsistently by different authors. Some investigators restrict the use

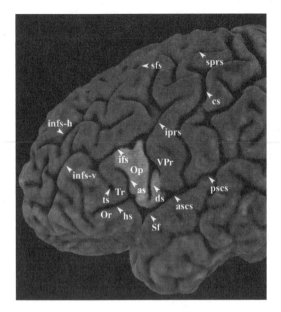

The ventrolateral surface of the human frontal cortex is dominated by the inferior frontal gyrus. It is delimited superiorly by the horizontally directed inferior frontal sulcus and inferiorly by the anterior part of the Sylvian (lateral) fissure (see Fig. 3–1). The inferior frontal gyrus can be divided into three parts: the pars opercularis, the pars triangularis, and the pars orbitalis. The pars opercularis, which is the most posterior part of the inferior frontal gyrus, lies immediately in front of the lower part of the precentral gyrus, where the orofacial motor/premotor region is repre-

FIGURE 3–1. Three-dimensional reconstruction of the lateral frontal lobe in the left hemisphere based on a magnetic resonance image of a single human brain. The shaded area shows the pars opercularis of the inferior frontal gyrus. as, ascending sulcus (i.e., vertical ramus of the Sylvian fissure); ascs, anterior subcentral sulcus; cs, central sulcus; ds, diagonal sulcus; ifs, inferior frontal sulcus; infs-h, intermediate frontal sulcus (horizontal part); infs-v, intermediate frontal sulcus (vertical part); iprs, inferior precentral sulcus; Op, pars opercularis of the inferior frontal gyrus; Or, pars orbitalis of the inferior frontal gyrus; pscs, posterior subcentral sulcus; Sf, Sylvian fissure; sfs, superior frontal sulcus; sprs, superior precentral sulcus; Tr, pars triangularis of the inferior frontal gyrus; ts, triangular sulcus; hs, horizontal sulcus (i.e., horizontal ramus of the Sylvian fissure); VPr, ventral precentral gyrus.

of this term to the pars opercularis that is the focus of the zone yielding dysphasic speech arrest upon electrical stimulation (see, e.g., Mohr et al., 1978; Rasmussen and Milner, 1975), whereas others use the term more broadly to include the pars opercularis and the pars triangularis (see, e.g., Amunts et al., 1999). Language disturbance following electrical stimulation can also occasionally be evoked by stimulation of the caudal part of the pars triangularis. This chapter first examines the gross morphology of the inferior frontal region of the human brain within which Broca's area lies and then examines the architectonic areas that are occupying this region and compares them with similar areas in the macaque monkey brain.

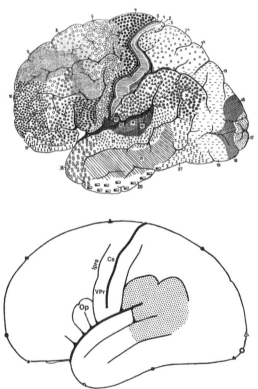

FIGURE 3–2. (*Top*) Cytoarchitectonic map of Brodmann (1909) with the pars opercularis (area 44) marked in yellow. (*Bottom*) Summary of electrical stimulation studies causing aphasic arrest of speech (adapted from Rasmussen and Milner, 1975). In the lateral frontal cortex, aphasic arrest of speech is obtained from stimulation of the pars opercularis (marked in yellow). Cs, central sulcus; Iprs, inferior precentral sulcus; Op, pars opercularis of the inferior frontal gyrus; VPr, ventral precentral gyrus.

sented. The inferior precentral sulcus separates the pars opercularis from the precentral region, and anteriorly, the vertical (ascending) ramus of the Sylvian fissure separates the pars opercularis from the pars triangularis. The pars triangularis lies between the ascending sulcus and the horizontal sulcus, that is, the horizontal ramus of the Sylvian fissure. Within the pars triangularis, there is usually a small sulcus, the triangular sulcus, also known as the incisura capitis. The pars orbitalis lies inferior to the horizontal sulcus and extends as far as the lateral orbital sulcus. Posteriorly, the inferior frontal sulcus originates close to the inferior precentral sulcus, and in many brains, there is a clear separation between these two sulci. In other cases, the narrow bridge of cortex that separates them may be submerged and thus the inferior frontal sulcus and the inferior precentral sulcus merge superficially. Eberstaller (1890) pointed out that the inferior frontal sulcus extends anteriorly until about the mid-portion of the dorsal edge of the pars triangularis of the inferior frontal gyrus. Our recent investigation of the frontal sulci of the human brain has confirmed Eberstaller's observations (Petrides and Pandya, 2004).

We examined in detail the morphology of the pars opercularis of the inferior frontal gyrus from the MR images of 54 normal adult human brains (Tomaiuolo et al., 1999). This region, which is defined as the part of the inferior frontal gyrus that lies between the inferior precentral sulcus and the vertical ramus of the Sylvian fissure, exhibits considerable morphological variability. The pars opercularis appears usually as a vertically oriented gyrus that may be subdivided into an anterior and a posterior part by the diagonal sulcus (Fig. 3–3, see color insert). In several brains, a variable extent of the posterior part of the pars opercularis may be submerged into the inferior precentral sulcus (see Tomaiuolo et al., 1999). An example of such a brain is shown in Figure 3–1, where the posterior part of the pars opercularis (i.e., the part behind the diagonal sulcus) is seen to be receding into the inferior precentral sulcus. Depending on the curvature of the pars opercularis and how much of it remains on the surface of the brain, the diagonal sulcus may appear to lie in the middle of the pars opercularis clearly separating it into two parts (i.e., two opercular convolutions) (Fig. 3–3), or it may appear to join any one of the surrounding sulci. This poste-

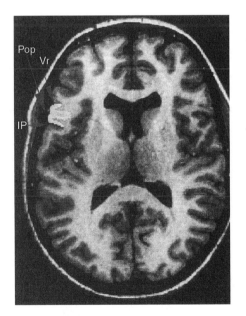
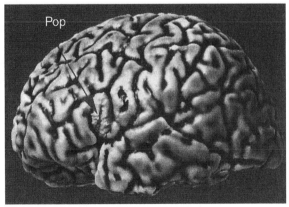

FIGURE 3–3. Three-dimensional reconstruction of the lateral surface of the left hemisphere based on a magnetic resonance image of a single human brain (right). A horizontal section through the pars opercularis is shown (left). The pars opercularis of the inferior frontal gyrus (Pop) is marked in yellow. Note that it is formed by two vertically oriented convolutions separated by the diagonal sulcus. IP, inferior precentral sulcus; Pop, pars opercularis of the inferior frontal gyrus; Vr, vertical ramus (ascending sulcus) of the Sylvian fissure.

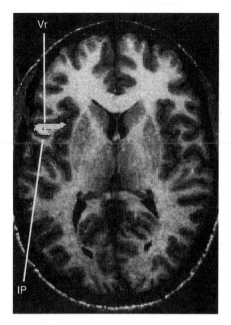
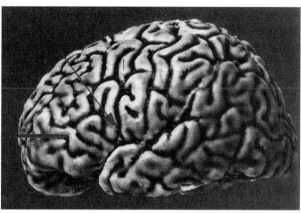

FIGURE 3–4. Three-dimensional reconstruction of the lateral surface of the left hemisphere based on a magnetic resonance image of a single human brain (*right*). A horizontal section taken at the level marked by the blue line is shown (*left*). The pars opercularis of the inferior frontal gyrus is marked in yellow. Note that it is mostly hidden within the inferior precentral sulcus. IP, inferior precentral sulcus; vr, vertical ramus (ascending sulcus) of the Sylvian fissure.

rior part of the pars opercularis may be completely or partially submerged in the inferior precentral sulcus. In some cases, we noted that the pars opercularis was formed by only one continuous convolution (i.e., it was not divided into anterior or posterior parts by a diagonal sulcus) and the gyrus was almost completely submerged (Fig. 3–4, see color insert). In such cases, the vertical (ascending) sulcus and the inferior precentral sulcus could not be distinguished on the lateral surface of the brain (red arrow, Fig. 3–4), but they could easily be identified on horizontal sections of the brain (white arrows, Fig. 3–4, left).

These findings have relevance to the identification of the anterior speech area (i.e., Broca's area) by means of electrical stimulation in patients undergoing brain surgery. Rasmussen and Milner (1975, p. 241) pointed out that speech arrest or interference with speech can occur as a result of electrical stimulation "from one or the other, or both of the two frontal opercular convolutions immediately anterior to the lower end of the precentral gyrus" (see Fig. 3–2B). Ojemann (1989) also emphasized that this region of the inferior frontal gyrus is the part from which speech arrest with brain stimulation can most reliably be elicited, but he went on to stress the variability of the precise location within this region from which speech arrest can occur. Although some of this variability may be due to the stimulation parameters and the nature of the behavioral response required, the possibility that this variability also reflects morphological differences must be seriously entertained. For instance, in brains in which all or a part of the pars opercularis is submerged, electrical stimulation of the lower precentral gyrus may evoke orofacial motor responses, but no or only minor dysphasic speech interference may be evoked from stimulation immediately in front of the precentral gyrus because the critical speech area may be lying largely hidden within the inferior precentral sulcus.

ARCHITECTONIC ORGANIZATION OF THE VENTROLATERAL FRONTAL CORTEX IN THE HUMAN AND THE MACAQUE MONKEY BRAIN

Cytoarchitectonic analyses have indicated that the pars opercularis is occupied by a distinct type of cortex that was labeled as area 44 by Brodmann (1908,

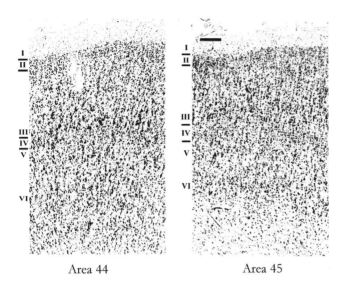

Area 44   Area 45

FIGURE 3–5. Photomicrographs of cortical areas 44 and 45 in the human frontal lobe. The calibration bar in layer I of area 45 indicates 1 mm.

1909) (Fig. 3–2) and as area FCBm by Economo and Koskinas (1925). The pars triangularis is occupied by another architectonic area that was labeled as area 45 by Brodmann (1908, 1909) (Fig. 3–2) and as area FDΓ by Economo and Koskinas (1925). Area 44, which is thought to constitute the main part of Broca's speech area (see Fig. 3–2), can be distinguished from the posteriorly adjacent cortical area 6, which lies on the precentral gyrus, by the presence of a layer IV that is lacking in the agranular area 6. Although layer IV is present in area 44, it is not well developed and, therefore, area 44 can be described as dysgranular (Amunts et al., 1999; Petrides and Pandya, 1994). Layer III contains mostly small and medium pyramidal cells in its upper part, and the lower part is occupied by deeply stained large and conspicuous pyramidal cells. Layer V also contains a number of rather large pyramidal cells (Fig. 3–5). Anteriorly, area 44 is replaced by Brodmann's area 45, which occupies the pars triangularis of the inferior frontal gyrus (Amunts et al., 1999; Brodmann, 1908, 1909; Petrides and Pandya, 1994; Sarkissov et al., 1955). In area 45, layer III contains small to medium pyramidal cells in its upper part, and in its lower part, it has clusters of deeply stained and densely packed large pyramidal neurons. Layer IV is well developed (Fig. 3–5). The defining feature of area 45 that distinguishes it clearly from all adjacent areas is that it has clusters of large and deeply stained pyramidal neurons in the deeper part of layer III in combination with the well-developed layer IV. Layer Va contains medium pyramidal cells and layer Vb is cell sparse; therefore, layer VI is clearly

separated from layer Va. Area 45 can be subdivided into an anterior and a posterior part, areas 45A and 45B, respectively (Fig. 3–6, see color insert). The subdivision of area 45 into areas 45A and 45B is based primarily on the relative development of layer IV, this layer being better developed in area 45A that in area 45B.

Thus, as one proceeds anteriorly within the ventrolateral frontal region of the human brain, starting from the central sulcus, one observes a series of architectonic areas arranged in an anterior-to-posterior direction (Figs. 3–2 and 3–6). At the most posterior extremity lies the lower part of area 4, representing the primary motor orofacial representation. Area 4 at this inferior level is almost entirely hidden in the rostral bank of the central sulcus. Area 4 is succeeded by another agranular area that occupies the crown of the precentral gyrus, namely ventral area 6, which can be divided into a caudal (area 6VC) and a rostral (area 6VR) part. Areas 4 and 6 are agranular frontal cortical areas, typical of the precentral motor region. The agranular areas are characterized by the absence of the granular layer IV. Area 6 is succeeded anteriorly by area 44 that occupies the pars opercularis of the inferior frontal gyrus. Area 44 exhibits a rudimentary layer IV above which are to be found the large and conspicuous pyramids of the deeper part of layer III (Fig. 3–5). Area 44 is replaced by area 45 that has a well-developed layer IV, a typical feature of prefrontal cortex, and a layer of large and deeply stained conspicuous pyramids in the deeper part of layer III (Fig. 3–5).

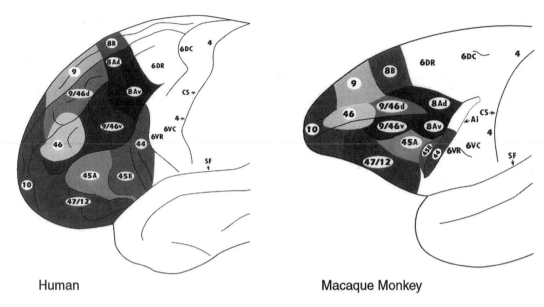

Human   Macaque Monkey

FIGURE 3–6. Comparative cytoarchitectonic maps of the lateral frontal lobe of the human and the macaque monkey brain by Petrides and Pandya (1994). Ai, inferior ramus of the arcuate sulcus; CS, central sulcus; SF, Sylvian fissure.

Although the presence of the agranular areas 4 and 6 in the ventrolateral frontal cortex of the monkey brain has not been the subject of debate, the identification of areas 44 and 45 in the monkey brain has been problematic. Most modern architectonic studies of the prefrontal cortex in the monkey have been influenced and were largely based on the map of the prefrontal cortex by Walker (1940). As can be seen in Figure 3–7, Walker identified a part of the monkey ventrolateral prefrontal cortex as area 45, but he only tentatively suggested that it might correspond to area 45 of the human brain, because he had not studied monkey and human architecture in a comparative manner (Walker, 1940, p. 67).

Given the confusion in identifying, in the ventrolateral frontal cortex of the monkey brain, areas comparable to areas 44 and 45 of the human brain, we carried out an architectonic investigation in which we compared the ventrolateral prefrontal cortex of the human brain with that of the macaque monkey (Petrides and Pandya, 1994, 2002; Petrides et al., 2005). The aim was to examine the question of whether areas 44 and 45 can be identified in the macaque monkey brain by applying the same architectonic criteria used to define these areas in the human brain. As is the case with the human brain, the lower part of the precentral gyrus of the monkey

brain, where the orofacial musculature is represented, is occupied by agranular areas 4 and 6 (Fig. 3–6). Area 4 lies very close to and extends into the anterior bank of central sulcus. Immediately anterior

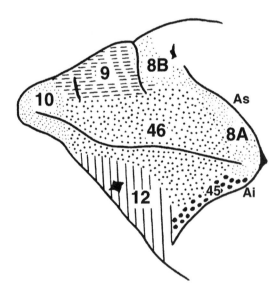

FIGURE 3–7. Architectonic map of the lateral surface of the macaque monkey prefrontal cortex according to Walker (1940). Ai, inferior ramus of the arcuate sulcus; As, superior ramus of the arcuate sulcus.

to area 4, on the crown of the precentral gyrus, area 6 replaces area 4. Two separate subdivisions of lower area 6 can be identified: a ventrocaudal area 6 (area 6VC) and a ventrorostral area 6 (area 6VR), which have been referred to as areas F4 and F5, respectively, by Matelli et al. (1985). The ventrorostral area 6 (area 6VR or F5) exhibits a better lamination than the caudoventral area 6 (area 6VC or F4) (Matelli et al., 1985; Petrides et al., 2000). Our architectonic studies showed that anterior to ventral area 6 and

buried mostly within the posterior bank and the fundus of the arcuate sulcus, a dysgranular area can be identified that exhibits a rudimentary layer IV and conspicuous deeply stained large pyramidal neurons in the deeper part of layer III. Because this area exhibits the same architectonic characteristics as area 44 in the human brain and occupies a comparable location (i.e., immediately anterior to the ventral agranular area 6), we consider this area to be comparable to human area 44 (Fig. 3–8).

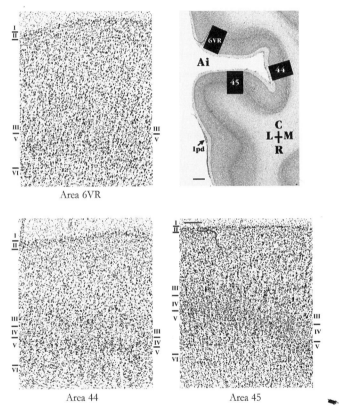

FIGURE 3–8 (see insert for enlarged Figure 3–8). Photomicrographs of cortical areas 6VR, 44, and 45 of the macaque monkey frontal lobe. The axial section perpendicular to the direction of the inferior ramus of the arcuate sulcus shows the location of the photomicrographs. Area 6VR is the anterior part of the ventral agranular premotor cortex and lacks layer IV. This area lies along the inferior ramus of the arcuate sulcus and continues for a variable distance within the upper part of the posterior bank of the sulcus. The dysgranular area 44 succeeds area 6VR within the caudal bank of the inferior ramus of the arcuate sulcus and continues within the fundus of the sulcus. Granular area 45 replaces area 44 at the lower part of the anterior bank of the inferior ramus of the arcuate sulcus. The Roman numerals indicate the cortical layers. Note the absence of layer IV in area 6VR (agranular), the emergence of a layer IV in area 44 (dysgranular), and the well-developed layer IV in area 45 (granular). Note also that in area 45 the granular layer IV happens to be inclined downward at this particular part of the section. Ai, inferior ramus of the arcuate sulcus; Ipd, infraprincipalis dimple. Directions: C, caudal; L, lateral; M, medial; R, rostral. The horizontal calibration bar placed in layer I in the photomicrograph of area 45 is 200 μm, and the calibration bar in the lower left side of the axial section indicates 1 mm.

In the human brain, area 44 is replaced, anteriorly, by area 45, which exhibits a well-developed layer IV; that is, it is a fully developed prefrontal cortex and has deeply stained and large neurons that are conspicuous in the deeper part of layer III. Indeed, this combination of architectonic features sets area 45 apart from all nearby architectonic areas. We therefore asked the question of whether, in the macaque monkey brain, there is an area that is comparable in cytoarchitecture to area 45 of the human ventrolateral prefrontal cortex. As pointed out, Walker (1940) designated as "area 45" a part of the cortex that lies along the anterior bank of the inferior ramus of the arcuate sulcus (see Fig. 3–7) and tentatively suggested that it may correspond to area 45 of the human brain. He was, however, uncertain about this correspondence because he had not explicitly compared monkey with human architecture (see Walker, 1940, p. 67). In addition, he was uncertain about its limits in the arcuate sulcus, pointing out that "the upper part of it merges with area 8 without definite line of demarcation" (Walker, 1940, p. 68, l. 3-5). Furthermore, Walker characterized the region he labeled as "area 45" as having "large pyramidal cells in the third and fifth layers" (p. 68, l. 1-2), whereas area 45 in the human brain is characterized by large neurons in layer III combined with pyramids of medium size in layer V.

Even more confusing, however, is the fact that the term "area 45" is sometimes used, in the field of oculomotor neurophysiology, to refer to the ventral part of the frontal eye field, from which small-amplitude saccades can be evoked with electrical microstimulation, whereas the part of the frontal eye field where large-amplitude saccades can be evoked is referred to as being in caudal area 8A (Schall et al., 1995). There are two problems with this use of the term "area 45" to define a part of the frontal eye field. First, there is no evidence that, in the human brain, area 45 is involved in any way with eye movement control. For instance, in the left hemisphere of the human brain, area 45 is involved in language processes and not eye movements. Second, in the monkey, the ventral part of the frontal eye field from which small-amplitude saccades can be evoked and which has been thought to lie in "area 45" is restricted to the anterior bank of the arcuate sulcus at a level just ventral to the caudal tip of the sulcus principalis. Thus, the ventral part of the frontal eye field would have to lie at the border of area 8 with the most dorsal part of area 45 as defined by Walker (1940), because oculomotor responses

from microstimulation have never been observed in the lower part of the inferior ramus of the arcuate sulcus where Walker's "area 45" extends (Bruce et al., 1985; Schall et al., 1995; Stanton et al., 1989).

These considerations gave rise to the following question. Is all or part of the strip of cortex that Walker (1940) labeled as "area 45" in the monkey arcuate cortex comparable in architectonic characteristics to area 45 in the human brain? Given that no part of area 45 in the human brain has ever been viewed as being involved in oculomotor control (i.e., as part of the "frontal eye field"), it is highly unlikely that, in the monkey, the part of the arcuate sulcus from which eye movements can be evoked is comparable to area 45 of the human brain. In our architectonic studies, we searched for an area that has architectonic characteristics similar to those of area 45 in the human brain. The definition of area 45 in the human brain is not controversial and is agreed on by all investigators who have examined this region (Amunts et al., 1999; Economo and Koskinas, 1925; Petrides and Pandya, 1994; Sarkissov et al, 1955). The striking characteristic of area 45 in the human brain that differentiates it very easily from surrounding areas is the presence of clusters of large deeply stained pyramidal neurons in the deeper part of layer III (i.e., layer IIIc) combined with a well-developed layer IV and medium-size neurons in layer V. The well-developed layer IV distinguishes area 45 from the caudally adjacent dysgranular area 44, where layer IV is rudimentary. We observed that only the inferiormost part of the anterior bank of the lower limb of the arcuate sulcus has architectonic characteristics comparable to those of area 45 of the human brain and that this cortex extends onto the adjacent ventrolateral prefrontal convexity for a considerable distance (i.e., as far as the infraprincipal dimple) (Figs. 3–6 and 3–8). As in the human brain, area 45 of the monkey can be distinguished, posteriorly, from the dysgranular area 44, which lies in the fundus and the posterior bank of the inferior ramus of the arcuate sulcus.

We were particularly concerned with the superior border of area 45 within the anterior bank of the inferior limb of the arcuate sulcus, that is, the part where the frontal eye field starts. As pointed out earlier, the frontal eye field region, as defined by low-threshold microstimulation, lies within the anterior bank of the arcuate sulcus in the region that curves just caudal to the sulcus principalis. In this microstimulation-defined frontal eye field region, the cortex exhibits large and dense pyramidal neurons in layer V (Stanton et al., 1989). These large layer V neurons diminish sharply as one proceeds into the lower part of the anterior bank of the inferior limb of the arcuate sulcus, that is, as one moves away from the region where eye movements can be evoked (Stanton et al., 1989). In the lower part of the inferior ramus of the arcuate sulcus that we consider to be comparable to area 45 of the human brain, we rarely encounter the very large pyramidal neurons in layer V that are typical in the dorsal part where the frontal eye field is located. We have included the upper part of the inferior limb of the arcuate cortex that exhibits large neurons in layer V as part of caudal area 8, as other investigators had previously done (e.g., Brodmann, 1905; Barbas and Pandya, 1989). Thus, the lower part of the anterior bank of the inferior ramus of the arcuate sulcus that we defined as area 45 (using the criteria of area 45 in the human brain) does not extend dorsally to the region where short-amplitude saccades are generated. In our architectonic scheme, both the large- and short-amplitude parts of the frontal eye field would lie within subdivisions of caudal area 8 and not in area 45. Furthermore, note that the area of the monkey brain that we defined as 45 (using the criteria of area 45 in the human brain) is not coincidental with the strip of cortex that Walker (1940) defined as area 45 and extends for a considerable distance anteriorly within the ventrolateral frontal cortex (see Fig. 3–6).

In conclusion, area 45 in the monkey ventrolateral prefrontal cortex when defined by criteria comparable to those of human area 45 is not coincidental with Walker's area 45 and does not include any part of the frontal eye field. When we injected retrograde fluorescent tracers into the part of the monkey prefrontal cortex that we identified as comparable to area 45 of the human cortex, we observed that its cortical inputs were from the supero temporal gyrus (i.e., the auditory system) and the multimodal areas of the superior temporal sulcus and *not* from areas that are known to be connected with the frontal eye field (Petrides and Pandya, 2002).

CORTICOCORTICAL CONNECTION PATTERNS OF AREAS 44 AND 45

The unique connectivity patterns of areas 44 and 45 in the human brain are not known. The traditional gross dissection methods of the pathways in the hu-

man brain identify the major fasciculi but cannot establish the precise origins and terminations of long association fibers. Modern methods of tracing connections in the human brain with diffusion tensor imaging are capable of demonstrating the fasciculi known from classic gross dissection methods, but they cannot yet reveal the precise origins and terminations of long association fibers that enter these fasciculi (e.g., Pajevik and Pierpaoli, 1999; Poupon et al., 2000). These methods, however, hold promise of eventually revealing the connections of the cortical architectonic areas of the human brain.

By contrast, experimental neuroanatomical methods used on macaque monkeys, such as the injection of radioactively labeled amino acids in particular cortical areas to show the precise trajectories and terminations of cortical association pathways or retrograde tracing of the cells projecting to an area with horseradish peroxidase or fluorescent tracers, can demonstrate the precise connections of cortical areas. Given the relatively conservative nature of connectivity patterns in brain evolution, one can assume that the connections of these areas in nonhuman primates reflect reasonably well the connectivity patterns in the human brain.

Figure 3–9 summarizes the corticocortical connections of area 44 in the macaque monkey brain. As can be seen, area 44, which is the transitional area between the lower premotor and the lower prefrontal cortex, is linked locally with ventral area 6, area ProM, area 9/46v, and area 47/12. This area is also connected with areas 11 and 13 of the orbital frontal cortex and areas 24 and 23 of the cingulate gyrus, as well as the supplementary motor area (MII). Its distant connections are with the Sylvian opercular cortex, that is, somatosensory areas 1 and 2 and the second somatosensory area (SII). There are also some connections with the dysgranular insula. Strong connections exist with area PFG of the anterior part of the intraparietal gyrus and anterior intraparietal sulcus (area AIT).

Area 45 is connected with many areas of the lateral prefrontal cortex: areas 8Av, 8Ad, 9/46v, 46, 10, 9, 8B, and 6DR (Fig. 3–10). Some connections exist between area 45 and medial frontal areas 10, 9, 8B, and 24. This area is also connected with nearby ventrolateral area 47/12 and areas 13 and 11 on the orbital frontal cortex. Long connections exist with the dysgranular and the granular insula, as well as areas PaI and ProK of the supratemporal plane. There are

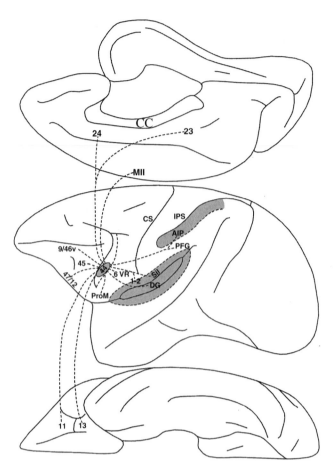

FIGURE 3–9. Diagrammatic representation of the medial, lateral, and orbital surfaces of the left cerebral hemisphere of the macaque monkey to illustrate the connections of area 44. The ventral bank of the intraparietal sulcus (*shaded area*) has been opened up to show connections with area AIP. The Sylvian fissure (*shaded area*) has been opened up to show connections with the second somatosensory cortex (SII) and dysgranular insula (DG). cc, corpus callosum; cs, central sulcus; ips, intraparietal sulcus.

major connections between the superior temporal region and area 45. There are also connections with the multimodal areas TPO and PGa in the superior temporal sulcus. Finally, there are connections with area SII in the parietal operculum and the mid-portion of the inferior parietal lobule (area PG).

IMPLICATIONS FOR FUNCTIONAL STUDIES OF BROCA'S AREA

The existence of areas 44 and 45 in the monkey ventrolateral frontal lobe implies that their fundamental functional contribution must not be limited to language production. These areas may play a more general role in cognition that, in the left hemisphere of the human brain, was adapted to serve linguistic processing as well. In other words, the monkey studies can provide important clues with regard to the fundamental aspects of information processing in areas

44 and 45, which, at the human level, came to contribute and be used for certain specific aspects of language processing.

As pointed out, the architectonic organization (see Fig. 3–8) and the connections of prefrontal areas 44 and 45 with other brain regions (see Figs. 3–9 and 3–10) are quite distinct. These differences in connectivity, as well as recordings of the properties of neurons in areas 44 and 45 of the monkey and in the posterior cortical areas with which they are connected, can provide important clues with regard to the cortical networks within which they are embedded and, therefore, their fundamental function. Area 44 is strongly connected with the anterior part of the inferior parietal lobule where the information processed is multimodal but nevertheless centered on the body. For instance, neurons in the anterior inferior parietal lobule exhibit complex body-centred responses (Hyvarinen and Shelepin, 1979; Leinonen et al., 1979; Robinson and Burton, 1980; Taira et al., 1990).

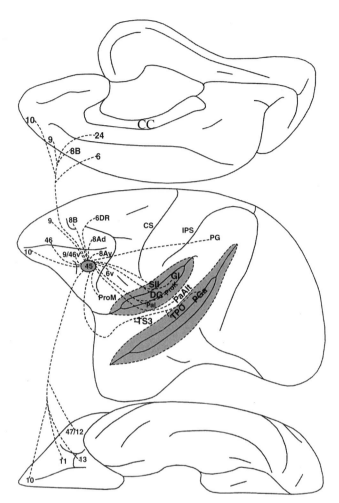

FIGURE 3–10. Diagrammatic representation of the medial, lateral, and orbital surfaces of the left cerebral hemisphere of the macaque monkey to illustrate the connections of area 45. The Sylvian fissure (*shaded area*) has been opened up to show connections with the second somatosensory cortex (SII), dysgranular insula (DG), and granular insula (GI). The banks of the superior temporal sulcus (*shaded area*) have been opened to show connections with multimodal areas TPO and PGa. cc, corpus callosum; cs, central sulcus; ips, intraparietal sulcus.

Within the frontal lobe, area 44 is connected with the rostral part of the ventral premotor cortex (area 6VR or F5) that has both orofacial (most ventrally) and hand/arm representations (more dorsally) and is, in turn, connected with the parts of the primary motor cortex (area 4) that control the orofacial and the arm/hand musculature. Area 44 is also connected with motor areas on the medial part of the hemisphere, such as the supplementary motor cortex. Furthermore, area 44, which lies at the interface between prefrontal and premotor cortex, is also bidirectionally connected with prefrontal areas 45 and 47/12 and ventral area 9/46. This connectivity pattern indicates that area 44 is embedded in a primarily somatomotor cortical network. Given its connectivity and its privileged position at the interface between prefrontal and premotor cortex, area 44 can exercise control over the orofacial and hand/arm musculature and therefore

can provide high-level control of certain aspects of the expression of communicative behavior. This contribution to the expressive aspects of communicative behavior may have preceded the evolution of linguistic ability in the human brain and may reflect a general function of area 44 in human and nonhuman primate behavior. With the evolution of linguistic ability in the human brain, area 44 may also have come to serve certain aspects of speech production. Indeed, there is strong evidence that communicative function in the human left hemisphere is closely related to its capacity for complex motor control (see Kimura, 1993, for review).

Clues regarding the special functional contribution of area 44 can be provided by examining what is known of the immediately adjacent anterior part of the ventral area 6 with which area 44 is closely interacting and, perhaps, controlling. Recordings of single-neuron activity in the anterior part of the premotor cortex (area 6VR, also referred to as F5) have demonstrated coding of action in abstract terms, rather than in terms of specific movements (Murata et al., 1997; Rizzolatti et al., 1988, 1996). Even more interesting is the demonstration of the class of neurons referred to as "mirror neurons" in the anterior part of the ventral premotor area 6. Mirror neurons are neurons that become active both when the monkey performs a particular motor action and when the monkey observes a similar action being made by another individual. Mirror neurons were originally observed for hand/arm movements (Rizzolatti et al., 1996) but have also been shown for orofacial movements (Ferrari et al., 2003). Thus, mirror neurons can be thought of as being part of a neural circuit that participates in the interpretation of another individual's action, perhaps by covertly replaying the observed action. These neurons have provoked considerable interest with regard to the evolutionary origins of language (Arbib and Rizzolatti, 1999) and have led to the suggestion that area F5, where they were originally recorded, may be the precursor of Broca's area. Our cytoarchitectonic analyses, however, have shown that the part of F5 where the mirror neurons have been recorded (i.e., the precentral gyrus caudal to the inferior ramus of the arcuate sulcus) is an agranular area that corresponds to the rostral part of ventral area 6 in the human brain and *not* to area 44. Area 44 in the monkey lies immediately anterior to the agranular part of area F5 where the mirror neurons have thus far been recorded. It remains to be determined whether mirror neuron activity can also be recorded in the lower part of the posterior bank and the fundus of the inferior ramus of the arcuate sulcus where dysgranular area 44 is located. If mirror neurons were to be discovered there, it would be of considerable interest to examine their similarities and differences with those recorded in the agranular premotor cortex (area F5/6VR).

What might be the role of area 44 in the higher order control of communicative behavior? Several investigators have suggested that speech evolved from gestural communication (Armstrong et al., 1995; Corballis, 2002; Kimura, 1993; MacNeilage, 1998). Communicative behavior may have been based, at least in part, on the mirror-system circuitry available in monkeys for action recognition, but this system had to adapt to serve intentional communication through gesture. The mirror neuron system in the premotor cortex of the monkey codes, primarily, object-directed actions, such as grasping, reaching, and manipulating

objects. However, sign articulations in gestural communication and in sign language are largely arbitrary. For instance, while the shape of the hand during grasping of a particular object is determined by the size and shape of that object, the hand shape for a particular gesture or a particular word in a sign language differs from the hand shape for another word in that sign language and also across different sign languages. Thus, a system that can control the arbitrary linkage between symbols and specific actions and their selection based on cultural (e.g., gestural communication) and lexical specification (e.g., sign language) would be necessary during the gradual evolution of the mirror system into language. Area 44 might have been critical in this respect. In monkeys, lesion studies of the periarcuate region that lies just dorsal to area 44 and, which is comparable in terms of level of anatomical organization, have shown that it is critically involved in the selection between competing actions based on conditional operations (see Petrides, 2004). Periarcuate lesions impair performance on conditional associative tasks in which the animals learn to select action X if cue A is presented and to select action Y if cue B is presented, although performance of these actions is completely intact. These conditional operations that depend on the periarcuate region provide enormous flexibility in the selection between different competing acts within a given context. Based on our earlier work with more dorsal periarcuate lesions, area 44 may therefore be thought of as exercising high-level control over orofacial and perhaps hand/arm actions, including those related to communicative acts, based on conditional and other types of rules, and that, in the human brain, area 44 came also to control certain aspects of the speech act on a similar basis. For instance, area 44 may be in a position to regulate the selection of alternative speech output based on conditional/contextual operations.

In sharp contrast to the primarily somatomotor connectivity of area 44 and its architectonic status as a transitional area between agranular premotor cortex and granular prefrontal cortex, area 45 is a clearly prefrontal granular area (see Fig. 3–8) that is connected with the superior temporal region and the adjacent multimodal areas of the superior temporal sulcus (see Fig. 3–10). Petrides (1994, 1996) has suggested that the mid-portion of the ventrolateral prefrontal cortex (areas 45 and 47/12) is critical for the active (i.e., strategic) regulation of information in posterior cortical association areas where information is perceived and coded in short-term and long-term form. This role of the mid-ventrolateral prefrontal cortex (areas 45 and 47/12) can be contrasted with that of the mid-dorsolateral prefrontal cortex (areas 9, 9/46, and 46), which is involved in the monitoring of mnemonic performance on the basis of the subject's current plans (Petrides, 1994, 1996). These functional contributions of the mid-dorsolateral prefrontal region (areas 9, 46, and 9/46) and the mid-ventrolateral prefrontal region (areas 45 and 47/12) are fundamental and true of the nonhuman, as well as the human, primate brain (see Petrides, 1994, 1996, for details). In the human left hemisphere, the specific role of area 45 for language processing may simply be an adaptation of the more general role of this mid-ventrolateral prefrontal region in primate brains for active retrieval based on the top-down regulation of information in posterior cortical association areas (Petrides, 1994, 1996).

Are these arguments consistent with the results of functional neuroimaging studies of the human brain? Paulesu et al. (1993), in a PET study, demonstrated the involvement of area 44 in the processing of articulatory/phonological information and, furthermore, its co-activation with the supramarginal gyrus during such processing. Note that this finding is consistent with the anatomical studies of the monkey area 44 that have shown that the strongest posterior cortical connections of area 44 are with the supramarginal gyrus and not with the posterior part of the superior temporal gyrus, as is often assumed. There is also other evidence suggesting that area 44 may be involved in articulatory/phonological processing (Fiez et al., 1996; Poldrack et al., 1999; Price et al., 1997), and these would be consistent with an area that is embedded in a primarily somatomotor network.

Consistent with the hypothesis regarding the functional role of mid-ventrolateral areas 45 and 47/12, based on nonhuman primate research (Petrides, 1994, 1996), we have provided functional neuroimaging evidence that, in the human brain, the mid-ventrolateral prefrontal cortex (areas 45 and 47/12) is involved in the active retrieval of information from memory. Active, controlled retrieval is required in situations where retrieval cannot be the result of automatic recognition or strong contextual and associative links (see Petrides, 1994, 1996). We have observed activation related to active retrieval primarily in the right hemisphere when the active retrieval involves nonverbal visual or visual-spatial information (Cadoret et al., 2001; Kostopoulos and Petrides, 2003; Petrides et al., 2002) and in the left hemisphere when it is verbal (Petrides et al., 1995). In the PET study in which we tested the prediction

that the mid-ventrolateral prefrontal cortex, in the left hemisphere, is involved in the active, strategic retrieval of verbal information from long-term memory, the main experimental condition involved the free recall of a list of arbitrary words that had been studied before scanning (Petrides et al., 1995). Free recall under these conditions is the result of active strategic retrieval processes, because the subject is asked to recall a specific set of arbitrary words that were presented on a particular occasion, namely the words studied before scanning. Because any recall task will require some degree of monitoring within working memory of the output from long-term memory, it was expected that during the performance of the above free recall task there would be significant activity in the mid-dorsolateral region of the frontal cortex, in addition to any ventrolateral activity that might be observed. Note that in our earlier functional neuroimaging work (e.g., Petrides et al., 1993), the mid-dorsolateral prefrontal cortex, but not the mid-ventrolateral, was shown to be specifically activated in relation to the monitoring of information within working memory. Two control conditions were therefore used to reveal the specific contribution of the left mid-ventrolateral prefrontal cortex to the active retrieval of verbal information. One of these scanning conditions required the simple repetition of auditorily presented words and was designed to control for processes involved in the listening, understanding, and production of words. The other control condition was designed to involve verbal retrieval that would be significantly easier than that of the free recall task but would also require monitoring, within working memory, of the retrieved verbal output. For this purpose, a verbal paired-associate task was used in which the pairs were well learned before scanning and were therefore easy to retrieve in comparison with the free recall task.

In relation to the repetition control task, the free recall task resulted in greater activation within both the mid-ventrolateral and the mid-dorsolateral prefrontal cortex, because both active retrieval and monitoring of the retrieved output within working memory were greater in the free recall task. The comparison between the free recall (i.e., difficult retrieval) and the highly learned paired-associate (i.e., easy retrieval) tasks revealed significantly greater activity in the left mid-ventrolateral prefrontal cortex in the free recall task but no difference between the two tasks in the mid-dorsolateral prefrontal cortex (Petrides et al., 1995). Thus, if postretrieval monitoring is controlled (i.e., the monitoring requirements are matched across two retrieval conditions that are being compared), no differences in activity will be observed in mid-dorsolateral prefrontal cortex. Retrieval per se will engage the mid-ventrolateral prefrontal cortex but primarily under circumstances that require disambiguation of information from short-term and long-term memory (Petrides, 1996).

A well-known and reliable finding from functional neuroimaging studies is the frequently observed increase in activity within the left ventrolateral prefrontal cortex during the performance of tasks that require semantic retrieval (e.g., Buckner et al., 1995; Klein et al., 1995; Petersen et al., 1988). Furthermore, the evidence suggests that the mid-ventrolateral prefrontal cortex (areas 47/12 and 45) may be more involved in the controlled retrieval of semantic information, whereas the posterior ventrolateral region (areas 44 and 6) may be more related to the control of phonological processing (Fiez et al., 1996; Poldrack et al., 1999; Price et al., 1997). One example of such a semantic retrieval task is the verbal fluency task in which the subject is required to produce words from a certain semantic category (e.g., animals). In functional neuroimaging studies, when activation in the semantic retrieval task (e.g., listing animals) has been compared with activation of highly automatic retrieval (e.g., listing the days of the week), greater activity is often observed within the part of the left ventrolateral prefrontal cortex involving area 45. This finding was recently confirmed in an fMRI study in which regions of interest within areas 44 and 45 were set up using cytoarchitectonic probabilistic maps (Amunts et al., 2004). The increases in activity during semantic retrieval were clearly shown to be focused within area 45, rather than area 44.

How can one reconcile the facts that area 45 in the human brain is involved in semantic retrieval and that a comparable area can be identified in a nonhuman primate brain, that of the macaque monkey? We argue that the role of area 45 in semantic retrieval is no different from that of its general role in the active retrieval of information stored in posterior cortical areas (Petrides, 1994, 1996). Obviously, in the nonhuman primate brain such active retrieval processing can operate only on nonverbal information stored in posterior cortical areas. In the human brain, however, and in particular in the left hemisphere, this same type of active retrieval processing can also operate upon verbal episodic memory, such as in listing words encountered in a particular study context (Petrides et al., 1995), as well as on semantic memory, such as in

listing items from a particular semantic category (e.g., Amunts et al., 2004; Poldrack et al., 1999) or finding synonyms to presented words or accessing semantic representations in other languages as in translation (Klein et al., 1995). The important claim here is that a fundamental functional contribution of the mid-ventrolateral prefrontal cortex across primate brains (nonhuman and human) is the active retrieval of information from short-term and long-term memory and that its role in semantic memory is simply the application of the same type of processing on semantic knowledge. The precise neural computations underlying active retrieval within the mid-ventrolateral prefrontal cortex and the posterior cortical areas with which it is interacting can be studied in the monkey brain using nonverbal stimuli.

ACKNOWLEDGMENTS   I would like to thank Scott Mackey for preparing the microphotographs in Figure 3–8. This work was supported by a grant from the Canadian Institutes of Health Research.

References

Alexander, M.P., Benson, D.F., & Stuss, D.T. (1989). Frontal lobes and language. *Brain and Language*, 37, 656–691.

Amunts, K., Schleicher, A., Burgel, U., Mohlberg, H., Uylings, H.B.M., & Zilles, K. (1999). Broca's region revisited: Cytoarchitecture and intersubject variability. *Journal of Comparative Neurology, 412*, 319–341.

Amunts, K., Weiss, P.H., Mohlberg, H., Pieperhoff, P., Eickhoff, S., Gurd, J.M., et al. (2004). Analysis of neural mechanisms underlying verbal fluency in cytoarchitectonically defined stereotaxic space- The roles of Brodmann areas 44 and 45. *NeuroImage*, 22, 42–56.

Arbib, M.A., & Rizzolatti, G. (1999). Neural expectations: A possible evolutionary path from manual skills to language. In P. Van Loocke (Ed.), *The nature of concepts: Evolution, structure and representation* (pp. 128–154). London: Routledge.

Armstrong, A.C., Stokoe, W.C., & Wilcox, S.E. (1995). *Gesture and the nature of language*. Cambridge: Cambridge University Press.

Barbas, H., & Pandya, D.N. (1987). Architecture and frontal cortical connections of the premotor cortex (area 6) in the rhesus monkey. *Journal of Comparative Neurology, 286*, 353–375.

Barbas, H., & Pandya, D.N. (1989). Architecture and intrinsic connections of the prefrontal cortex in the rhesus monkey. *Journal of Comparative Neurology, 286*, 353–375.

Brodmann, K. (1905). Beitraege zur histologischen Lokalisation der Grosshirnrinde. III. Mitteilung: Die Rindenfelder der niederen Affen. *J. Psychol. Neurol. (Lzp)* 4, 177–226.

Brodmann, K. (1908). Beitraege zur histologischen Lokalisation der Grosshirnrinde. VI. Mitteilung: Die Cortexgliederung des Menschen. *J. Psychol. Neurol. (Lzp.)*, 10, 231–246.

Brodmann, K. (1909). *Vergleichende Lokalisationslehre der Grosshirnrinde in ihren Prinzipien dargestellt auf Grund des Zellenbaues.* Leipzig: Barth.

Bruce, C.J., Goldberg, M.E., Fushnell, M.C., & Stanton, G.B. (1985). Primate frontal eye fields: II. Physiological and anatomical correlates of electrically evoked eye movements. *Journal of Neurophysiology, 54*, 714–734.

Buckner, R.L., Raichle, M.E., & Petersen, S.E. (1995). Dissociation of human prefrontal cortical areas across different speech production tasks and gender groups. *Journal of Neurophysiology, 74*, 2163–2173.

Cadoret, G., Pike, G.B., & Petrides, M. (2001). Selective activation of the ventrolateral prefrontal cortex in the human brain during active retrieval processing. *European Journal of Neuroscience, 14*, 1164–1170.

Corballis, M.C. (2002). *From hand to mouth. The origins of language.* Princeton: Princeton University Press.

Déjerine, J.J. (1914). *Sémiologie des Affections du Système Nerveux.* Paris: Masson et Cie.

Duffau, H., Capelle, L., Denvil, D., Gatignol, P., Sichez, N., Lopes, M., et al. (2003). The role of dominant premotor cortex in language: a study using intraoperative mapping in awake patients. *Neuroimage, 20*, 1903–1914.

Eberstaller, O. (1890). *Das Stirnhirn.* Wien: Urban & Schwarzenberg.

Economo, C., & Koskinas, G.N. (1925). *Die Cytoarchitektonik der Hirnrinde des erwachsenen Menschen.* Wien: Springer.

Ferrari, P.F., Gallese, V., Rizzolatti, G., & Fogassi, L. (2003). Mirror neurons responding to the observation of ingestive and communicative mouth actions in the monkey ventral premotor cortex. *European Journal of Neuroscience, 17*, 1703–1714.

Fiez, J.A., Raife, E.A., Balota, D.A., Schwarz, J.P., Raichle, M.E., & Petersen, S.E. (1996). A positron emission tomography study of the short-term maintenance of verbal information. *J. Neurosci., 16*, 808–822.

Geschwind, N. (1970). The organization of the language and the brain. *Science, 170*, 940–944.

Grodzinsky, Y. (2000). The neurology of syntax: Language use without Broca's area. *Behavioral and Brain Sciences, 23*, 1–71.

Hyvarinen, J., & Shelepin, Y. (1979). Distribution of visual and somatic functions in the parietal associative areas 7 of the monkey. *Brain Research, 169*, 561–564.

Klein, D., Milner, B., Zatorre, R.J., Meyer, E., & Evans, A.C. (1995). The neural substrates underlying word generation: A bilingual functional-imaging study. *Proceedings of the Natural Academy of Science USA, 92*, 2899–2903.

Kimura, D. (1993). *Neuromotor mechanisms in human communication.* New York: Oxford University Press.

Kostopoulos, P., & Petrides, M. (2003). The mid-ventrolateral prefrontal cortex: insights into its role in memory retrieval. *European Journal of Neuroscience, 17*, 1489–1497.

Leinonen, L., Hyvarinen, J., Nyman, G., & Linnankoski, I. (1979). Functional properties of neurons in lateral part of associative area 7 in awake monkeys. *Experimental Brain Research, 34*, 299–320.

Matelli, M., Luppino, G., & Rizzolatti, G. (1985). Patterns of cytochrome oxidase activity in the frontal agranular cortex of the macaque monkey. *Behavioral and Brain Research, 18*, 125–136.

MacNeilage, P.F. (1998). The frame/content theory of evolution of speech production. *Behavioral and Brain Science, 21*, 499–511.

Mohr, J.P., Pessin, M.S., Finkelstein, S., Funkenstein, H.H., Duncan, G.W., & Davis, K.R. (1978). Broca aphasia: Pathologic and clinical. *Neurology, 28*, 311–324.

Murata, A., Fadiga, L., & Fogassi, L. (1997). Object representation in the ventral premotor cortex (area F5) of the monkey. *Journal of Neurophysiology, 78*, 2226–2230.

Ojemann, G.A., Ojemann, J.G., Lettich, E., & Berger, M.S. (1989). Cortical language localization in left, dominant hemisphere. An electrical stimulation mapping investigation in 117 patients. *Journal of Neurosurgery, 71*, 316–326.

Pajevik, S., & Pierpaoli, C. (1999). Color schemes to represent the orientation of anisotropic tissues from diffusion tensor data: Application to white matter tract mapping in the human brain. *Magnetic Resonance Medicine, 42*, 526–540.

Paulesu, E., Frith, C.D., & Frackowiak, R.S.J. (1993). The neural correlates of the verbal component of working memory. *Nature, 362*, 342–345.

Penfield, W., & Roberts, L. (1959). *Speech and brain mechanisms.* Princeton: Princeton University Press.

Petersen, S.E., Fox, P.T., Posner, M.I., Mintun, M., & Raichle, M.E. (1988). Positron emission tomography studies of the cortical anatomy of single word processing. *Nature, 331*, 585–589.

Petrides, M. (1994). Frontal lobes and working memory: Evidence from investigations of the effects of cortical excisions in nonhuman primates. In F. Boller and J. Grafman (Eds.), *Handbook of neuropsychology, Vol. 9* (pp. 59–82). Amsterdam: Elsevier.

Petrides, M. (1996). Specialized systems for the processing of mnemonic information within the primate frontal cortex. *Phil. Trans. Royal Society, London B, 351*, 1455–1462.

Petrides, M. (2005). The rostral-caudal axis of cognitive control within the lateral frontal cortex. In S. Dehaene, G.R. Duhamel, M. Hauser, & G. Rizzolatti (Eds.), *From monkey brain to human brain* (pp. 293–314). Cambridge, MA: MIT Press.

Petrides, M., & Pandya, D.N. (1994). Comparative cytoarchitectonic analysis of the human and the macaque frontal cortex. In Boller, F., & Grafman, J. (Eds), *Handbook of Neuropsychology, Vol. 9* (pp. 17–58). Amsterdam: Elsevier.

Petrides, M., & Pandya, D.N. (2002). Comparative cytoarchitectonic analysis of the human and the macaque ventrolateral prefrontal cortex and corticocortical connection patterns in the monkey. *European Journal of Neuroscience, 16*, 291–310.

Petrides, M., & Pandya, D.N. (2004). The frontal cortex. In G. Paxinos & J.K. Mai (Eds.), *The human nervous system*, 2nd edition (pp. 950–972). San Diego: Elsevier Academic Press.

Petrides, M., Alivisatos, B., Meyer, E., & Evans, A.C. (1993). Functional activation of the human frontal cortex during the performance of verbal working memory tasks. *Proceedings of National Academy of Science USA, 90*, 878–882.

Petrides, M., Alivisatos, B., & Evans, A.C. (1995). Functional activation of the human ventrolateral frontal cortex during mnemonic retrieval of verbal information. *Proceedings of National Academy of Science USA, 92*, 5803–5807.

Petrides, M., Alivisatos, B., & Frey, S. (2002). Differential activation of the human orbital, mid-ventrolateral and mid-dorsolateral prefrontal cortex during the processing of visual stimuli. *Proceedings of National Academy of Science USA, 99*, 5649–5654.

Petrides, M., Paxinos, G., Huang, X.-F., & Pandya, D.N. (2000). Delineation of the monkey cortex on the basis of the distribution of a neurofilament protein. In G. Paxinos, X.-F. Huang, & A.W. Toga (Eds.), *The rhesus monkey brain in stereotaxic coordinates* (pp. 155–165). San Diego: Academic Press.

Petrides, M., Cadoret, G., & Mackey, S. (2005). Orofacial somatomotor responses in the macaque monkey homologue of Broca's area. *Nature, 435*, 1235–1238.

Poldrack, R.A., Wagner, A.D., Prull, M.W., Desmond, J.E., Glover, G.H., & Gabrieli, J.D.E. (1999). Functional specialization for semantic and phonological processing in the left inferior prefrontal cortex. *NeuroImage, 10*, 15–35.

Poupon, C., Clark, C.A., Frouin, V., Regis, J., Bloch, I., LeBihan, D., et al. (2000). Regularization of diffusion-based direction maps for the tracking of brain white matter fasciculi. *NeuroImage, 12*, 184–195.

Price, C.J., Moore, C.J., Humphreys, G.W., & Wise R.S.J. (1997). Segregating semantic from phonological processes during reading. *Journal of Cognitive Neuroscience, 9*, 727–733.

Rasmussen, T., & Milner B. (1975). Clinical and surgical studies of the cerebral speech areas in man. In K.J. Zulch, O. Creutzfeldt, & G.C. Galbraith (Eds), *Cerebral localization* (pp. 238–257). Berlin: Springer-Verlag.

Rizzolatti, G., Camarda, R., & Fogassi, L. (1988). Functional organization of inferior area 6 in the macaque monkey: II. Area F5 and the control of distal movements. *Experimental Brain Research, 71*, 491–507.

Rizzolatti, G., Fadiga, L., & Gallese, V. (1996). Premotor cortex and the recognition of motor actions. *Cognitive Brain Research, 3*, 131–141.

Robinson, C.J., & Burton, H. (1980). Organization of somatosensory receptive fields in cortical areas 7b, retroinsula, postauditory, granular insula of M. fascicularis. *Journal of Comparative Neurology, 192*, 69–92.

Sarkissov, S.A., Filimonoff, I.N., Kononowa, E.P., Preobraschenskaja, I.S., & Kukuew, L.A. (1955). *Atlas of the cytoarchitectonics of the human cerebral cortex*. Moscow: Medgiz.

Schall, J.D., Morel, A., King, D.J., & Bullier, J. (1995). Topography of visual cortex connections with frontal eye field in macaque: Convergence and segregation of processing streams. *Journal of Neuroscience, 15*, 4464–4487.

Stanton, G.B., Deng, S.-Y., Goldberg, M.E., & McMullen, N.T. (1989). Cytoarchitectural characteristic of the frontal eye fields in macaque monkeys. *Journal of Comparative Neurology, 282*, 415–427.

Taira, M., Mine, S., Georgopoulos, A.P., Murata, A., & Tanaka, Y. (1990). Parietal cortex neurons of the monkey related to the visual guidance of hand movement. *Experimental Brain Research, 83*, 29–36.

Thompson-Schill, S., D'Esposito, M., Aguirre, G.K., & Farah, M.J. (1997). Role of left inferior prefrontal cortex in retrieval of semantic knowledge: A reevaluation. *Proceedings of the National Academy of Science USA, 94*, 14792–14797.

Tomaiuolo, F., McDonald, J.D., Caramanos, Z., Posner, G., Chiavaras, M., Evans, A.C., et al. (1999). Morphology, morphometry and probability mapping of the pars opercularis of the inferior frontal gyrus: An in vivo MRI analysis. *European Journal of Neuroscience, 11*, 3033–3046.

Walker, A.E. (1940) A cytoarchitectonic study of the prefrontal area of the macaque monkey. *Journal of Comparative Neurology, 73*, 59–86.

II

MATTERS LINGUISTIC

4

Weak Syntax

Sergey Avrutin

Why should linguists be interested in the study of Broca's region? There are, in my view, several reasons why such investigation is mutually beneficial to linguists and aphasiologists alike. Not only does linguistic theory provide a tool for the proper characterization of the function of Broca's area's, but also studies of this area, especially research with aphasic speakers, may contribute to a proper formulation of a linguistic theory. Indeed, the computational theory of mind, an approach widely accepted in today's cognitive science, views the relationship between language and the brain as analogous to the relationship between software and hardware. For any computer to function properly—and the human brain is, in some sense, a natural biological computer—there must be well-functioning hardware capable of running particular (domain-specific) software. Theoretical linguistics can thus be characterized as a study of the natural, language-related software, a study that aims at giving a precise characterization of the rules the language areas of the brain should be able to support. Aphasiology, on the other hand, can contribute to the proper

formulation of a linguistic theory in at least the following way. Assume two competing linguistic theories, one of which lumps together two linguistic observations (e.g., two different types of linguistic constructions), while the other suggests that the observed facts are to be explained by different principles. The two theories would make different predictions about the linguistic performance of brain-damaged patients: the first one would predict a similar performance on the two constructions (both good or bad), while the other would predict a possible differentiation.[1]

Another reason involves the division of labor between various components of language system. Correct comprehension (and production) involves interplay of various domains, such as morphology, syntax, and discourse. To properly characterize the function of Broca's region, researchers need to have a clear picture of what kind of linguistic processes are involved in interpreting a particular structure under investigation. In this sense, developments in linguistic theory may have significant consequences for our understanding of the function of Broca's region. A rather characteristic example in this sense is the pattern of errors observed in experiments with aphasic patients in their offline comprehension of pronominals (e.g., Grodzinsky et al., 1993) or in aphasics' errors in on-line studies (e.g., Love et al., 1998). While investigating somewhat different constructions, both of these studies observed an abnormal pattern of comprehension or activation in these patients. The explanations proposed in these studies, however, were based mostly on the theory of anaphora available at that time, that is, Chomsky's binding theory (Chomsky, 1986). Specific conclusions about the function of Broca's region were drawn on the basis of that theory, but it appears clear now that the theory was inadequate and conceptually problematic (for review, see Reuland, 2003). More specifically, it has been argued that syntax (or the "narrow syntax," in current terms) is unrelated to the constraints on pronominals of the type investigated in the above-mentioned studies. Thus, the pattern of errors observed experimentally calls for a non-syntactic explanation, and, consequently, the function of Broca's region (at least in this regard) needs to be reconsidered as including operations beyond narrow syntax.

The next problem follows immediately. If Broca's aphasics demonstrate some kind of comprehension deficiency, such as interpretation of passive constructions or object relative clauses, is it reasonable to attribute this deficit to the disruption of their syntactic machinery? This question arises because the function of Broca's region in this case becomes rather undifferentiated: it would have to support processes that, according to theoretical linguistics, belong to different parts of language architecture.

All else being equal, a characterization of the function of Broca's region should be able to account for a variety of dysfunctions in a more or less unified way. It seems to me that researchers often provide a detailed linguistic characterization of some particular comprehension errors in aphasia without attempting to connect their explanation with the well-known difficulties in speech production in these patients. The two modalities—production and comprehension—are treated as if they had nothing to do with each other and as if it were a pure coincidence that one and the same patient (with a particular brain damage in Broca's region) has an effortful, telegraphic speech, with multiple omissions (or substitutions), while in comprehension he or she demonstrates a chance performance on passive constructions.

Finally, a proper formulation of a linguistic theory can explain to what extent "agrammatism" often attributed to Broca's aphasics represents a case of producing truly "ungrammatical" utterances. In other words, there is a distinction between an *unacceptable* utterance and an *ungrammatical* one. An utterance can be unacceptable because of variety of reasons, only some of which are syntactic in nature. As is demonstrated soon, what we often judge as ungrammatical represents, in fact, a case where certain (required) contextual conditions are satisfied. The sentence is, indeed, unacceptable in a particular case, but it has nothing to do with grammar: it *is* grammatically well formed. This is perhaps a question of terminology, but if we take the notion of "ungrammatical" to mean something that violates the rules/principles of the narrow syntax (as I believe researchers often do), we cannot ignore the fact that some "ungrammatical" expressions typical for Broca's aphasics are often observed in unimpaired populations as well. To give a brief example (a more detailed discussion follows), frequent omission of subjects in the speech of English-speaking aphasics is a typical characteristic of the diary style register in unimpaired English (for discussion and examples see Haegeman, 1990). Nonfinite main clauses, frequently observed in the speech of Dutch and German Broca's aphasics (e.g., Dutch *hij lachen*! 'he to-laugh!') are fully productive (and fully acceptable) in some special registers in these languages (e.g., Kolk and Heeschen, 1992; Blom, 2003; Tesak and Ditman, 1991; Avrutin, 2004; among others). Indeed, the range of contextual circumstances when such utterances are used by normal and aphasic speakers differs significantly, but the point is that by itself such omissions do not go beyond what is allowed, under certain conditions, in unimpaired language. If so, a proper formulation of an aphasic syndrome, and hence a better understanding of Broca's area's functions, has to be provided in such terms that could explain why allegedly ungrammatical utterances are allowed in unimpaired speech as well, *provided the contextual conditions are satisfied.*

The Model

What Does the Model Seek to Account for?

As a first step, the proposed model seeks to provide an explanation for the following observations:

1. Omission of some functional categories, such as determiners and tense, is allowed in unimpaired speech in many languages that are traditionally assumed to require these elements. Importantly, however, such omissions are allowed only when specific contextual conditions are satisfied. Thus, the model needs to show why such omissions are in principle possible, and why they are restricted to special (context-related) registers.

2. Optional omission of functional categories is a characteristic feature of Broca's aphasics' speech in languages such as Dutch, German, English, and Swedish. The model seeks to provide an explanation for why these elements are omitted in aphasic speech and why such omission is optional (i.e., the same patient sometimes omits and sometimes produces a determiner). In addition, the model needs to explain what role the context plays in the omission pattern in aphasic speech, given that such omissions are allowed in special registers (see earlier).

3. Aphasic speakers demonstrate significantly more errors with tense than with agreement. The model needs to explain why there is such difference.

4. As discussed later, there is a correlation between omission of determiners and tense in a given utterance of an aphasic speaker. This correlation needs to be accounted for within the proposed model.

5. The above observations have to do with speech production. Well-known phenomena of comprehension (e.g., poor comprehension of passive constructions and object relative clauses) need to be explained within the same model.

6. The proposed model seeks to connect the above-mentioned linguistic observations with more low-level facts about brain damage, specifically with lower-than-normal brain activation. In other words, the goal is to show how diminished available brain resources result in what may appear to be a structural deficit.

7. As an illustration for the last point, the model seeks to account for recent results on comprehension of pronouns by Dutch Broca's aphasics. As discussed later in Economy in Broca's Aphasia, these patients demonstrate a significantly worse performance precisely in those cases where the processing economy hierarchy is at stake.

It has to be acknowledged, of course, that at this point it is perhaps impossible to come up with a truly unifying theory that would connect all experimental and theoretical dots in a scientifically harmonious way. Clearly, this is not my intention here. Nevertheless, I will attempt to outline a new approach to the investigation of aphasics' linguistic errors. This model represents a further development of ideas outlined in Avrutin (1999); its application to the child data is provided in Avrutin (2004).

Special Registers in Unimpaired Speech

As mentioned, omission of functional categories is allowed in unimpaired language, although only in some restricted contexts. Consider, for instance, example 1. Taken out of context, this sentence is unacceptable in English:

(1) *John dance.

However, as noticed, for example, by Akmaijan (1984), Tesak and Dittmann (1991), Schütze (1997), among others,[2] this construction becomes acceptable in the so-called Mad Magazine register:

(2) John dance???!!! Never!

Similar examples exist in Russian and Dutch. A tenseless clause example (3) is unacceptable if produced "out of the blue," but it becomes fully "normal" when it follows, in a given discourse, a completed event [as in (4)]:

(3) *Deti prygat' ot radosti.   [Russian]
    Children to-jump[INF] of joy
    'children started jumping out of joy'

(4) Ded Moroz prinjos podarki. Deti prygat' ot radosti! Santa Clause has brought gifts. Children to-jump[INF] of joy!

(5) Maria vertelde Peter een mop. Hij *lachen*.
                                           [Dutch]
    Mary told Peter a joke he laugh-inf

Omission of determiners in a language that normally requires them is also possible in a specific context, as illustrated by the following Dutch examples (from Baauw et al., 2002; see also Tesak and Dittmann, 1991).

(6a) Q: Wie heeft jou gisteren gebeld?
       'Who called you yesterday?'

A: Oh, *meisje* van   school
    Oh, girl   from school
(6b) Leuk *huisje* heb je.
    nice house have you

Such expressions are fully acceptable and productive, both in Russian and Dutch; however, they do require specific contextual conditions. For example, Russian nonfinite clauses are possible only if they follow a completed event [see earlier example (4)]. Dutch determinerless NPs are acceptable only in specific contexts where there is a sufficient presupposition with regard to the referent of the NP. Thus, what these examples suggest is that the function of a functional category can be sometimes taken over by the context. When such conditions are not satisfied, functional elements must be provided in order to make an utterance interpretable. In the next section, I outline a model to capture the interaction among the narrow syntax, information structure, and context. I begin with how the proposed model explains the omission pattern in special registers in unimpaired speech and what role the context plays in this case. I extend the application of the model to aphasia in Economy in Broca's Aphasia.

From the Narrow Syntax to Information Structure and Beyond

Following the basic tenets of the Minimalist Program (Chomsky, 1995), I assume that narrow syntax is a computational system that is isolated and encapsulated with respect to meaning; that is, that such system conducts symbolic operations on lexical items, putting them together in some specific order that is allowed in a given language. The output of this system must be eventually interpretable. The meaning of lexical items by themselves is clearly not always sufficient; for example, the interpretation of a pronominal element depends on the information in the linguistic discourse. Thus, the output of the narrow syntax is submitted to what Chomsky calls conceptual–intentional interface (C-I). In my view, this is precisely the same level as linguistic discourse, or information structure (as in Vallduví, 1992), as it is precisely here that the information about topic, focus, specificity, and pronominal anaphora is encoded.

As shown shortly, I distinguish between the notions of linguistic discourse and the context. The linguistic discourse for me is a level of representation responsible for resolving (at least some) anaphoric dependencies, identifying topic and focus, determining an appropriate antecedent for a logophoric element,[3] and performing other operations usually referred to as "discourse operations." This system is constructed dynamically in the course of a given conversation and operates by rules that go beyond a sentence level. What I mean by context, on the other hand, is a nonlinguistic system of thought that can be modified by different means, including, but not limited to, linguistic ones. Thus, the way the term "discourse" is sometimes used in the literature is, in my view, somewhat confusing as it encompasses both purely linguistic operations ("linguistic discourse" in my terminology) and the context. To avoid confusion, I use the terms "information structure" and "context" throughout this article.

The information structure is part of the computational system involved in language. Like the narrow syntax that operates on syntactic symbols according to its specific principles, the information structure operates on its own symbols and in accordance with its own rules. Depending on a particular theory, these symbols can be represented as a discourse representation structure (DRS) (Kamp and Reyle, 1993) or a file card (Heim, 1982). The point is that there is, at this level, a basic unit, a chunk of information, that must be made completely interpretable. This, in fact, may be a nonlinguistic requirement: After all, any communication system, and language is such a system, should be designed in such a way that it transmits *interpretable* chunks of information.

In Avrutin (2004), I discuss some constraints (and a possible reason for their existence) that ensure the well-formedness of the information structure. The central idea is that the units of this system consist of two parts: a frame and a heading. They are introduced, respectively, by functional and lexical projections from the narrow syntax. The units of information structure must contain both parts in order to be fully interpretable. A frame ensures that information units are separated from each other, and a heading provides the information necessary for interpretation. The diagram below illustrates relationship between narrow syntax, information structure, and other, nonlinguistic cognitive faculties, such as context.[4] The frame of the unit is supplied by determiner 'a', and the heading is supplied by noun 'dog'. This entity represents what we may call an individual unit of information

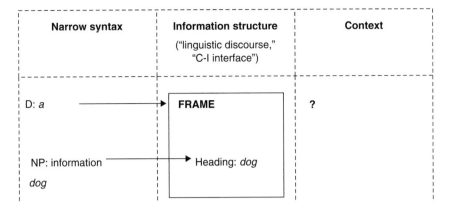

FIGURE 4–1. Normal way of introducing an individual information unit for DP "a dog".

(or an individual file card, adapting Heim's 1982 terminology) (Fig. 4–1).

Similarly, a TP in example (7) contains a functional element T and its lexical complement VP.

(7)   TP
       / \
      T   VP
     +fin run

As a result of the translation from the narrow syntax into the information structure, we obtain an event unit of information (or an event file card) represented in Figure 4–2 (T supplies the event heading, and V supplies the heading).

Let us look again at the special register exemplified in examples 1 through 6. Characteristic of these examples is that they represent a case where functional categories are missing. Thus, at the level of information structure, such expressions are unable to introduce frames. At the same time, as mentioned, they are fully acceptable, provided certain contextual conditions are satisfied. That means that certain contextual conditions can take over the function of functional categories, specifically to introduce a frame. In principle, this should not be surprising, as the information structure is an intermediate level between the narrow syntax and our general cognitive capacity, which is involved in constructing the context representation. Thus, it is reasonable that this interface level may be subject to impact from either side. This would make information structure qualitatively different from narrow syntax, which is fully isolated, autonomous, and encapsulated. As such, external conditions cannot influence the well-formedness of a structure in narrow syntax; however, such influence

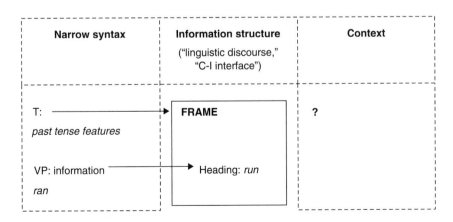

FIGURE 4–2. Normal way of introducing an event unit of information.

is possible in information structure. Consider again example (6a). The response is a determinerless expression, so the narrow syntax does not supply the material necessary for introducing an individual frame. However, the specific contextual circumstances—the fact that the text is a question–answer pair with strong presupposition by the speaker—allows the listener to "rescue" the incomplete information unit by alternative means, namely by inference about speaker's presupposition.

Notice that Figures 4–1 and 4–2 represent the process of speech comprehension: the information units are constructed by the listener on the basis of narrow syntax (e.g., on the basis of the parser's output). In the case of special registers, the model should look slightly different. Indeed, in this case it is more appropriate to describe the process of *encoding of a message* by the speaker. Adapting Levelt's (1989) model of speech production, we can represent the information unit as a message that needs to be encoded by the speaker (normally through morphosyntax) in order to be transmitted to the listener. I suggest that in case of special registers, some information is presupposed on the basis of a given context, and therefore does not need to be encoded by linguistic means. In terms of information transfer,

we can say that some information is transmitted through context (Fig. 4–3).

A tenseless main clause is similar. As mentioned, the necessary condition in Russian seems to be that there is a specific temporal point introduced in the previous linguistic discourse, to which the new event can be anchored (in terms of Enç, 1991). If the speaker has provided such a point in the linguistic discourse, it will be part of the context. The encoding of the temporal information by morphosyntax thus becomes unnecessary, as the listener will be able to infer the temporal information about the tenseless clause and to introduce the event frame by nonsyntactic means (Fig. 4–4).

Crucially, if the discourse condition is not satisfied, a tenseless main clause is unacceptable because the event information unit has no frame: it has not been provided either by the narrow syntax or by the context.

Notice that the proposed model makes clear what the context can and cannot do. Specifically, when a certain element is needed because of the requirements of the narrow syntax, it cannot be omitted (i.e., supplied by the context), because the narrow syntax is an independent, modular system. Reliance on context is possible only in those cases where the require-

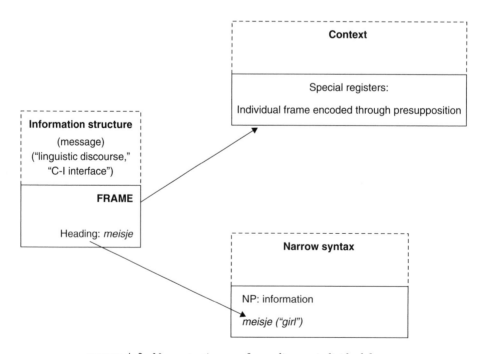

FIGURE 4–3. Nonsyntactic way of encoding an individual frame.

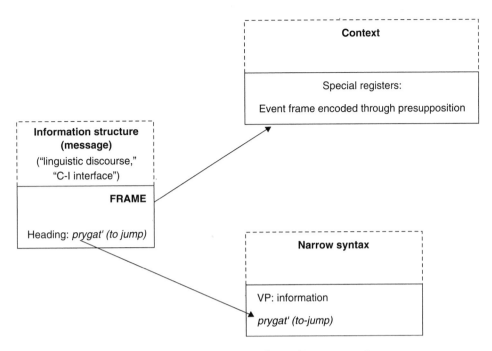

FIGURE 4–4. Nonsyntactic way of encoding an event frame.

ments of the information structure are at stake. A clear example of this distinction is the respective roles of agreement and tense. As a morphosyntactic characteristic, agreement must be present because of the narrow syntax requirements. Tense, on the other hand, is required to make a connection (anchoring) of an utterance to the linguistic discourse (e.g., Enç, 1991). Thus, the model predicts that there will be no register that would allow for omission of agreement. Indeed, this seems to be the case: while many languages allow a nonsyntactic encoding of the event frame (e.g., nontensed main clauses), they do not allow omission of agreement (e.g., no register in Russian would allow a sentence like *deti prygnul 'children[PL] jumped[SING]'). This feature of the model is important because it makes further predictions about errors in aphasic speech, discussed later. Briefly, it predicts that problems with tense should be observed significantly more often than problems with agreement in the speech of these patients.

A question that arises at this point is why "special" conditions would be necessary for "special registers." In other words, if the possibility of encoding an event or an individual frame by nonsyntactic means is in principle available in natural languages, why do speakers not always omit functional categories and rely on (often quite reliable) context in order to build the information units? I would like to propose that the answer is related to economy considerations. I hypothesize that in normal adult speakers, narrow syntax is the cheapest, most economical way of encoding individual and event frames and that this is the most economical way of building information structure.[5] This is in line with the theory formulated in Reuland (2001) for unimpaired language. He argues that operations that take place at different levels (syntax, semantics, discourse) form an *economy hierarchy*, the syntactic ones being the cheapest and the discourse ones being the most expensive. Thus, the use of narrow syntax in unimpaired language for encoding messages follows from its position in the hierarchy.

Economy in Broca's Aphasia

The cheapest, most economical option in unimpaired language does not necessarily enjoy the same status in the language of brain-damaged patients. If Broca's region is involved with syntactic computations, it is only natural that damage to this area would make these operations more resource consuming. The economy hierarchy will then be different: what used to be the easiest way of building information structure, or encoding messages, will now become more expensive than (or at least equally expensive as) other options in principle available to the language system. The straightforward reflection of such change in the economy hierarchy will be noticeable precisely in those cases where, in unimpaired language, alternative options are avoided because of their relatively higher cost.

What I propose therefore is a possible way of what a theory of complexity may look like if it is to explain certain omissions in production and some specific errors in comprehension. The main idea is that the resources necessary for conducting syntactic operations are diminished in Broca's aphasia, with consequences reflected both in the production pattern and in comprehension errors of these speakers.[6]

Production   In production, the use of narrow syntax ("the syntactic channel") becomes less efficient because it is no longer the most economical option available. Rather, an alternative option is now used—specifically, reliance on the context. Importantly, this option is also available for unimpaired speakers in special registers. In other words, damage to Broca's region does not create a new information-processing system. Depending on the degree of severity of damage, or perhaps on other factors still to be investigated, the two means—syntactic and nonsyntactic—may become comparable with each other in the amount of information they can encode and transmit. We would then expect to see occasional use of the syntactic channel and occasional use of the nonsyntactic one. The result is the well-known phenomenon of variability in aphasic speech.

The proposed model also makes an interesting prediction about the correlation between omission of determiners and tense. Because such omissions represent the use of nonsyntactic means of transmitting information, the prediction is that once this alternative is selected by Broca's aphasics, it is likely to be selected for both functional categories. This prediction is borne out. Baauw et al. (2002) presented evidence that there is a correlation between omissions of these two functional elements. For the utterances of a group of Dutch-speaking Broca's aphasics, it was shown that the more likely a sentence was to contain tense, the more likely it was that a determiner would also be produced. And the other way around: tenseless clauses are more likely to contain determinerless NPs. The authors argue that this correlation is due to

the optional reliance on nonsyntactic means for introducing information units: if a nonsyntactic root is chosen (as the easiest in the sense discussed earlier), it is more likely to fulfill all functions with regard to encoding a message, both for individual and for event information units.[7]

As discussed earlier, the ability of the context to compensate for what has not been encoded morphosyntactically is limited. If a certain element of the structure is required because of the requirements of the narrow syntax (a modular, independent computational system), this element cannot be omitted. Again, for example, there is no register such that allows mismatch in agreement. The prediction about Broca's aphasics is then that these patients would make significantly fewer errors with agreement than with tense, because there is no alternative way to encode agreement rather than by means of morphosyntax. Indeed, as many authors have argued, there is a difference in aphasics' performance with respect to these two elements. Friedmann (1999), Benedet et al. (1998), Kolk (2000), and Wenzlaff and Clahsen (2005), among others, show that Hebrew-, Dutch-, and German-speaking Broca's aphasics are more impaired with tense than with agreement. Given that in many cases these patients produce a nonfinite verb, the results support the proposed model.

To continue this line of argument about what the context can and cannot do, it is important to remember that the speech of Broca's aphasics is not overall impaired. It has been demonstrated that these patients are sensitive to some subtle syntactic constraints. Bastiaanse and Zonneveld (1998), for example, show that the use of nonfinite forms in aphasics is restricted to the main clause (the authors' claim being that agrammatics have problems with verb movement that takes place in Dutch only in the main clause; see however, Lonzi and Luzzatti, 1993). When asked to complete a sentence with a missing verb, agrammatics produced finite forms only 49% of the time; in embedded clauses, however, their performance increased to 86%. Avrutin (1999) suggests that these findings demonstrate patients' sensitivity to what Gueron and Hoekstra (1995) label "the tense chain," the requirement on the coindexation of Comp and T. Thus, they preserve the subtle syntactic knowledge that in the presence of overt Comp, only finite T can participate in the tense chain. Further support for this view comes from the observation that these speakers always produce tensed auxiliary verbs and modals (even in the main clause), the elements that head TP and therefore occur in the tense chain (e.g., Bastiaanse and Jonkers, 1998; De Roo, 1999; Kolk, 1998).[8]

Broca's aphasics also demonstrate subtle syntactic knowledge of the relationship between verb movement and finiteness. Kolk and Heeschen (1992) show that if a nonfinite verb is produced by a Dutch or German (V2 languages) aphasic speaker, this verb, in the vast majority of cases, is in the clause final position; a finite verb is always correctly placed in the second position. Lonzi and Luzzatti (1993) report similar results for Italian Broca's aphasics. The authors observe that when the verb is nonfinite, it either precedes or follows the adverb (both positions are correct in Italian), but when the verb is finite, the adverb always follows it.

As for comprehension, which I discuss shortly, Broca's aphasics do not differ from normal speakers in their sensitivity to a verb's representational complexity. Thus, as Shapiro et al. (1987) demonstrate, it takes longer for normal speakers to process verbs that have more possible argument structures (e.g., alternating datives such as 'send' take more resources than a transitive verb such as 'fix'). Following up on this study, Shapiro and Levine (1990) showed that Broca's aphasics exhibit a similar pattern of performance: while their reaction, overall, is significantly slower than normal, the same distinction between verbs with regard to the argument structure complexity can be detected in these patients.

Interestingly, these findings represent precisely those cases where the context cannot serve as an alternative. Verb movement, for example, is triggered by the principles of narrow syntax and has no direct consequences for building of information structure. Moreover, there is no register in unimpaired Dutch or German that would allow a nonfinite verb in the second position. These observations further support the claim that the "agrammatic" performance exhibited by Broca's aphasics does not constitute impairment of grammar (taken here to mean principles of narrow syntax). Their errors are restricted to those cases that can be characterized as reliance on alternative means of building information structure (in comprehension) or encoding a message (in production). If this alternative is not available, these patients will produce, perhaps slower than in unimpaired speech, syntactically well-formed utterances.

A natural question is why functional categories are more vulnerable than lexical ones. First, notice that omission of functional categories is compatible with some registers in unimpaired language, while there is no register that would allow optional omission of a lexical element (e.g., even if we know from a given context that the conversation is about a specific boy who read some book, it is impossible to say "the . . . read a . . ."). Simply speaking, lexical elements are too informative to be omitted. In terms of Shannon's information theory (Shannon, 1948), these elements are selected from a larger set compared with the functional categories, which makes them, in the technical sense, "more informative." Avrutin (in preparation) provides more discussion of how a formal information theory can be integrated into current psycholinguistic research. Suffice it to say that the amount of information of an element is proportional to the degree of activation it receives and therefore is less likely to be omitted. The same kind of reasoning explains why in some languages aphasic patients demonstrate substitution patterns rather than omissions. These are usually morphologically rich languages; thus, each form is to be selected from a larger set of related elements (a somewhat similar, processing-based account is offered in Lapointe, 1985). This fact makes them more informative, with direct consequences for processing cost and activation (for more discussion of such relationship in unimpaired speech, see, for example, Kostic et al. [in press]).

Comprehension   In order to illustrate how the proposed model explains comprehension deficiency in Broca's aphasia, I now discuss some experimental findings that can be straightforwardly explained in terms of a competition between two systems. It is certainly beyond the scope of this article to address all findings in aphasia; the ones presented later simply serve as an illustration of the application of the model.

A typical case where economy considerations determine a possible interpretation is the so-called exceptional case marking (ECM) constructions illustrated in Dutch example (8) (SE stands for 'simplex expression': a monomorphemic element that is always referentially dependent on an antecedent in the same sentence).

(8) Jan$_i$ zag [zich$_i$ / *hem $_i$ dansen]
John saw [SE/him dance]

Reuland (2001), in his *Primitives of Binding* framework, argues that various types of anaphoric dependencies form an economy hierarchy in such a way that a more costly dependency is disallowed, provided a cheaper alternative is available. For example, Dutch anaphor 'zich' can enter a syntactic dependency with its antecedent as a result of feature checking. Pronouns, on the other hand, are unable to participate in this type of dependency because, unlike simplex expression 'zich', they possess a number feature that cannot be deleted. Thus, no syntactic dependency can be formed for a pronoun. There are, of course, other dependencies in natural language, such as discourse dependency where 'Jan' and 'hem' would receive the same value from discourse storage[9]:

(9) Jan zag hem dansen ———→ zag (x, (dansen (y));
x = y
John saw him dance

However, according to Reuland's hierarchy, a discourse dependency is more expensive than a syntactic one. Thus, it is disallowed on the basis of economy considerations.

If the narrow syntax is "weakened" and is no longer the most economical option, the hierarchy proposed by Reuland changes. If so, there should be no prohibition against establishing a nonsyntactic dependency between the antecedent and a pronoun in example (9). Ruigendijk et al. (2003) demonstrated that indeed Dutch-speaking Broca's aphasics show an impaired pattern of responses. In a picture selection task, subjects were presented with sentences such as in example 10 and three pictures corresponding to the correct choice of an antecedent, an incorrect one, and a filler. Each sentence began with an introductory clause of the form 'First the boy and the man drank something and . . .' (in order to make two possible antecedents available) and concluded with the following:

(10) . . . daarna zag de man hem voetballen [Dutch]
. . . then the man saw him playing soccer

The correct picture showed a boy playing soccer in front of the mirror and a man looking at the boy. The incorrect picture showed a man playing soccer in front of the mirror looking at himself. Thus, if a listener disallows coreference between 'him' and 'the man', he or she should choose the correct picture. If he or she allows 'him' to refer to the matrix subject, the incorrect picture could be chosen.

Adult controls correctly chose the picture where the man sees the boy in the mirror. Aphasic speakers, however, incorrectly pointed to the picture where the boy sees himself around 50% of the time, which is not different from chance.[10] In other words, they quite often allowed a local dependency relation between the pronoun and the matrix subject. The authors argue that because the syntactic dependency is the less economical one for this population, they sometimes allow a semantic or discourse dependency between the matrix subject and the pronoun. Notice that such allowance is once again "optional"—it is not the case that subjects always select this picture. This is not surprising, however, because, as in the case of production, the errors result from the competition between two systems—the narrow syntax and an alternative that is the context. For some speakers, one system can win on some occasions, and the other will take over in other cases, which results in an overall chance performance.[11]

These results show that Broca's aphasics sometimes fail to establish a dependency relation between an antecedent and a pronoun correctly. Other results concerning dependency between two positions involve passive constructions and object relatives. The abnormal, chance-level comprehension of agrammatic Broca's aphasics on passive constructions is well known. As discussed extensively in Grodzinsky (1990),[12] a typical observation is that Broca's aphasics choose at a more or less chance level between 'the cat' and 'the dog' as the agent of the chasing event in the following sentence.

(11) The cat was chased by the dog.

Grodzinsky's *trace-deletion hypothesis* suggests that aphasic patients are unable to represent traces, so a trace in the object position of the verb 'chase' is deleted. As a result, the subject DP does not receive the agent theta-role (as it should in an unimpaired linguistic structure), and because each DP must have a theta role in order to be interpreted, the subject receives an interpretation by means of some kind of strategy that assigns, at least in English, the agenthood to the first DP in the sentence. Alternative explanations for this phenomenon were offered, among others, by Piñango (1999), who argues that the impairment is restricted to mapping between syntactic and semantic structures.

Notice, however, that the phonologically empty element in the object position (a trace or a copy) normally enters a syntactic dependency with the subject. This dependency may be represented as a syntactic chain or as some other mechanism that would link the two positions in narrow syntax. I suggest that such dependency must be established in a timely fashion, that is very fast, in a normal case, in order to function as a reliable source of interpretation. Syntactic operations, however, are slowed in aphasia, as demonstrated convincingly by Zurif et al. (1993) and Swinney (2003).[13] These researchers showed that Broca's aphasics show priming for an antecedent significantly later than normal controls. The main point thus is that the syntactic dependency is, in principle, intact in aphasia; however, the necessary syntactic connection is significantly slowed.[14] In terms of the proposed model, we can interpret these findings as evidence for the lack of necessary resources for conducting syntactic operations in time because, as in any other physical system, speed is a function of available energy; in other words, it is proportional to the available brain activation. As the syntactic system is no longer the most economical (and hence the cheapest one) for these patients, they may sometimes avoid reliance on narrow syntax when interpreting passive constructions. As the first DP in a passive construction is usually the most prominent element, a topic, and as there is a general correlation between topichood and agency (as also pointed out by Grodzinsky in his formulation of aphasics strategy), the information unit introduced by the first DP may end up marked as the agent. Once again, there is a competition between the two systems. Depending on which system wins, patients will either choose a correct interpretation (subject = patient), or an incorrect one (subject = agent.) Overall, we observe a chance performance.[15]

Finally, the proposed model makes the prediction that the chance performance in comprehension will be observed in Broca's aphasics only in cases where competition between the syntactic and discourse-related operations may take place. As discussed earlier for production, when no alternative is possible and the application of a syntactic operation is required, these patients are predicted to show an above-chance performance. A clear example of such a situation in comprehension is the case of *wh-* questions. Hickok and Avrutin (1995) and Tait et al. (1995) show that Broca's aphasics performed above chance on object WHO-questions (as in example 12) but around chance on object WHICH-questions (as in example 13).[16]

(12) Who did the cat chase?
(13) Which dog did the cat chase?

WHO-questions differ from WHICH-questions in that only the latter is discourse linked. Specifically, the *wh-* phrase 'who' functions as a pure operator and is not represented by a discourse referent. The *wh-*phrase 'which dog', on the other hand, does have such a representation, because it presupposes the existence of a known set of dogs. Importantly, thus, only in example (13) is a discourse link between the object position and the *wh*-phrase possible; for WHO-questions the only option is to establish the connection in syntax. Broca's aphasics demonstrated a good performance on the "pure syntactic" question, while showing a chance performance on the condition where a competition between two systems (syntactic and nonsyntactic) was in principle possible. Given that their syntactic system was weakened, they would occasionally rely on a nonsyntactic one, which resulted in a an overall chance performance in the same way as in the case of interpreting ECM constructions or passive sentences.

SUMMARY

As a result of damage to Broca's region, the amount of resources necessary for conducting operations involving narrow syntax is diminished. This causes a slowdown in the process of speech production. Moreover, reduced power of this system (a direct consequence of diminished resources) may result in the situation where alternative systems become more powerful and therefore are used for the purposes of building information structure in comprehension or encoding a message (in production: an option available, in principle, in unimpaired language[17]).

Impairment in Broca's aphasia is not limited to structures involving constituent movement (e.g., passive constructions, object relative clauses). Comprehension of pronouns and other determiners causes difficulties as well. Slow, effortful, telegraphic speech is characteristic of the same patients who demonstrate problems with comprehension of certain elements. The unified explanation of these phenomena presented here is based on the claim that the power of the damaged Broca's region is diminished, with direct consequences for both production speed and economy-based errors in comprehension.

In order to produce speech in normal time and to rely on narrow syntax for the purposes of conveying and processing information, speakers need to have strong, powerful syntactic apparatus capable of performing required operations in time. As a result of brain damage, the power available to this system is reduced, and the syntax becomes weak.

ACKNOWLEDGMENTS   The preparation of this publication was supported by the Dutch National Science Foundation (NWO) as part of the Comparative Psycholinguistics research program. I thank Sergio Baauw, Yosef Grodzinsky, Joke de Lange, Esther Ruigendijk, Nada Vasic, and Shalom Zuckerman for their comments. Special thanks are due to Jocelyn Ballantyne for proofreading the manuscript.

Notes

1. For example, Grodzinsky et al. (1991) used evidence from Broca's aphasics to distinguish between two theories of passive constructions. They demonstrated that these patients are selectively impaired in those constructions that, according to one of the competing theories, involve syntactic transformations.

2. Haegeman (1990) also shows that omission of subjects in a non–pro drop language such as English is possible in some specific "diary-style" registers.

3. Recent work by Cole et al. (2001) is particularly interesting in this regard as it shows that the choice of an antecedent for a logophor can be parameterized with value of parameters differing in different dialects. This evidence demonstrates that the level of "discourse" is, indeed, linguistic in nature and that the term "linguistic discourse" is rather appropriate.

4. I put a question mark under "context" as I remain agnostic with regard to the type of symbols and the structure of context as a cognitive system.

5. In this sense, the notion of economy that has played a major role in recent theoretical work (e.g., Chomsky, 1995; Reuland, 2001) is more than a formal notion. In my view, it should reflect, at some level, the amount of resources used by the brain when performing a specific computation. In Avrutin (2000), I discuss experimental evidence supporting the claim that the narrow syntax operations are the cheapest. For further evidence, see also Piñango et al. (2001).

6. The reduction of resources, and a consequent slowdown of the syntactic machinery, is most likely due to problems with lexical access in Broca's aphasia, as argued by many researchers (e.g., Shapiro and Levin, 1990; Swinney et al., 1989; Zurif, 2003, among others.)

7. For a somewhat different explanation of these data, see Ruigendijk (2002).

8. The same approach explains the omission of complementizers in aphasics' speech. Because Comp and T form a chain, omission of one element necessitates omission of the other in order to avoid an invalid chain formation.

9. Once again, there is a discrepancy in terminology. What Reuland (2001) refers to as "discourse dependency" is, in my terminology, a dependency at the level of information structure ("linguistic discourse") established by reliance on contextual information. Reuland's notion of "discourse storage" should be viewed as part of the context in the present terminology.

10. When in the same construction the pronoun is replaced with 'zichzelf', the patients demonstrated an almost perfect performance. Thus, their problem is not related to ECM constructions per se but rather to the interpretation of a pronoun in such constructions.

11. Another reason is that there is always a choice between two pictures; that is, even if subjects allow for a discourse dependency between the matrix subject and the pronoun, they do not have to make this choice: it is always possible to interpret the pronoun as referring to an external antecedent.

12. Grodzinsky (1999) provides a more general picture of the role of Broca's area in comprehension of structures involving transformations. For expository purposes, I focus here on passive constructions, although, I believe, the account can be extended to relative clauses and clefts.

13. Other results that are relevant are reported in Swinney et al. (1989), who showed that Broca's aphasics exhibit abnormal pattern of activation of word meaning. In a study with ambiguous words, these researchers show that Broca's aphasics are capable of accessing only the most frequent meaning of the word within the initial, short period of time. Later on, however, both meanings become available.

14. Further evidence that Broca's aphasics maintain a normal ability to connect two positions in a syntactic tree but in a slower-than-normal way is presented in Piñango and Burkhardt (2001).

15. The same explanation also holds for the chance performance observed in object relative clauses, as in the pioneering work of Caramazza and Zurif (1976).

16. Performance on both types of subject *wh*- questions was above chance, as predicted because in this case the information about the thematic role of the unmoved object is sufficient to obtain a full interpretation.

17. Another population that exhibits performance similar to that of Broca's aphasics is normally developing children. See Avrutin (2004) for more discussion and the application of the proposed model to child speech.

References

Akmaijan, A. (1984). Sentence type and form-function fit. *Natural Language and Linguistic Theory, 2,* 1–23.

Avrutin, S. (1999). *Development of the syntax-discourse interface.* Dordrecht: Kluwer Academic Publishers.

Avrutin, S. (2000). Comprehension of D-linked and non-D-linked wh-questions by children and Broca's aphasics. In Y. Grodzinsky, L. Shapiro, & D. Swinney (Eds.), *Language and the brain* (pp. 295–313). San Diego: Academic Press.

Avrutin, S. (2004). Optionality in child and aphasic speech. *Lingue e Linguaggio, 1,* 67–89.

Baauw, S., de Roo, E., & Avrutin, S. (2002). Determiner omission in language acquisition and language impairment: Syntactic and discourse factors. *Proceedings of the Boston University Conference on Language Development* (pp. 23–35). Boston: Cascadilla Press.

Bastiaanse, R., & Jonkers, R. (1998). Verb retrieval in action naming and spontaneous speech in agrammatic and anomic speech. *Aphasiology, 12,* 951–969.

Bastiaanse, R., & van Zonneveld, R. (1998). On the relation between verb inflection and verb position in Dutch agrammatic aphasics. *Brain and Language, 64,* 165–181.

Benedet, M.J., Christiansen, J.A., & Goodglass, H. (1998). A cross-linguistic study of grammatical morphology in Spanish- and English-speaking agrammatic patients. *Cortex, 34,* 309–336.

Blom, E. (2003). *From root infinitive to finite sentences.* Doctoral dissertation. the Netherlands: Utrecht University.

Caramazza, A., & Zurif, E. (1976). Dissociation of algorithmic and heuristic processes in language comprehension: Evidence from aphasia. *Brain and Language, 3,* 572–582.

Chomsky, N. (1981). *Lectures on government and binding,* Dordrecht: Foris.

Chomsky, N. (1986). *Knowledge of language.* New York: Praeger.

Chomsky, N. (1995). *The minimalist program.* Cambridge, MA: MIT Press.

Cole, P., Hermon, G., & Huang C.-T.J. (2001). Long distance reflexives. In P. Cole, G. Hermon, & C.-T.J. Huang (Eds.), *Syntax and Semantics Series 33.* New York: Academic Press.

De Roo, E. (1999). *Agrammatic grammar.* Doctoral dissertation, The Netherlands: Leiden University.

Enç, M. (1991). Anchoring conditions for tense. *Linguistic Inquiry, 18,* 633–657.

Friedmann, N. (1999). *Functional categories in agrammatic production: A cross-linguistic study.* Doctoral dissertation. Tel Aviv: Tel Aviv University.

Grodzinsky, Y. (1990). *Theoretical perspectives on language deficit.* Cambridge, MA: MIT Press.

Grodzinsky, Y., Pierce, A., and Marakowitz, S. (1991). Neuropsychological reasons for a transformational derivation of syntactic passive. *Natural Language and Linguistic Theory, 6,* 431–453.

Grodzinsky, Y. (1999). The neurology of syntax: Language use without Broca's area. *Brain and Behavioural Science, 23,* 47–117.

Grodzinsky, Y., Wexler, K., Chien, Y.-C., Marakovitz, S., & Solomon, J. (1993). The breakdown of binding relations. *Brain and Language, 45,* 371–395.

Gueron, J., & Hoekstra, T. (1995). *The temporal interpretation of predication.* In A. Cardinalletti & T. Guasti (Eds.), *Syntax and semantic.* San Diego: Academic Press.

Haegeman, L. (1990). Understood subjects in English diaries: On the relevance of theoretical syntax for the study of register variation. *Multilingua, 9,* 157–199.

Heim, I. (1982). *The semantics of definite and indefinite noun phrases.* Doctoral dissertation. Amherst: University of Massachusetts.

Hickok, G., & Avrutin, S. (1995). Representation, referentiality, and processing in agrammatic comprehension: Two case studies. *Brain and Language, 50,* 10–26.

Hofstede, B. (1992). *Agrammatic speech in Broca's aphasia; Strategic choice for the elliptical register.* Doctoral dissertation. Nijmegen Institute for Cognition and Information, Holland.

Kamp, H., & Reyle, U. (1993). *From discourse to logic.* Dordrecht: Kluwer Academic.

Kolk, H. (2000). Canonicity and inflection in agrammatic sentence production. *Brain and Language, 74,* 558–560.

Kolk, H.H.J., & Heeschen, C. (1992). Agrammatism, paragrammatism and the management of language. *Language and Cognitive Processes, 7,* 89–129.

Kolk, H.H.J. (1998). *Disorders of syntax in aphasia.* In B. Stemmer & H. Whitaker (Eds.), *Handbook of neurolinguistics* (pp. 249–260). San Diego: Academic Press.

Kolk, H.H.J. (1995). A time-based approach to agrammatic production, *Brain and Language, 50,* 282–303.

Kostic, A. (in press). *The effects of the amount of information on processing of inflected morphology.* Belgrade: University of Belgrade.

Levelt, W.J.M. (1989). *Speaking: From intention to articulation.* Cambridge, MA: MIT Press.

Lapointe, S. (1985). A theory of verb form use in the speech of agrammatic aphasics. *Brain and Language, 24,* 100–185.

Lonzi, L., & Luzzatti, C. (1995). Omission of prepositions in agrammatism and universal constraint of recoverability, *Brain and Language, 51,* 129–132.

Love, T., Nicol, J., Swinney, D., Hickok, G., & Zurif, E. (1998). The nature of aberrant understanding and processing of pro-forms by brain-damaged populations. *Brain and Language, 65,* 59–62.

Piñango, M. (1999). Syntactic displacement in Broca's aphasia comprehension. In Y. Grodzinsky & R. Bastiaanse (Eds.), *Grammatical disorders in aphasia: a neurolinguistic perspective* (pp. 75–87). London: Whurr.

Piñango, M.M. (2000). *Neurological underpinnings of binding relations.* Paper presented at the linguistic society of Germany, Marburg, Germany, March 2.

Piñango, M., Burkhart, P., Brun, D., & Avrutin, S. (2001). *The architecture of the sentence processing system: The case of pronominal interpretation.* Paper presented at SEMPRO meeting, Edinburgh, UK.

Piñango, M., & Burkhardt, P. (2001). Pronominals in Broca's aphasia comprehension: the consequences of syntactic delay. *Brain and Language, 79, 1,* 167–168.

Reuland, E. (2003). A window into the architecture of the language system. *GLOT International, 7,* No. 1/2.

Reuland, E. (2001). Primitives of binding. *Linguistic Inquiry, 32,* 439–492.

Ruigendijk, E. (2002). *Case assignment in agrammatism.* Doctoral dissertation. Groningen: Groningen University.

Ruigendijk, E., Baauw, S., Zuckerman, S., Vasić, N., de Lange, J., and Avrutin, S. (2003). *A cross-linguistic study on the interpretation of pronouns by children and agrammatic speakers: Evidence from Dutch, Spanish, and Italian,* Paper presented at CUNY sentence processing conference, Boston.

Schutze, C. (1997). *The empirical base of linguistics: Grammaticality judgments and linguistic methodology.* Chicago: University of Chicago Press.

Shannon, C.E. (1948). A mathematical theory of communication. *Bell System Technical Journal, 27,* 379–423, 623–656.

Shapiro, L., & Levine, B. (1990). *Verb processing during sentence comprehension in aphasia. Brain and Language, 38,* 21–47.

Shapiro, L., Zurif, E., & Grimshaw, J. (1987). Sentence processing and the mental representation of verbs. *Cognition, 27,* 219–246.

Swinney, D., Nicol, J., & Zurif, E. (1989). The effects of focal brain damage on sentence processing: An examination of the neurological organization of a mental module. *Journal of Cognitive Neuroscience, 1,* 25–37.

Swinney, D. (2003). *Psycholinguistic approaches.* Paper presented at the Fourth Science of Aphasia Conference, Trieste.

Tait, M.E., Thompson, C.K., & Ballard, K.J. (1995). Subject-object asymmetries in agrammatic comprehension of four types of wh-questions. *Brain and Language, 51,* 77–79.

Tesak, J., & Dittmann, J. (1991). Telegraphic style in normals and aphasics. *Linguistics, 29,* 1111–1137.

Vallduví, E. (1992). *The informational component.* New York: Garland.

Zurif, E.B. (2003). The neuroanatomical organization of some features of sentence processing: Studies of real-time syntactic and semantic processing. *Psychologia, 32,* 13–24.

Zurif, E.B., Swinney, D., Prather, P., Solomon, J., & Bushell, C. (1993). An on-line analysis of syntactic processing in Broca's and Wernicke's aphasia. *Brain and Language, 45,* 448–464.

Wenzlaff, M., & Clahsen, H. (2005). *Finiteness and verb-second in German agrammatism. Brain and Language, 92,* 33–34.

5

Speech Production in Broca's Agrammatic Aphasia: Syntactic Tree Pruning

Naama Friedmann

Agrammatic aphasia, a deficit that usually occurs following brain lesion in Broca's area and its vicinity in the left hemisphere, causes individuals to lose their ability to produce syntactically well-formed sentences. They can no longer inflect verbs correctly for tense, use subject pronouns, form relative sentences, produce subordination conjunctions, or construct a well-formed Wh question. Even more striking is the fact that at the same time they retain their ability to inflect verbs for subject agreement, use object pronouns, form reduced relatives, and produce coordination conjunctions, and they are still able to form yes/no questions in some languages. This pattern is also open to cross-linguistic variability: for example, individuals with agrammatic aphasia who speak Arabic and Hebrew can produce well-formed yes/no questions, but speakers of Dutch, English, and German with the same impairment cannot.

The study of this intricate pattern of dissociations is promising for both the exploration of the functional characterization of various brain areas and for the inquiry of the psychological reality of linguistic constructs. In the realm of brain and function, it suggests a window through which the role of brain areas that are involved in speech production, and specifically the syntactic aspects of production, can be viewed. Once a selective deficit in a specific syntactic function can be described in fine functional details, it can then be related to the brain area that was damaged, with the possible result of the description of brain areas that subserve this specific function.

The selective nature of impairment also makes the exploration of agrammatic aphasia valuable for syntactic theories, as the selectivity of the impairment imposes constraints on the theory of normal functioning of the relevant cognitive ability: linguistic theory. For example, a selective deficit in one type of verb inflection, such as tense (the inflection of the verb for past, present, or future tense), which can occur without a deficit in other types of inflection, such as agreement (the inflection of the verb for person, gender and number), suggests that syntactic theory should treat tense and agreement inflections as distinct constructs and as functions that are represented or processed by different modules. Therefore, such a finding can be useful when two different linguistic models are suggested for verb inflection: one in which tense and agreement inflections form a single natural class, and one in which tense and agreement belong to two different classes. A finding from aphasia that shows a dissociation between tense and agreement can support the latter model and bring support for it from a neuropsychological angle. Such a dissociation is presented in the current study.

For many years, the standard view concerning agrammatic speech production has been that the deficit is very broad. Many researchers in the field claimed that syntactic ability is completely lost in these individuals and that they merely lean on non-linguistic strategies to concatenate words into a sentence (cf., for instance, Berndt and Caramazza, 1980; Caplan, 1985; Goodglass, 1976; Goodglass and Berko 1960; Saffran et al., 1980). Later, the impairment has been presented as a more circumscribed deficit, and attempts have been made to account for it using linguistic terms. In this framework, Kean (1977) suggested ascribing the deficit to phonological factors such as the fact that grammatical morphology is generally unstressed. Grodzinsky (1984, 1990) convincingly argued that the underlying deficit is syntactic, rather than phonological. He used the distinction between languages that allow "zero morphology," namely, languages in which omission of morphemes is licit, and languages in which it is illicit, to account for the finding that morphology is omitted in some languages and substituted in others. Still, even these accounts that used grammatical terms to explain the pattern of agrammatic impairment in production assumed a very vast deficit in grammatical elements. Grodzinsky (1984, 1990; see also Ouhalla, 1993), for example, suggested that all functional elements are impaired in agrammatic speech production.

However, empirical evidence regarding agrammatic aphasia has accumulated in recent years, suggesting that the deficit is actually finer-grained and that not all functional elements are impaired in agrammatic production. Some syntactic abilities were found to be intact, and some other structures were found to be differentially impaired in different languages following the same lesion. In sentence production, the empirical investigation of different syntactic structures through constrained tests has shown that the impairment in agrammatic production does not involve all grammatical structures and function words. To give just a few examples of elements that have been shown to be intact in agrammatic production, case was shown to be spared in Finnish and Polish (Menn and Obler, 1990), and in Dutch and Hebrew (Ruigendijk and Friedmann, 2002), coordination conjunctions were shown to be spared and even overused (Menn and Obler, 1990), and negation markers and their position relative to adverbs were studied in Italian and French by Lonzi and Luzzatti (1993) and proved to be intact. Even in the domain of verb inflection, some intact abilities were found: De Bleser and Luzzatti (1994) examined past participle agreement in a structured production task and found a considerable preservation of this inflection. Their participants performed at around 90% correct on most of the tasks in nonembedded sentences. These results called for a systematic exploration of the impaired and unimpaired syntactic abilities in agrammatic production, as well as for an account that will explain why some functions are impaired and what separates them from the unimpaired functions. But before such systematic explorations of various syntactic domains and the syntactic generalization are presented, let us start with a short presentation of the syntactic terms that will be required.

According to syntactic theories within the generative tradition (e.g., Chomsky, 1995; Pollock, 1989), when we produce and understand sentences, they are represented as *phrase markers* or *syntactic trees*. In these syntactic trees, content and function words are represented in different nodes (Fig. 5–1). Functional nodes include inflectional nodes: an agreement phrase (AgrP), which represents agreement between the subject and the verb in person, gender and number, and a tense phrase (TP), representing tense inflection of the verb. Finite verbs move from V, their original position within the verb phrase (VP), to Agr and then to T in order to check (or collect) their inflection. Thus, the ability to correctly inflect verbs for agreement and tense crucially depends on the inflectional nodes, AgrP and TP. The highest phrasal node in the tree is the complementizer phrase (CP), which hosts complementizers, which are embedding elements like "that," and *Wh* morphemes such as "where" and "what." Other elements that move to CP are verbs and auxiliaries in Germanic languages that require the verb to be in second position in the sentence and in yes/no questions in languages like Eng-

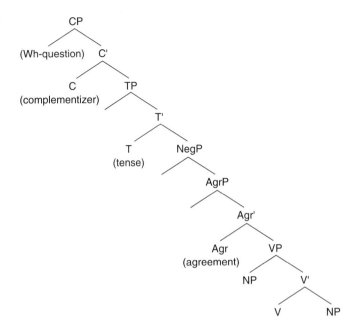

FIGURE 5–1. Syntactic tree (from Pollock, 1989).

lish, German, and Dutch, which require movement of the auxiliary or the verb to the beginning. Thus, the construction of embedded sentences, *Wh* questions, and the position of the verb in some languages depend on the CP node being intact and accessible. The nodes are hierarchically ordered in the syntactic tree—the lowest node is the VP, the nodes above it are the AgrP and the TP (in this order according to Pollock, 1989), and the CP is placed in the highest point of the syntactic tree. This hierarchical order was suggested on the basis of purely linguistic grounds such as arguments from the relative order of elements of various types (subjects and verbs, inflected verbs and negation, infinitive verbs and adverbs, etc.).

The following sections present a set of experiments that systematically explored the status of syntactic structures that relate to these functional nodes in agrammatic production, proceeding from the bottom to the top nodes: AgrP and TP and then various structures that relate to CP.

The study encompassed a variety of tasks that were administered to 18 individuals with agrammatism following brain lesion in the left hemisphere, 16 speakers of Hebrew and 2 Palestinian Arabic-speaking agrammatic aphasics. Following these studies, a portrait of the selective syntactic impairment in agrammatic production with respect to these functional nodes and a syntactic characterization are presented. The spared and impaired abilities are shown to form

two natural classes when looking at them from the point of view of syntactic trees. It will be suggested that what underlies the syntactic deficit in agrammatic production is the inability to project syntactic trees up to their highest nodes (the Tree Pruning Hypothesis, Friedmann, 1998, 1999; Friedmann and Grodzinsky, 1997, 2000). This has implications for syntactic theory, and at a later stage it would also allow conclusions regarding the brain areas that subserve various syntactic functions.

VERB INFLECTIONS

A Study in Hebrew and Arabic

Hebrew and Palestinian Arabic serve as excellent testing ground for verb inflection ability, because their inflection is rich: For every finite verb produced, the speaker has to choose between three tenses—past, present, and future—and 12 agreement forms—agreeing in person, gender, and number with the subject.

All of these inflection forms were examined using two simple tasks—verb completion and sentence repetition. In the completion task, two simple sentences were presented. The first included a verb inflected for tense and agreement. In the second sentence, the participant had to supply the correctly inflected verb. In the **tense** condition, the temporal adverb was changed,

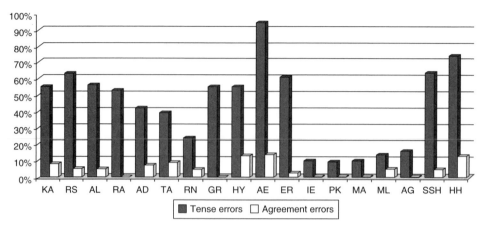

FIGURE 5–2. Performance of individual participants in the agreement and tense completion task. Shown is percent errors.

and the missing verb differed from the supplied verb in tense only (example 1); in the **agreement** condition the subject was changed, so that the missing verb differed from the existing verb in one agreement feature only—person, gender, or number (example 2). Another type of sentence completion test required completion of a verb inflected for both tense and agreement, without a temporal adverb (example 3).

(1) Tense:
axshav ha-yeled holex. gam **etmol** ha-yeled _____.
(halax)
now the boy walks. **Yesterday** too the boy _____.
(walked)
(2) Agreement:
axshav ha-**yeled** holex. berega ze gam ha-**yeladim** _____. (holxim)
now the **boy** walks. Right now the **boys** also _____.
(walk -plural)
(3) Tense and Agreement:
ha-yalda racta likfoc, az hi amda al ha-makpeca ve _____. (kafca)
The girl wanted to-jump, so she stood on the diving-board and _____. (jump-past, 3rd, fem, sg)

In the repetition task, participants repeated short simple sentences of three or four words that included a verb inflected to one of the 30 inflection forms (for detailed description of participants, method, and results, see Friedmann, 1998).

The results showed remarkable dissociation between the production of tense and agreement inflections. While tense was severely impaired, agreement was relatively intact both in Hebrew and in Arabic (see Fig. 5–2 for the results of the completion task; the Arabic-speaking participants were HH and SSH). Participants made tense substitution errors, but almost no agreement errors. This pattern was consistent for all participants, and each one of them showed significantly better performance on the agreement tests than on the tense tests. Even in the simple repetition task (which was only administered in Hebrew), participants made tense errors, repeating the sentence with the correct verb in a wrong tense inflection. They made no agreement errors (Table 5–1).[1]

Tense was significantly poorer than agreement in both the completion and the repetition tasks, using Wilcoxon signed rank test, $W = 6$, $P < 0.0001$, for both comparisons in Hebrew. In Arabic, we used χ^2 because there were only two participants, and the difference was significant, too, $\chi^2 = 34.82$, $P < 0.0001$.

In contrast to Germanic languages, in which the infinitives are the preferred substituting forms (Kolk and Heeschen, 1992), in Hebrew the infinitive was not used instead of the finite verb. In the repetition task, 0% of the errors were toward the infinitival form.

TABLE 5–1. Sentence Repetition Task Showing Percent Errors (Number of Inflection Errors/Total Number of Inflected Verbs)

Hebrew (n = 12)	Tense Errors	Agreement Errors
Repetition	16% (143/912)	0% (4/912)

An additional completion task with half infinitives and half finite verbs as target forms was administered to 12 of the Hebrew-speaking patients. In this test, only 2% of the substitutions were from finite to infinitive verbs, and the large majority of errors was within the finite paradigm. (See Friedmann, 2000, for a possible account for this cross-linguistic difference.)

Inflection in Other Languages

Studies in other languages point in the same direction. In Spanish, too, verb agreement was found to be much better preserved than tense inflection: using a sentence completion procedure, Benedet et al. (1998) reported that the six Spanish-speaking agrammatics they tested produced only 5.5% correct verbal tense but produced 63.8% correct subject-verb agreement. They found a similar pattern of results in English for the seven agrammatics they examined but with a smaller difference: the English-speaking agrammatics produced 42% correct agreement and about 15% correct tense. The same was found in French: the agrammatic patient Mr. Clermont reported in Nespoulous et al. (1988, 1990) had only tense errors in spontaneous speech but no verb agreement errors. Ferreiro (2003) tested 14 agrammatic aphasics in Catalan and Spanish, with the same completion and repetition tasks described above, and reported a similar pattern of dissociations: tense was more impaired than agreement in Catalan and Spanish. Wenzlaff and Clahsen (2004) tested seven German-speaking agrammatics using forced-choice completion of inflection and also showed a dissociation between completion of agreement, which was similar to that of the control subjects (greater than 90% correct) and completion of tense, which was at chance level (68% correct).

Based on these results, two main conclusions can be drawn. First, not all functional categories are impaired in agrammatic production. Agrammatism is neither a complete loss of syntax nor a complete loss of grammatical morphemes or functional categories, as has been claimed in different versions by many researchers of agrammatism over the years (Caplan, 1985; Caplan and Futter, 1986; Grodzinsky, 1984, 1990; Kean, 1977; Ouhalla, 1993). Second, a clear dissociation has been demonstrated between two types of verb inflection: tense and subject agreement. Tense is severely impaired, whereas agreement is relatively intact.

What Can Account for the Dissociation Between Tense and Agreement?

The split inflection syntactic tree suggested by Pollock (1989) (see Fig. 5–1) seems to offer a natural syntactic way to capture the dissociation found between good agreement and poor tense. In this tree, tense and agreement are represented in two different functional phrases, TP and AgrP. This allows for a selective impairment of one but not the other. The finding that agreement is always better than tense, and never vice versa, can also be explained by this syntactic representation. As TP is situated higher than AgrP on the syntactic tree, we might suggest that higher nodes are harder for agrammatic aphasics to access or project. Thus, while agreement node is accessed appropriately, and therefore subject-verb agreement is intact, tense is higher and therefore less accessible, and tense errors follow. Thus, two properties of Pollock's tree allow for an explanation of the dissociation found in agrammatic speech. The split of the inflectional phrase into two inflectional nodes allows for the selectivity in impairment, and the hierarchical order accounts for the asymmetry of this impairment.[2]

Based on these results, Friedmann (1994, 1998, 2000, 2001) and Friedmann and Grodzinsky (1997) suggested the tree pruning hypothesis (TPH), according to which the syntactic tree of agrammatic aphasics is pruned and higher nodes are inaccessible in agrammatism.[3] The dissociation in verb inflection follows from this: Agrammatic aphasics can project AgrP; therefore, agreement is intact, but they frequently fail to project (or access) TP, which causes tense errors.

If indeed individuals with agrammatism are impaired in getting as high up as the tense node, this would have rather radical empirical consequences, as it would mean that they would fail to access nodes above TP as well. This implies that all structures that depend on the highest node of the tree, the CP, are predicted to be impaired in agrammatism.

Therefore, the next step was to examine structures that require the CP. Recall that the CP hosts Wh elements of Wh questions, complementizers of embedded clauses, and verbs and auxiliaries that move to second position of the sentence. The study thus proceeded with examining the production of questions, embedding, and verb position in Hebrew and Palestinian Arabic as well as with perusal of the cross-linguistic literature. If agrammatic aphasics are unable to project the syntactic tree up to its highest nodes, the prediction is twofold. First, Wh questions, embedding structures and verbs in second position, are expected to be impaired. Furthermore, while questions and embeddings that require the high node would be impaired, questions and embedded clauses that do not require CP should be unimpaired (in the absence of additional impairments).

PRODUCTION OF QUESTIONS

The first step toward evaluating the status of the CP node in agrammatic production was to assess patients' ability to produce questions. A *Wh* question such as (4) below is formed from (5), by means of movement of the *Wh* morpheme to the beginning of the sentence (to spec CP). Because the production of *Wh* questions involves CP, the highest node of the tree, an impairment in CP should entail a deficit in *Wh* questions. Studies by Shapiro and Thompson and their group (see Chapter 8) focused on treatment of the production of *Wh* questions in English and reported very poor baseline abilities to produce questions (Thompson et al., 1993, 1996, 1997; Thompson and Shapiro, 1995). Thompson and Shapiro (1995) reported that all of the 17 Broca's aphasics who participated in five different studies were unable to produce *Wh* questions before the onset of treatment.

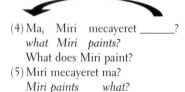

(4) Ma$_i$ Miri mecayeret _____?
   what Miri paints?
   What does Miri paint?
(5) Miri mecayeret ma?
   Miri paints   what?

Wh Questions in Hebrew and Arabic

To assess patients' ability to form questions, we used analysis of spontaneous speech as well as two constrained tasks: question repetition and question elicitation. Spontaneous speech was collected from 12 Hebrew-speaking agrammatic patients and from 1

Arabic-speaking agrammatic patient, from free conversation between the subjects and the experimenter. The structured tests were administered to 10 Hebrew- and 1 Arabic-speaking agrammatic patients and to matched control subjects without neurological deficit.

In the question repetition task, participants were asked to repeat simple four- or five-word Wh questions. In the elicitation task, participants heard a declarative sentence with a missing detail, signified by nonspecific words like "someone" or "something," and were required to ask a question about the missing detail (see example 6). (For more details on the tests, the individual results, and discussion see Friedmann, 2002.)

(6) Experimenter: Danny ate **something**. You want to ask me about this thing. So you ask. . . .
   Target: ma   dani   axal?
        what Danny ate?
        'What did Danny eat?'

The results showed a severe impairment in Wh question production across all types of assessment. In spontaneous speech, most Wh questions that were produced were ill formed. Of 2272 utterances in Hebrew and Arabic, attempts for 100 Wh questions were made. Of these 100 Wh questions, only 13 were grammatical. In the elicitation task, all agrammatic participants showed a clear deficit in Wh question production (see Fig. 5–3). The matched control participants were 100% correct in this task.

Even in the relatively easy repetition task, all participants showed a clear deficit in Wh question production. Table 5–2 presents the performance on the repetition task. In this analysis, inflectional errors and lexical substitutions were disregarded, and are included in the correct responses if the syntactic structure of the question was well preserved.

An analysis of the errors the participants produced while trying to produce a *Wh* question shows that the most common error types were production of yes/no questions instead of Wh questions (example 7), production of only the *Wh* morpheme without the rest of the question (example 8), various ungrammatical questions, and Wh in situ (example 9).

Example 7

(7) **Yes/no questions** instead of Wh questions (in the elicitation task):
   Experimenter: The sun rose today at a certain hour. You want to know about the hour.
   So you ask . . .
   Patient: beshesh . . . hashemesh zarxa . . . hashemesh hayom . . . lo yodaat.   Hashemesh zarxa hayom?
        at-six . . .   the-sun rose . . .   the-sun   today . . .(I) don't know. The-sun   rose   today?

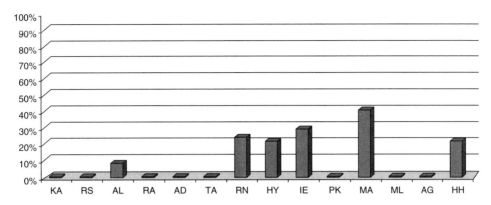

FIGURE 5–3. Performance of individual participants in the Wh questions elicitation task. Shown is percent correct.

(8) **Wh morpheme sequence** (in spontaneous speech)
  ma . . . lama? ma, lama?
  what . . . why? what, why?
(9) **Wh in situ** (in the question repetition task)
  Target : *eifo dani sam et hamafteax?*
      where Dani put ACC the-key?
  Patient: *dani sam et hamaftex eifo?*
      Dani put ACC the-key where?

These errors offer two important hints regarding the nature of the agrammatic deficit in question production. The production of *Wh* morpheme sequences and of *Wh* in situ shows that it is not a lexical problem of *Wh* morpheme retrieval that underlies the difficulty in question production. The *Wh* in situ errors suggest that the deficit is structural, and that the movement of the *Wh* element to the beginning of the sentence cannot take place.

Wh versus Yes/No Questions in Hebrew and Arabic

In contrast to *Wh* questions, yes/no questions in Hebrew and Palestinian Arabic do not require the highest node as they do not require any overt morpheme in CP (in the beginning of the sentence). In Hebrew, for example, unlike in English, a yes/no question like "Do you like hummus?" can be asked without any morpheme in the beginning of the sentence (see example 10).

(10) *at ohevet xummus?*
   you like hummus?

So if the deficit that underlies the impairment in Wh question production is indeed the inaccessibility of the high syntactic nodes and not a general problem with questions, then the production of yes/no questions in Hebrew and Arabic should show a completely different pattern from that of Wh questions. In fact, they are expected to be unimpaired. A first hint that this was indeed the case could be seen in that patients often provided yes/no instead of Wh questions. In order to examine this prediction empirically, we compared the production of yes/no questions with that of Wh questions in spontaneous speech, in the same corpus of 2272 utterances produced by 13 of the participants, and in the question elicitation test.

The performance in spontaneous speech and in the elicitation task confirmed this prediction. Yes/no question production was much better than Wh question production. Both in spontaneous speech and in elicitation, a much higher percentage of yes/no questions was produced correctly (Table 5–3). Using Wilcoxon signed-rank test, Wh questions were elicited significantly worse than yes/no questions, $W = 45$, $P = 0.002$).

Thus, the deficit cannot be ascribed to a general problem with the speech act of asking questions as

TABLE 5–2. Wh Question Repetition Task Showing Percent Correct (Correct/Total)

Repetition (n = 10)	Wh Questions
Agrammatic	57% (188/327)
Control	100% (200/200)

TABLE 5–3. Question Production in Spontaneous Speech and in Question Elicitation Task Showing Percent Correct (Correct/Total)

	Wh Questions	Yes/No Questions
Spontaneous speech (n = 13)	13% (13/100)	96% (81/84)
Elicitation (n = 11)	22% (64/285)	87% (148/170)

some have claimed, but it is rather a structural deficit. A dissociation is found between Wh questions, which require the highest nodes, and therefore are impaired, and yes/no questions, which can be produced without the high nodes in Hebrew and Arabic, and thus are spared.

Question Production in English Dutch and German—The Dissociation Disappears

A completely different pattern is expected in languages in which yes/no questions *do* require the high nodes. In English, for example, yes/no questions start with an auxiliary (example 11), and the auxiliary resides in the high node C. If the C node is impaired, yes/no questions are expected to be impaired in such a language.

(11) Do you like pasta?

In fact, several studies indicate that yes/no questions are impaired in the speech of English-speaking agrammatic aphasics. Goodglass, Gleason, Bernholtz, and Hyde (1972) tested the production of various sentence structures in English—among them, yes/no questions. Their patient made errors on all his yes/no questions trials (0 of 14 correct). Thompson et al. (1993) observed that the English-speaking agrammatic aphasics they examined produced mainly questions that did not include movement of any kind—neither Wh movement nor subject/auxiliary inversion. Their patients only used rising inflection to express a question. These English-speaking patients were impaired also in yes/no questions and produced them without the initial "do" (e.g., "You like eggplant?"). The same tendency was reported by Myerson and Goodglass (1972). Although they did not refer specifically to yes/no questions, they remarked that their three English-speaking agrammatics used intonation alone to indicate a question in their spontaneous speech.

We also administered the same tests we used in Hebrew and Arabic for the elicitation of Wh and yes/no questions to one English-speaking individual with agrammatism. He failed to produce both Wh and yes/no questions (Friedmann, 2002). Similarly, data from Dutch and German indicate that individuals with agrammatic aphasia fail to produce both Wh- and yes/no questions (De Bleser and Friedmann, 2003; Ruigendijk et al., 2004). To conclude, the data on question production in languages in which yes/no questions require the CP node indicate that in English, Dutch, and German, unlike in Hebrew and Arabic, yes/no questions are also impaired.

We see that whether a structure involves high nodes is the critical factor for its status in agrammatic speech production. Wh questions in Hebrew, Arabic, Dutch German, and English and yes/no questions in English, Dutch, and German require high nodes and thus are impaired, whereas yes/no questions in Hebrew and Arabic do not require high nodes and therefore are spared.

EMBEDDING

The next function of CP we studied was embedding—the ability to embed one sentence to the other, usually using "that." We tested the ability of the agrammatic aphasics to produce embedded structures, while comparing embeddings that require the CP with embeddings that do not. Again, two types of analysis were used. First, we analyzed spontaneous speech in Hebrew and in Palestinian Arabic and searched for embeddings in order to obtain general information regarding embedding ability. Later, in order to receive a quantitative and accurate measure in which the target sentence can be controlled, structured tests were devised—embedded sentence repetition and relative clause elicitation.

Spontaneous Speech Analysis

The spontaneous speech of 11 Hebrew-speaking and one Palestinian Arabic–speaking agrammatic aphasics

TABLE 5–4. Subordination Production in Spontaneous Speech—CP Embedding Versus Untensed Embedding Showing Percent Correct (Correct/Total Embeddings Produced)

Spontaneous Speech (n = 12)	CP Embedding	Untensed Embedding
1,950 utterances	12% (13/110)	99% (93/94)

was analyzed for embedded sentences of two types: embeddings that require full CP such as sentential complements and full relative clauses and embeddings that involve lower structures such as untensed embeddings like infinitival complements and reduced relatives. For each type of embedding, the number of grammatical versus ungrammatical sentences was reckoned.

This analysis of spontaneous speech showed that embedding was impaired whenever CP was involved. Compared with speakers without language impairment, very few CP-embedded structures were present, and the embedded structures that did appear were ill formed (Thompson et al. [1994] report a 1.1:1 rate of complex/simple sentences for normal speakers of English; our counting in normal Hebrew yielded an even higher rate of 1.8:1, whereas the spontaneous speech of our patients included an extremely low rate of 1:18). On the other hand, untensed embeddings that do not require any morpheme in CP were almost always grammatical (Table 5–4).

Structured Tasks: Embedded Sentence Repetition and Elicitation

Repetition and elicitation tasks were used to quantitatively assess subordination production in agrammatic speech. The repetition task included repetition of relative clauses (example 12) and sentential complements of nouns and verbs (example 13).

(12) Yoxanan ra'aa et ha-ish she-hit'atesh.
　　　John　　saw　the-man that-sneezed.
(13) Yoxanan ra'aa she-ha-ish　hit'atesh.
　　　John　　saw that-the-man sneezed.

In the subject-relative clause elicitation task, patients were shown two drawings of a person involved in some action and were asked to depict each picture in one sentence in a specific way. Example 14 shows the (translated) experimenter presentation of the question, and example 15 is the target relative clause response. The control condition for this test was elicitation of adjectival modification, using the same type of elicitation method ("This is the red fish, this is the blue fish").

(14) Here are two men. One man is playing tennis, another man is rowing a boat. Which man is this? Start with "This is the man. . ."
(15) Target: ze　ha-'ish　**she**-xoter besira.
　　　　　 this the-man that-rows in-boat

　'This is the man **who** rows a boat.'

The results of the two tests again indicated a severe deficit in embedding production. In repetition, both sentential complements and relative clauses were impaired, with a mere 33% correct in the simple repetition task (Table 5–5).

This lack of difference between relative clauses and sentential complements indicates that the agrammatic deficit in production is a structural deficit that involves the CP node rather than a movement deficit. Given that only relative clauses include a movement, a movement deficit entails that only relative clauses, not sentential complements, be impaired. Structural impairment of the CP node, on the other hand, accounts for the impairment of both structures, which involve CP.

In the elicitation test, full subject relative clauses were very poorly produced, both in Hebrew and in Arabic (see Fig. 5–4 for the performance of individ-

TABLE 5–5. Embedded Sentence Repetition Showing Percent Correct (Correct/Total)

Repetition (n = 10)	Relative Clauses (Mary knew the man that sneezed)	Sentential Complements (Mary knew that the man sneezed)
Agrammatic	33% (50/152)	33% (29/87)
Control	100% (100/100)	100% (100/100)

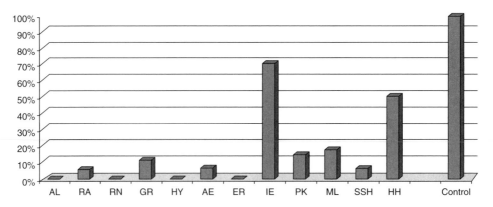

FIGURE 5–4. Performance of individual participants in the relative clause elicitation task. Shown is percent correct.

ual participants). Adjectival modifications were significantly better than the relative clauses, with an average 98% correct compared with 22% for the relative clauses. The good performance in the adjectival modification control items shows that the failure in relative clauses was not due to lack of comprehension of the task or a general deficit of predication.

In order to further compare the production of embedded structures that involve CP to embedded structures that do not involve CP, we included these two types of embedding in an additional repetition test. In this test, patients were asked to repeat comparable sentences with tensed (example 16) or untensed (example 17) sentential complements of verbs.

The results, presented in Table 5–6, again show a clear dissociation between tensed and untensed sentences. This dissociation cannot be related to sentence length, because sentence length was identical in the two conditions, nor can it be ascribed to meaning. Rather, it relates to the different syntactic properties of the two types of subordination—untensed sentences are analyzed syntactically as structures that do not involve CP or TP nodes of the syntactic tree; the tensed sentences in the study require CP.

The most frequent error types in the spontaneous speech and the structured tests were use of direct instead of indirect speech; no embedded sentence after the complementizer (in sentential complements); ungrammatical CP: filled trace, unrelated embedded etc.; complementizer omission; "and" instead of a complementizer—all indicating inability to use CP to embed one sentence to the other.

Another interesting type of response that appeared in the repetition and elicitation tasks in Hebrew was the use of participial relative (example 18) or semi-relative instead of a full relative. According to Siloni (1994, 1997) and Friedemann and Siloni (1997), reduced relatives do not contain either CP, AgrsP, or TP. This probably allows the agrammatic aphasics to produce subordination even when CP is inaccessible.

Example 16

(16) Tensed: yoxanan xashav she-Sharon rakda
     John   thought that Sharon danced

Example 17

(17) Untensed: yoxanan ra'a et   Sharon rokedet
     John   saw ACC Sharon dance-participle

TABLE 5–6. Repetition of Tensed and Untensed Embedding in Hebrew Showing Percent Correct (Correct/Total)

Repetition (n = 6)	Tensed Embedding	Untensed Embedding
Agrammatic	31% (50/162)	92% (130/141)
Control	100% (120/120)	100% (120/120)

(18) zo   ha-yalda ha-roxevet   al ofanayim
     This the-girl the-riding-participle on bicycle.

A similar preference for "low" relatives can also be found in the data of Ni et al. (1997) in English. In a relative clause elicitation task, their patients did not produce a single correct full relative clause, but instead they produced 12/32 reduced relatives. A study we conducted with an English-speaking agrammatic aphasic showed similar results: K.C.L. was unable to repeat sentences with CP embeddings. He repeated only 3 of 56 relative clauses and sentential complements (5% correct). In marked contrast, he could repeat sentences with small clauses much better: he repeated correctly 29 of 41 comparable sentences with small clauses (71% correct) (Friedmann and Taranto, 2000). The spontaneous speech of agrammatic aphasics in French and Japanese tells a similar story: while their CP embeddings are scarce and ill formed, they produce untensed embeddings correctly (Nespoulous et al., 1988, 1990; Sasanuma et al., 1990).

The deficit in embedding is a very robust phenomenon that occurs across all languages in which agrammatic production was studied. Data from spontaneous speech in various languages show the same picture: agrammatics have severe difficulties in the production of embeddings, which manifest in their avoidance of complex sentence and in errors when they do try to produce them. This was found in English (Thompson et al., 1994, 1996, 1997; Bates et al., 1988), in Italian and German (Bates et al., 1988), in French, (Nespoulous et al., 1988, 1990), in Japanese (Hagiwara, 1995), in Hindi (Bhatnagar, 1990; Bhatnagar and Whitaker, 1984), and in Dutch, Swedish, Polish, and Finnish (Menn and Obler's [1990] corpora).

To summarize, embedding is severely impaired in agrammatic production, but, just like in the production of questions, the impairment is selective. In Hebrew and Arabic, embeddings that do not involve CP are better preserved than CP embeddings. Indications for the same dissociation can be found also in English, French, and Japanese. The impaired structures are those that involve the highest nodes of the syntactic tree (TP, CP), whereas embedded structures that do not include these nodes are intact. Thus, full relatives and tensed sentential embeddings that require a complementizer in C and a finite verb are impaired. Semirelatives, reduced relatives, and untensed embeddings do not include TP and CP and are therefore spared.

VERB INFLECTION AND POSITION IN GERMANIC LANGUAGES

Another structure that requires access to CP is the inflected verb that moves in some languages to the second position of the sentence, which, on the tree, is a movement of the verb to C. This happens obligatorily in Germanic languages such as Dutch, German, and the Scandinavian languages, and it is optional in Hebrew. In Germanic languages, the finite verb in every main clause moves to the second position of the clause, following the first constituent—the subject or any other constituent (see examples 19 and 20 in Dutch). Nonfinite verbs (participles and infinitives), do not move, and in Dutch and German, they remain in sentence-final position (example 21). This phenomenon of finite verb in second position (V2) is analyzed syntactically (at least in the case of nonsubject first constituent) as a movement of the verb from its base-generated position at the end of the VP to C (Koster, 1975).

(19) Vfin 2nd: De boer   **melkt** de koe
                  the farmer milks the cow
(20) Vfin 2nd: Langzaam **melkt** de boer   de koe
                  slowly   milks the farmer the cow
(21) Vinf final: De boer   wil   de koe **melken**
                  the farmer wants the cow milk-inf

Consider how a deficit in the high nodes of the syntactic tree might affect verb production in such V2 sentences. If TP and CP are not accessible, the verb will not be able to move to C (through T). Thus, the prediction is that in V2 languages, the verb will not appear in second position but rather in final position. Given the close relation between verb inflection and verb movement (Pollock, 1997), whenever a verb cannot move to the high nodes it will also be uninflected. Therefore, although main verbs in sentences without auxiliaries should always be inflected, many matrix verbs can be expected to appear uninflected in sentence final position, instead of inflected in second position. In sentences in which the speaker succeeds in moving the verb, the verb will be inflected and in second position.

Data from structured tests and spontaneous speech verify this prediction: Many matrix verbs in German and Dutch appear in an infinitival form in sentence final position (when they are supposed to be finite, and in second position), and when finite verbs are produced, they appear in second position. This has been found for Dutch and German (Bastiaanse and van Zonneveld, 1998; Kolk and Heeschen, 1992), and some indications for verb position implication were also found for Swedish and Icelandic (see Friedmann, 2000, for a review).

A study of verb movement to C in Hebrew yielded similar results. In modern Hebrew, the basic word order is SVO (subject, verb, object) (example 22).

(22) etmol   ha-yalda axla xumus
yesterday the-girl ate hummus
'The girl ate hummus yesterday.'

However, in Hebrew it is also possible to move the verb to the second position of the sentence, immediately after a nonsubject phrasal constituent. This movement creates an XVSO structure such as (23) (Shlonsky 1987, 1997; Shlonsky and Doron, 1992).

(23) etmol   axla ha-yalda xumus.
yesterday ate the-girl hummus
'The girl ate hummus yesterday.'

According to Shlonsky and Doron (1992) and Shlonsky (1997), the XVSO structure in Hebrew is created by a nonsubject constituent at spec CP, which triggers the movement of the verb to C. Thus, XVSO and XVSO structures in Hebrew form a minimal pair with respect to movement to CP. The comparison of the two structures might suggest an additional indi-

cation about whether movement to CP is possible in agrammatism. If indeed agrammatic aphasics are unable to access the high nodes of the syntactic tree, they are expected to fail on the XVSO structure that involves movement to these nodes.

The production of verb movement to CP was assessed using a sentence repetition task that included 40 sentences. Half were XVSO, that is, structures with verb movement to CP, and the other half were XSVO. The XSVO and XVSO sentences were matched for length (Friedmann and Gil, 2001).

The results were that the repetition of sentences with verb movement to CP was profoundly impaired in all agrammatic participants, as seen in Figure 5–5. Repetition of the XVSO structures was significantly worse than of the XSVO structures (for the group, paired t test, one-tailed, $t(4) = 12.17$, $P = 0.0001$, M = 24% and 83%, respectively; and for each individual participant, using the Fisher exact test, $P < 0.002$).

The two most common error types in repeating XVSO sentences were inversion of verb-subject order to subject-verb order, and verb omission. Inversion errors were far more frequent in XVSO (56 inversions) than in XSVO (only two inversions) $[t(4) = 4.43, P = 0.005]$. Verb omissions occurred more frequently in XVSO sentences than in XSVO sentences: There were 17 verb omissions in the sentences containing verb movement, compared with 6 verb omissions in the sentences without verb movement. These results also have an implication for the nature of verb omission in agrammatism. Many studies have reported that agrammatic aphasics have difficulties in verb production (Luzzatti et al., 2002). There are different ex-

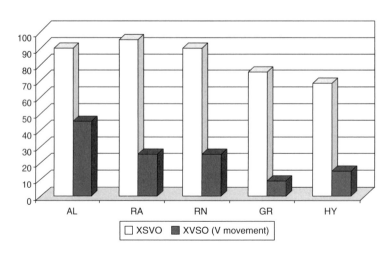

FIGURE 5–5. Percent correct repetition of sentences with and without verb movement to second position.

planations of this deficit: Some researchers hold that agrammatic aphasics have a selective deficit in the lexical retrieval of verbs (Kim and Thompson, 2000; Zingeser and Berndt, 1990). Others have suggested that the deficit is syntactic rather than lexical (Friedmann, 2000). The results of the current study further confirm that the syntactic deficit is involved in verb omissions, as sentences that were similar in all but the movement of a verb yielded a different rate of verb omission—verbs were omitted three times more often from sentences with verb movement to C than from sentences without verb movement. These results are similar to those of Bastiaanse and van Zonneveld (1998) and Zuckerman, Bastiaanse, and van Zonneveld (2001) in Dutch, who used a verb completion test and found a clear difference between verb retrieval in verb-second position and sentence-final position. Their patients retrieved significantly fewer verbs in second position (when the verb was to be positioned in C) than when they had to complete a sentence-final verb. In addition, data from treatment studies indicate an improvement in verb retrieval following treatment of syntactic domains such as movement to CP (Friedmann et al., 2000) and tense inflection (Weinrich et al., 1997). These results confirm that verb retrieval failure in agrammatic aphasia has syntactic underpinnings. When, due to syntactic tree pruning, agrammatics fail to raise their verbs to inaccessible nodes in the tree, they either drop them or leave them unraised in a low node. When the accessibility of high nodes is improved following treatment, verb retrieval improves as well.

To conclude, data from V2 in Hebrew and in Germanic languages support the claim that the highest node of the syntactic tree, the CP, is impaired in agrammatic production, and this impairment causes the agrammatic speakers not to be able to move their verbs to second position of the sentence, before the subject. This also causes the agrammatic aphasics to frequently produce uninflected verbs at their base-generated position at the end of the sentence, and to omit verbs.

INTERIM SUMMARY—IMPAIRED AND INTACT SYNTACTIC STRUCTURES

Where do we stand now? It definitely seems that not all functional elements are impaired in agrammatic production; furthermore, it seems that the dissociations, both within and between languages, behave very

regularly along syntactic lines that are drawn by the syntactic tree. In the realm of inflections, a dissociation was found between tense and agreement inflection: tense is impaired, but agreement seems to be intact. This can be accounted for by the hierarchy of the syntactic tree: the node in which agreement is checked (or collected) is located lower than the node that is responsible for tense inflection. Therefore, if the syntax of an individual with agrammatism allows only access to lower node, agreement might be fine, but tense is impaired. Another cluster of findings relates to all structures that require the highest node, CP. These structures, embedding, Wh questions, yes/no questions in Germanic languages, and verb movement to second sentential position, are impaired for all the participants. Importantly, when a question or an embedded structure does not involve the highest node (such as yes/no questions in Hebrew and Arabic, or reduced relative clauses), it is produced correctly, pointing to the CP node as the source of difficulty in the production of these structures.

DEGREES OF AGRAMMATIC SEVERITY AND THE TREE

Do all individuals with agrammatism show the same pattern of impairment? The next step was to look at the performance of each of the individual participants on structures that relate to the three syntactic levels. Several researchers in the field have pointed to the variability that exists between individuals with agrammatism, to the point that there were calls to dispense with the concept of a neuropsychological syndrome of agrammatic aphasia altogether. This makes the intrasyndrome variability another important target to study.

For this aim, the performance of the 18 participants on agreement completion, on tense completion, and an average score of Wh question and relative clause elicitation was pitted together in Figure 5–6. When looking at the performance of each individual patient, two very clear patterns emerge. One pattern, manifested by the more severe patients, is that of intact agreement, impaired tense, and impaired Wh questions and embedded sentences. The milder patients (shown on the right hand side of the chart) show a different pattern. In their production, both tense and agreement are relatively intact (with agreement at 100% and tense at around 90% correct), but Wh-questions and embedded sentences are impaired.

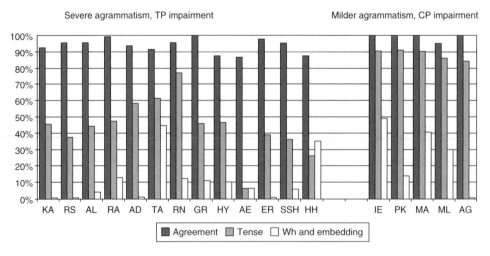

FIGURE 5–6. Individual performance in agreement, tense, Wh questions, and embedding tests.

This difference in severity is easily captured by the height of the deficit on the tree. The severe patients are impaired both in TP and in CP; the milder impaired patients are only impaired higher up, in CP (Fig. 5–7). Crucially, none of the patients showed a deficit in TP without a deficit in CP, or a deficit in AgrP without a deficit in TP and CP. So a deficit at a specific level on the tree entails a deficit in all levels above it. The higher a patient can access (the higher the pruning site), the milder is the impairment, because more functional nodes can be accessed. The lower the impaired node is on the syntactic tree, the more severe is the clinical manifestation of agrammatism, because less functional nodes are available.

In every other respect, except the functional categories C, T, and Agr, these patients share all the standard clinical sign of agrammatism. The speech of all of them is nonfluent and impaired in aspects of their grammar—they have short phrase length, they produce ungrammatical sentences, and, in particular, they cannot embed or ask questions. So it seems that indeed the impairment of all of these participants be-

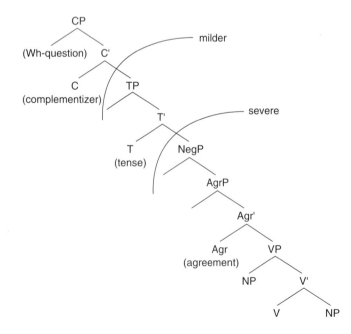

FIGURE 5–7. Degrees of agrammatic severity: pruning at CP describes a milder impairment than pruning at TP.

longs to the same general clinical generalization but in different degrees of severity. The crucial point here is that there is a single principle that distinguishes them from one another—the level in the syntactic tree at which the pruning occurs. This is how the tree pruning hypothesis provides a flexible conception of a neuropsychological syndrome that may have more than a single manifestation. Yet this generalization is highly constrained, as it has strong predictions with respect to what is *not expected* as a pattern of agrammatic production. Specifically, given that inaccessibility to a certain node prevents access to higher nodes, we do not expect to find individuals with impaired functions that relate to TP (subject case, tense inflection, subject pronouns) but with intact CP functions such as Wh question production and production of CP-embedded sentences. Similarly, if agreement-related structures are impaired, we expect both TP and CP to be impaired.[4]

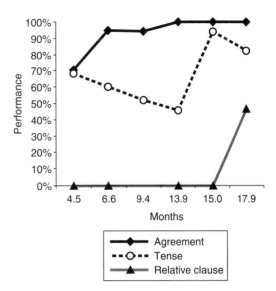

FIGURE 5–8. The spontaneous recovery of SB in agreement, tense, and relative clause production.

RECOVERY ON THE SYNTACTIC TREE

So far, the syntactic performance of the participants was assessed in one point in time, after spontaneous recovery is completed. But what is the path that spontaneous recovery follows? Can it also be captured by the hierarchical order on the syntactic tree? A study we recently conducted asked this exact question (Friedmann, 2005). We continuously tested the production of functional elements and syntactic structures of S.B., a young woman with agrammatic aphasia following traumatic brain injury, and left craniotomy that resulted (according to a computed tomography scan obtained 4 months later) in a vast hypodense area in the left hemisphere, including temporal, parietal, and frontal lobes, enlarged lateral ventricle, and right hemiplegia. S.B. was 20 years old and a native speaker of Hebrew who had 12 years of education.

Her syntax was systematically tested since she started speaking again, 4.5 months after her injury, and then regularly until 18 months post-injury. Her abilities that are related to Agr, T, and C were tested: she was tested in agreement inflection, tense inflection, and relative clause and question production. The results, as can be seen in Figure 5–8, are that during the first stage, 4.5 months postinjury, all of the tested functions were impaired. She had both agreement and tense inflection substitutions in production tasks, and she was completely unable to construct either Wh

questions or embedded relative clauses (neither subject nor object relative clauses). Two months later, 6.6 months post-injury, she was already able to inflect verbs for agreement but still had many errors of tense inflections and could not construct embedding and Wh questions. Tense inflection recovered around 15 months post-injury, at which point relative clauses were still not produced. At 18 months post-injury, relative clauses started to emerge in elicitation tasks, indicating the occasional access to the highest node of the tree, CP. At this time she could also produce some Wh questions and some sentential complements of verbs.

Thus, it seems that the recovery of S.B. can be described as gradual climbing on the syntactic tree, at each stage obtaining access to a higher node of the tree (Fig. 5–9). First, AgrP, TP, and CP are not accessible. Then, around 6 months after injury, AgrP becomes available, and TP and CP are still not accessible. Then, 15 months after the injury, TP becomes available, but CP is still out of reach. The final stage is characterized by access to AgrP and TP, and partial access to CP.

Apart from indicating that syntactic recovery might be described by the hierarchy on the syntactic tree, these results also have another important contribution. Recall that in the last section all participants had either TP and CP impairment or only CP impairment. S.B. shows an additional pattern that goes very

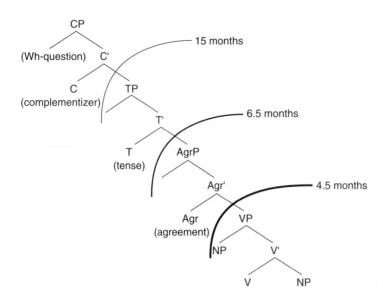

FIGURE 5–9. SB—gradual recovery on the syntactic tree.

well with the severity generalization. At 4.5 months post-onset, she had a deficit that included also AgrP (as well as TP and CP). This suggests that the fact that only individuals with a tree pruned at TP or pruned at CP were reported in the initial study of 18 participants (see section on degrees of severity), may have resulted from the fact that we included in the initial study only individuals at a stable stage who had sentences of two words and more. It might be that the individuals who are impaired in agreement too are either not yet in a stable condition, or produce very short sentences. These results also show the three different degrees of severity, characterized by three different pruning sites, AgrP, TP, and CP in one and the same patient, during recovery from very severe to mild agrammatism.

SUMMARY

The study of speech production in Broca's agrammatic aphasia showed that not all functional elements and not all syntactic structures are impaired and that the deficit is highly selective. This selective pattern can be captured using theoretical syntactic notions such as the hierarchical structure of various functional nodes on the syntactic tree. The tree pruning hypothesis suggests that individuals with agrammatism fail to project their syntactic tree all the way up to the treetop. This leads to the dissociations between the production of structures that depend on high parts of

the tree, which are impaired, and lower structures, which are preserved. This approach also enables an account for the way the same deficit manifests differently in different languages.

Thus, within a language, dissociations are found between structures, depending on their position on the syntactic tree. For example, a deficit in TP impairs the production of structures that require TP or the node above it, CP, but leaves the structures that relate to AgrP intact. Thus, tense inflection, full relatives and embeddings, Wh questions, yes/no questions in English and German, and verbs in second position are impaired. On the other hand, agreement inflection, reduced relatives, infinitival sentential complements, yes/no questions in Hebrew and Arabic, and nonfinite verbs can make do with the lower part of the syntactic tree and therefore are produced correctly. Thus, these seemingly unrelated deficits are all part and parcel of the same underlying deficit—the inability to project the syntactic tree up to its highest nodes, and the site of pruning determines which structures can be produced and which structures are impaired. Differences between languages for individuals with the same structural deficit are accounted for by the difference in the syntactic structure similar sentence types have between languages. For example, when one language requires the use of an impaired node and the other language suffices with a lower node for a certain structure, only speakers of the first language would be impaired in this structure, as is the case with yes/no questions.

The hierarchical nature of the syntactic tree also accommodates findings regarding differences in performance between individuals. While some patients are impaired both in TP-related abilities (like tense inflection) and in CP-related abilities (such as Wh questions and embedding), others are impaired only in CP-related abilities. If, with linguistic theory, we assume that CP is higher than TP, this pattern follows: milder patients can access higher parts of the tree, and thus can access TP but not CP, but more severe patients cannot even reach TP and thus are impaired both in TP and in CP. The most severely impaired patient, at the first stage of her agrammatism, was unable to access either AgrP, TP, or CP. Crucially, the hierarchy of the functional nodes on the tree forms a perfect Guttman scale (Guttman, 1944); namely, when a lower node is impaired, all nodes above it are always impaired, too. When a node is intact, it means that all nodes below it are intact.

This hierarchy has been shown as a possible description for spontaneous recovery of syntactic abilities after brain damage as well. A longitudinal study of the syntactic abilities of a woman with agrammatism has shown that she started without being able to access any functional node, failing in agreement and tense inflection as well as in the production of embedded sentences. The next step brought her to access AgrP but not TP or CP; then she could access both AgrP and TP but not CP, and the final step involved partial recovery of CP.

Apart from allowing for an accurate description of the agrammatic deficit, these findings offer support for the psychological reality of syntactic trees from a neuropsychological angle. That is to say, the finding that tense and agreement can be selectively impaired indicates that tense and agreement are indeed checked (or affixed) in distinct nodes, as was originally suggested by Pollock (1989). Furthermore, the finding that some agrammatic individuals are impaired in Wh questions and subordinations but not in tense inflection suggests that tense resides in a different functional node than Wh questions and embeddings. Thus, we have support for three phrasal nodes, parallel to AgrP, TP, and CP, that have been assumed in the linguistic literature for independent reasons. The pattern of asymmetric dissociations also supports a specific hierarchical order of these nodes.

The possibility to characterize the selective pattern of agrammatic impairment by terms of functional nodes and their hierarchical order on the syntactic tree argues for the psychological reality of the syntactic tree. But the syntactic tree is not only psychologically real: it is also neurologically real. The findings and accounts presented in this chapter suggest that the brain areas implicated in agrammatic aphasia, which are typically Broca's area and its vicinity, are involved in the structuring and projection of the syntactic tree. It might be that a lesion in these area restricts the number of phrasal nodes that can be projected (represented or processed) in the syntactic tree.

ACKNOWLEDGMENT The research was supported by the National Institute for Psychobiology in Israel (Friedmann 2004-5-2b).

Notes

1. The repetition task yielded better performance than the completion task. This means that repetition is easier than completion and that completion is a more sensitive task for verb inflection assessment. These methodological considerations are not at the focus of this paper, but although this difference between different tasks prevents us from directly comparing performance in different tasks, it allows for a comparison within a task: for example, in both completion and repetition tasks, tense was significantly more impaired than agreement. This should also be borne in mind in the next sections with respect to the comparisons between different tasks: the exact rate of success in question elicitation task cannot be compared with the rate in the relative clause elicitation task, which was different in nature, but conclusions can be drawn on the basis of general success or failure in the tasks.

2. Tense above Agr is the order proposed by Pollock (1989, 1993) for English and French and by Demirdache (1988) and Ouhalla (1994) for Arabic. It is, nevertheless, the opposite of the relative order suggested by Belletti (1990) for Romance and by Chomsky (1995), who later gave up the representation of Agr on the tree altogether. At this point, it seems that there is no definitive linguistic argument for either order (especially given that checking and inflection collection yield opposite results), and it might be that results from neuropsychological studies, of the sort suggested here, can be taken as argument for the tense-above-agreement ordering.

3. See section on degrees of agrammatic severity for two such degrees: patients whose syntactic tree is pruned at TP, who are impaired in structures related to TP and CP, and milder patients whose syntactic tree is pruned at a higher point, at CP, who are impaired only in structures related to CP.

4. Note that morphophonological impairments that also induce verb inflection errors (such as the one

witnessed in reproduction conduction aphasia) are not expected to be characterized by the syntactic tree and therefore can appear with unimpaired CP.

References

Bastiaanse, R., & van Zonneveld, R. (1998). On the relation between verb inflection and verb position in Dutch agrammatic aphasics. *Brain and Language, 64*, 165–181.

Bates, E.A., Friederici, A.D., Wulfeck, B.B., & Juarez, L.A. (1988). On the preservation of word order in aphasia: Cross-linguistic evidence. *Brain and Language, 33*, 323–364.

Belletti, A. (1990). *Generalized verb movement: Aspects of verb syntax.* Torino, Italy: Rosenberg & Sellier.

Benedet, M.J., Christiansen, J.A., & Goodglass, H. (1998). A cross-linguistic study of grammatical morphology in Spanish- and English-speaking agrammatic patients. *Cortex, 34*, 309–336.

Berndt, R.S., & Caramazza, A. (1980). A redefinition of Broca's aphasia: Implications for a neuropsychological model of language. *Applied Psycholinguistics, 1*, 225–278.

Bhatnagar, S. (1990). Agrammatism in Hindi: A case study. In L. Menn & L. Obler (Eds.), *Agrammatic aphasia: A cross-language narrative sourcebook.* Philadelphia: John Benjamin.

Bhatnagar, S., & Whitaker, H.A. (1984). Agrammatism on inflectional bound morphemes: A case study of a Hindi-speaking aphasic patient. *Cortex, 20*, 295–301.

Caplan, D. (1985). Syntactic and semantic structures in agrammatism. In M.-L. Kean (Ed.), *Agrammatism.* New York: Academic Press.

Caplan, D., & Futter, C. (1986). Assignment of thematic roles by an agrammatic aphasic patient. *Brain and Language, 27*, 117–134.

Chomsky, N. (1995). *The minimalist program.* Cambridge, MA: MIT Press.

De Bleser, R., & Friedmann, N. (December 2003). A cross-linguistic study of syntactic disorders in aphasia: From theory to therapy. Presented at BMBF-MOS Cooperation in Medical Research 2nd Status Seminar in Neurosciences, Eilat, Israel.

De Bleser, R., & Luzzatti, C. (1994). Morphological processing in Italian agrammatic speakers syntactic implementation of inflectional morphology. *Brain and Language, 46*, 21–40.

Demirdache, H. (1988). *Nominative NPs in modern standard Arabic.* Unpublished.

Ferreiro, S.M. (2003). *Verbal inflectional morphology in Broca's aphasia.* Thesis. Barcelona: Universitat Autonoma de Barcelona.

Friedemann, M.A., & Siloni, T. (1997). AGRobject is not AGRparticiple. *The Linguistic Review, 14*, 69.

Friedmann, N. (1994). *Morphology in agrammatism: A dissociation between tense and agreement.* Thesis. Tel Aviv: Tel Aviv University.

Friedmann, N. (1998). *Functional categories in agrammatic production: A cross-linguistic study.* Doctoral dissertation. Tel Aviv: Tel Aviv University.

Friedmann, N. (1999). 'That' and 'what' in agrammatic production. *Brain and Language, 69*, 365–367.

Friedmann, N. (2000). Moving verbs in agrammatic production. In R. Bastiaanse & Y. Grodzinsky (Eds.), *Grammatical disorders in aphasia: A neurolinguistic perspective* (pp. 152–170). London: Whurr.

Friedmann, N. (2001). Agrammatism and the psychological reality of the syntactic tree. *Journal of Psycholinguistic Research, 30*, 71–90.

Friedmann, N. (2002) Question production in agrammatism: The Tree Pruning Hypothesis, *Brain and Language, 80*, 160–187.

Friedmann, N. (2005). Degrees of severity and recovery in agrammatism: Climbing up the syntactic tree. *Aphasiology, 19*, 1037–1051.

Friedmann, N., & Gil, M. (2001). *Verb movement in agrammatic comprehension and production.* A paper presented at the Second "Science of Aphasia" conference, Giens, France.

Friedmann, N., & Grodzinsky, Y. (1997). Tense and agreement in agrammatic production: Pruning the syntactic tree. *Brain and Language, 56*, 397–425.

Friedmann, N., & Grodzinsky, Y. (2000). Split inflection in neurolinguistics. In M.-A. Friedemann & L. Rizzi (Eds.), *The acquisition of syntax: Studies in comparative developmental linguistics* (pp. 84–104). Geneva, Switzerland: Longman Linguistics Library Series..

Friedmann, N., & Taranto, G. (2000). *Small clauses are better than big ones: The production of embedding in an English-speaking individual with agrammatism.* Ms. University of California, San Diego.

Friedmann, N., Wenkert-Olenik, D., & Gil, M. (2000). From theory to practice: Treatment of agrammatic production in Hebrew based on the Tree Pruning Hypothesis. *Journal of Neurolinguistics, 13*, 250–254.

Goodglass, H. (1976). Agrammatism. In H. Whitaker & H.A. Whitaker (Eds.), *Studies in Neurolinguistics, Vol. 1.* (pp. 237–260). New York: Academic Press.

Goodglass, H., & Berko, J. (1960). Agrammatism and inflectional morphology in English. *Journal of Speech and Hearing Research, 3*, 257–267.

Goodglass, H., Gleason, J.B., Bernholtz, N.A., & Hyde, M.R. (1972). Some linguistic structures in the speech of Broca's aphasic. *Cortex, 8*, 191–212.

Grodzinsky, Y. (1984). The syntactic characterization of agrammatism. *Cognition, 16*, 99–120.

Grodzinsky, Y. (1990). *Theoretical perspectives on language deficits.* Cambridge, MA: MIT Press.

Guttman, L. (1944). A basis for scaling qualitative data. *American Sociological Review, 9*, 139–150.

Hagiwara, H. (1995). The breakdown of functional categories and the economy of derivation. *Brain and Language, 50*, 92–116.

Kean, M.L. (1977). The linguistic interpretation of aphasic syndromes. *Cognition, 5*, 9–46.

Kim, M., & Thompson, C.K. (2000). Patterns of comprehension and production of nouns and verbs in agrammatism: Implications for lexical organization. *Brain and Language, 74*, 1–25.

Kolk, H.H.J., & Heeschen, C. (1992). Agrammatism, paragrammatism and the management of language. *Language and Cognitive Processes, 7*, 89–129.

Koster, J. (1975). Dutch as an SOV language. *Linguistic Analysis, 1*, 111–136.

Lonzi, L., & Luzzatti, C. (1993). Relevance of adverb distribution for the analysis of sentence representation in agrammatic patients. *Brain and Language, 45*, 306–317.

Luzzatti, C., Raggi, R., Zonca, G., Pistarini, C., Contardi, A., & Pinna, G.–D. (2002). Verb–noun double dissociation in aphasic lexical impairments: The role of word frequency and imageability. *Brain and Language, 81*, 432–444.

Menn, L., & Obler, L. (Eds.). (1990). *Agrammatic aphasia: A cross-language narrative sourcebook.* Philadelphia: John Benjamin.

Myerson, R., & Goodglass, H. (1972). Transformational grammars of three agrammatic patients. *Language and Speech, 15*, 40–50.

Nespoulous, J.-L., Dordain, M., Perron, C., Ska, B., Bub, D., Caplan, D., et al. (1988). Agrammatism in sentence production without comprehension deficits: Reduced availability of syntactic structures or of grammatical morphemes? A case study. *Brain and Language, 33*, 273–295.

Nespoulous, J.-L., Dordain, M., Perron, C., Jarema, G., & Chazal, M. (1990). Agrammatism in French: Two case studies. In L. Menn & L. Obler (Eds.), *Agrammatic aphasia: A cross-language narrative sourcebook.* Philadelphia: John Benjamin.

Ni, W., Shankweiler, D., Harris, K.S., & Fulbright, R.K. (October 1997). Production and comprehension of relative clause syntax in nonfluent aphasia: A coordinated study. Presented at the Academy of Aphasia Conference, Philadelphia.

Ouhalla, J. (1993). Functional categories, agrammatism and language acquisition. *Linguistische Berichte, 143*, 3–36.

Pollock, J.Y. (1989). Verb movement, universal grammar and the structure of IP. *Linguistic Inquiry, 20*, 365–424.

Pollock, J.Y. (1993). *Notes on clause structure.* Amiens: Universite de Picardie.

Ouhalla, J. (1994). Verb movement and word order in Arabic. In N. Hornstein & D. Lightfoot (Eds.), *Verb movement.* Cambridge: Cambridge University Press.

Pollock, J.Y. (1997). Notes on clause structure. In L. Haegeman (Ed.), *Elements of grammar* (pp. 237–280). Dordrecht: Kluwer.

Ruigendijk, E., & Friedmann, N. (2002). Not all grammatical morphemes are impaired in agrammatism: Evidence from the production of case in Hebrew and Dutch. *Israeli Journal of Language, Speech and Hearing Disorders, 24*, 41–54 (in Hebrew).

Ruigendijk, E., Kouwenberg, M., & Friedmann, N. (2004). Question production in Dutch agrammatism. *Brain and Language, 91*, 116–117.

Saffran, E., Schwartz, M.E., & Marin, O. (1980). The word-order problem in agrammatism: II. Production. *Brain and Language, 10*, 263–280.

Sasanuma, S., Kamio, A., & Kubota, M. (1990). Agrammatism in Japanese: Two case studies. In L. Menn and L. Obler (Eds.), *Agrammatic aphasia: A cross-language narrative sourcebook.* Philadelphia: John Benjamin's.

Shlonsky, U. (1987). *Null and displaced subjects.* Thesis. Cambridge, MA: MIT.

Shlonsky, U. (1997). *Clause structure and word order in Hebrew and Arabic.* New York: Oxford University Press.

Shlonsky, U., & Doron, E. (1992). Verb second in Hebrew. In *Proceedings of the West Coast Conference on Formal Linguistics 10* (pp. 431–446). Stanford, CA: Stanford Linguistics Association, Stanford University.

Siloni, T. (1994). *Noun phrases and nominalizations.* Thesis. University of Geneva.

Siloni, T. (1997). Noun phrases and nominalizations: The syntax of DPs. In *Studies in natural language and linguistic theory, 40*. Dordrecht: Kluwer.

Thompson, C.K., & Shapiro, L.P. (1995). Training sentence production in agrammatism: Implications for normal and disordered language. *Brain and Language, 50*, 201–224.

Thompson. C.K., Shapiro, L.P., Ballard, K.J., Jacobs, B.J., Schneider, S.S., & Tait, M.E. (1997). Training and generalized production of Wh- and NP-movement structures in agrammatic aphasia. *Journal of Speech, Language, and Hearing Research, 40*, 228–244.

Thompson, C.K., Shapiro, L.P., & Roberts, M. (1993). Treatment of sentence production deficits in aphasia: A linguistic-specific approach to Wh-interrogative training and generalization. *Aphasiology, 7,* 111–133.

Thompson, C.K., Shapiro, L.P., Schneider, S.S., & Tait, M.E. (1994). *Morpho-syntactic and lexical analysis of normal and agrammatic aphasic language production.* Paper presented at TENNET V, Montreal, Canada.

Thompson, C.K., Shapiro, L.P., Tait, M.E., Jacobs, B.J., & Schneider, S.L. (1996). Training Whquestion production in agrammatic aphasia: Analysis of argument and adjunct movement. *Brain and Language, 52,* 175–228.

Weinrich, M., Shelton, J.R., Cox, D.M., & McCall, D. (1997). Remediating production of tense morphology improves verb retrieval in chronic aphasia. *Brain and Language, 58,* 23–45.

Wenzlaff, M., & Clahsen, H. (2004). Tense and agreement in German agrammatism. *Brain and Language, 89,* 57–68.

Zingeser, L.B., & Berndt, R.S. (1990). Retrieval of nouns and verbs in agrammatism and anomia. *Brain and Language, 39,* 14–32.

Zuckerman, S., Bastiaanse, R., & van Zonneveld, R. (2001). Verb movement in acquisition and aphasia: Same problem, different solutions—evidence from Dutch. *Brain and Language, 77,* 449–458.

6

A Blueprint for a Brain Map
of Syntax

Yosef Grodzinsky

THE MULTIFUNCTIONALITY OF
BROCA'S REGION

Broca's region on the left in humans can do many things. While this multifunctionality has long been recognized, distinctions are becoming finer with time. Broca viewed it as the locus (*siége*) of the *faculté du langage articulé* (which he aptly distinguished from other aspects of linguistic capacity, see [this volume, Chapter 18]). The distinctness of the language faculty did not gain universal acceptance (this volume, Chapter 19), but Broca nonetheless had influential successors who placed language production in the area they named after him, and proceeded to localize other linguistic activities (i.e., comprehension, repetition, reading, writing and naming) elsewhere in additional "language" regions (see Wernicke, 1874, Lichtheim, 1885, Geschwind, 1979 [this volume, Chapters 20 and 26]. See Basso [2003] for a recent historical review). When this clinical scene was later invaded by psychologists and linguists, the focus of investigation into brain/language

relations shifted: the borders of Broca's region—now known as left inferofrontal gyrus (LIFG), or areas 44 and 45, in Brodmann's nomenclature—were now aligned not only with activities/modalities but also with linguistic concepts such as phonology, lexicon, and syntax (e.g., Blumstein, 1973; Goodglas and Hunt, 1958 [Chapter 25]; Zurif, 1980). Some of these functions, gleaned almost exclusively through analyses of aberrant linguistic behavior in Broca's aphasia, were at times imputed neither to deficiencies in activities, nor to loss of linguistic knowledge but rather to impaired "psychological mechanisms," such as fluency (Goodglass et al., 1967), general sensory motor failures (e.g., Schuell and Sefer, 1973), or memory (Paulesu et al., 1993). The bag of descriptive tools used in accounts of brain–language relations was growing, containing now a mixed vocabulary of activities/modalities, sensory/motor and cognitive concepts, and, finally, linguistic terminology. Matters were getting complicated.

With time, the amount of relevant data and analyses grew. More experimentation and enhanced methods led to refined perspectives on the role of Broca's region in linguistic behavior. The advent of functional neuroimaging technologies made the picture even richer. That is where we now stand. This chapter is about some of these intriguing complexities and the way they might bear on our understanding of the nature of language and its relation to neural tissue.

Current literature underscores the multifunctionality of Broca's region: It is implicated in phonology (Blumstein, 1998) and in the way words are handled (see Cappa & Perani, this volume, Chapter 12); it is also said to contain resources that are recruited in working memory tasks (Smith and Jonides, 1999); there is even some evidence linking it to mental imagery (Binkofski et al., 2002). Many things seem to happen, then, in this relatively small portion of the left cerebral hemisphere. Finally, Broca's region seems to be crucial for syntactic analysis (see Chapters by Avrutin, Friederici, Friedmann, and Shapiro, this volume, Chapters 4, 5, 8, and 13). This chapter is about the role this brain area plays in receptive syntax and its place in the broader context—within a brain map for syntax.

More specifically, as it is becoming increasingly clear that Broca's region plays a limited role in receptive syntax (see Grodzinsky [2000a] for a recent review), an attempt to draw a full-blown syntax brain map must go beyond this area. Based on new findings that seem to localize pieces of syntax in other parts of the brain (particularly in the right hemisphere), I try to provide a rough sketch (based on the sparse available evidence) and consider its potential significance to neuroscience and linguistics.

A syntax map locates syntactic operations in brain space. However, a map merely points to the anatomical addresses of distinct operations, remaining a chapter in phrenology (albeit new and refined). I aim for more intricate properties that a syntax map might have, from which clues can be obtained regarding the character of principles of syntax. The idea is to harness the spatial geometry of the cerebral representation of syntactic operations for theoretical purposes. Drawing on results obtained in vision and in somatosensory physiology, I consider the theoretical significance that a syntax map might have. I entertain the following idea:

Syntacto-Topic Conjecture (STC)
a. Major syntactic operations are neurologically individuated.

b. The organization of these operations in brain space is linguistically significant.

Part a of the STC conjectures that formal properties of the linguistic signal are neurologically significant, that is, they reside in distinct brain loci and align with anatomically defined borders; the study of the functional neuroanatomy of syntax thus must make use of linguistic tools. Part b supposes that the spatial properties of this organization in neural tissue are linguistically significant. If supported, this conjecture would add an anatomical, perhaps even a quantitative, dimension to the theory of syntax.

The STC is a very general framework and is formulated against the background of current approaches to the visual, auditory and sensory motor systems. To give it life (i.e., empirical content) requires a long journey. Currently, there seems to be more questions than answers, yet a first step is to examine the current experimental record and to see whether relevant information can be gleaned for a syntactic brain map. I begin with a short review of two current methods for the study of brain language relations (next section) and move on to syntactic deficits in Broca's aphasia, which I argue are restricted to syntactic movement (*a k a* grammatical transformations). Next, I review the current experimental record in neuroimaging of the healthy brain in Broca's region and seek convergence with the aphasia results.

The next section looks beyond this region. It reviews two rather surprising recent findings that have located certain intrasentential dependency relations in different portions of the right hemisphere. These results drive the conclusion that a rough brain map for syntax may be within reach. Finally, I propose dimensions along which the STC may be explored by examining how visual maps are currently investigated.

NEW PHRENOLOGICAL TOOLS: ERRORS IN APHASIA, FMRI IN HEALTH

Of the plethora of experimental techniques currently in use, two seem to have contributed the most toward an understanding of brain–language relations: (1) the study of linguistic behavior in aphasic patients who have focal lesions in Broca's region and (2) functional imaging investigations of language in neurologically intact adults.[1] In aphasia, various types of linguistic stimuli and tasks are used, the typical dependent measure being error level. Erroneous performances are then correlated with lesion location. In neuroimaging of healthy language users, normal behavior is correlated with both anatomical locus and relative intensity of activation per a stimulus contrast (in a given task). As results obtained with these methods constitute the empirical backbone of this chapter, I now review some of their properties, in an attempt to understand the nature of the inference from data to theory that can later be made.

Componential analysis of behavior. In health, functional imaging measures brain correlates of normal behavior. Units of behavior can be identified on the basis of loci and relative intensity of blood oxygen level–dependent (BOLD) response. In aphasiology, behavioral abnormalities (errors) help discover neurologically natural classes of behavior—those affected and those spared by focal brain damage. This is done through the construction of deductive accounts that map the theory of the normal onto the pathological.

The nature of the inference. We map health onto pathology by removing components that seem to underlie the observed aberrant behavior subsequent to focal brain lesion. A success in deducing the absolute level of errors points to the crucial role of the removed component in the processing of the relevant stimulus in health. Such deficit analyses identify the role that the missing neural tissue plays in health. Such accounts are difficult to construct on the basis of fMRI data, because these data typically come in the form of contrasts in relative, rather than absolute, activation level. Activation of a brain region by some stimulus contrast is thus at best indicative of that region's participation in processing, but not necessarily of a critical role it plays (see Jezzard et al., 2001).

Analysis of brain activity. Remote and poorly understood as the index of brain activation that imaging currently provide may be, it does provide a measure of neural activity. No such measure is made in lesion studies discussed later.

Anatomical accuracy. Neuroimaging technologies are hailed as a technological breakthrough that enables unprecedented anatomical accuracy. This may be true, yet in the context of language it should be considered against three facts: (1) Interindividual variation in the language regions is great, a finding that repeats with every known anatomical mapping method (see Chapters 2 and 3). (2) It appears that, as Brodmann (1909 [this volume]) proposed, the anatomical method that produces borders that align best with functional distinctions is the cytoarchitectonic mapping method (Mattelli et al., 1991). Yet, cytoarchitectonic borders (not visible on fMRI) do not align well with topographic borders (visible on fMRI). As a result, our ability to localize linguistic processes precisely is constrained by the biology (see Amunts et al., 1999). (3) Lesion size and lesion variation in aphasic patients are thought to be on average larger than the corresponding measures in fMRI in health. This may be true, yet it is important to note that no study that compares lesion volume with volume of activations in health has ever been conducted.

Anatomical constraints. Neuroimaging methods are not limited to a specific brain area, because, unlike aphasia, they are not lesion dependent. As a consequence, a broader view of the brain is possible. Here, we see how significant is this feature. In at least one case, aphasia results exclude the involvement of Broca's area, yet only fMRI investigations localize them elsewhere. Table 6–1 summarizes the main points of comparison.

TABLE 6–1.

Dimension	Method	
	Lesion Studies (Aphasia)	fMRI in Health
A. Type of measured behavior	Errors	Normal performance
B. Possibility for a deductive account	Yes	No
C. Measured brain activity	None	Blood flow
D. Degree of anatomical precision	Up to lesion size and inter individual lesion overlap	Up to resolution of functional image and individual variation
E. Possibility of a broad view of the brain	No	Yes

FOCAL INSULT TO BROCA'S AREA RESULTS IN A SYNTACTIC MOVEMENT FAILURE—TRACE-DELETION HYPOTHESIS

Common wisdom is that Broca's area on the left hemisphere is entrusted with syntactic responsibilities. However, it is becoming increasingly clear that these are limited and do not encompass all of syntax. Remove Broca's area from a person, and she or he will be left with quite a lot of syntax; create a functional image of this area during syntactic analysis, and you will find that it remains silent on many syntactic tasks. Thus, important parts of syntax must be elsewhere in the brain, if they are to have neurological existence.

Focusing on receptive abilities in Broca's aphasia, I first present a view of the role Broca's region plays in supporting syntactic computations. I assume no prior knowledge in neuroimaging or in linguistics, although occasional [bracketed] hints and comments for imagers and linguists are included.

Focal insult to the vicinity of the left inferior frontal gyrus (i.e., the area that "encompass[es] most of the operculum, insula, and subjacent white matter," Mohr, 1978, p. 202) impairs linguistic ability in highly specific ways. The etiology of this condition may be stroke, hemorrhage, protrusion wound, tumor, or excision of tissue. As we look into syntax, only studies that use minimal pairs can be of use. That is, although many studies incorporate varieties of syntactic considerations into their design, I discuss only studies that contrast syntactic types with other syntactic types. This restricted domain has been a focus of intense study in recent years, and a rich body of data is currently available. Work carried out in many laboratories, through varied experimental methods and on several languages, has indicated that the receptive abilities of Broca's aphasics at the sentence level are selectively compromised. When tested in comprehension, grammaticality judgment as well as receptive timed tasks, they yield mixed results, success or failure (or aberrant performance) depending on sentence type. The goal of this section is to uncover a pattern in their performance.

Let me get to the bottom line right away: When core results are scrutinized, the deficit seems to encompass all and only sentences that contain syntactic movement. This deficit may have different faces when tapped by the various task types, but overall, syntactic movement operations (*a k a* grammatical transforma-

tions) are the heart of the receptive deficit and hence constitute the central syntactic function of Broca's area. A brief syntax tutorial follows.

Some Basics of Syntactic Movement

Simply put, syntactic movement is an operation that changes the relative sequential order of elements in a sentence. It is thus an abstract relation between two positions—an element's original position in a sentence and its "landing site." This operation may affect the visible (or audible) nature of a sentence, but it can also be invisible/covert, with empirical consequences that are sometimes detectable only through subtle tests. Overt movement of an element in the sentence (our current focus) implies that it has a split existence: as a phonetic entity, it is located in one position in the sentence (the landing site), yet its semantic interpretation is elsewhere (its original position, now phonetically empty but thematically active). Movement is the relation between the two positions. Consider the distinction between a declarative sentence and a corresponding question:

(1)

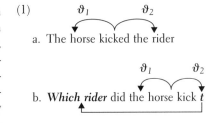

    a. The horse kicked the rider

    b. **Which rider** did the horse kick *t*

In the declarative sentence (example 1a), the predicate *kick* assigns thematic (θ)-roles to the argument immediately preceding it, *horse*, and to the one immediately following it, *rider*. Verb semantics determine which role (drawn out of a universal inventory of labels that specify possible argument denotations, such as agent, patient, experiencer, goal, source, and instrument) is assigned to each argument (ϑ_1 = agent, ϑ_2 = patient, in example 1a). In the corresponding question (example 1b), however, the elements ⟨kick, rider⟩ are nonadjacent, and their sequential order is reversed. Still, as the verb *kick* has not changed, only its surroundings, the manner by which it assigns its ϑ-roles, must remain fixed–ϑ_1 to the left and ϑ_2 to the right. Yet *rider* remains recipient-of-action or patient under this major change. To maintain ϑ-constancy despite the sequential change, a transmission mechanism is posited (which will be then shown to have additional functions): *'the rider'* not only becomes *'which rider'* but also is copied to the front of the sentence, and its token in its previous position is deleted and replaced by a symbol *'t'* for *trace* of movement. In the question, *'kick'* assigns a patient ϑ-roles rightward to the position marked by *'t'*. This means that phonetically, *'which rider'* is sentence-initial, but its ϑ-role is downstream in *'t'*. The two positions ⟨*'which rider'*, *'t'*⟩ are related by a link that ensures that the ϑ-role is transmitted from *t* to *'which rider'*, so that interpretation will be carried out properly.

Movement is a generalized, yet highly constrained, relation between positions in a sentence. From a ϑ-perspective, example 1 and the English passive construction (example 2) are somewhat similar, in that they contain one indirect assignment that a trace mediates:

(2)

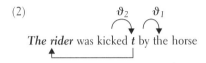

This presentation (in which accuracy is sacrificed for clarity and accessibility to a broader audience) has thus far adopted a thematic perspective to movement. This choice is made because the relevant comprehension studies on Broca's aphasics are mostly about the manner by which they interpret ϑ-roles. Yet traces of movement have syntactic functions that go beyond the mediation of ϑ-roles. They are also crucial for the determination of the grammatical status of strings. Movement operations are highly constrained: Allowing constituents to move around freely would result in a very large number of ungrammatical strings (cf. the pair I *believe that it is likely that John is a fool* and **John is believed that it is likely to be a fool*). We must set conditions to prevent such eventuality. Many of these restrictive conditions are predicated over traces. For example, while movement from subject position to create a multiple question is possible in English (example 3a), such a question is impossible to formulate if the object is fronted (example 3b).

(3) a. I don't know *who* [*t* saw *what*]

b. *I don't know *what who* [*t* saw *t*]

Ungrammaticality seems to occur when the link connecting a moved question word to its traces crosses another question word (example 3b). If true, this observation suggests that traces are involved in the determination of grammaticality of sentences, and thus have purely syntactic functions. On this view, traces of movement have a dual role: They are involved in interpretation through their function in transmitting ϑ-roles to moved arguments, and they are embedded in constraints on movement. [Notice that as presented, movement may be "vacuous," as it may occur without overt changes (example 3a). I return to this issue later.]

With these basic tools at hand, we can now examine the mixed performance of Broca's aphasics in both comprehension and grammaticality judgment tests, to start searching for a pattern in their behavior.

Some Core Data on the Syntactic Comprehension Deficit in Broca's Aphasia

When asked to match the sentences (in example 4) to depicted scenarios in binary choice experiments (i.e., on 'who did X to whom' tasks that require correct matching of two arguments in a sentence to two actors in a scenario, which amount to ϑ-role assignment), Broca's aphasic patients perform well above chance (as measured by tests that typically consist of 10 to 30 trials per sentence type). In example 5, however, their comprehension performance drops dramatically to a level that is around chance (see Drai and Grodzinsky, 2006, and Drai, this volume, Chapter 7 for discussion of this measure). These form the basic data array from which we start, which is presented next in an annotated form [traces of subject movement from VP-internal position are ignored; more on that later]:

(4) *Above-chance comprehension*
   a. The woman is chasing the man
   b. ***The woman*** who *t* is chasing the man is tall
   c. Show me ***the woman*** who *t* is chasing the man
   d. It is ***the woman*** that *t* is chasing the man
   e. ***Which man*** *t* touched Mary?

(5) *Chance comprehension*
   a. ***The man*** that the woman is chasing *t* is tall
   b. Show me ***the man*** who the woman is chasing *t*
   c. It is ***the man*** that the woman is chasing *t*
   d. ***The man*** is chased *t* by the woman
   e. ***Which man*** did Mary touch *t*?

This pattern of performance is intricate, and its connection to syntactic movement as described earlier is not immediately apparent. That is, traces feature in many (if not all) sentence representations in examples 4 and 5, and thus their presence or absence does not place the cases in the correct performance groupings. Still, syntactic movement and traces do function as critical building blocks in various incarnations of a deficit analysis known as the trace-deletion hypothesis (TDH) (Grodzinsky, 1984, 1986, 1995, 2000a), which attempts to account for these data. The idea behind the TDH is that the core receptive deficit in Broca's aphasia inheres in an inability to represent traces of movement in syntactic representations. If true, this theory would mean that the central role of Broca's area in sentence perception is to support syntactic movement. Next, I present the logic behind the TDH and show it at work.

Mapping Deficient Representations Onto Performance

Suppose that traces of movement are deleted from syntactic representations in Broca's aphasia, as the TDH would have it. On minimal expectations, it is not clear how any behavior can be derived from such a supposition. On the one hand, if every trace deletion is to affect performance, more comprehension failures than observed are expected, because most cases not only in example 5, but also in example 4, contain traces, and their deletion is supposed to cause comprehension problems. On the other hand, it is not clear why the deletion of traces would impact patients' success rate in comprehension tasks in the first place. This account, then, seems to be both too strong and too weak.

An example will help elucidate the problem. Consider ϑ-assignment in subject (example 6a) and object (example 6b) relative clauses in English, measured in aphasia through the typical sentence-to-picture matching task, in which correct ϑ-assignment is critical for errorless performance. In both examples 6a and 6b, a [bracketed] relative clause modifies the subject of an italicized main clause. From here, the cases diverge. In example 6a, *the woman* is the subject of the relative clause (i.e., of the verb *chase*), hence linked to a trace in subject position; in example 6b, *the man* is the object of the relative and is linked to an object trace.

The transitive verb *chase* assigns two roles, $\langle \vartheta_1 =$ agent; $\vartheta_2 =$ patient$\rangle$, to the subject on its left and to the object on its right, respectively. The verb in both sentences is one and the same, and hence its ϑ-assigning properties are unaffected by sentential context (i.e., position of the trace) and remain fixed. In both instances, one ϑ-role is mediated by a trace. If trace deletion diminishes performance, then Broca's aphasics' success rates should be low for both examples 6a and 6b. Yet, their performance is split: they are above chance on example 6a and at chance levels on example 6b. But even if we could derive this split, we would still have to say why the deletion of the trace would bring about the particular performance level observed for example 6b. Mere deletion of traces thus neither singles out object relatives for impairment nor accounts for the particulars of this divergent pattern.

These observations may help us formulate preliminary requirements that a deficit analysis must satisfy: It must have a descriptive device that would set the impaired behaviors apart from the preserved ones, and it must offer an account from which the aberrant behavioral pattern can be deduced—an explicit mapping from normal to pathological behavior. An understanding of the deficit behind the behavior presupposes an explicit mapping from structural deficiency to measured behavior (= error rate).

Example 6

(6) **Normal ϑ-representation**   **Aphasic performance**

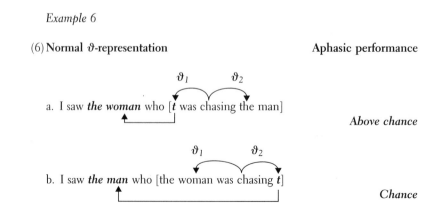

Above chance

Chance

Next, the quest for a deductive account leads us to ponder the quantitative nature of aberrant behavior. Earlier, no concrete numerical value was given to the aphasics' performance level, only its relation to chance. This stems from the recognition that a syntax-based approach does not have quantitative scales. The unavailability of an implementation (performance model) with such scales, and the binary nature of the experiments at issue, leave us with three performance types only: A patient performing a binary-choice comprehension (ϑ-assignment) task that contains multiple tokens can either get it right (= above chance level) or wrong (= below chance), or guess (= chance).

Finally, comprehension tasks require that referential elements have an interpretation. The task thus forces the deficient system to label each referential element with a ϑ-role. Our desiderata from an account can be summarized in the following premises:

(7) **Premises for deducing error data in error-measuring experiments**

P1. Transparency: Error rates must be derived deductively.
(explicit mapping from representation to error-rate on each sentence type)

P2. Restricted Outcomes: Experimental paradigm determines the range of discernible error types.
(In a binary-choice, ϑ-assignment paradigm, unless quantitative parameters are introduced to the interpretive framework, outcomes can only be related to chance.)

P3. Full Interpretation Under Duress (FIUD): Interpretive forced-choice tasks require every referential element to have a semantic role.
(When grammatical ϑ-assignment fails, a ϑ-less referential element acquires a semantic role via extra-grammatical means.)[2,3]

With these premises in our pocket, we can now try to account for the experimental results in example 6 through the TDH. If all traces in example 6 are deleted, example 8a becomes the deficient representation of example 6a, whereas example 8b represents example 6b.

Premises *P1* and *P2* enter first into play: An account of Broca's aphasia must deduce the patients' performance levels from deficient representations (*P1*), and error rates are given in terms of their relation to chance (*P2*). Moving to the results, we begin with the virtually normal comprehension performance in example 8a. The relative object 'the man' is assigned ϑ_2 (= patient) directly. The story is different for the moved subject ***the woman***: Assignment of ϑ_1 is normally mediated by a trace, now deleted (annotated by "*"); the subsequent disruption of the link between ϑ_1 and the moved constituent ***the woman*** (annotated by a perforated line) leads to a ϑ_1-assignment failure, in violation of premise *P3* (FIUD).

How can *P3* be satisfied? Notice that the direction of ϑ_1-assignment is toward ***the woman***; moreover, no referential element intervenes between ***the woman*** and "*". As example 8a depicts it, this peculiar configuration allows the thematic gap caused by trace-deletion to be bridged, as the assignment of ϑ_1 may stretch leftward. Call this operation **ϑ-bridging**. Now both arguments of the verb have ϑ-roles, as ϑ_2 is assigned normally, and ϑ_{1-} by ϑ-bridging (hence bolded); this thematic representation is correct, and normal performance follows. A somewhat similar approach to ϑ-roles in subjects in the absence of a trace-antecedent link is independently considered in the context of developing children (see Fox and Grodzinsky, 1998) [Note that the ϑ-bridging mechanism also provides a solution to a potential problem that arises regarding gaps in ϑ-transmission that are created due

Example 8

(8) **Broca's aphasics' ϑ-representation**   **Performance level**

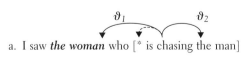

a. I saw ***the woman*** who [* is chasing the man]

                                                          Above chance

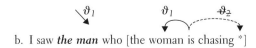

b. I saw ***the man*** who [the woman is chasing *]

                                                          Chance

to the deletion of traces of movement from VP-internal position and their subject antecedents. That is, despite trace deletion, the ϑ-role assigned to the subject VP-internally can reach the subject in its IP position by ϑ-bridging in a manner similar to what we have seen. We ignore this issue for ease of exposition.]

Now consider example 8b. Here, ϑ_1 is assigned correctly, having no interaction with the TDH (again, traces of movement from VP-internal subject position notwithstanding). The problem assignment is that of ϑ_2: The mediating trace is deleted by the TDH, which creates a gap between ϑ_2 and *the man*. Like before, P3 requires each referential element to have a ϑ-role; unlike before, ϑ_2 cannot reach its assignee through ϑ-bridging, because its bridging operates on linear sequences, and here the direction of assignment is not toward *the man*, but away from it. ϑ_2 is stranded (hence struck through), *the man* remains ϑ-less in the relative clause, and P3 is again violated.

The failure of grammatical devices forces the system to resort to knowledge acquired through experience, in an attempt to satisfy P3. Bever (1970) observed that in most of the world's languages, the most frequent linear order of semantic roles in transitive sentences is $\langle \vartheta_1 = \text{agent}, \vartheta_2 = \text{patient} \rangle$. Suppose that in order to satisfy P3, a link—driven by an extra-grammatical default strategy—is established between the ϑ-less NP and the role that is most frequently associated with its linear position in the string. A clause-initial NP that has not obtained its ϑ-role grammatically would thus become agent.

Consider now the thematic representation that a Broca's aphasic patient has for a sentence with movement under the TDH. It is based on two knowledge sources: an incomplete grammar, and the strategy. In example 8b, the resulting representation contains two arguments, both associated with $\vartheta_1 = \text{agent}$. In a task that requires ϑ-assignment, a ϑ-conflict arises, and chance performance is forced. The grammar-based strategic ϑ-assignment pulls in opposite directions (e.g., given two arguments and an $\langle \text{agent}, \text{patient} \rangle$ ϑ-representation of the predicate, grammar dictates that argument$_1$ = agent, and strategy dictates that argument$_2$ = agent). Note that chance performance follows only if the thematic output of the deficient grammar and the thematic dictum of the strategy have equal weights. Whether this is true remains to be empirically investigated (see Chapter 7).

Many of these ideas have been around for a while. What is new here is the explicit formulation of interpretive principles (example 7) that link syntactic representations to numerical results of experiments. P1 posits a general requirement, that an account derive aberrant performance deductively. P2 sets up a range of possible experimental outcomes for the specific task under consideration, and P3 connects deficient representations to compensatory mechanisms that may be involved when deficient comprehenders perform this task. Hopefully, these premises will help shed new light not only on the structure of neurolinguistic explanation but also on the interpretation of similar experiments with language-deficient populations in general (e.g., developing children).

Next, it is important to distinguish the TDH from an apparently simpler, canonicity-based account of deficient performance (e.g., Frazier and Friederici, 1992; Zurif, 1995). This approach suggest that canonical sentences, in which the linear order of overt arguments corresponds to their order in the lexicon, yield normal comprehension in Broca's aphasia, whereas deviation from canonicity leads to comprehension difficulties. As the TDH relies on directionality of ϑ-role assignment—itself an expression of the canonical arrangement of arguments around a predicate (agent to its left, patient to its right, etc.)—it is important to compare the two accounts.

To begin with, the canonicity account is incommensurate with interpretive premise P1, transparency. While it may partition the cases correctly into those that induce error (example 5) and those that do not (example 4), it says nothing about why errors are observed and why performance is at these levels. The TDH, by contrast, is transparent.

Second, the two approaches are empirically distinguishable. Consider multiclausal sentences with movement (example 9a) and their array of ϑ-roles and predicates (example 9b).

When linearized, the ϑ-arrays of the two verbs are interwoven: the agent argument of 'say', 'the girl', intervenes between '*pushed*' and '*which boy*'. However, the precedence relations between *push* and its arguments—*which boy* >>pushed>> the old man—do correspond to the order of ϑ-roles in the lexicon. This correspondence seems to be the rationale behind a canonicity-based account of the comprehension deficit in Broca's aphasia, which contends that patients who succeed use lexical knowledge to compensate for a syntactic deficit (of an unspecified nature). In (example 9a), however, similarity in precedence relations does not mean congruence with

Example 9

(9)

$$\vartheta_1 \quad \vartheta_2$$

a. **Which boy** did the girl say [* *pushed the old man*]
b. $<\vartheta_{1\text{-}push}>$ $<\vartheta_{1\text{-}say}>$ say $<\vartheta_{2\text{-}say}>$ = [push $<\vartheta_{2\text{-}push}>$]>

order in the lexicon. Reliance on lexical information—as a canonicity-based account would have it—may not be sufficient, and a comprehension failure would follow.

By contrast, a straightforward construal of the TDH predicts normal comprehension in Broca's aphasia: *which boy* is dissociated from its agent ϑ-role due to trace-deletion, but because it is clause-initial, this deficiency is expected to be correctly compensated for by the default strategy.

The TDH Cross-Linguistically

We move to languages whose structural properties differ from English in ways that interact with the deficit in Broca's aphasia. Results from a variety of language types seem to bear on the TDH. In Chinese, an SVO language, heads (bold) follow their relative clause (examples 10a and 11a), unlike English, in which they precede it (examples 10b and 11b).

This structural difference leads to a remarkable prediction for Broca's aphasia: Opposite English/Chinese performance patterns are expected. In English subject relatives (example 10b), trace-deletion deprives the relative head 'cat' of its agent ϑ-role; correct assignment—hence, above chance performance—is obtained through ϑ-bridging. In the Chinese subject relative (example 10a), the link between the relative head **mau** is to the right of the verb but ϑ-assignment is to the left. The trace is deleted, yet unlike its English counterpart, ϑ-bridging cannot work because ϑ_1-assignment is in a direction contralateral to its argument. Premise P3 forces default assignment, and given the clause-final position of the ϑ-deficient argument, it now receives the patient role. The resulting representation has $2 \times \vartheta_2$ = patient ('dog' and *cat*), and guessing follows. Similar considerations hold in object relatives (examples 11a and 11b) and are left to the reader who will notice the mirror ϑ-images. This prediction is confirmed: the results in Chinese form a remarkable mirror image of the English ones (Grodzinsky, 1989; Law, 2000; Su, 2000), and correlate with the contrasting position of the relative head in the two languages. The phenomenon of

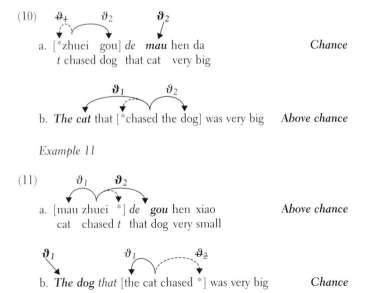

Example 10

(10) ϑ_1 ϑ_2 ϑ_2

     a. [*zhuei   gou] *de* **mau** hen da   *Chance*
         t chased dog that cat   very big

             ϑ_1 ϑ_2

     b. **The cat** that [*chased the dog] was very big   *Above chance*

Example 11

(11) ϑ_1 ϑ_2

     a. [mau zhuei *] *de* **gou** hen xiao   *Above chance*
        cat   chased *t*   that dog very small

ϑ_1 ϑ_1 ϑ_2

     b. **The dog** *that* [the cat chased *] was very big   *Chance*

Example 12

(12) a. *English*

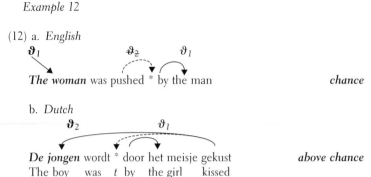

The woman was pushed * by the man   *chance*

b. *Dutch*

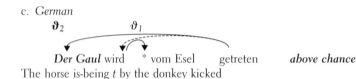

De jongen wordt * door het meisje gekust   *above chance*
The boy   was   *t* by   the girl   kissed

c. *German*

Der Gaul wird   * vom Esel   getreten   *above chance*
The horse is-being *t* by the donkey kicked

ϑ-conflict is thus generalized, manifesting as agent versus agent in English and as patient versus patient in Chinese.

Further intriguing cross-linguistic contrasts are also found. Take passive: In many languages, its comprehension by Broca's aphasics is at chance level, yet this is not universally true. Performance levels of Dutch and German Broca's aphasics are above chance (e.g., Burchert et al., 2002; Friederici and Graetz, 1987; Kolk and van Grunsven, 1985; see Drai and Grodzinsky, 2006, for quantitative analyses contrasting English and Dutch/German). Consider how ϑ-assignment in Broca's aphasia works for passive in these languages.

How the *by*-phrase is assigned a ϑ-role by the predicate (thin line) is orthogonal to the current discussion. For simplicity, we assume that ϑ_1 = agent is to the assigned object of the *by/door/vom*-phrase (see Baker et al., 1989; Fox and Grodzinsky, 1998, for some discussion of the problems in this assignment).

We now focus on the assignment of ϑ_2 = patient, the locus of a critical difference between English and Dutch/German: Only the latter are verb final languages (i.e., their basic word order is SOV). That is, objects in English are canonically to the right of the verb, whereas in Dutch/German they are to the left. Given that ϑ-roles (such as agent and patient) are assigned by a predicate (verb) to its arguments, this cross-linguistic contrast has two relevant implications to the thematic identity of the moved argument: (a) in English, ϑ-assignment to the internal argument (the one canonically in object position but now fronted) is to the right (example 12a); in Dutch/German, it is to the left (examples 12b and 12c); (b) in English passive, movement of the object to subject position crosses the verb; in Dutch/German passive, the object only crosses the auxiliary when it moves. It stays on the same side of the main verb as in active.

As a consequence, normal ϑ-assignment to object position in English passive (perforated arrow in example 12a) is in a direction *contralateral* to the position of the moved argument **the woman**. The aphasia result follows, in a manner similar to the object relatives: the ϑ-role fails to reach its target, and a strategically assigned agent role is forced on the moved subject by the default strategy, which leads to a ϑ-conflict, hence chance performance; in Dutch/German, by contrast, ϑ-bridging is possible: the moved constituent **De jongen** or **Der Gaul** is *ipsilateral* to the ϑ-role is should receive, and no intervener stands between the ϑ-role and its target. A uniform cross-linguistic view of the deficit in Broca's aphasia follows, which may actually provide critical hints regarding the correct analysis of passive in Dutch and German.

ϑ-Bridging has been repeatedly invoked here, and it needs some elaboration. A ϑ-role fails to reach its target argument only if the direction of assignment is contralateral to the direction of movement. Otherwise, ϑ-bridging works both in the subject-versus-object trace contrast in English and the cross-linguistic contrast in passive we have just seen. While this might make intuitive sense, there are puzzles that remain. Specifically, there are cases in which movement leaves an NP ipsilateral to its ϑ-role and, still, aphasic performance is at chance. This is the case in scrambling constructions in SOV languages. They might shed light on ϑ-bridging.

Many languages have a scrambling rule that moves the object across the subject in simple declarative sentences. In Japanese, a subject-object-verb language, this rule transforms a sentence with an SOV word order (example 14a) into OSV (example 14b). This movement operation yields a representation with a trace. The two sentence configurations are otherwise on a par, yet performance in Broca's aphasia splits (Fujita, 1977; Hagiwara and Caplan, 1990):

(13)

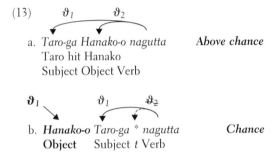

    a. *Taro-ga Hanako-o nagutta*   **Above chance**
       Taro hit Hanako
       Subject Object Verb

    b. **Hanako-o** *Taro-ga* * *nagutta*   **Chance**
       Object   Subject *t* Verb

A remarkable result was obtained in German. That is, patients who perform successfully on passive (example 12) fail on the German analogue of scrambling in a manner identical to the Japanese one (Burchert et al., 2001). Analogous results have also been obtained in Hebrew, Spanish, and Korean (Beretta et al., 2001; Friedmann and Shapiro, 2003). As the graphics make clear, movement and ϑ-assignment in (example 13b) go in the same direction—leftward—and still, patients are at chance. Recall that in example 12, the explanation of the performance contrast between English and Dutch/German on passive exploited the fact that although in English the displaced argument moved leftward and ϑ-assignment went rightward, in Dutch/German they both go in the same direction. Yet, in Japanese they go in the same direction, and patients are still at chance. Why cannot the TDH-induced gap between ϑ_2 and **Hanako-o** be ϑ-bridged? How can these seemingly contradictory cross-linguistic results be reconciled?

Observe that in Dutch/German passive, no thematically active element (i.e., predicate, argument) intervenes between the position of the trace and the

argument to which a ϑ-role must reach. That is, the gap that trace-deletion creates between ϑ-role and argument can be bridged effortlessly. In Japanese scrambling constructions, by contrast, the subject intervenes between the trace and the moved object and blocks the ϑ-role from bridging the gap that trace deletion created.[4]

Informally speaking, the consequence is that in Broca's aphasia, ϑ-assignment to a moved element may succeed despite trace-deletion if two conditions are met: (a) movement is in the same direction as ϑ-assignment and (b) there is no thematically relevant *intervener* between the trace and the antecedent. These conclusions are important: they indicate that scrambling and cases of XP-movement form a neurological natural class.

Finally, a recent important study by Luzzatti and colleagues (2001) is a test of the default strategy from another angle. Italian-speaking Broca's aphasics, who give the typical comprehension pattern in active/passive, exhibit a complex pattern when clitic movement is at issue. In active sentences with transitive verbs, they perform above chance not only on simple sentences like example 14a but also, on their cliticized analogues (example 14b), even though the object clitic *le/la* moves across the verb (see, e.g., Sportiche, 1995) and is dissociated from its ϑ-role. Furthermore, while the patients' comprehension is similarly near-normal on ditransitives (example 14c), their performance drops significantly, to chance level, when they are faced with cliticized versions of these sentences (example 14d)[5]:

(14) a. *Mario cerca Flora*   **Above chance**
      Mario seeks Flora

    b. *Mario la cerca t*   **Above chance**
      Mario *her* seeks *t*
      'Mario seeks her'

    c. *Mario dà un regalo a Flora*   **Above chance**
      Mario gives a present to Flora

    d. *Mario le dà un regalo t*   **Chance**
      Mario her gives a present
      'Mario gives her a present'[6]

How can we cut these results correctly? Performance does not seem to split the pie along familiar lines. The good performance on (examples 14a and 14c) follows from the TDH straightforwardly, as they contain no movement. Next, the paradigm contains two sentence types with movement (examples 14b and 14d), and yet patients have trouble only with example 14d. Consider example 14b first: Cliticization moves the object across the verb, producing an $SO_{(clitic)}V$ sequence. The verb normally assigns ⟨agent, theme⟩ left and right, respectively. In Broca's aphasia, S is assigned agent grammatically, whereas the object clitic—located to the left of the verb—is dissociated from its ϑ-role due to the deletion of its trace that is to the verb's right. Yet, being second in the linear sequence, this clitic is assigned the theme role by the default strategy, and correct compensation, hence normal performance, follows.

By the same logic, the strategy assigns the theme role to the clitic in example 14d. Yet here, matters are different: The verb is ditransitive, and its ϑ-grid is ⟨agent, theme, goal⟩. The output of the cliticization process is $SO^{1}_{(clitic)}VO^{2}$. The moved element should normally be goal, being the result of cliticizing the recipient of the gift Flora in example 14c. In Broca's aphasia the trace is deleted, and the string-second $O^{1}_{(clitic)}$, now dissociated from its goal ϑ-role, receives the theme role from the strategy. But this role cannot be assigned to animate arguments; moreover, there are now two themes, as one is already assigned to O^{2} grammatically. A conflict ensues, resulting in the observed performance drop.

The logic underlying the TDH, as well as its implementation in a range of fairly complex cases, is thus demonstrated. It can be summarized thus:

(15) **TDH**
  a. *Trace-deletion*: Delete all traces of phrasal movement
  b. *Interpret referential elements*: A ϑ-argument satisfies P3 either by ϑ-bridging, or by a linear default strategy that assigns it a role

Statement 15a specifies the syntactic deficit; statement 15b proposes a mechanism to satisfy P3 (FIUD). Limiting myself to an informal account, I offer no precise definitions, and only note that the linear default strategy is defined relative to the sequence of ϑ-roles around the predicate and that ϑ-bridging enables an argument that is adjacent to a deleted trace to acquire the latter's ϑ-role in the absence of an intervener (whose precise nature awaits definition). These principles are obviously related, perhaps reducible to a single statement. As they are predicated over the linear order of elements, one can perhaps imagine a reformulation of (at least parts of) the TDH, as a pathological modification of conditions on the linearization

of syntactic representations in normal speakers (*cf.*, Fox and Pesetsky, in press, for one framework that may be a candidate platform for this idea).

If this type of account is on the right track, we can conclude that the core syntactic deficit in Broca's aphasia—hence the central role of Broca's region in sentence reception—is the computation of syntactic movement. Next, I present additional converging evidence from aphasic performance in experimental tasks that do not require ϑ-assignment and show that this conclusion is not task dependent.

Pathological Performance Across Experimental Methods

Grammaticality Judgment

When patients are requested to indicate whether the sentences in example 16 are grammatical (a task for which training is necessary), these patients are quite agile, performing at near-normal levels. By contrast, when asked about the sentences in example 17, they vacillate, failing to distinguish the grammatical (i) cases from the ungrammatical ones (ii) (Grodzinsky and Finkel, 1998; see Lima and Novaes, 2000, for a replication in Brazilian Portuguese).

(16) *Successful Determination of Grammatical Status*
  a. (i) The children sang
     (ii) *The children sang the ball over the fence
  b. (i) The children threw
     (ii) *The children threw the ball over the fence
  c. (i) Could they have left town?
     (ii) *Have they could leave town?
  d. (i) John did not sit
     (ii) *John sat not

(17) *Failed Determination of Grammatical Status*
  a. (i) It seems that John is likely to win
     (ii) John seems likely *t* to win
     (iii) *John seems that it is likely to win
  b. (i) Which woman did David think *t* saw John?
     (ii) *Which woman did David think that *t* saw John?
  c. (i) I don't know who *t* saw what
     (ii) *I don't know what who *t* saw *t*

All of the well-judged sentences do not contain movement (i.e., if we restrict our attention to XP-movement), whereas the poorly judged ones do (except example 18a, i). Deleted traces preclude the aphasics from determining the grammatical status of these sentences—whether grammatical or not—and the observed failure follows. Similarly, when patients are required to make judgments of semantic plausibility, and these crucially depend on traces, errors follow. Such results have been obtained through different experimental methods and in different languages (*cf.*, Dickey and Thompson, 2004; Mikelič et al., 1995; Schwartz et al., 1986; Wilson and Saygın, 2004).

Real-time Processing

It has long been known that neurologically intact subjects access the antecedents of traces at the gap position in real-time. This is demonstrated by Cross-Modal-Lexical-Priming (CMLP) tests, in which subjects listen to sentences such as example 18a and watch a screen, onto which a visual probe of the types in i through iii may be projected at points 1, 2, or 3 in the sentence. Their task is to make a lexical decision on the visually presented item:

(18) a. The passenger smiled at **the baby**[1] that the woman[2] in the pink jacket fed[3] *t* at the train station
   b. The passenger smiled at **the baby**[1] in the blue pajamas[2] who *t*[3] drank milk at the train station
     i. *Diaper* (related)
     ii. *Horse* (unrelated)
     iii. *Strile* (non-word)

In both sentences, access to (i), the related target, at position (1) – immediately after the prime – is facilitated, and reaction times are shorter when compared to (ii); at position (2), a decay of this effect is monitored, as the distance from the prime increases; surprisingly, at (3), there appears to be facilitation – after the decay, the prime reawakens, becomes reactivated at the gap position, and reaction time to (i) is decreased again, relative to (ii) (Love and Swinney, 1996).

If Broca's aphasics suffer from a deficit that the TDH describes, they should be unable to reactivate traces properly. Indeed, when confronted with this task, they do not show normal priming at the gap (Zurif et al., 1993).

The CMLP technique provides an important cross-task angle on subject traces. In comprehension, the deletion of subject traces is circumvented by ϑ-bridging. In the CMLP task, trace deletion should preclude antecedent reactivation. CMLP tests of Broca's aphasics with subject relative clauses (Zurif et al., 1993) confirmed this view (example 18b). The pattern of performance observed was indistinguishable from that found for object relatives (example 18a)—the patients failed to prime the relevant target at point 3, indicating that they did not reactivate the antecedent at trace position. Thus, Broca's aphasics evidence split performance in subject relative clauses: this sentence type yields near-normal comprehension but pathological performance in CMLP. Once again, a curious contingency is revealed, where the same sentence type may yield different results, depending on how the particular experimental task interacts with the patient's deficit.

MOVEMENT IN HEALTHY BROCA'S AREA: AN FMRI PERSPECTIVE

Imaging Syntactic Analysis

The study of syntax in the healthy brain through functional brain imaging seeks to tease apart syntactic operations by monitoring an index of regional brain activity (usually done through the measurement of changes in regional cerebral blood flow) during syntax tasks. To this end, stimuli made of minimal pairs of sentences are used, to make possible the isolation of the relevant syntactic operations. This reduces the number of currently available studies that can be discussed, because many, if not most, imaging investigations at the sentence level are designed with more general goals in mind (e.g., whether syntactic and semantic processes are distinct [Dapretto and Bookheimer, 1999; Vandenbergh et al., 2002; see Grodzinsky, 2002, for a critical review]). Still, the few relevant results that are available provide preliminary hints regarding the relevance of this endeavor to the STC. Before these are presented, a short digression to experimental issues is necessary.

Effects in fMRI experiments are always difficult to obtain, due to a relatively poor signal-to-noise ratio (see Jezzard et al., 2001, for tutorials). In experiments that feature syntactic contrasts, matters are considerably harder: Sentence stimuli are typically of exceedingly long duration, about 4 seconds per stimulus, compared with about 300 to 400 milliseconds in vision experiments. To isolate a syntactic operation, a difference in brain response between members of a minimal syntactic pair needs to be detected. Like in vision experiments, we compare the difference in the strength of the BOLD response between experimental conditions. Yet, unlike vision, the effect that such contrasts produce is weak relative to the overall BOLD response generated by the cognitively taxing analysis of long sentence stimuli.

The most compelling evidence for regional activity in the brain that correlates with a stimulus contrast is provided through statistical maps (e.g., Worsley et al., 2001). These maps are constructed through an exhaustive search across the whole brain for a significant difference in BOLD response between experimental conditions. Signal intensity that each contrast induces is compared on every brain volume (voxel) that the technology defines. This method thus involves multiple statistical comparisons. The nature of statistical comparisons opens way to spurious effects in such cases, for which we must control (i.e., correct for accidental effects obtained simply by the multiplicity of statistical tests). As a consequence, the threshold for each comparison is elevated, requiring more power to be significant. Syntactic effects, whose size is typically small, rarely pass the required threshold, making the direct construction of syntax maps difficult.

An alternative approach is the regions of interest (ROI) approach, which seeks to increase signal intensity and at the same time reduce the number of statistical comparisons. It focuses on those parts of the brain that interest us and ignores the rest; at the same time, it pulls together all voxels within this region and treats them as one unit. The result is higher signal intensity, with less correction. Weaker effects may surface to the forefront. These gains do not come for free: anatomical resolution is sacrificed for statistical power. Moreover, as an *a priori* anatomical choice is made, ROI analyses need motivation, as well as a method for the delineation of the chosen brain areas. Most (although not all) of the data I present come from ROI analyses.

Currently, three findings can be reported. (1) A series of studies in English, German, and Hebrew in multiple contrasts and tasks correlate a movement effect with increased BOLD response in Broca's region of the left cerebral hemisphere. These results converge on the findings for Broca's aphasia; most, but not all, of these contrasts also activate left (and perhaps right) Wernicke's region. (2) Reflexive binding uniquely activates the Superior frontal gyrus of the

right hemisphere. (3) Dative shift uniquely activates the anterior insula and the ventral portion of the precentral sulcus, both in the right hemisphere, and does not activate Broca's region. The remainder of this section reviews the movement studies; the rest are described in the subsequent one.

Relative versus Complement Clauses

Initial imaging studies of syntax contended that Broca's region is entrusted with the task of processing complex sentences (see Caplan, 2001, for a review). Among the contrasts tested were many that involved syntactic movement. For a variety of reasons, it seemed worthwhile to try and tease apart the two notions—movement and complexity.[7]

The first study to do so (Ben-Shachar et al., 2003) used Hebrew auditory stimuli that were identical on a large number of commonly used complexity measures (length, number of words, propositions, embeddings, verbs, ratio of functional to lexical categories, and more) and differed only with respect to syntactic movement. Object relative clauses (example 19a) with an embedded transitive verb were pitted against sentences with sentential (CP) complements that contained an intransitive verb (example 19b). This setup produced a minimal ± movement contrast.

Each sentence had an ungrammatical counterpart, created by switching the embedded verbs—*meet* for *sleep* and vice versa. Subjects were asked to make grammaticality judgments.

Weak effects forced an ROI approach. Four ROIs on which the analysis was focused were defined on each hemisphere anatomically (based on past aphasia results) and functionally (through a "filler-sentences minus silence" localizer and a minimum of 100 contiguous activated voxels). Each definition led to an independent analysis. Anatomical ROIs were (1) inferior frontal gyrus (BA 44,45); (2) posterior superior temporal sulcus, the posterior third of STS; (3) anterior insula—the anterior third of the insula, bordering the IFG; and (4) Heschl's complex, Heschl's gyrus and sulcus (BA 22).

Analysis revealed a movement effect in Broca's region (LIFG). On the functional definition of ROIs, effects in both left and right IFG and pSTS were found, but none in the anterior insula or HC. Yet, only in IFG was the effect lateralized to the left hemisphere. All effects were in the "movement" direction (i.e., +Movement > −Movement). Over and above

Example 19

(19) a. *Relative (+movement)*
    'azarti   *la-yalda* [Še-Rina pagŠa *t* ba-gina]
    helped-I to-**the-girl** that-Rina met *t* in-the-garden
    "I helped the girl that Rina met in the garden"
  b. *Embedded complement (–movement)*
    'amarti le-Rina [Še-ha-yalda yaŠna ba-gina]
    told-I to-Rina that-the-girl slept in-the-garden
    "I told Rina that the girl slept in the garden"

Example 20

(20) a. *Declarative (−movement)*
    Dani natan 'et   ha-sefer ha-'adom la-professor   me-Oxford
    Dani gave ACC. the-book the-red   to-the-professor from-Oxford
    "Danny gave the red book to the professor from Oxford"
  b. *Topicalized (+movement)*
    'et ha-sefer ha-'adom Dani natan *t* la-professor   me-Oxford
    ACC. the-book the-red   Dani gave *t* to-the-professor from-Oxford
    "To the professor from Oxford, Danny gave the red book"

Example 21

(21) a. *Wh-questions (+movement)*
    (i) ha-meltzar sha'al *'eyze tayar t* hizmin avocado ba-boker (**subject question**)
      The waiter asked **which tourist** *t* ordered avocado in the morning
    (ii) ha-meltzar sha'al *'eyze salat* ha-tayar ha-shamen hizmin *t* ba-boker (**object question**)
      The waiter asked **which salad** the fat tourist   ordered *t* in the morning
  b. *Yes/no questions (−movement)*
    ha-meltzar sha'al 'im ha-tayar   hizmin salat avocado ba-boker
    The waiter asked if the tourist ordered avocado salad in the morning

any potential "complexity" effects, a movement effect is thus recorded in Broca's region, thereby providing direct imaging evidence that converges on the lesion data.

Topicalization and Questions

Encouraged by this finding, as well as by results obtained for the contrast between subject and object cleft sentences in English (Caplan et al., 2000), Ben-Shachar and colleagues proceeded to lead the fMRI investigation into other movement contrasts, to test the TDH-based claim that Broca's area is the central locus for movement in general (Ben-Shachar et al., 2004). The next experiment featured two new ±Movement contrasts in Hebrew: declarative versus topicalized sentences (example 20) and embedded questions with and without movement (example 21).

Syntactically, the contrast falls under the same syntactic generalization as the first study (i.e., syntactic movement), although sentence materials are different. The task was modified, to see whether the movement effect holds not only across constructions, but also across tasks (as was done in the lesion studies). Rather than judge grammaticality, subjects now listened for comprehension (and answered interleaved yes/no questions to ensure that they were attending).

ROIs were defined anatomically and functionally (roughly, on the basis of an "all sentences—silence" localizer, and a volume criterion [>300 contiguous voxels]). At the groups level, a movement effect for both contrasts in examples 20 and 21 was found in LIFG. The functional definition also revealed activations in (roughly) Wernicke's regions in both hemispheres. Another region (the ventral portion of the precentral sulcus) was activated as well (see Meyer et al.,

2000, for discussion). All effects were in the "movement" direction (i.e., +Movement >> −Movement).

When the results of individual subjects for the two contrasts are examined, they reveal a similar activation pattern for examples 20 and 21. While no numerical analysis of the degree of overlap between the contrasts has thus far been carried out (although it is currently in preparation by Drai and colleagues), visual inspection is rather suggestive, which indicates that movement is a syntactic operation whose strong link to Broca's region had wide reflections not only in disease but also in health.

German Scrambling Contrasts

To the picture that has emerged, one might add another intriguing finding, also related to the lesion-based results: fMRI results from German scrambling contrasts converge on the above data. While this contrast produces chance performance in Broca's aphasia in many languages, an fMRI experiment in healthy adults (Röder et al., 2001) yielded convergent results. It tested several types of sentences containing double-object verbs. The idea was to see whether contrasts between different orderings of the subject, direct object, and indirect object would activate the language areas. Röder and colleagues used the well-known verb-second property of German to create uninterrupted sequences of these three NPs in different orders (example 22).

In German, when there is a combination between an auxiliary (*wird*) and a main verb (*beschreiben*), the former is inflected and occupies the second position (here, second to the adverbial *jetzt*), while the latter remains uninflected in sentence-final position. This allows for a sequence of three NPs (*der Astronaut, dem Forscher, den Mond*), which can be reordered by a scrambling rule that can scramble one or two objects out of the VP and over the subject. Thus, example 22b is derived from example 22a by scrambling an object (*dem Forscher*) across the subject, while meaning

remains unchanged. The contrasts reported by Röder and colleagues provide a coherent (if partial) picture: When −scrambling (example 22a) sentences are subtracted from +scrambling (example 22b), activation is detected in the same areas for which we found activations in the Hebrew fMRI experiments, that is, mostly in LIFG, with some bilateral temporal activation (similar results are reported by Fiebach et al., 2001).

These findings provide an important imaging angle on the receptive role of LIFG but also on the nature of scrambling. Convergent on the lesion data, Broca's area is activated by contrasts between scrambled and nonscrambled simple active declarative sentences (for an indication that well-formed German sentences without movement are *not* computed in Broca's area see Friederici et al., 2003). Neurologically, the centrality of Broca's region in movement is thus repeatedly demonstrated for a variety of sentence types in different languages. Linguistically, these data show that scrambling is a species of syntactic movement, as the two align in both diseased and healthy brains.

SYNTAX IN THE RIGHT HEMISPHERE

Reflexive Binding in the Left IFG and the Right SFG

A movement impairment in Broca's aphasia and movement-related activity in the corresponding brain region in health are only a first hint. It is still possible that this brain region handles not just movement but in fact all intrasentential dependency relations. There is evidence that generic working memory resources are housed in the same locus (Smith and Jonides, 1999). Thus our findings could result from the fact that movement is a dependency relation that holds among two potentially nonadjacent positions in a sequence. Linking such positions requires some

Example 22

(22) a. −*Scrambling*
Jetzt wird der Astronaut   dem Forscher den Mond beschreiben
Now will the astronaut [to] the scientist the moon describe
"The astronaut will now describe the moon to the scientist"
b. +*Scrambling*
Jetzt wird **dem Forscher** der Astronaut *t* **den Mond** beschreiben

kind of a temporary store, which makes this working memory a prime candidate explanation to the observations made in both health and disease.

To examine this possibility, one might test intrasentential dependency relations that hold among nonadjacent constituents (and hence need working memory support) but are not governed by syntactic movement. The first test that comes to mind involves the binding theory, governing the relationship between referentially dependent elements (pronouns and reflexives) and the expressions on which they depend (antecedents). Preliminary clues suggested that Broca's aphasics are capable of handling intrasentential dependency relations when these pertain to the binding relation between reflexives, pronouns, and their antecedents (Blumstein et al., 1983; Grodzinsky et al., 1993).[8] Contrasting the two types of dependency relations directly—in both disease and health—might help us distinguish the two theoretical possibilities.

To this end, we conducted a lesion-based grammaticality judgment experiment that tested movement and reflexive binding (Grodzinsky, 2000c; Grodzinsky and Santi, 2004). Patients' were asked to detect agreement violations in sentences that pitted reflexive binding against movement (example 23). Every case involved a dependency relation between a reflexive and an antecedent in sentences with two NPs as potential antecedents that differed in gender. Each sentence contained a sequence of the form ⟨NP1, NP2, reflexive⟩, where gender$_{NP1}$ ≠ gender$_{NP2}$. In the grammatical sentences, the antecedent was either local (examples 23 and 24a) or moved (examples 23 and 24c); in the ungrammatical sentences, the gender of the reflexive was changed, so that it did not match the proper antecedent and matched an NP that could not function as its antecedent (examples 23, 24b, and 24d). The necessary knowledge is (a) condition A of the binding theory that essentially says that a reflexive must have a local antecedent and (b) that movement leaves a trace that may serve as a local antecedent. After some training with the task, subjects were asked to decide whether the reflexive matched NP1 or NP2. The sentences divide along the ±Movement, ±Grammatical dimensions.

(23) a. The woman believes the man likes **himself** —M,+G

b. *The woman believes the man likes **herself** —M, —G

c. **Which man** does The woman believe *t* likes **himself** +M, +G

d. ***Which man** does The woman believe *t* likes **herself** +M, —G

(24) a. It seems to Sally that the father rewards **himself** —M,+G

b. *It seems to Sally that the father rewards **herself** +M, —G

c. **The father** seems to Sally *t* to reward **himself** +M, +G

d. ***The father** seems to Sally *t* to reward **herself** +M, —G

We tested Broca's-, Wernicke's-, and right hemisphere–lesioned patients and carried out between- and within-group comparisons. The performance of the right hemisphere patients was near ceiling on all conditions. The performances of Broca's and Wernicke's patients were not distinguishable on the basis of this test. For both groups, the performance on movement conditions was lower than on the reflexive conditions (which were all above chance level).While these results are suggestive, they are somewhat weak.

The quest for converging evidence from the intact brain led us to adapt this test for fMRI in healthy adults who were asked to judge the grammaticality of sequences as in example 25, in order to tease apart neural responses to movement and to binding (Grodzinsky and Santi, 2004). The basic logic was the same as above.

As before, special care was taken to ensure that the subjects who participated in the experiment understood the fine nature of the task (all subjects were right-handed monolingual English-speaking linguists or students of linguistics). Only data from the grammatical sentences were analyzed. The effects we got were stronger than most: We were able to construct a GLM-based statistical map (that is, one that makes no *a priori* selection of brain ROIs), which revealed a significant reflexive effect ($P < 0.005$, uncorrected for multiple comparisons). That is, when conditions con-

Example 25

(25) a. [$_{NP1}$**Which man**] does [$_{NP2}$The woman] believe *t* likes **himself/*herself**

b. [$_{NP1}$The woman] believes [$_{NP2}$the man] likes **himself/*herself**

c. [$_{NP1}$**Which man**] does [$_{NP2}$The woman] believe *t* likes/*slept Mary

d. [$_{NP1}$The woman] believes [$_{NP2}$the man] likes/*slept Mary

taining reflexives were compared with the rest, activations were detected in the right superofrontal gyrus (a frontal region above Broca's and in front of the ventral portion of the precentral sulcus). No movement effect was detected in this region. In the left hemisphere, three effects were detected (also at $P < 0.005$, uncorrected): In LIFG, we detected both a movement and a reflexive effect; a movement effect was also detected in the left inferior posterior central sulcus.

An ROI approach delineated an ROI functionally, through the use of a fairly standard "all sentences—silence" localizer, and captured a contiguous area that spanned over the posterior part of Broca's region (BA 44), as well as the ventral portion of the precentral sulcus. An analysis of variance revealed a significant difference between the movement and reflexive conditions (movement > reflexive).

We thus have two results: First, reflexives, but not movement, activated the right SFG. Second, an ROI analysis revealed a mail effect of movement.

The results obtained thus far are not clear cut and are open to a variety of criticisms. An improved version of this test, designed by Andrea Santi, is currently under way. It parameterizes the distance between the reflexive, the trace, and their antecedents, to control for potential distance effects. The overall picture suggests a limited role for Broca's region in the processing of dependencies other than movement.

Dative Shift in the Left Anterior Insula and the Right Ventral Portion of the Precentral Sulcus

Preliminary evidence is now available about an additional syntactic dependency relation—dative shift.

This is a regular relation (studied extensively; see, e.g., Aoun and Li, 1989; Beck & Johnson, 2004; Larson, 1988) that holds among two orderings of objects in sentences containing triadic predicates, hence two objects ($O1$, $O2$), such as *give, send, mail* (example 26).

The change in the relative order suggests a movement relation (note that the annotation of objects as $O1$, $O2$ and the exclusion of the preposition *to* are just for expository purposes). Indeed, two recurrent questions have concerned linguists:

(*I*) What type of movement (if any) is involved?
(*II*) If there is movement, which complement order is base generated and which is derived? Is it $O1$ $O2$ or vice versa?

A neuroimaging perspective on these questions was recently attempted by Ben-Shachar and Grodzinsky (2002). We tried to see whether it is possible to use the location and intensity of the fMRI signal as a tool for the examination of these questions. To this end, we conducted a comprehension test of Hebrew double objects, aimed to get an imaging perspective on the linguistic analysis of this construction. While Hebrew is somewhat different from English, linguistic tests suggest that its dative (example 27a) is like its English counterpart (example 26a); likewise, Hebrew example 27b is comparable to example 26b.

We embedded these materials in the above topicalization experiment: Sentences like examples 26a and 26b were mixed with their topicalized and untopicalized counterparts (examples 27a and 27b).

Question (*I*) can be resolved when the activation pattern of the dative contrast is compared to that of the topicalization contrast. That is, an activation-by-

Example 26

(26) a. *Dative*
    Danny gave/sent/mailed [$_{O1}$ a book] to [$_{O2}$ Donna]
  b. *Double Object*
    Danny gave/sent/mailed [$_{O2}$ Donna] [$_{O1}$ a book]

Example 27

(27) *Dative Shift*
    a. Dative: Dani natan 'et   [$_{O1}$ ha-sefer ha-'adom] la-[$_{O2}$ professor me-Oxford]
       Dani gave ACC.   the-book the-red   to-the-professor from-Oxford
    b. Double Object: Dani natan [$_{O2}$ la-professor me-Oxford] 'et [$_{O1}$ ha-sefer ha-'adom]
       Dani gave to-the-prof. from-Ox.   ACC   the-book the-red

Example 28

(28) *Topicalization*
　　a. *'et　　ha-sefer　ha-'adom* Dani natan la-professor　　me-Oxford
　　　　ACC. the-book the-red　　Dani gave　to-the-professor from-Oxford
　　b. *la-professor me-Oxford* Dani natan 'et　　ha-sefer　ha-'adom
　　　　To-the-prof. from-Ox.　Dani gave　ACC. the-book the-red

region interaction between the dative-shift contrast (examples 27a and 27b) and the topicalization contrast (examples 28a and 28b) would imply that the two relations are computed in different regions and thus are neurologically distinct. Question (*II*) can be resolved when the relative intensity of the signal in examples 27a and 27b is compared. That is, the derived sentence should produce a stronger signal than the base configuration. Our study used two types of empirical argument: *the anatomical locus* of the fMRI signal as reflecting uniformity or distinctness of operations (topicalization versus dative shift), and *the relative intensity* of the fMRI signal within an anatomical region as reflecting more mental computation (double object versus dative).

We obtained two results: First, regarding question *I*, our results indicated a spatial pattern quite different for dative shift compared with the topicalization contrast. Specifically, the comparison between examples 27a and 27b activated two frontal regions in the right cerebral hemisphere and none of the topicalization-related regions 28a versus 28b, which like other movement contrasts activated Broca's area on the left and Wernicke's area bilaterally. This difference suggests that a different type of operation is involved.

Second, regarding question *II*, the intensity of the BOLD signal was measured in the two right frontal regions that are sensitive to the dative-shift contrast. The result for double objects (example 27b) was significantly higher than for datives (example 27a), suggesting that Hebrew double objects are more demanding than datives and providing an indication of their derived nature. Dative shift, then, is a distinct dependency relation that appears to be computed outside Broca's area. Finally, it is surprising, perhaps that the dative shift contrast activates anterior regions of the right hemisphere.

Dative shift and reflexive experiments activated different regions in the right hemisphere – the former in Superior Frontal Gyrus, the latter in vPCS and anterior Insula. This provides preliminary hints that syntax is not exclusively on the left side of the brain.

Wernicke's Area in Brief

It has been recurrently observed that Wernicke's area is engaged in similar activity—similar, but not identical. In aphasia studies of syntax, initial striking differences (e.g., Zurif, 1980) in functional role gave way to findings that indicated overlap. Some studies conducted over the years have found the performance of Wernicke's aphasics to hold great individual variation and present a blurry picture that is not quantitatively discernible from that of the Broca's aphasics (e.g., Grodzinsky and Finkel, 1998; Grodzinsky and Santi, 2004). At the same time, important syntactic differences between Broca's and Wernicke's aphasics have been demonstrated (Shapiro et al., 1993; Zurif, 2003; Zurif et al., 1993). While it is fairly clear that the role of these areas in syntax is not identical, providing a precise account that would tease apart their functions has turned out to be quite difficult.

In this respect, the empirical record obtained by fMRI is not that clear either: Some, but not all, experiments have detected activation not only in the left Wernicke's area but also on the right (Ben-Shachar et al., 2003, 2004; Friederici et al., 2003; Röder et al., 2001). The paucity of data and analyses at this point— from both lesion and imaging studies—precludes a more thorough assessment of the role of Wernicke's area, yet this clearly is a question that warrants careful attention and should be investigated.

A BLUEPRINT FOR A SYNTAX MAP

I hope the reader has become convinced that the beginnings of a brain map for syntax are starting to surface, as three seemingly distinct syntactic operations are supported by mechanisms in distinct brain areas— movement in Broca's (perhaps to an extent in Wernicke's) areas; dative shift in posterior portions of the right frontal lobe (vPCS, aINS); and reflexive-antecedent binding in an anterior part of the right frontal lobe (SFG). It is time now to come full circle and return to the STC:

Syntacto-Topic Conjecture (STC)

a. Major syntactic operations are neurologically individuated.
b. The organization of these operations in brain space is linguistically significant.

We have seen that the use of descriptive tools from linguistics is beneficial for brain mapping; we have also seen some evidence that suggests the brain honors fine syntactic distinctions in both aphasia and fMRI. In aphasia research, this is not new: correspondence between neurological and syntactic natural classes has been found several times in the past 60 years, since Jakobson (1941) first hinted at the possibility (Avrutin, 2001; Friedmann and Grodzinsky, 1997; Goodglass and Hunt, 1958; Grodzinsky et al., 1991, 1993).

The STC seeks to go beyond these results and to determine whether the manner by which syntax is organized in the brain is theoretically meaningful. There is a large set of related questions: Is the arrangement of syntactic components in the brain haphazard or orderly? Is the representation of language similar for all humans, whose experiences vis-à-vis language are so diverse? Why would the cerebral arrangement of grammatical abilities be in different places in the brain? Is there, in other words, any significance to the spatial arrangement of the neural patches that support certain central syntactic computations? And if so, what are the relevant parameters, and how can they be studied?

Looking at adjacent domains might actually help. Since the sensorimotor homunculi discovered by Penfield and Rasmussen (1950), much neurophysiological work—in vision, audition, and the sensorimotor domain—has charted the spatial arrangement of functional systems in the brain. Thus, somatotopy in sensory and motor cortex has long been investigated (e.g., Beisteiner et al., 2004), as has retinotopy in visual cortex (e.g., Tootel et al., 1997) and tonotopy in auditory cortex (e.g., Pantev et al., 1989; Zhang et al., 2001). Diesch et al. (1996) even attempted (not very successfully) to detect for the spatial organization of vowels.

Moreover, some have gone beyond mere functional localization and tried to harness the anatomy to the quest of constitutive principles. To this end, efforts have been made to see whether the topological arrangement of neural systems that support behavior is theoretically meaningful or arbitrary. One salient example comes from vision, where there have been recent attempts to identify overarching principles that govern the organization of cortical maps for vision. Take visual maps, for example. For a while it has been known that these are composed of receptive fields, each having separate maps for orientation, spatial frequency, direction of motion, color, ocular dominance, and perhaps more (see Swindale, 1996, for a review). Yet is the topographic organization of these maps within a receptive field accidental, or does it have some meaning? Moreover, is there any significance to the manner by which the various functions are laid on the receptive fields and superimposed on one another?

Until very recently, no definitive answer could be given to this type of question, although it has long occupied the minds of vision scientists. The advent of optical and magnetic resonance imaging methods has led to several discoveries regarding the spatial geometry of visual functions. Thus, it was found that orientation columns, that mark orientation preference of cells, are organized in cycles around orientation centers, known as singularities, or "pinwheels" (Bonhoeffer and Grinvald, 1991); it was also found that some of these systems are superimposed on one another in geometrically regular ways (Huebener et al., 1997). While the reason for this type of arrangement is not immediately clear, its regularity is quite striking and calls for an explanation. Indeed, there have been attempts to discover general organizing principles for the visual system through the study of the neural geometry of its subsystems (see Swindale et al., 2000, for a formalization and an empirical test of general principles proposed by Hubel and Wiesel, 1977).

Given the findings just presented, it seems reasonable to explore whether such an arrangement exists in the language domain. Why would syntactic abilities be localized in the first place, and if so, why would certain parts be in the left hemisphere and others in the right? We are coming to a point when such questions can actually be formulated. In particular, I think that the following questions can now begin to be asked:

1. Can specific rule systems be characterized by the volume of tissue involved in their implementation? More concretely, when we compare the volume of tissue in Broca's region ac-

tivated during the computation of movement to that activated on the right SFG during binding, can the result have implications to the relation between movement and binding?

2. Does spatial arrangement matter? Do relative proximity and hemisphericity of specific grammatical components have theoretical significance? What are we to make of the fact that dative shift and binding are anatomically adjacent?

3. Does signal intensity matter? Why do certain syntactic contrasts produce stronger signals than others?

4. How much individual variation is there for each principle, and is there a cerebral reflection of parametric variation observed in grammatical systems?

5. Are there more abstract spatial relations couched within the anatomy that are linguistically relevant?

It is, of course, possible that the emerging topological arrangement of syntactic principles is arbitrary and that nothing can be learned from a syntax map, which would be meaningless, its geometry being of no consequence.

Yet if the preliminary clues I presented above are a lead, then the biology is actually telling us something important: That an attempt to make sense of those vague patches we see in those images is a key to a future understanding of the language faculty. And while it is difficult to predict how far we can get, to my mind this is an opportunity that should not be missed.

ACKNOWLEDGMENTS   This work was supported by Canada Research Chairs, Canada Foundation for Innovation, and a McGill VP-research grant. This author thanks Dan Drai, Lew Shapiro, and especially Na'ama Friedmann and Andrea Santi for their helpful comments.

Notes

1. Space limitations led me to focus on core data from aphasia and fMRI. Many important results were unfortunately omitted (e.g., Hickok and Avrutin, 1995, Thompson et al., 1999); also absent is discussion of other experimental techniques (e.g., ERP—Friederici et al., 1996; Hahne and Friederici, 1999; Neville et al., 1991). Future work will hopefully incorporate these into the discussion.

2. *P3* refers to a semantic role, rather than a ϑ-role because this requirement may be met outside the language faculty. That is, it may be that the forced assignment (unconscious as it is) takes place once the thematically deficient representation is matched against the task. As ϑ-role is a designated term for a syntactically sensitive semantic role, I worded P3 thus. Yet, the reader will see below that I label the semantic roles assigned by extragrammar as ϑ_i. This is done for simplicity.

3. Premise (P3) is formulated over referential elements because it is formulated in the context of forced-choice interpretive experiments, where every NP corresponds to character, and where the subject's task is to either establish or to check the match between characters and NPs. In the context of experiments that do not necessarily require interpretation, i.e., certain judgment tests (see below), *P3* does not apply.

4. One important piece of data that remains a mystery is the performance of Japanese- and Korean-speaking Broca's aphasics on passive. These are SOV languages, and unless a reason is given, their passive construction is analyzed as the German and Dutch ones. And yet, contrary to Dutch/German, Korean and Japanese patients perform at chance. While properties of passive may differ cross-linguistically, I am currently unaware of a way to capture this fact. One possible direction to explore may capitalize on the fact that in Korean/Japanese, passive sentences contain no auxiliary verb, only a passive morpheme, while Dutch/German require an auxiliary verb, just like English.

5. The characterization of these results here differs from Luzzatti et al.'s. The reason is a somewhat different approach I took to their data. Three of their 11 Broca's aphasics were at ceiling on all conditions, as can be seen from the raw individual subject results that the paper provides. As we are looking for pathological patterns, the inclusion of these normally performing patients in the sample mitigates the results. The results as described in the text reflect the statistical analysis on Luzatti et al.'s data, carried out through an ANOVA and a series of t-tests after these three patients were excluded from the sample.

6. Luzzatti et al.'s experiment had another level, using subject pronouns instead of name. Our ANOVA detected no subject pronoun effect, hence this aspect of the study—that is orthogonal to present purposes—is ignored here.

7. This might be true to an extent, yet as complexity—even if made precise—is at best a property of constructions, it is not clear how to formulate a mechanism that handles it. More importantly, it is not clear how this putative role of Broca's region is related to its role in syntactic movement, as evidenced in aphasia.

8. I am ignoring for the moment certain deficiencies in the way the patients treat pronouns, as these may not follow from sentence level. See Grodzinsky et al., 1993; Avrutin, this volume, Chapter 4.

References

Amunts, K., Schleicher, A., Bürgel, U., Mohlberg, H., Uylings, H., & Zilles, K. (1999). Broca's region revisited: Cytoarchitecture and intersubject variability. *Journal of Comparative Neuroogy*, 412, 319–341.

Aoun, J., & Li, A. (1989). Scope and constituency. *Linguistic Inquiry* 20, 141–172.

Hickok, G., & Avrutin, S. (1995). Representation, referentiality, and processing in agrammatic comprehension: Two case studies. *Brain and Language*, 50, 10–26.

Avrutin, S. (2000). Comprehension of Wh-questions by children and Broca's aphasics. In Y. Grodzinsky, L.P. Shapiro, & D.A. Swinney (Eds.), *Language and the brain: Representation and processing* (pp. 295–312). Academic Press, San Diego.

Avrutin, S. (2001). Linguistics and agrammatism. *Glot International*, 5.3, 1–5.

Baker, M., Johnson, K., & Roberts, I. (1989). Passive arguments raised. *Linguistic Inquiry* 20, 219–251.

Basso, A. (2003). *Aphasia and its therapy*. New York: Oxford University Press.

Beck, S., & Johnson, K. (2004). Double objects again. *Linguistic Inquiry*, 35, 97–123.

Beisteiner, R., Gartus, A., Erdler, M., Mayer, D., Lanzenberger, R., & Deecke, L. (2004). Magnetoencephalography indicates finger motor somatotopy. *European Journal of Neuroscience* 19, 465–472.

Ben-Shachar, M., Hendler, T., Kahn, I., Ben-Bashat, D., & Grodzinsky, Y. (2003). The neural reality of syntactic transformations: Evidence from fMRI. *Psychological Science*, 14.5, 433–440.

Ben Shachar, M., & Grodzinsky, Y. (2002). On the derivation of Hebrew double objects—a functional imaging investigation. Paper presented at NELS 33, MIT.

Ben-Shachar, M., Palti, D., & Grodzinsky, Y. (2004). Neural correlates of syntactic movement: Converging evidence from two fMRI experiments. *NeuroImage*, 21, 1320–1336.

Beretta, A., Schmitt, C., Halliwell, J., Munn, A., Cuetos, F., and Kim, S. (2001). The effects of scrambling on Spanish and Korean agrammatic interpretation: why linear models fail and structural models survive. *Brain and Language*, 79, 407–425.

Bever, T. (1970). The cognitive basis of linguistic structures. In J.R. Hayes (Ed.), *Cognition and the development of language*. New York: Wiley.

Binkofski, F., Amunts, K., Stephan, K.M., Posse, S., Schormann, T., Freund, H.-J., Zilles, K., & Seitz, R. (2000). Broca's region subserves imagery of motion: A combined cytoarchitectonic and fMRI study. *Human Brain Mapping*, 11, 273–285.

Blumstein, S. (1973). *Phonological investigations of aphasia*. The Hague: Mouton.

Blumstein, S. (1998). Phonological aspects of aphasia. In M. Sarno (Ed.), *Acquired aphasia* (pp. 157–185). New York: Academic Press.

Blumstein, S., Goodglass, H., Statlender, S., & Biber, C. (1983). Comprehension strategies determining reference in aphasia: A study of reflexivization. *Brain & Language*, 18, 115–127.

Bobaljik. J. (2002). A-chains at the PF-interface: Copies and 'covert' movement. *Natural Language and Linguistic Theory*, 20, 197–267.

Bonhoeffer, T., & Grinvald, A. (1991). Iso-orientation domains in cat visual cortex are arranged in pinwheel-like patterns. *Nature* 353, 429–431.

Burchert, F., de Bleser, R., & Sonntag, K. (2001). Does case make the difference? *Cortex* 37, 700–703.

Caplan, D. (2001). Functional neuroimaging studies of syntactic processing. *Journal of Psycholinguistic Research* 30, 297–320.

Caplan, D., Vijayan, S., Kuperberg, G., West, C., Waters, G., Greve, D., & Anders, D. (2002). Vascular responses to syntactic processing: Event-related fMRI study of relative clauses. *Human Brain Mapping* 15, 26–38.

Caplan, D., & Waters, G. (1999). Verbal working memory and sentence comprehension. *Behavioral and Brain Sciences*, 22, 77–126.

Chomsky, N. (1995). *The minimalist program*. Cambridge, MA: MIT Press.

Dapretto, M., & Bookheimer, S. (1999). Form and content: Dissociating syntax and semantics in sentence comprehension. *Neuron*, 24, 427–432.

Dickey, M.W., & Thompson, C. (2004). The resolution and recovery of filler-gap dependencies in aphasia: Evidence from on-line anomaly detection. *Brain and Language*, 88, 108–127.

Diesch, E., Eulitz, C., Hampson, S., & Ross, B. (1996). The neurotopography of vowels as mirrored by evoked magnetic field measurements. *Brain & Language*, 53, 143–168.

Drai, D., & Grodzinsky, Y. (2006). Stability of functional role in Broca's region: Quantitative neurosyntactic analysis of a large data set from Aphasia. *Brain & Language*, 76.

Fiebach, C., Schlesewsky, M., & Friederici, A. (2001). An ERP investigation of syntactic working memory during the processing of German wh-questions. *Journal of Memory and Language*.

Fox, D. (2002). Antecedent contained deletion and the copy theory of movement. *Linguistic Inquiry, 33*, 63–96.

Fox, D., & Pesetsky, D. (in press). Cyclic Linearization of Syntactic Structure. *Theoretical Linguistics*, special issue on Object Shift in Scandinavian; K.É. Kiss (Ed).

Friederici, A., & Frazier, L. (1992). Thematic analysis in agrammatic comprehension: Syntactic structures and task demands. *Brain and Language, 42*, 1–29.

Friederici, A., & Graetz, P. (1987). Processing passive sentences in aphasia: Deficits and strategies. *Brain and Language, 30*, 93–105.

Friederici, A., Hahne, A., & Mecklinger, A. (1996). The temporal structure of syntactic parsing: Early and late event-related brain potential effects elicited by syntactic anomalies. *Journal of Experimental Psychology: Learning, Memory, and Cognition, 22*, 1219–1248.

Friederici, A., Rueschemeyer, S.-A., Hahne, A., & Fiebach, C. (2003). The role of left inferior frontal and superior temporal cortex in sentence comprehension: Localizing syntactic and semantic processes. *Cerebral Cortex, 13*, 170–177.

Friedmann, N., & Grodzinsky, Y. (1997). Tense and agreement in agrammatic production: Pruning the syntactic tree. *Brain & language, 56*, 397–425.

Friedmann, N., & Gvion, A. (2003). Sentence comprehension and working memory limitation in aphasia: A dissociation between semantic-syntactic and phonological reactivation. *Brain & language, 86*, 23–39.

Friedmann, N., & Shapiro, L. (2003). Agrammatic comprehension of simple active sentences with moved constituents: Hebrew OSV and OVS structures. *Journal of Speech and Hearing Research, 46*, 288–297.

Fujita, I., Miyake, T., Takahashi, Y., Sakai, K., & Akitake, M. (1977). Shi tsugoshyoosha no koobunn no rikai [syntactic recognition in aphasics]. *Onse Gengo Igaku* [The Japan Journal of Logopedics and Phoniatrics], *18*, 6–13.

Gabrieli, J., Poldrack, R., & Desmond, J. (1998). The role of left prefrontal cortex in langauge and memory. *Proceedings of the National Academy of Sciences USA, 95*, 906–913.

Geschwind, N. (1979). Specializations of the human brain. *Scientific American*, September.

Goodglass, H., Fodor, I., & Schulhoff, C. (1967). Prosodic factors in grammar—evidence from aphasia. *Journal of Speech and Hearing Research, 10*, 5–20.

Goodglass, H., and Hunt, J. (1958). Grammatical complexity and aphasic speech. *Word, 14*, 197–207.

Grodzinsky, Y. (1984). *Language deficits and linguistic theory*. Doctoral dissertation, Brandeis University.

Grodzinsky, Y. (1986). Language deficits and the theory of syntax. *Brain & Language, 27*, 135–159.

Grodzinsky, Y. (1990). *Theoretical perspectives on language deficits*. Cambridge, MA: MIT Press.

Grodzinsky, Y. (2000a). The neurology of syntax: Language use without Broca's area. *Behavioral and Brain Sciences, 23.1*, 1–71.

Grodzinsky, Y. (2000b). *Syntactic dependencies as memorized sequences in the brain*. A paper presented at the TENNET XI annual conference on theoretical and experimental neuropsychology, Montreal, Canada. Available at http://freud.tau.ac.il/~yosef1.

Grodzinsky, Y. (2002). Neurolinguistics and neuroimaging: Forward to the future, or is it back? *Psychological Science, 13*, 189–193.

Grodzinsky, Y. (2004). Variation in Broca's region: Preliminary cross-methodological comparisons. In Lyle Jenkins (Ed.), *Variation and universals in biolinguistics*. Oxford: Elsevier.

Grodzinsky, Y., & Finkel, L. (1998). The neurology of empty categories. *Journal of Cognitive Neuroscience, 10.2*, 281–292.

Grodzinsky, Y., Pierce, A., & Marakovitz, S. (1991). Neuropsychological reasons for a transformational analysis of verbal passive. *Natural Language & Linguistic Theory, 9*, 431–453.

Grodzinsky, Y., & Santi, A. (2004). An fMRI investigation into reflexive binding vs. movement. Cognitive Neuroscience Society, April, San Francisco.

Grodzinsky, Y., Wexler, K., Chien, Y.-C., Marakovitz, S., & Solomon, J. (1993). The breakdown of binding relations. *Brain & Language, 45*, 396–422.

Hagiwara, H., & Caplan, D. (1990). Syntactic comprehension in Japanese aphasics: Effects of category and thematic role order. *Brain & language, 38*, 159–170.

Hahne, A., & Friederici, A. (1999). Electrophysiological evidence for two steps in syntactic analysis: Early automatic and late controlled processes. *Journal of Cognitive Neuroscience, 11*, 194–205.

Hickok, G., & Avrutin, S. (1995). Comprehension of Wh-questions by two agrammatic Broca's aphasics. *Brain & Language, 51*, 10–26.

Hubel, D., & Wiesel, T. (1977). Functional architecture of macaque monkey visual cortex. *Proceedings of the Royal Society, London, B 198*, 1–59.

Huebener, M., Shoham, D., Grinvald, A., and Bonhoeffer, T. (1997). Spatial relationships among three columnar systems in cat area 17. *Journal of Neuroscience, 17*, 270–9284.

Hughlings-Jackson, J. (1878/1932). *Selected writings of John Hughlings Jackson* (2 Vols.). Edited by J. Taylor. London: Hodder and Stoughton.

Jezzard, P., Matthews, P.M., and Smith, S.M. (Eds.) (2001). *Functional MRI: An introduction to method.* Oxford: Oxford University Press.

Kluender, R., & Kutas, M. (1993). Bridging the gap: Evidence from ERPs on the processing of unbounded dependencies. *Journal of Cognitive Neuroscience, 5,* 196–214.

Kolk, H., and van Grunsven, M. (1985). Agrammatism as a variable phenomenon. *Cognitive Neuropsychology, 2,* 347–384.

Larson, R. (1988). On the double object construction. *Linguistic Inquiry, 19,* 335–391.

Law, S.-P. (2000). Structural prominence hypothesis and Chinese aphasic sentence comprehension. *Brain and Language, 74,* 260–268.

Lichtheim, L. (1885). Über Aphasie. *Deutsches Archiv für klinische Medicin, Leipzig, 36,* 204–268. [Engl.: On Aphasia, *Brain, 7,* 433–484].

Lima, R., & Novaes, C. (2000). Grammaticality judgments by agrammatic aphasics: Data from Brazilian-Portuguese. *Brain and Language, 74,* 515–551.

Love, T., & Swinney, D. (1996). Coreference processing and levels of analysis in object relative constructions; Demonstration of antecedent reactivation with the cross modal paradigm. *Journal of Psycholinguistic Research, 25,* 5–24.

Luzzatti, C., Toraldo, A., Guasti, M.T., Ghirardi, G., Lorenzi, L., & Guarnaschelli, C. (2001). Comprehension of reversible active and passive sentences in agrammatism. *Aphasiology, 15,* 419–441.

Matelli, M., Luppino, G., & Rizzolatti, G. (1991). Architecture of superior and mesial area 6 and the adjacent cingulate cortex in the macaque monkey. *Journal of Comparative Neurology, 311,* 445–462.

Meyer, M., Friederici, A.D., von Cramon, D.Y. (2000). Neurocognition of auditory sentence comprehension: Event related fMRI reveals sensitivity to syntactic violations and task demands. *Cognitive Brain Research, 9,* 19–33.

Mikelič, S., Boskovic, Z., Crain, S., & Shankweiler, D. (1995). Comprehension of nonlexical categories in agrammatism. *Journal of Psycholinguistic Research, 24,* 299–311.

Mohr, J.P. (1978). Broca's area and Broca's aphasia. In H. Whitaker (Ed.) *Studies in neurolinguistics* (Vol II, pp. 201–235). San Diego: Academic Press.

Neville, H., Nicol, J., Barss, A., Forster, K., & Garrett, M. (1991). Syntactically based sentence processing classes: Evidence from event-related potentials. *Journal of Cognitive Neuroscience, 3,* 151–165.

Pantev, C., Hoke, M., Lütkenhöner, B., & Lehnertz, K. (1989). Tonotopic organization of the auditory cortex: Pitch versus frequency representation. *Science, 246,* 486–488.

Paulesu, E., Frith, C., & Frackowiak, R. (1993). The neural correlates of the verbal component of working memory. *Nature, 362,* 342–345.

Penfield, W., & Rasmussen, T. (1950). *The cerebral cortex of man.* A *clinical study of localization of function.* New York: Macmillan.

Röder, B., Stock, O., Neville, H., Bien, S., & Rösler, F. (2001). Brain activation modulated by the comprehension of normal and pseudo-word sentences of different processing demands: A functional magnetic resonance imaging study. *NeuroImage, 15,* 1003–1014.

Schuell, H., & Sefer, J.W. (1973). *Differential diagnosis of aphasia with the Minnesota test.* Minneapolis: University of Minnesota Press.

Schwartz, M., Linebarger, M., Saffran, E., & Pate, D. (1987). Syntactic transparency and sentence interpretation in aphasia. *Language and Cognitive Processes, 2,* 85–113.

Shapiro, L.P., Gordon, B., Hack, N., & Killackey, J. (1993). Verb-argument structure processing in complex sentences in Broca's and Wernicke's aphasia. *Brain & Language 45.3,* 423–447.

Su, Y.-C. (2000). Asyntactic thematic role assignment: Implications from Chinese aphasics. Paper presented at the LSA Meeting, Chicago.

Smith, E., & Jonides, J. (1999). Storage and executive processes in the frontal lobes. *Science, 283,* 1657–1661.

Sportiche, D. (1995). Clitic constructions. In R. Johan & L. Zaring (Eds.), *Phrase structure and the lexicon.* Bloomington, IN: IUCL Press.

Swindale, N. (1998). Modules, polymaps and mosaics. *Current Biology, 8,* R270–R273.

Swindale, N., Shoham, D., Grinvald, A., Bonhoeffer, T., & Hübener, M. (2000). Visual cortex maps are optimized for uniform coverage. *Nature Neuroscience 3,* 822–826.

Thompson, C.K., Tait, M.E., Ballard, K.J., & Fix, S.C. (1999). Agrammatic aphasic subjects' comprehension of subject and object extracted Wh-questions. *Brain and Language, 67,* 169–187.

Tomaiuolo, F., MacDonald, J.D., Caramanos, Z., Posner, G., Chiavaras, M., Evans, A.C., & Petrides, M. (1999). Morphology, morphometry and probability mapping of the pars opercularis of the inferior frontal gyrus: an *in vivo* MRI analysis. *European Journal of Neuroscience, 11,* 3033–3046.

Tootel, R., Mendola, J.D., Hadjikhani, N.K., Ledden, P.J., Liu, A.K., Reppas, J.B., et al. (1997). Functional analysis of V3A and related areas in human visual cortex. *The Journal of Neuroscience*, *17*, 7060–7078.

Vandenberghe, R., Nobre, A.C., & Price, C.J. (2002). The response of left temporal cortex to sentences. *Journal of Cognitive Neuroscience 14*, 550–560.

Wernicke, C. (1874). *Der Aphasische Symptomenkompleks*. Breslau: M. Crohn und Weigert.

Wilson, S., & Saygın, A.P. (2004). Grammaticality judgment in aphasia: Deficits are not specific to syntactic structures, aphasic syndromes, or lesion sites. *Journal of Cognitive Neuroscience*, *16*, 238–252.

Worsley, K., Liao, C., Aston, J., Petre, V., Duncan, G.H., Morales, F., et al. (2002). A general statistical analysis for fMRI data. *NeuroImage*, *15*, 1–15.

Zhang, L., Bao, S., and Merzenich, M.M. (2001). Persistent and specific influences of early acoustic environments on primary auditory cortex. *Nature Neuroscience*, *4*, 1123–1130.

Zurif, E.B. (1980). Language mechanisms: A neuropsychological perspective. *American Scientist*, May.

Zurif, E.B. (1995). Brain regions of relevance to syntactic processing. In L. Gleitman & M. Liberman (Eds.), *An invitation to cognitive science* (2nd ed., Vol. I). Cambridge, MA: MIT Press.

Zurif, E.B. (2003). The neuroanatomical organization of some features of sentence comprehension: Studies of real-time syntactic and semantic composition. *Psychologica*, *32*, 13–24.

Zurif, E.B., & Caramazza, A. (1976). Linguistic structures in aphasia: Studies in syntax and semantics. In H. Whitaker and H.H. Whitaker (Eds), *Studies in neurolinguistics* (Vol. 2). New York: Academic Press.

Zurif, E.B., Swinney, D., Prather, P., Solomon, J., & Bushell, C. (1993). An on-line analysis of syntactic processing in Broca's and Wernicke's aphasia. *Brain and Language*, *45*, 448–464.

7

Evaluating Deficit Patterns of Broca Aphasics in the Presence of High Intersubject Variability

Dan Drai

A sensible strategy for studying the functional role of a brain area is to analyze the performance deficits of people affected by a lesion of that area. The hope, of course, is that the performances of the affected subjects will show a differential pattern. Ideally, some function will be isolated such that the performance of a task requiring it is abnormal for affected subjects, while the performance of those tasks not requiring it is normal. Broca's area is not an exception in this respect, and there is a rather large body of data on the linguistic performances of subjects with a lesion in Broca's area. A series of studies (all referenced in Drai and Grodzinsky, 2006) focus on a single aspect of aphasic performance: relative pattern of success and failure on comprehension of sentences of different structural types. The relevant data were gathered in sentence–to–picture matching tests in which sentences were constructed that could not be understood solely on the basis of the mapping between the meanings of single words and what is normally the case in the real world. That is, the comprehension tests used

semantically reversible sentences in which either of (at least) two nouns could logically fill the role of agent of the described action. A data point in such a study is simply a couple (number of trial sentences, number of successes in the comprehension task), and each study typically involves a few patients (i.e., 5 to 10 data points). Summarizing the data from theses studies, for each putative contrast between sentences, we are given two sets of performances of a relatively large number of subjects (30 to 60 data points, depending on the contrast) on the two different types of sentences, and we are to determine whether the performances on the two sets of sentences show a differential pattern.

An hypothesis about the existence of a computation for which Broca's area is indispensable would thus take the following form: identify two classes of sentences such that one involves the relevant computation and the other does not, then form a motivated prediction on the way a deficit in this computation should affect the performance of the Broca aphasics. The concluding step should be, of course, to evaluate the prediction in light of the empirical record of performances of Broca aphasics. This chapter is exclusively concerned with this last step. Indeed with respect to a specific hypothesis of the form just described, the trace-deletion hypothesis (TDH) (Grodzinsky 1986, 1990, 2000), there has been a longstanding controversy over the meaning of the empirical record, some claiming the record confirms the hypothesis (Grodzinsky et al., 1999; Grodzinsky, 2000) and others arguing that the variability of performances across patients precludes the drawing of any stable conclusion or even refutes the TDH (Berndt et al., 1996; Caramazza et al., 2000). The debate has been to some extent about the choice of patients to be included in the empirical database to be evaluated, but (and we believe crucially) the debate also stems from the lack of a precise quantitative methodology for analyzing group data of performances in the presence of high interindividual variability. Our aim in this chapter is to propose such a methodology. In particular, we shall look for a way of modeling the data that leaves room for sharp statistical claims, such as: "The performances of Broca aphasics on sentences of type A are significantly different from their performances on sentences of type B" while taking into account the high variability of the data. Accordingly, the plan of this chapter is as follows:

1. *Data collection.* We report on the principles that have guided the compilation of performance data to which we shall apply our methodology.
2. *TDH.* We briefly explain the TDH and its prediction concerning patterns of performance of Broca aphasics.
3. *Binomial view and its intuitive meaning.* We present a very simple stochastic model for the performances of a given subject and deduce a way of summarizing one individual's performance on a set of sentences.
4. *Variability.* We illustrate the high individual variability of performance data viewed through the above statistics.
5. *Framework for group analysis.* We present a model for evaluating group performances (the beta binomial).
6. *Results of group analysis.* We apply the described framework to the evaluation of the TDH, showing a contrast in accordance with the prediction of TDH.

7. *Was this tautological?* We present the results of our analysis on an alternative division of the stimulus sentences and show that it does not yield a contrast of performances.
8. *Conclusion.* TDH rephrased.

THE DATA COLLECTION

Scores were selected from the published literature by a sieve of five highly restrictive criteria. A patient's score was admitted into the database only if all of the following requirements were met[1]:

1. Positive diagnosis of Broca's aphasia is made with a well-established test[2] and sound neurological considerations (i.e., imaging when available, clinical workup otherwise).
2. Tests investigate comprehension at the sentence level, through a forced binary-choice task ('who did what to whom') with multiple 'semantically reversible' sentences, and with scenario pairs that depict thematic reversals <"*a* does X to *b*", "*b* does X to *a*">.
3. Detailed descriptions of experimental conditions and procedures are available.
4. Raw individual patient scores are available.
5. Identifying information is available (to avoid multiple counting of patients who participated in more than one study).

TRACE DELETION HYPOTHESIS (TDH)

The TDH is discussed in detail in (Grodzinsky, this volume, Chapter 6), and we shall keep the present discussion fairly abstract, referring the reader to Grodzinsky's chapter in this volume for theoretical flesh while we stick to the statistical bones.

From the present point of view, all that matters is that TDH entails the claim that there exists a certain feature of syntactical structure of sentences (called Movement) such that Broca aphasics have to *guess* thematic roles when processing sentences that possess this feature, whereas they can compute these roles in a more or less normal way for sentences that do not possess the feature (other things being equal of course, see Chapter 6 for experimental details). Movement is an abstract feature, and it can exist within many linguistic constructs; in Drai and Grodzinsky, 2006 the approach described in the present chapter was ap-

Movement

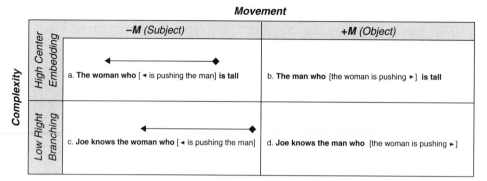

		−M (Subject)	**+M (Object)**
Complexity	**High Center Embedding**	a. **The woman who** [◄ is pushing the man] **is tall**	b. **The man who** [the woman is pushing ►] **is tall**
	Low Right Branching	c. **Joe knows the woman who** [◄ is pushing the man]	d. **Joe knows the man who** [the woman is pushing ►]

FIGURE 7–1. Two levels of contrast in English relative clauses. Each sentence contains a main clause (bold), and a relative clause (bracketed, set in Courier subscript). Rows constitute the complexity level: The relative can either modify the subject of the main clause (resulting in the more complex center embedding a, b) or the object (in the less complex right branching c, d). Columns constitute the movement level: In the bracketed relative clause, the grammatical function of the head (the woman, the man) can be either subject (◄) (a, c) or object (►) (b, d). In subject relative constructions (a, c), the blue relative head connects to an empty proximal position (◄), located on the left edge of the relative clause. The link (the woman–◄) crosses no part of the relative and is analyzed as −movement.* In object-relative constructions (b, d) by contrast, the red relative head connects to ►, a distal, non–left-edge, empty position. The +movement link (the man–►), depicted by the arrow, crosses both the verb and the subject of the relative clause. (*The relative pronoun *who* is viewed here as being in-between the clauses, belonging to neither; we assume irrelevance of "vacuous movement" for the perspective developed here [or a "±vacuous movement" contrast]).

plied to several linguistic constructs (relative clauses, monoclausal passive/actives) that involve a contrast between sentences involving movement and sentences not involving movement. Here, we confine ourselves to the relative clauses construct, because the emphasis of the present chapter is on the quantitative methodology. The syntactic motivation for the contrast between Movement relative clauses and non-Movement relative clauses is summarized in Figure 7–1, as well as an alternative dichotomy between relative clauses sentences. Both dichotomies are analyzed with the tools presented in this chapter.

The original formulation of the TDH (e.g., Grodzinsky, 1990) is that Broca aphasics will perform *at chance level* on Movement sentences and *above chance level* on non-Movement sentences (other things being equal). The obvious interpretation is a binomial one, in which one expects that all patients (albeit with variations in performances) will display a performance consistent with a binomial with probability parameter of 0.5 for Movement sentences and not so for non-Movement sentences.

A BINOMIAL VIEW AND ITS INTUITIVE MEANING

We model the forced binary choice task of a subject as a binomial experiment; that is, we assume there is such a thing as the probability that this subject understands a given sentence of a given type. Given such a (subject-specific) probability parameter P, we can write an explicit expression for the probability that the subject understands correctly m sentences among n trials:

$$\text{Binom}[\{n,m\}; P] := \binom{n}{m} P^m \cdot (1 - P)^{n-m}$$

This formulation simply means that we consider the successive choices of a given patient as independent binary choices driven by an underlying individual probability of success P on any given sentence. Each value of P entails a certain probability of observing m successes among n trials, given by the usual binomial formula. But we can also reverse the way we look at this and ask for the probability of a certain value of P

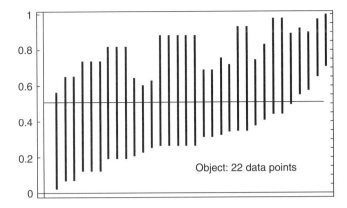

FIGURE 7–2. Display of 99% confidence intervals for the probability parameter of a population of subjects. Each vertical line represents the performance of a patient on object relative clause sentences, on the y-axis are possible values for the parameter $P_{X,S}$. The vertical segment for each patient X is the interval $[P_{LX,S}, P_{UX,S}]$. The horizontal line signals the probability = 0.5 value.

given an observed couple {n,m}. In other words we can give an α-level confidence interval $[P_L, P_U]$ for the value of the underlying probability parameter given an observation {n,m}; this amounts to solving the following equations:

$$\sum_{k=0}^{m} \binom{n}{k} p_U{}^k (1 - p_U)^{n-k} = \alpha/2$$

$$\sum_{k=0}^{m-1} \binom{n}{k} p_L{}^k (1 - p_L)^{n-k} = (1 - \alpha)/2$$

So for a given type of sentences X, and a given patient A, we get a couple $[P_{LXA}, P_{UXA}]$ that describes an α-level confidence interval for the value of the probability parameter of A on sentences of type X. In brief, we view the performance as an indication of the value of the underlying probability parameter and evaluate a lower bound (P_{LXA}) and an upper bound (P_{UXA}) on the "reasonably plausible" values of the probability parameter given the observed performance. We can now summarize the performances of each patient on a given type of sentence. Notice that simply summarizing a performance by a percentage of success would not be proper in view of the fact that data are collated from experiences in which the numbers of trials are not necessarily equal.

THE VARIABILITY

We chose to summarize the performances at the 0.01 confidence level, and this enables us to graphically display the intersubject variability inherent in the performance data. Let us consider, for instance, the performance data for relative clauses constructions with

movement (object relative clauses, see the previous section 3), and display the confidence intervals for the probability parameter as explained above (Fig. 7–2).

This graphic display calls for a few comments, as it does not seem to comply with the prediction of the TDH. Recall that object relative clauses are those relative clauses constructions that involve movement, so under a strict interpretation, the prediction of the TDH is that patients should perform at chance level on such sentences. Indeed, notice the horizontal line that signals the $P = 0.5$ value; one can readily see that there are four patients for whom the hypothesis that they perform at chance level can be rejected at the 0.01 confidence level, and quite a few others for which $P_{X,A} = 0.5$ is in the lower range of plausible options for the interpretation of the performances. Moreover, it can be seen that the intersection between the ranges of the more extreme vertical lines is empty, so no single value of P (even different from 0.5) can simultaneously accommodate all of the data as a set of binomial trials.

FRAMEWORK FOR GROUP ANALYSIS

As we have just seen, there is a wide variability in the performances of subjects on a given type of sentences. This variability precludes summarizing the group performance on a type of sentence as a single number. For example, as we have remarked, a typical $P = 0.5$ value for the binomial model will not account for the variety of performances (neither will any other value of P). Does this mean that we should renounce the idea of showing a difference in patterns of performances between two types of sentences? The variability of the data certainly shows that the naïve in-

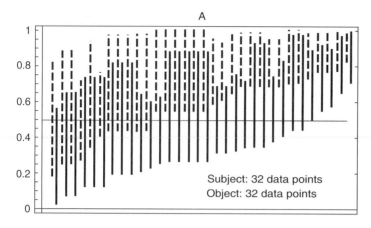

FIGURE 7–3. Binomial confidence interval analysis subject by subject, as in Figure 7–2, for both sets of performances. Dashed vertical lines correspond to performances on subject relative clauses, and solid black vertical lines, to performances on object relative clauses.

terpretation of the quantitative implication of the TDH (binomial performance with $P = 0.5$ for +Movement sentences and $P >> 0.5$ for −Movement sentences) is not tenable. But the naïve quantitative interpretation is not the only possible one. If we follow the overall logic of the argumentation, we see that what is essential to assess, at the group level, is whether there is a significant difference between the group performances on +Movement sentences and on −Movement sentences, the former being poorer on the whole than the latter. In other words, what is important is the existence of a contrast, not the uniformity of the binomial probability parameter. An immediate illustration of this point is given in Figure 7–3, top.

In Figure 7–3, we see that although the confidence intervals on +Movement and on −Movement sentences are both highly variable, there is a clear overall tendency. What we need then is a way of rigorously assessing whether this tendency is within the bounds of chance fluctuations or indicative of a true contrast.

To carry such an analysis, we need a framework that suits the binomial nature of the data, while leaving room for the possibility that the probability coefficient in the corresponding binomial distribution varies among subjects.

In other words, we need a way of describing the probability distribution of the probability parameter $P_{x,S}$ for a population X and a set of sentences S. Let us elucidate this last phrase a little bit, as it is not common procedure in psychological studies. What we are doing is the following: We assume there is some well-

defined entity called "the probability that a patient x will understand correctly a sentence from S"; we admit that this entity has a stochastic character, and we seek a way of describing the way in which the value of this entity is distributed in the population. That is, for each possible value p_0 of $P_{X,S}$ (i.e., each number between 0 and 1), we would like to say what is the probability, when x is picked randomly in the population X, of obtaining $P_{x,S} = p_0$.

Actually the situation is slightly more complicated: because the possible values for $P_{x,S}$ span the whole continuum of values from 0 to 1, the probability of obtaining any particular value is 0 and we have to use what is called a probability density function (pdf). A probability distribution of the possible values for $P_{x,S}$ is of a function f such that:

$$\int_0^1 f(x)dx = 1 \text{ (The probability of obtaining}$$
$$\text{a value in the whole 0–1 range is 1)} \quad (1)$$

$$\Pr\{p_0 - h \leq P_{X,s} \leq p_0 + h\} = \int_{p_0 - h}^{p_0 + h} f(x)dlx \quad (2)$$

That is, for any h bigger than 0, the probability of obtaining a value in the range [$p_0 - h$, $p_0 + h$] is given by the area under the curve f between the bounds $p_0 - h$, $p_0 + h$.

A pdf for $P_{x,S}$ thus specifies the way in which the probability of obtaining a particular value varies. One can think about it as a generalization of the idea of assigning a probability to each possible outcome of an experiment (e.g., the roll of a dice), when the set of possible outcomes is continuous.

Now our original question about the patterns of performances on two sets of sentences, S_1 and S_2, can be specified thus:

Let f_1 be the probability density function for $P_{X,S1}$ and f_2 be the probability density function for $P_{X,S2}$. Is the hypothesis that f_1 is not different from f_2 tenable in view of the observed performances?

The only remaining problem is to have a way of carrying out hypothesis testing of the above kind. Fortunately, the conceptual tools for implementing such an approach have already been invented by mathematicians (Skellam, 1948) and even applied to biological data by statisticians (Williams, 1975). We need a framework in which the probability distribution of our probability parameters, $P_{X,S}$, can be described by a probability density function that can be determined from the observed performances. This is provided by the beta binomial family of distributions, a natural generalization of the binomial distribution, in which the probability parameter (fixed in the binomial) is allowed to vary according to a parametric law $B(\alpha,\beta)$. The $B(\alpha,\beta)$ family plays in the present context the role played by Gaussian family of distributions in more usual hypothesis testing. Namely, it is a finitely parameterized family of functions such that we have some grounds for assuming that the probability distribution of the quantity we are measuring is well approximated by a member of the family. In the case of the Gaussian family, this assumption is, of course, founded on a mathematical theorem (the central limit theorem). In the case of the $B(\alpha,\beta)$ family, more modestly, the belief that nothing important empirically is lost by restricting ourselves to this family comes from the fact that when the parameters α and β are varied, the $B(\alpha,\beta)$ function can assume a wide variety of shapes (see Fig. 7–4).

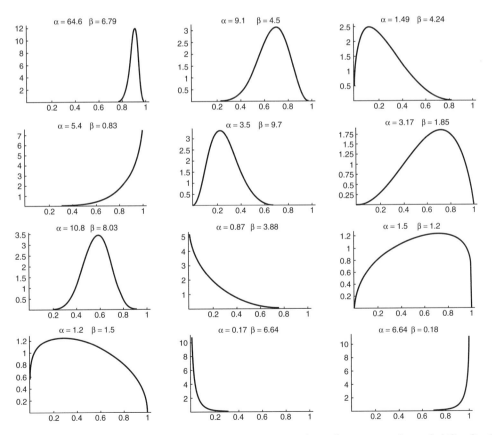

FIGURE 7–4. Some of the shapes that can be assumed $B(\alpha,\beta)$. Each graph represents the probability distribution function for a given couple of values for α and β. The x-axis values are the possible values for the random variable, and the y-axis values are arbitrary units chosen so that the total area under the curve equals 1.

In the context of the beta binomial model, we can, for each set of subject's performance, determine the best-fitting value for the parameters α, β. Furthermore, for the performances of a set of subjects on two types of sentences, we can test the null hypothesis that the whole data set comes from one distribution against the hypothesis that they come from two distinct distribution. The analogy to the hypothesis-testing procedure with which our reader is probably familiar runs thus:

1. Given the empirical data (the performances on two sets of sentences), one determines, for each data set, the best-fitting (most likely) beta function, which amounts to finding two couples of numbers (α_1, β_1), (α_2, β_2).

   This corresponds to the way one would evaluate the (most likely) means and standard deviations from two data sets assumed to follow Gaussian distributions.
2. One computes a quantity that depends on the two couples (α_1, β_1), (α_2, β_2).

   This corresponds to the computation of the *t* statistic.
3. Finally, the hypothesis that the two distributions are in fact equal is tested by comparing the obtained value with the known distribution of the previously computed statistic in case the hypothesis is true.

   This corresponds to the determination of a *P* value for the hypothesis that the means of the two populations are equal. This *P* value is obtained from the known distribution of the *t* statistic when the two populations indeed come from the same underlying Gaussian process.

Note that a Gaussian approach is not appropriate here, for several reasons:

- Summarizing the performances of each patient as a percentage of success gives an empirical distribution of a number in the [0,1] range, which does not square with the range of the normal distribution assumption underlying the *t* test.
- This move is unwarranted also because the number of trials for different patients/studies (and even for different contrasts for a given patient) is not fixed. This means that the percentage values cannot be pooled safely.
- More conceptually, we are trying to determine the distribution over the population of Px for a given type of sentence X, and there is no reason to assume *a priori* that this distribution is bell shaped (in fact, some of the empirical analyzes

in Drai and Grodzinsky 2006 show a best-fitting distribution that is J-shaped).

In order to specify the analytical details of the scheme, we now have to go into specific formulas, which the reader who is adverse to equations can skip to go directly to the next section, in which the method is applied to empirical results.

Formally, under the $B(\alpha, \beta)$ model, the probability of m successes in n trials is

$$P(x = m|n) = \binom{n}{m} B(\alpha + m, n + \beta - m)/B(\alpha, \beta);$$

with

$$B(\alpha, \beta) = \Gamma(\alpha) * \Gamma(\beta)/\Gamma(\alpha + \beta).$$

The function Γ being defined by the integral

$$\Gamma(z) = \int_0^\infty t^{z-1} e^{-t} \, dt$$

In order to compute the maximum likelihood parameters given the data, it is convenient to reparameterize the distribution, setting

$$\mu = \alpha/(\alpha + \beta)$$
$$\theta = 1/(\alpha + \beta)$$

Then μ is the expectation of the distribution, while θ is a parameter that determines the shape of the curve. Under these notations the variance σ^2 is given by $\sigma^2 = \mu(1 - \mu)\theta/(1 + \theta)$ (Williams, 1975).

Ignoring constants involving only the observations, the log-likelihood for a set of results $\{(n_1, m_1) \ldots (n_k, m_k)\}$ is given by

$$(*)$$
$$L(\mu, \theta|\{(n_1, m_1) \ldots (n_k, m_k)\}) =$$
$$\sum_{j=1}^{k} \left(\sum_{r=0}^{m_j - 1} \log[\mu + (r * \theta)] \right.$$
$$+ \sum_{r=0}^{n_j - m_j - 1} \log[1 - \mu + (r * \theta)]$$
$$\left. - \sum_{r=0}^{m_j - 1} \log[1 + (r * \theta)] \right)$$

Note that this likelihood depends on the full information concerning the number of trials and of successes of each subject so that no concern over unduly pooling incomparable percentages arises. If $\{(n_1, m_1) \ldots (n_k, m_k)\}$, represents the performances of subjects on one type of sentence and $\{(n_{k+1}, m_{k+1}) \ldots (n_{k+q}, m_{k+q})\}$ represents their performances on an other type, we can proceed to test the hypothesis that the performances are similar using the following:

If L_1 is the maximal value of

$$L(\mu, \theta | \{(n_1, m_1) \ldots (n_k, m_k),$$
$$(n_{k+1}, m_{k+q}) \ldots (n_{k+1}, m_{k+1} \, q)\})$$

and L_2 is the maximal value of

$$L(\mu, \theta | \{(n_1, m_1) \ldots (n_k, m_k)\})$$
$$+ L(\mu, \theta | \{(n_{k+1}, m_{k+1}) \ldots (n_{k+q}, m_{k+q})\})$$

Then an asymptotically valid test of the similarity of performance for the two types of tasks is given by comparing $2(L_2 - L_1)$ with upper percentage points of the χ^2 distribution with 2 degrees of freedom (Williams, 1975).

We are now in position to assess whether the pattern of performance of Broca aphasics on one set of sentences S_1 is distinct from that on set S2. Given the sets of performances we can compute the μ and θ parameters for each set of sentences and the values of L_1 and L_2 by maximizing the expression (*) for each set of results. Our hypothesis testing now consists of computing $2(L_2 - L_1)$ and asking where it stands on the χ^2 distribution with 2 degrees of freedom: if the probability of obtaining a value as high as the one we actually obtain is very small, we must reject the hypothesis that the two sets of performances correspond to the same underlying distribution of values for the probability parameters.

RESULTS OF GROUP ANALYSIS

Let us now apply the contrastive scheme we described in the preceding section and check whether despite the variability of the performances, and hence of the binomial probability parameter, a contrast can still be established. To check this, we apply the hypothesis-testing procedure of the previous section to a comparison of performances on object relative clauses (+Movement) with subject relative clauses (−Movement). Figure 7–5 summarizes the situation.

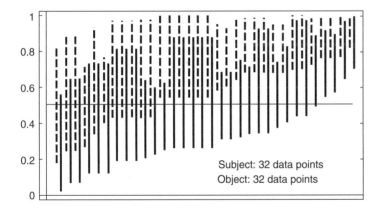

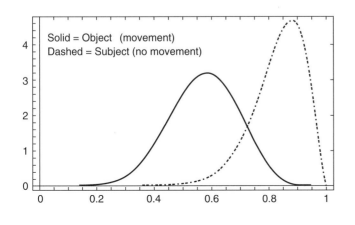

FIGURE 7–5. (*Top*) binomial confidence interval analysis subject by subject, as in Figure 7–3, for both sets of performances. Dashed vertical lines correspond to performances on subject relative clauses, and solid vertical lines, to performances on object relative clauses. (*Bottom*) Corresponding beta models probability distributed functions (pdf's) for both sets of performances. The x-axis represents the possible values for the probability parameter, and the units on the y-axis are arbitrary numbers ensuring that the total area under each curve equals 1.

Applying the computations detailed at the end of the last section, we obtain the following values for the parameters:

	+Movement	−Movement
μ	0.573	0.835
σ	0.119	0.09
P value		2.4×10^{-8}

The intuitive impression that the two sets of performances are distinct is reflected in the fact that the two curves corresponding to the two sets of parameters obtained from the two sets of performances look different. Moreover, this impression can be quantified by computing the relevant statistic and here we obtain a P value of 2.4×10^{-8}, thereby enabling us to reject with very high confidence the hypothesis that the performances for +Movement and −Movement on sentences with relative clauses come from the same underlying distribution of probabilities of success.

WAS THIS TAUTOLOGICAL?

If we allow taking the intrinsic variability of performances into account, are we not bound to be able to accommodate any counterexample? Or, in other words, are we not turning the TDH (albeit under a modified quantitative form) into a tautology? The short answer is no. Like any other statistical discrimination claim, the alleged contrast between +Movement and −Movement sentences is open to refutation in at least two ways: one could bring massive group evidence that points in another direction, so that the discrimination (here between +Movement and −Movement performances) disappears after all. Alternatively, one may come up with a new, more interesting distinction, one that has better theoretical justifications and that separates the data in an even better way. In any case, we do not have to remain at this philosophical level; the TDH as tested here is not circular, at least not in the sense of tautologically yielding a distinction in performances. Indeed, we can reanalyze the same data set by dividing the sentences in an alternative manner, not informed by the concept of movement but current in psycholinguistic methodology. We did, and the result is a lack of contrast in the performances (i.e., performing the same analysis as before one could not reject the relevant

null hypothesis). Recall from Figure 7–1 two possible ways of categorizing the relative clause sentences used in the experiments:

1. Through the Movement/non-Movement distinction
2. Through a complexity distinction in which center embedding is contrasted with branch embedding

The contrasts in both cases are presented in Figure 7–6.

The results for the two contrasts are summarized as follows:

	High (CE)	Low (RB)	+Movement	−Movement
μ	0.716	0.687	0.573	0.835
σ	0.16	0.17	0.119	0.09
P value	0.84		2.4×10^{-8}	

In brief, the +Movement-versus-−Movement contrast yields a very significant contrast, whereas the high complexity–versus–low complexity contrast yields no contrast.

CONCLUSION: TDH REPHRASED

Grodzinsky's analysis of the mechanism that generates the faulty performances of Broca aphasics in the case of Movement sentences posits a competition between two computational strategies for the assignment of thematic roles (see Grodzinsky, this volume, Chapter 6 for details). Following a kind of principle of parsimony, he therefore predicted that performances for Movement sentences should be *at chance level* (the two strategies have equal influences, and all one can do is randomly guess). This prediction, in such a wording, is not confirmed by the data because the overall structure of the data for all patients taken collectively cannot be accounted by a $P = 0.5$ binomial. Our analysis shows that the TDH is confirmed by the empirical record, albeit in a slightly modified form: The group performances on +Movement sentences is significantly poorer than that on −Movement sentences, in the sense that the distribution of probability parameters that summarizes +Movement group perfor-

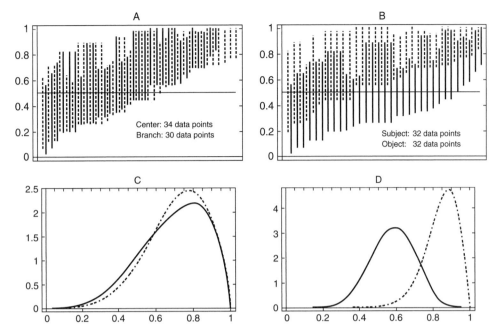

FIGURE 7–6. Individual confidence intervals and beta distribution for relative clauses. (A) The center embedding (dashed lines) versus right branch (solid lines) contrast is represented by a vertical display of the confidence intervals for all patients. Each vertical line represents the confidence interval for a given patient. (B) Same as A, except −movement is shown by dashed lines and +movement is shown by solid lines. (C) The beta model for CE (dashed lines) and RB (solid lines). The x-axis represents possible values of the probability parameter, and the y-axis units are such that the area under the curve equals 1. (D) Same as C, except −movement is shown by dashed lines, and +movement is shown by solid lines. The complexity contrast (A and C) discerns no structure; movement was vastly superior—the contrast was highly significant, indicating that movement, but not complexity, is a linguistic factor supported by Broca's region.

mance is markedly concentrated on smaller values than the probability distribution for −Movement sentences. The present approach also enables us to have a fresh look at some objections to the TDH and to understand whether they affect what, it seems, is the real heart of the matter: Can (should) group studies be used to understand aphasic comprehension data and are the contrasts in performance predicted by TDH (poorer performance on +Movement than on −Movement)?

One objection to the TDH was voiced by Druks and Marshall (1995); specifically, a case was reported in which a Broca aphasic performed better on +Movement than on −Movement sentences (actually the contrast was active versus passive but in the context considered the two contrasts coincide). Ignoring all possible polemics on the validity of classifying that specific patient as a Broca aphasic, we can

now see that such an isolated result is perfectly consistent with the population structure we have uncovered, and the overall difference between the performances on the two categories of sentence can leave peacefully one data point showing the inverse relation. Actually this remark leads to a more serious argument: Quite a few patients are not at chance on +Movement sentences, some patients are at chance on −Movement: doesn't this refute the TDH?

Notice for instance that in Figure 7–5 the curves corresponding to +Movement and −Movement overlap and have quite a sizeable width. Therefore, as pointed out in Berndt et al. (1996) and in Caramazza et al. (2000), the pattern of performance has some variability. For example (see Fig. 7–3), some patients are provably above chance level on +Movement, and many perform on −Movement in a way that does not allow us to exclude the possibility that they perform at chance level. So indeed, if one hoped to summarize all performances by a single binomial parameter, or through the dichotomy *at chance/above chance*, the situation looks hopeless. This fact has led some to contest the value of group studies and to argue that the variability is so great that the results are meaningless. In the present context, this is seen to be a much too extreme conclusion. If we try to quantitatively characterize the variability in performance—as we did here—we are led to an empirical assessment that not only gives meaning to group study data but can ONLY be performed in the context of group study data. If there is some intrinsic variability in the performances of patients, the only way to still assess whether there is a pattern in the performances is to compare the curves that describe the varying performances and to assess whether it is reasonable to assume that they come from the same underlying process.

The logical conclusion of our analysis is that the dichotomy between +Movement and −Movement captures an aspect of linguistic processing that crucially involves Broca's area. The assumptions underlying the stochastic model that enables the hypothesis testing procedure do, however, leave open a question about the source of the variability of performance.

Here we must confess to a relative ignorance of the precise mechanisms that create the variability. Obviously the size and severity of the lesions are variable, and the brains within which they occur are variable to start with. Moreover, we do not know if there is a systematic structure to the variability itself. For instance, is the variance dependent (in an interesting way) on the kind of linguistic construct in which Movement is studied? The kind of explanation proposed originally in the TDH, that is, the existence of a computational strategy orthogonal to syntax, which takes over when syntax fails, could be modified to accommodate a model with variability, for instance by postulating that given the conflicting information from syntax and from the general strategy, each individual brain weights the sources of information differently. But this is purely programmatic. The theory at its present stage is not entirely mute about implementation, though; it implies that whatever the implementation of the processing of sentences turns out to be, it must have the property of degrading in a way that yields the observed stochastic behavior when deprived of one of its components (the one corresponding to Broca's area).

ACKNOWLEDGMENTS Dan Drai's research at the Weizmann Institute of Science is supported by the Golda and Dr. Yehiel Shwartzman and by a Sara and Haim Medvedi Families Postdoctoral Fellowship.

Notes

1. The references to the study used in compiling the complete data matrix appear as an appendix in Drai and Grodzinsky (2006).

2. For example, Boston Diagnostic Aphasia Examination, Western Aphasia Battery, Aachen Aphasia Test, and others.

References

Berndt, R.S., Mitchum, C.C., & Haedinges, A.N. (1996). Comprehension of reversible sentences in "agrammatism": A meta-analysis. *Cognition, 58,* 289–308.

Caramazza, A. (1986). On drawing inferences about the structure of normal cognitive processes from patterns of impaired performance: The case for single-patient studies. *Brain and Cognition, 5,* 41–66.

Caramazza, A., Capitani, E., Rey, A., & Berndt, R. (2000). Agrammatic Broca's aphasia is not associated with a single pattern of comprehension performance. *Brain and Language, 76,* 158–184.

Drai, D., & Grodzinsky, Y. (2006). Stability of functional role in Broca's region: Quantitative neurosyntactic analysis of a large data set from Aphasia *Brain and Language, 96,* 1.

Druks, J., & Marshall, J.C. (1995). When passives are easier than actives: Two case studies of aphasic comprehension. *Cognition, 55,* 311–331.

Grodzinsky, Y. (1986). Language deficits and the theory of syntax. *Brain and Language, 27,* 135–159.

Grodzinsky, Y. (1990). *Theoretical perspectives on language deficits.* Cambridge, MA: MIT Press.

Grodzinsky, Y. (2000). The neurology of syntax: Language use without Broca's area. *Behavioural Brain Sciences, 23,* 1–21.

Grodzinsky, Y., Pinango, M.M., Zurif, E., & Drai, D. (1999). The critical role of group studies in Neuropsychology: Comprehension deficits in Broca's aphasia. *Brain and Language, 67,* 134–147.

Skellam, J.G. (1948). A probability distribution derived from the binomial distribution by regarding the probability of success as variable between the sets of trials. *Journal of the Royal Statistical Society. Series B (Methodological), 10.2,* 257–261.

Williams, D.A. (1975). The analysis of binary responses from toxicological experiments involving reproduction and teratogenicity. *Biometrics, 31.4,* 949–952.

Treating Language Deficits in Broca's Aphasia

Lewis P. Shapiro
Cynthia K. Thompson

This chapter describes a research program investigating treatment of sentence production and comprehension deficits found with individuals who have Broca's aphasia. The purpose of this program is to investigate the efficacy of a treatment approach that is based on evidence from a variety of sources, including linguistic, psycholinguistic, and neurolinguistic investigations. Our intent also is to use treatment and recovery data to reveal brain–language relations. To get to the approach and its fruits, we need to take you through its empirical origins. We then describe, in relative detail, the treatment approach and its experimental products.

Our interest in how linguistic theory and psycholinguistic experimentation can inform learning, and therefore treatment, began empirically on two separate fronts. One of us (Shapiro and colleagues) ran a small experiment that examined how argument structure might serve as a point of connection between linguistic and nonlinguistic conceptual information (Canseco-Gonzalez et al., 1990, 1991). Our single participant had incurred a stroke that yielded a left

hemisphere lesion involving most of Broca's area, the insular region, and putaminal area with superior extension into premotor, motor, and sensory cortical areas.[1] He evinced severely nonfluent speech as well as sentence comprehension difficulties on noncanonical structures, that is, on sentences where the direct object noun phrase had been displaced from its typical post-verb position (e.g., passives, object relatives). We trained our participant on c-VIC, a visually based, computerized artificial language (see, for example, Kleczewska et al., 1987).[2] We taught our subject to associate either one or two visual symbols that corresponded to the natural language equivalent of "sentences" containing either obligatory two-place or optional three-place predicates.

We found that the ease with which c-VIC symbols were learned was predicted by the number of argument structure entries for natural language verbs that equivalently referred to the depicted actions. So, for example, our subject performed better when learning two symbols for the possibilities inherent with natural language dative verbs (those that allowed either a two-place or three-place possibility) than for learning the symbols that represented the natural language equivalent of pure two-place verbs (with or without adjuncts). Additionally, we found that "verbs" that allowed an optional third argument yielded better performance when they were inserted in more complex, three-argument "sentences" than when inserted in two-place equivalents. Our interpretation of these findings suggested that knowledge of argument structure might be spared by the damage underlying Broca's aphasia because it serves a translation function between language and conceptual structure, the computation of the latter which is considered to be intact. The work also suggested that the sparing of argument structure might be exploited in developing treatment programs for sentence-level deficits in aphasia.

At approximately the same time that we were investigating the processing of argument structure in aphasia (see Sentence Processing, for more details), Thompson and Wambaugh (1989) were directly initiating investigations of treatment for the sentence production difficulties observed in Broca's aphasia. In the initial report, a treatment experiment was described whereby Broca's aphasic individuals were trained on *wh*-question production, a problematic structure for these individuals (baseline levels of performance approached 0% correct). It was found that training a set of *what*-questions generalized to untrained *what*-questions but did not generalize to untrained *when*-questions. It became apparent to both of us that this lack of cross-generalization could be explained by the argument structure properties of the verbs used to form the two question types. The verbs used for *what* questions, for example, were two-argument verbs like *eat*, whereas those used to generate *where* questions were one-argument verbs like *sleep*. Simply put, because of the verb's argument structure properties, movement in *who* questions involves displacement of an argument of the verb (e.g., a direct object); that involved in *where* questions involves movement of an adjunctive phrase (e.g., a locative prepositional phrase). This result led us to surmise that generalization should be forthcoming if the questions trained and those tested for generalization were structurally similar. Later, we flesh out what is meant by "structural similarity." More generally, we predicted that controlling for those lexical and syntactic properties that form the basis for language processing in neurologically intact as well as individuals with brain damage could result in efficacious treatment for the language disorders inherent in Broca's aphasia. Keeping

these initial findings in mind, we now fill in some of the details of the background to our treatment work.

LINGUISTIC BACKGROUND

In most theories of grammar, there is an intimate relation between lexical representations and syntax. This relation as well has been the focus of much work in psycholinguistics and investigations of brain language.

Argument Structure

The information that seems most clearly relevant to the interaction between lexical properties and syntax is argument structure. Borrowing from logic, a sentence can be considered analogous to a proposition, which can be organized into a set of arguments that "revolve around" an event described by the predicate. In its essence, argument structure simply describes the number and type of participants entailed by, typically, a verb. For example, consider the English verb *defeat*:

1. *Kerry will defeat Bush in November.*
    In example 1, there are two NPs—subject and complement (direct object)—that contribute to the event described by the verb. The remainder of the material—the prepositional phrase—although adding to the syntax and interpretation of the sentence, does not form part of the verb's contribution and is therefore considered an adjunct. Thus, the verb *defeat* is said to be a two-place predicate.

There is a limited range of argument structures allowed in English as well as in other languages. Consider the following examples:

2. *Joelle slept easily last night. Sleep* is a one-place (intransitive) predicate, where the subject NP is the sole argument selected by the verb.
3. *Zack discovered that the ball went over the fence. Discover*, in this case, is a two-place predicate with the second argument syntactically realized as a complement phrase.
4. *Dillon threw/sent/lent the ball to the umpire.* These verbs allow three arguments, with the third argument contained within the prepositional phrase.

Arguments can be required or optional. For example, in *Dillon threw the ball*, there are only two arguments specified by the verb. In this case, it could be argued that the verb *throw* is an optional three-place verb, and in its present realization only two of the arguments are apparent. On the other hand, verbs like *put* and *give* require three arguments for a sentence to be well formed, as in *Joelle put the makeup on the shelf* (**Joelle put the makeup*) and *Dillon gave the ball to the umpire* (**Dillon gave the ball*).

Further consideration of the argument structures for sentences 1 through 4 reveals that the arguments play different semantic roles in relation to their verbs. So, in example 1, the subject argument lexically filled by the NP *Kerry* is playing the role of "agent of the action" and the direct object argument *Bush* is playing the role of "patient" or "theme." In example 2, the subject argument *Joelle* is the "experiencer" of the action described by the verb. In example 3, the clausal argument *that the ball went over the fence* is a "proposition." In example 4, the NP argument *the umpire* that is embedded in the prepositional phrase *to the umpire* plays the role of the "goal" of the action.

The array of these roles, idiosyncratically selected by each verb, forms the verb's thematic grid. The verb *defeat* bears an (agent theme) grid; the verb *give* an (agent theme goal), the verb *discover* an (agent proposition), and so on. Within the principles and parameters framework (see Chomsky and Lasnik, 1993; Haegeman, 1994; Radford, 1997), thematic information interacts with syntax via theta theory. Briefly, a lexical head (e.g., verb) assigns its thematic roles to argument positions in the sentence in its underlying representation. So, for example, considering the verb *give* and its thematic grid (agent theme goal), agent is assigned to the subject argument position, theme is assigned to the direct object position, and goal is assigned to the oblique object position. In this way, thematic information forms a lexically based constraint on well-formedness. That is, if all of the thematic roles for a particular verb are discharged to their appropriate argument positions, the sentence that is generated is grammatical; if they are not, or if there is an argument position where a thematic role is not assigned, the sentence that is generated is ill formed.

In more recent accounts based on *minimalist* considerations (Chomsky, 1995; 1998, see also Adger, 2003), there is no role for modules or subtheories of any sort; the architecture of the grammar is said to be driven by methodological economy (i.e., fewer primitives, relations, and assumptions). A basic syntactic operation is *Merge*, which selects an item from the lexicon that has a rich set of features (a *lexical array*)

and combines it with another such selected item, yielding a higher-order category. Simplifying, a series of such merger operations builds the syntactic structure of the sentence.

Still, the facts that arguments can play any one of a number of thematic roles, and that verbs idiosyncratically select a set of such roles, should be understood within the grammar. Thus, we might claim that theta-assignment occurs as part of merge (Radford, 2004). Consider, then, how thematic roles are assigned in a simple SVO structure, exemplified as *Kerry will defeat Bush*:

5.

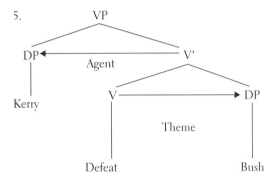

Here, as V is merged with DP to yield V′, the theta role of theme is assigned to the direct object argument position; as V′ is merged with DP to form a VP, the theta role of agent is assigned to the subject (note that the subject is internal to the VP and raises to the specifier position of TP, which we discuss later). The VP in example 5 is merged with a T′ constituent, and so on up the tree.[3] In some extended accounts of the lexicon, thematic information is considered an abbreviation for a more richly specified conceptual or event structure in which the verb plays a central role (e.g., Jackendoff, 1990; Pustejovsky, 1995).

Movement

Within the theory we are considering here, sentences are derived from two operations: one, described above, is merge: two categories merge to yield a higher-order category, and a series of such merge operations builds constituent structure or the syntactic tree (see Friedmann, this volume, for details of the tree, particular those that have relevance for accounts of production in agrammatic Broca's aphasia). It was suggested above that thematic role assignment is part of the merge operation, allowing lexical features to percolate to syntax. The second operation is *move*. It has long been recognized that there are three subtypes of movement. One is head movement (seen in English in "subject-Aux inversion"; e.g., "Dillon is playing soccer" → "Is Dillon playing soccer"?); the others are *wh*-movement (or A-bar movement, written as A′; in English object-extracted wh-questions, clefts, and object relatives) and NP- or A-movement (seen in English passives, unaccusatives, and subject raising). In the following we briefly describe the latter two movement operations, most relevant to the empirical work described later in this paper.

wh-Movement (A′ Movement)

Consider the following sentences:

6. The soldier pushed the woman
7. Which woman did the soldier push?

It is apparent that examples 6 and 7 are related. Each sentence contains the same two-place predicate with the same lexical items filling the argument slots (ignoring the *wh*-word in example 7). The NP playing the agent in the event in example 6 plays the same role in example 7; the NP playing the role of patient plays that same role in both sentences as well. Given the relation between these constructions, it is likely that the question form in example 7 is somehow derived from the underlying event stated in example 6. One way of describing this relation is to suggest that, in the question form, the direct object argument is transferred from its base position occurring after the verb to a position higher in the syntactic tree:

8.

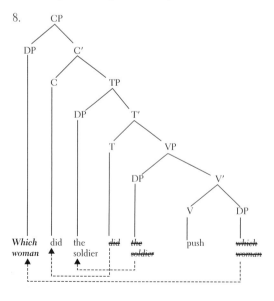

The structure in example 8 shows the derivation of the wh-question. The complement of *push*—*which woman*—is represented in its base, direct object, position. It moves to Spec-CP, and as a result it leaves a clone or copy of itself, also known as a trace in the principles and parameters framework. The thematic role of theme is assigned to the complement position via merge of V and DP. The subject DP—*the soldier*—raises out of VP into the Spec-TP position (for reasons not germane to the current discussion); agent is assigned to the subject constituent via merge of DP with V′. The copies of the moved constituents are deleted (or rather, given a null status phonetically) before they are sent off to the level of representation concerned with phonetic form.[4]

NP-Movement (A Movement)

The other type of move operation relevant to the work described here derives passives as well as raising constructions. Consider the passive:

9.

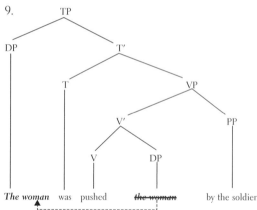

Here, the complement of the verb *push*—*the woman*—is moved to Spec-TP from its canonical complement position, leaving a copy that is subsequently deleted. Thus, an argument is moved to another argument position, unlike the case of *wh*-movement described in example 8, where the landing site for movement is a nonargument position (Spec-CP).

Interim Summary

In this section we have described some basic linguistic notions (admittedly skipping many details) that turn out to have important implications for the treatment work that we soon discuss. Argument structure is a type of lexical property (or set of features; e.g., thematic roles) that characterizes the number and types of participants in an event described by the verb. This property interacts with the syntax, particularly the syntactic tree, and thus places constraints on the well-formedness of sentences. Sentences are derived from the output of two operations: merge, which takes two syntactic objects selected from the lexicon, combines them and yields a higher-order category, and move, which displaces a category to another position in the syntactic tree. In the following, we briefly describe the processing consequences of these linguistic operations.

SENTENCE PROCESSING

In a series of online experiments, we have found that normal listeners—when encountering a verb during the temporal unfolding of a sentence—exhaustively activate their argument-taking properties (e.g., Shapiro et al., 1987, 1989, 1993). Once active, these properties are then used by the processing system—perhaps during a secondary routine—to establish thematic relations among the arguments in the sentence, allowing for final interpretation. Indeed, regardless of theoretical orientation, most sentence processing accounts claim a privileged role for the constraints established by argument structure in both sentence production and comprehension (e.g., Bock, 1995; Bock and Levelt, 1994; Levelt 1999; Shapiro et al., 1991, 1993; Trueswell and Kim, 1998).

Wernicke's aphasic individuals, those who have typically incurred damage to posterior cortical regions, do not show normal online sensitivity to these argument structure properties, suggesting that the conceptual-semantic aspects of these lexical properties influence the types of "semantic-like" deficits observed in these individuals. Yet, Broca's aphasic individuals perform just like the neurologically intact population; that is, when they encounter a verb in a sentence, they activate its argument structure properties.

There is also a large body of evidence suggesting that normal listeners/readers respect movement operations (e.g., Garnsey et al., 1989; Hickok et al., 1993; Nicol and Swinney, 1989; Shapiro and Hestvik, 1995). In a series of online experiments, Swinney and colleagues (1987) have shown that a moved complement is reactivated at its base position. In sentences like "The policeman saw the boy who the crowd at

the party accused of the crime", where the complement of *accused* (i.e., *the boy*) has been moved up the tree to Spec-CP and leaves a copy in the direct object position, listeners show activation for the moved argument at the copy position (and not at a position before the copy). We have recently found such "gap-filling" effects in wh-questions (Shapiro and Thompson, in preparation), VP-ellipsis constructions (Shapiro and Hestvik, 1995; Shapiro et al., 2003), and NP-movement constructions (Friedmann et al., submitted).

Importantly, in constructions derived by movement, individuals with Broca's and Wernicke's aphasia show the reverse pattern observed with argument structure. Broca's aphasic individuals do not show normal "gap-filling" effects, yet those individuals with Wernicke's aphasia do (e.g., Zurif et al., 1993[5]). This double-dissociation—that individuals with Broca's aphasia show normal lexical processing routines involving argument structure but aberrant structural routines involving movement, and those with Wernicke's aphasia show disordered lexical processing but relatively normal online structural routines—strongly suggests that lexical and structural processing are independent. And, indeed, there is a recent neuro-imaging evidence to support this possibility. Ben-Shachar et al. (2003) found that Broca's region (left inferior frontal gyrus) is activated during processing of movement structures, yet argument structure complexity revealed activation only in left posterior superior temporal sulcus. Thompson et al. (submitted) reported a similar finding, comparing activation patterns for verbs by argument structure. Verbs with a greater number of arguments, such as three-argument versus two- or one-argument verbs, yielded bilateral posterior, superior temporal gyri/sulci activation. These findings support the deficit patterns seen in aphasic patients.

It is now a well-established fact that individuals with Broca's aphasia have difficulty understanding and producing sentences that are "noncanonical." A more precise definition of what that means inevitably brings us to detailed aspects of movement (see, for example, Grodzinsky, Friedmann, this volume). Grodzinsky has described a detailed account (the trace-deletion hypothesis [TDH]) that explains a host of sentence comprehension patterns evinced by Broca's aphasic individuals involving constructions derived by movement. Remediation of sentence-level deficits requires a treatment program that takes these linguistic notions seriously. Before we describe such a program, we briefly ground our work in the extant treatment literature.

TREATMENT OF LANGUAGE DEFICITS IN APHASIA: A BRIEF REVIEW

Our intention, then, was to develop a treatment program based on linguistic theory, psycholinguistic findings, and what we knew about the deficit patterns in aphasia, and critically, we also required that this program be testable using the right kinds of experimental designs (Shapiro and Thompson, 1994; Thompson and Shapiro, 1994). The literature on recovery and treatment of sentence deficits resulting from brain damage prior to the initial Wambaugh and Thompson (1989) effort consisted primarily of case studies and uncontrolled group studies (and to some extent, this continues to be the case). Very few studies considered the relevance of linguistic or psycholinguistic variables, even broadly defined. One exception is an approach developed by Schwartz et al. (1994; see also Byng, 1988; Jones, 1986), based on the "mapping hypothesis," which holds that agrammatic performance reflects an impaired mapping between grammatical constituents (subject, object) and thematic roles (agent, theme) (Schwartz et al., 1987). Using color-coded materials corresponding to sentence constituents, participants were trained to recognize the thematic roles of noun phrases set around the verbs in sentences in both canonical (active NP-V-NP sentences) and noncanonical sentences by responding to questions of the form "Who did what to whom." Treatment outcomes were mixed, with generalization within sentence types claimed for some participants, and sparse evidence for generalization across sentence types.

Although the intent of these studies was laudable, the experimental designs have fallen short of those required in a controlled treatment study. For example, simple pretest, posttest designs are often implemented (e.g., Schwartz et al., 1994; for a more recent example, see Beveridge and Crerar, 2002), or the case study approach is taken; neither can unambiguously attribute any potential gains to the treatment itself. Byng (1988), for example, presented case studies for two subjects, reporting only pretreatment and posttreatment data, without control for potentially extraneous factors. Further, in the Schwartz et al. program, a pretraining phase was instituted whereby patients were

trained to understand *wh*-questions necessary for the subsequent training phase. But as noted by the investigators, *wh*-questions are problematic for these patients. Indeed, according to the "mapping" hypothesis, the same deficit contributes to the problems these patients have in understanding *wh*-questions and the sentences that were targets for treatment; that is, both sentence types are derived from noncanonical thematic role assignment. Yet to reap the benefits of the treatment, the patients had to understand the *wh*-questions in the pretraining phase.

Another treatment program that has considered linguistic variables was "Cueing verb treatment" (CVT) (e.g., Loverso et al., 1986). This program used case grammar (Fillmore, 1968) as a basis for treatment targeting production of simple sentence structures. Case grammar, whose constructs found their way into more current approaches to lexical representation, considers the verb as the "motor" of the sentence's propositional structure. Loverso et al. designed a treatment program that first trained the verb and then, in a series of graduated steps, attempted to expand the verb to include both its subject and, depending on the type of verb, either its object or a location, adverbial of time, instrument, etc. The sentence expansion was produced by clinician-controlled use of *wh*-words (e.g., "who run" written on index cards yields patient-initiated "I run," "who run when" yields "I run yesterday," "who hit" yields "I hit," etc.). The investigators claimed generalization because of increases on formal aphasia test measures (although, so far as we are aware, generalization to untrained verb and verb-argument combinations was not assessed in their experimental design. Whether these subjects would show such generalization remains unanswered).

The generalization issue aside, from our present perspective Loverso and colleagues (1986) should be commended for devising perhaps the first treatment program that considered the influence of lexical properties on sentence generation. Their approach, however, was limited to the production of simple sentences, and, not unlike the Schwarz et al. program, the use of *wh*-words to elicit the simple sentences was quite likely to be problematic for some participants. And although their materials were controlled for frequency of occurrence, imagery, and concreteness, the verbs themselves were not controlled for the number and types of arguments they entailed. Again, we know from the psycholinguistic literature that the lexical properties of verbs have direct consequences for syntax, and for sentence comprehension and production, and thus it may be necessary to control for these properties when devising treatment programs.

So, to the best of our knowledge, the treatment literature contains few instances of studies that have seriously considered the linguistic and psycholinguistic underpinnings of sentence targets, and those that have have used research designs that limit the generalizability of any positive results. As you will soon see, there is some underlying similarities between our approach and the mapping/cueing verb treatment approaches described earlier. One important similarity is the reliance on verb-argument structure. However, one critical difference is the acknowledgment of movement operations involved in the derivation of noncanonical structures, as Grodzinsky and colleagues have so clearly shown may be at the heart of the sentence interpretation patterns evinced by Broca's aphasic individuals. With these rather lengthy preliminaries out of the way, we now describe our treatment program.

TREATMENT OF UNDERLYING FORMS

We have labeled our treatment program "Treatment of Underlying Forms" for good reason: We take advantage of the underlying, abstract, properties of language. We assume that training such properties will allow for more effective generalization. The properties we exploit are lexical—argument structure—that appears to be spared in some individuals with agrammatic Broca's aphasia, and syntactic—movement—that is compromised in these same individuals. Our treatment investigations use small numbers of subjects but with controlled experimental designs; we assess, and find, generalization to untrained structures that share similar underlying properties to those structures that are trained, and in some cases we find generalization to overall language performance as well.

Our first collaborative empirical effort (Thompson et al., 1993) sought to accomplish two things: (1) establish pilot data using the treatment of underlying forms approach and (2) examine if training one type of question would generalize to another type of question if we controlled for verb argument structure and the type of movement involved. We began with two participants; each suffered a single left-hemisphere cerebrovascular accident. Both participants were diagnosed with nonfluent aphasia with agrammatism.

Briefly, sentence production was characterized by short phrases and simple sentences consisting primarily of major lexical categories, with inflectional morphemes compromised. Using elicited production, both participants could produce simple SVO sentences relatively accurately (again, with inflectional morphology compromised) but were unable to produce grammatically correct wh-questions or passive constructions. Auditory comprehension of active SVO constructions was above-chance levels, and comprehension of reversible passives was at chance.

We examined whether training who-questions would generalize to untrained who- and untrained what-questions (and vice versa), and whether training wh-questions based on more complex underlying forms (NP-V-NP-PP; e.g., "What is the man giving to the boy?") would generalize to wh-questions based on less complex forms (NP-V-NP; e.g., "What is the man fixing?"). A single-subject multiple-baseline across behaviors and subjects was used to examine acquisition and generalization effects of treatment. Subject 1 was trained to first form what-questions, and subject 2 was trained to first form who-questions.[6]

Baselines of one subject were extended into the treatment phases of the other subject, and, for each subject, one question type was trained at a time to allow us to examine generalization to the other question form. This type of design—a multiple baseline across subjects (and behaviors)—allows one to establish effects that can be unambiguously assigned to treatment variables rather than to extraneous, uncontrolled variables. That is, in the multiple baseline across subjects approach, treatment is initiated for each participant after baselines varying in length. If stable baselines are observed for participant 2 during the time participant 1 is undergoing treatment, and then treatment is instituted for participant 2 and increased performance is observed, a good argument can be made that it is the treatment itself that is responsible for the change in behavior. The multiple baseline across behaviors portion of the design involves training one question form at a time for each participant. In all cases, probes designed to assess generalization to untrained versions of the same behavior (e.g., complex what-questions for subject 1; complex who-questions for subject 2), and untrained versions of the other behaviors (e.g., simple and complex what-questions, and simple and complex who-questions), were assessed throughout treatment. In this way, we could scrutinize individual subject data, carefully inspecting the relation between trained and untrained question types.

We predicted that training what-questions would generalize to untrained who-questions and vice versa because both structures are derived from wh-movement, and their only difference is the wh-morpheme that heads the question form. In this initial effort, we found that some of our predictions were borne out. First, we observed that both participants evinced increased performance on wh-questions after treatment. At baseline, neither subject could produce well-formed wh-questions. Participant 1 showed 2% correct production of wh-questions at baseline with 68% of the sentences produced consisting of rising intonation without the appropriate wh-morpheme, 22% consisting of utterances with no wh-morpheme and no evidence of movement, and 9% including the correct wh-morpheme but no movement. At posttreatment, this participant produced 82% correct. Participant 2 showed similar performance, with only 2% correct at baseline and 96% at posttreatment. Second, and more specifically, when treatment was applied to what-questions for participant 1, generalization to untrained exemplars of what-questions was observed. However, acquisition of who-questions was not observed until treatment was applied to those structures, not supporting our prediction. For participant 2, however, training of who-questions resulted in generalization to untrained what-questions, supporting our prediction. In addition, this participant showed generalization from complex to simple exemplars of both who- and what-questions. This latter finding encouraged us to move forward in our treatment work.

Training Movement of Arguments Versus Movement of Adjuncts

Following up on the initial study just described (Thompson et al., 1993), we further examined the relation between those wh-questions that required movement of an argument and those that required movement of an adjunctive phrase (Thompson et al., 1996). Recall that who- and what-questions refer to, typically, a moved direct object argument of the verb (as in "The soldier pushed *the woman* into the street. *Who* did the soldier push _____ into the street?"), while, for example, where-questions refer to movement of an adjunct (as in "The soldier pushed the woman into *the street*. *Where* did the soldier push the woman _____?"). Seven individuals with aphasia

participated in the experiment. All incurred a single left-hemisphere infarct; five became aphasic secondary to a cerebrovascular accident in the distribution of the left middle cerebral artery, one suffered a left middle cerebral artery from a ruptured aneurysm in the temporoparietal region, and one had a mass excised from the left frontal lobe. The results of a series of formal and informal tests revealed that production was more compromised than comprehension and that speech was nonfluent, consisting of primarily short phrases and sentences, most of them simple structures that were, nevertheless, ungrammatical. In an analysis of verb-argument structures produced in discourse situations, significantly fewer verbs and less complex argument structures relative to normal controls were observed. Sentence comprehension was compromised as well. For example, all the participants performed from 70% to 100% correct on active SVO sentences as well as on subject relatives; on passives and object relatives, they performed from 50% to 70% correct.

A single-subject multiple-baseline design across behaviors was used to examine generalization patterns across wh-questions. As one structure was treated, generalization to the other structures was examined. For each participant, once the initial structure reached criterion, treatment ensured for a second structure. The order of wh-questions entered into treatment was counterbalanced across the participants. For example, participant 1 was first trained on when-questions that rely on movement of an adjunct, and generalization was tested to untrained where-questions that also relied on movement of the adjunct and to untrained who- and what-questions, both of which rely on movement of the direct object argument. In a second phase, what-questions were entered into treatment, and generalization to untrained who-questions was assessed. For participant 2, who-questions were first trained and generalization to untrained what-, where-, and when-questions was assessed. In the second phase for participant 2, when-questions were entered into treatment and generalization to untrained where-questions was assessed, and so on.

We predicted that training sentences derived from movement of an argument (e.g., who-questions) would only generalize to untrained material using a different set of wh-questions (e.g., what-questions) that also relied on movement of an argument, and not to sentences derived from movement of an adjunct phrase (e.g., when- and where-questions). Relatedly, we predicted that training sentences derived from movement of an adjunctive phrase would not generalize to those derived from movement of an argument.

Overall results indicated that for every participant, treatment yielded improved production significantly above baseline levels for all wh-questions entered into treatment. Further observation revealed two patterns of results. First, three participants evinced patterns in line with our initial predictions. When these individuals were trained on wh-questions derived from movement of an argument, generalization to untrained forms was restricted to those materials that also rely on movement of an argument. A similar pattern was observed within questions derived from movement of adjunctive phrases. Importantly, generalization across structures derived from movement of an argument and movement of an adjunct did not occur. Interestingly, these participants' error patterns revealed a correct wh-question pattern but with what has been called a "filled gap" (e.g., when required to respond with "Who is the soldier pushing into the street?" a participant would attempt "Who is the soldier pushing the woman"). Referring back to the Linguistic Background section, it seems that the participants may have failed to delete the copy of the moved constituent.

A second pattern was revealed for four other participants. Training of a particular question (e.g., when-questions) yielded generalization to untrained materials of the same question type but did not generalize to untrained materials of other question types, whether they were derived by the same type of movement. An examination of the error patterns was quite revealing; these participants primarily evinced errors of wh-morpheme selection (e.g., instead of producing "who is the soldier pushing?" they would produce "where is the soldier pushing?"), while at the same time reducing errors of co-reference that were observed during baseline testing. We then entered these individuals into supplemental wh-morpheme discrimination and production training. Once initiated, these individuals evinced generalization to all wh-question forms, and their wh-morpheme selection errors significantly decreased there.

The story does not stop there. For three of these four individuals, if we ignored errors of wh-morpheme selection, the patterns revealed that training wh-questions relying on movement of an argument did indeed increase performance on other untrained wh-questions relying on argument movement, and later

adjunct movement improved (and vice versa). That is, the within-question type generalization observed for the first three participants was also revealed in these other three participants, but the latter's performance was masked by the errors of wh-morpheme selection. These two patterns suggest two putatively distinct operations involved in the production of wh-questions. One has to do with processing routines enabling co-reference; the other has to do with selection of the correct lexical item that fills the functional category. Regarding the latter, it is interesting to note that more than 10 years ago, Grodzinsky (1990) suggested that sentence production deficits observed in agrammatic Broca's aphasia might be partially explained by a deficit to the features inherent in functional categories and that such individuals randomly select items to fill these categories.

Finally, in this study (and in others as well), we examined pretreatment and posttreatment discourse patterns. We found significantly improved sentence production across the board. Our participants produced significantly more verbs post-relative to pretreatment, more correct argument structures, more adjuncts, a great number of wh-questions, a greater proportion of complex sentences, and more embeddings per utterance. One interpretation of these impressive gains is that because our training program targets lexical and structural properties that are involved in many aspects of sentence production, significant and pervasive changes may occur to the more broadly conceived language system.

Wh- (A′ Movement) Versus NP-Movement (A Movement)

As described previously, a distinction can be made between two types of movement. One type is Wh-movement, which displaces a complement from its underlying position after the verb (in English) to Spec-CP, a nonargument (A′) position. Object extracted wh-questions, as well as cleft structures and object relatives, involve this type of movement. The other is NP-movement, which moves elements into the subject argument (A) position. Two types of sentences indicative of this operation are passives and raising constructions. Given this theoretical distinction—and our premise and earlier findings that generalization should occur only among constructions that have like-structural properties—we addressed the following question: Will training sentences that rely on one type of movement generalize to only those constructions also relying on that type of movement, or, alternatively, will any type of movement generalize to any other type of movement? This is a much stronger test of our underlying forms premise than the argument/adjunct distinction, because the spell-out forms of sentences generated from Wh-movement (e.g., wh-questions; object clefts and relatives) cannot be said to be similar in any analogical way to each other or to sentences generated by NP-movement (e.g., passives, raising).

In our first effort addressing this issue (Thompson et al., 1997), we tested two participants with language production and comprehension patterns consistent with agrammatic Broca's aphasia. Both participants had aphasia resulting from a single left hemisphere stroke; both had damage to regions involving the pars triangularis and opercular parts of the inferofrontal lobe. Both revealed nonfluent production, with short and primarily ungrammatical sentences. In terms of auditory comprehension, both participants performed relatively well on active SVO and subject relative constructions and poorer on passives and object relatives.

We again used a single-subject multiple-baseline design across subjects and behaviours. Following baseline testing, participant 1 was trained to produce object cleft sentences that relied on wh-movement. During training, generalization to untrained who-questions, also relying on wh-movement, was assessed. Constructions derived by A movement (passives, subject raising) were also tested. Next for this participant, subject-raising sentences were entered into treatment while generalization to untrained passives was tested. The order of training was counterbalanced for participant 2 who was first trained on passives while generalization to untrained subject-raising was tested, as were object clefts and wh-questions. Finally, for participant 2, object clefts were trained. Again, we predicted that training sentences derived from wh-movement (e.g., object clefts) would only generalize to untrained object clefts and wh-questions, and training sentences derived from A movement (e.g., passives) would only generalize to other A movement constructions (e.g., subject raising).

The data revealed the following patterns: For both participants, the sentences entered into treatment were acquired very quickly once treatment began and remained significantly above baseline performance levels throughout the study. Observed generalization patterns aligned with our predictions: For participant 1, training on object cleft constructions yielded significantly increased performance on untrained who-questions (from 0% at baseline to 48% during object cleft training). Yet, this training did not influence production of passives or subject-raising constructions. For participant 2, training on passives yielded significantly improved performance on subject-raising constructions (0% at baseline; 80% during training of passives) but no generalization to untrained object cleft constructions was noted. Thus, these patterns corroborated and extended the results from our studies examining argument and adjunct distinctions in wh-movement; that is, generalization occurs only to constructions that have similar underlying properties as those trained. In follow-up studies, we have found similar patterns (Ballard and Thompson, 1999; Jacobs and Thompson, 2000).

We also assessed sentence production through narrative discourse samples, collected pretreatment, immediately after treatment, and 4 weeks posttreatment. We put these samples through our sentence production analysis coding system (Thompson et al., 1995). The results showed that both participants significantly increased the proportion of sentences that were grammatical. Participant 1, for example, evinced 26% grammatical sentences in the sample taken pretreatment. At immediate posttreatment, grammatical sentences rose to 36%, and to 39% at 4 weeks posttreatment. Participant 2 evinced only 19% grammatical sentences at pretreatment; at immediate posttreatment grammatical sentences increased to 31% and remained stable (31%) 4 weeks posttreatment. We believe that these are impressive gains, and we attribute them to the nature of the treatment and the possibility that the entire language system may be facilitated if the right kinds of linguistic variables are targeted.

The reader may detect that we have been primarily describing work that examines sentence *production* treatment. However, our production treatment requires aspects of sentence interpretation as well. As pointed out previously, the details of our treatment take the participant through an underlying structure where arguments are in their canonical positions and then trains the participant on thematic relations and, importantly, on how each sentence (e.g., a wh-question) is derived through movement. These are the critical features of this treatment program, and these are the operations shared by the computation of producing or understanding sentences. We note, however, that in a study directly examining the relation between production and comprehension, we (Jacobs and Thompson, 2000) found little improvement in comprehension of complex sentences even though the patients showed improved ability to produce complex sentences when provided with treatment of underlying forms. For this reason, we added more explicit comprehension components to our treatment. Indeed, the bulk of the participants who are included in our studies show both impoverished production and sentence comprehension patterns indicative of Broca's aphasia. Therefore, we surmised that focusing more on comprehension would help to ameliorate both deficits. Indeed, this is what we have found. This additional comprehension component has resulting in improvements in both production and comprehension in these patients (see, for example, Thompson et al., 2003, described later).

Complexity Effects

The final set of treatment studies to discuss here describes our proposal that initially training complex structures yields more efficacious and wide-ranging treatment effects than using simpler structures as a starting point for treatment. Note the following patterns: (1) in our attempt to train an aphasic individual on an artificial visual symbol system designed to mimic natural language predicates, we discovered that learning was facilitated when the symbols were acquired in the context of more complex structures (Canseco-Gonzalez et al., 1990); (2) in our initial collaborative treatment effort (Thompson and Shapiro, 1993), we found that training wh-questions that relied on "denser" underlying phrase structure configurations generalized to wh-questions based on less-dense structures; and (3) in a closer analysis of response patterns from our previous studies that examined wh-questions and object clefts (Thompson and Shapiro, 1994; Thompson et al., 1997), we found that several of our participants evinced better generalization when first trained on object clefts relative to when first trained on wh-questions. As the reader will soon observe, these patterns tie together quite nicely when viewed from a complexity perspective. A more detailed test of the complexity proposal was thus required.

The syntax of object cleft constructions involves movement of a direct object NP from an underlying complement position to Spec-CP. Movement takes place within an embedded relative clause; the maximal projection (CP) of this clause is dominated by another TP in the matrix clause. In simple wh-questions, the wh-phrase moves to Spec-CP as well, but this CP dominates all other nodes in the construction. Thus, the syntax of a simple wh-question forms a *subset* of the entire phrasal configuration of an object-cleft construction (as an important aside, we recognize that it is critical to define, in detail, what is meant by *complexity*).

Given this complexity metric, and assuming that such a notion can be transferred to the processing routines underlying sentence production and comprehension, we conducted some formal tests of this complexity hypothesis. In one of our efforts (Thompson et al., 1998), we tested three agrammatic Broca's aphasic individuals who were trained on object clefts (e.g., *It was the artist who the thief chased*) and wh-questions (e.g., *Who did the thief chase?*). Using, again, a single-subject experimental design, participants were trained to produce either object-clefts or simple wh-questions in counterbalanced order, while generalization to untrained structures was assessed.

The results of this study showed that for participant 1, performance on wh-questions increased dramatically during baseline testing, that is, without treatment, likely related to repeated opportunity to practice target items during the baseline period. However, simultaneous improvement of object-clefts did not occur during this period when wh-questions were emerging. Rather, object clefts required direct training. For participant 2, who received object cleft training initially, object cleft production increased significantly above baseline levels, and so, too, did wh-question production (indeed, the learning curves for both constructions looked remarkably similar). Finally, for participant 3, who received training initially on wh-questions, these question forms emerged quickly, but no increase on untrained object clefts was observed until object cleft training was initiated. For all three participants, the production of passives, generated from the application of A movement, did not increase above initial baseline levels. These patterns align with our complexity predictions: treatment effects are more pronounced when treatment is initiated on complex structures; in such a case simpler structures appear to come along for the ride. The reverse—that it is best to begin treatment with simpler structures and progressively increase complexity— appears to be falsified by this, and indeed, other similar treatment experiments. Our results, therefore, turn conventional clinical wisdom on its head. In our most recent effort (Thompson et al., 2003), we replicated and extended this work. Briefly, our participants revealed both sentence production and comprehension deficits, particularly on noncanonical constructions (wh-questions, passives, object relatives) compared with canonical structures (actives, subject relatives). In this experiment we added an additional structure — object relative constructions. Note that object relatives (e.g., *The man saw the artist who the thief chased*) and object clefts (e.g., *It was the artist who the thief chased*) are similar in that one cannot be said to be a subset of the other, unlike matrix wh-questions (e.g., *Who did the thief chase?*), which are in a subset relationship with both object clefts and relatives. Yet, object relatives and clefts are (obviously) different structures. In the matrix clause of object relatives (e.g., *The man saw the artist . . .*), the subject is base-generated in Spec-VP (refer to example 8) and moves to Spec-TP. Furthermore, the subject acquires the agent role when the V′ (*saw the artist*) merges with the DP (*the man*) (refer to example 5). In the matrix clause of the object cleft (e.g., *It was the artist . . .*), however, on a standard analysis the subject is represented by a pronoun (*It*) that lacks semantic content, and is base generated in its surface position, that is, in Spec of TP.

We were thus in a position to examine whether the syntactic subset relation is the only complexity metric responsible for the patterns we observed in our previous work or if we should extend our notion of complexity to other factors that influence structure and interpretation. First, as pointed out earlier, in this experiment we tracked both sentence comprehension and production; we found improvements in both. The results showed that training object relatives resulted in significant generalization to untrained object clefts and wh-questions, while training wh-questions did not show generalization to untrained object relatives and clefts. Furthermore, when object clefts were entered into treatment, generalization was not observed for untrained object relatives. These patterns suggest, then, that the subset relationship cannot be the sole contributor to generalization effects and that, in object relatives, the addition of the subject that moves from its base position in the VP (requiring a theta-role) contributes as well.[7]

The complexity hypothesis is buttressed by mounting evidence from multiple sources. For example, Eckman and colleagues (1988) have found that teaching relative clauses to L2 learners of English generalizes to untrained canonical structures (actives and subject relatives), much like what we have found with our Broca's aphasic participants. Gierut and colleagues, in numerous studies, have shown that unmarked phonological structures replace marked structures in the error patterns observed in children with phonological disorders. Furthermore, training marked structures (e.g., defined in terms of sonority or cluster formation) results in greater systemwide changes than training unmarked structures (see, for example, Gierut, 1998; Gierut and Champion, 2001; see also Archibald, 1998; Barlow, 2001; Eckman and Iverson, 1993, for evidence from L2 phonological acquisition). This, again, is similar to the systemwide changes we observed when analyzing speech in discourse for our aphasic individuals after treatment on complex syntactic forms. We have also observed such complexity training effects with adult individuals with apraxia of speech (Maas et al., 2002) and those with fluent aphasia and naming deficits (Kiran and Thompson, 2003). Finally, evidence for the complexity hypothesis also comes from domains outside of language (e.g., in math learning, Yao, 1989; in motor learning, Schmidt and Lee, 1999).

SUMMARY AND CONCLUSIONS

To summarize, we have found that the sentence production and comprehension deficits observed subsequent to Broca's aphasia lend themselves to remediation and that if the materials to be trained are of the right kind, pervasive changes can be observed. These changes occur when underlying lexical and syntactic properties are considered. Furthermore, similarity breeds generalization. Structures that share fundamental properties generalize; those that do not share such properties do not generalize. And this generalization effect occurs in like-structures with spell-out forms that are dissimilar (as in the case of A′ movement-derived structures or A movement structures). Importantly, there is a variable superimposed on these findings: training more complex forms generalizes to less complex forms, but the reverse does not work as well. Thus, consideration of both the linguistic similarity of forms and their complexity (based on linguistic principles as well as sentence-processing evidence) are important for efficacious treatment of language disorders. These patterns follow from the thesis that linguistic theory can and should be used to deduce what goes awry in the aphasias and then should form the basis for the design of treatment programs.

Our work suggests, indeed, requires, that the brains of our treatment patients have undergone change. Thompson and colleagues (submitted) have recently embarked on a program to image brains of individuals with aphasia that have or have not undergone "treatment of underlying forms" (through functional MRI). In their first effort, three participants received treatment and three acted as controls. For the three treated participants, changes were noted in activation patterns in the right hemisphere homologue of Wernicke's and surrounding areas and, for two of those three, the right hemisphere homologue of Broca's area. Posttreatment recruitment of spared left hemisphere areas was also observed in two of the participants. This is just a small step; there is much more to do and it would not be surprising if activation patterns, initially, are idiosyncratic and difficult to interpret. Nevertheless, the foundation of the research program—an efficacious treatment based on linguistic and psycholinguistic evidence—appears to be in place.

We end, now, with some brief comments regarding how our work reflects on the functional role of Broca's region. Our participants were chosen because they had particular kinds of deficits that we believed might be amendable to a linguistically focused treatment program. A large majority of these individuals revealed classic signs of Broca's aphasia: in production, halting, and effortful speech, with a paucity of functional categories, short utterance lengths, and a limited repertoire of sentence "types"; in comprehension, a clear distinction between SVO constructions and those derived by movement.

Nevertheless, the lesion data were not as consistent. Many of our participants evinced classic Broca's region damage. But there were considerable exceptions. Should we be concerned, therefore, that the functions of language are not so easily localized in our work? We do not think so. It is likely that the impairments our participants exhibit cannot be explained by a minimalistic syntactic deficit. That is, they likely did not exhibit deficits that can be described solely in terms of trace deletion, of tree pruning, of resource limiting binding principles, and the like. We did not chose our participants for any one of these deficits. Rather, it is likely that a (limited) range

of functional deficits were typical of our patients, and therefore it is quite likely that the normal operations that were impaired recruit brain tissue from sources beyond Broca's region.

Relatedly, although our treatment might appear to be narrowly focused, it is not, to our minds, too narrowly focused, nor is it too broadly conceived. We targeted argument structure properties of verbs, movement operations, and wh-morpheme selection. There is good evidence that each of these has independent processing reflections (e.g., lexical operations targeting argument structure properties are functionally and perhaps even neurologically independent of movement operations). It is therefore perhaps not surprising that our approach has thus far been so successful, given that we targeted a reasonable range of processing operations in our treatment program. Likewise, it is not surprising that we find generalization effects in language beyond what we targeted in treatment. It remains to be seen whether we can successfully modify our approach to encompass an even wider range of deficits found in aphasia; if we do, it will likely be because the modifications respect the linguistic and psycholinguistic operations underlying the deficits.

ACKNOWLEDGMENTS   We would like to thank the participants and their families for their support; we hope that in some small way our work will contribute to a higher quality of life for them. We also acknowledge the support of the NIH, from grants R01DC00494 and R01DC01948.

Notes

1. Our reliance on Broca's aphasia in this and other studies can serve two independent roles. The first is to mine the syndrome of Broca's aphasia to help inform language studies, and in turn to reflect back on the syndrome to help further define its behavioral range and to generalize findings to various theoretical claims (see Avrutin, Grodzinsky, and Friedmann, this volume). The second is to use Broca's aphasia for its lesion localizing value (see, again, Chapter 6). It is apparent from the literature that Broca's aphasia encompasses more cortical (and subcortical) regions than suggested by classical Broca's area. Yet, exploiting Broca's aphasia for its lesion localizing value has still borne considerable empirical fruit.

2. c-VIC, developed by Richard Steele and colleagues (Steele, Weinrich, Wertz, Kleczewska, & Carlson, 1989), was a computerized version of a low-tech

VIC, a visual communication system developed at the Boston Aphasia Research Center (Gardner, Zurif, Berry, and Baker, 1976) and designed for individuals with global aphasia. The electronic version used on-screen decks of cards with pictures or symbols that could be manipulated by the patient via a mouse. The version we used contained a "lexicon" for noun-like objects and a lexicon for "actions" (i.e., verbs), which could be combined to form rudimentary sentence-like communication.

3. The assumption that it is the V′ that assigns a thematic role to its subject rests on the fact that the type of thematic role assigned to the subject is determined by the composition of the verb and its object, and not by the verb alone. For example, in the sentence "Bush broke his promise," the subject of the verb plays the role of Agent, yet in "Bush broke his toe" the subject *Bush* plays the role of the Experiencer (on the interpretation that *his toe* refers to *Bush* and that the event was accidental).

4. Note also that there is another movement operation in (8), where the head of TP (e.g., *did*) moves to the head of CP; this is known as head movement.

5. The aphasic participants used in the Zurif et al. studies overlapped with those participants used in the Shapiro et al. studies. Arguments that there is too much variability inherent in the syndrome approach for it to be useful for uncovering brain-language relations won't hold here.

6. The treatment procedures for most of these studies involved several steps. These included presenting picture pairs depicting reversed actions (e.g., a man pushing a woman and a woman pushing a man) and asking the participant to point to the correct picture, and correcting an error while pointing out the Agent and Patient; asking the participant to produce a sentence by being primed with one of the pictures (e.g., "In this picture you want to know who the man is pushing so you ask . . . "?); using anagram cards, each with a written word from the sentence. The examiner moves the direct object to the front of the sentence, replaces it with a "wh-card," inverts the subject-aux if necessary. In essence, the procedures involve "meta-linguistic" knowledge of verb properties and movement.

7. Sentence length cannot be a serious contender for contributing to our complexity effects given that our object relatives and clefts were controlled for length. Furthermore, the number of propositions expressed in the sentences cannot explain the observed patterns, since both matrix wh-questions and object clefts could be argued to entail only one proposition, yet object clefts and wh-questions did not pattern together. Nevertheless, we take it as an open question as to the set of factors that might contribute to a complexity metric.

In this regard, currently one of the most serious attempts to connect detailed aspects of linguistic theory to sentence production patterns in Broca's aphasia comes from the work of Friedmann (e.g., Friedmann, 2002; see Chapter 5). Friedmann suggests that the underlying deficit in agrammatism is best explained by reference to the syntactic tree. Friedmann, Wenkert-Olenik, and Gil (2000) trained an agrammatic speaker on structures relying on higher levels of the tree and found significant improvement on related structures that weren't trained but that relied on lower levels. Relatedly, Friedmann (Chapter 5) describes the spontaneous recovery of a single aphasic patient; the types of sentences the patient produced over time could be explained by reference to higher and higher levels of the tree. If these patterns can be replicated with additional participants and structures, it supports the case that the syntactic tree can also be used as a complexity metric for treatment.

References

Adger, D. (2003). *Core syntax: A minimalist approach.* New York: Oxford University Press.

Archibald, J. (1998). Second language phonology, phonetics, and typology. *Studies in Second Language Acquisition, 20,* 189–212.

Ballard, K.J., & Thompson, C.K. (1999). Treatment and generalization of complex sentence structures in agrammatism. *Journal of Speech, Language, and Hearing Sciences, 42,* 690–707.

Barlow, J.A. (2001). Individual differences in the production of initial consonant sequences in pig Latin. *Lingua, 111,* 667–696.

Ben-Shachar, M., Hendler, T., Kahn, I., Ben-Bashat, D., & Grodzinsky, Y. (2003). The neural reality of syntactic transformations: Evidence from fMRI. *Psychological Science, 14,* 433–440

Beveridge, M.A., & Crerar, M.A. (2002). Remediation of asyntactic sentence comprehension using a multimedia microworld. *Brain and Language, 22,* 243–295.

Bock, J.K., & Levelt, W.J.M. (1994). Language production: Grammatical encoding. In M. Gernsbacher (Ed.), *Handbook of psycholinguistics* (pp. 945–984). New York: Academic Press.

Bock, J.K. (1995). Sentence production: From mind to mouth. In J. Miller & P. Eimas (Eds.), *Handbook of Perception and Cognition: Speech, Language, and Communication* (pp. 181–216). New York: Academic Press.

Byng, S. (1988). Sentence processing deficits: Theory and therapy. *Cognitive Neuropsychology, 5,* 629–676.

Canseco-Gonzalez, E., Shapiro, L.P., Zurif, E.B., & Baker, E. (1990). Predicate-argument structure as a link between linguistic and nonlinguistic representations. *Brain and Language*, 39, 391–404.

Canseco-Gonzalez, E., Shapiro, L.P., Zurif, E.B., & Baker, E. (1991). Lexical argument structure representations and their role in translation across cognitive domains. *Brain and Language*, 40, 384–392.

Chomsky, N. (1995). *The minimalist program*. Cambridge, MA: MIT Press.

Chomsky, N. (1998). Some observations of economy in generative grammar. In P. Barbosa, D. Fox, P. Hagstrom, M. McGinnis, & D. Pesetsky (Eds.), *Is the best good enough? Optimality and competition in syntax* (pp. 115–127). Cambridge, MA: MIT Press.

Chomsky, N. & Lasnik, H. (1993). The theory of principles and parameters. In J. Jacobs, A. von Stechow, W. Sternefeld, & T. Vennemann (Eds.), *Syntax: An international handbook of contemporary research* (pp. 506–569). Berlin: de Gruyter.

Eckman, F.R., & Iverson, G.K. (1993). Sonority and markedness among onset clusters in the interlanguage of ESL learners. *Second Language Research*, 9, 234–252.

Eckman, F.R., Bell, L., & Nelson, D. (1988). On the generalization of relative clause instruction in the acquisition of English as a second language. *Applied Linguistics*, 9, 1–20.

Fillmore, C. (1968). The case for case. In E. Bach & R. Harms (Eds.), *Universals in linguistic theory* (pp. 1–88). New York: Holt, Reinhart, and Winston.

Friedmann, N. (2002). Question production in agrammatism: The tree pruning hypothesis. *Brain and Language*, 80, 160–187.

Friedmann, N., Taranto, G., Shapiro, L.P., & Swinney, D. (submitted). The leaf fell (the leaf): The on-line processing of unaccusatives. *Language*.

Friedmann, N., Wenkert-Olenik, D., & Gil, M. (2000). From theory to practice: Treatment of agrammatic production in Hebrew based on the tree pruning hypothesis. *Journal of Neurolinguistics*, 13, 250–254.

Gardner, H., Zurif, E., Berry, T., & Baker, E. (1976). Visual communication in aphasia. *Neuropsychologia*, 14, 275–292.

Garnsey, S., Tanenhaus, M., & Chapman, R. (1989). Evoked potentials and the study of sentence comprehension. *Journal of Psycholinguistic Research*, 18, 51–60.

Gierut, J.A., & Champion, A.H. (2001). Syllable onsets. II: Three-element clusters in phonological treatment. *Journal of Speech, Language, and Hearing Research*, 44, 886–904.

Gierut, J.A. (1998). Treatment efficacy: Functional phonological disorders in children. *Journal of*

Speech, Language, and Hearing Research, 41, S85–S100.

Grodzinsky, Y. (1990). *Theoretical perspectives on language deficits*. Cambridge, MA: MIT Press.

Haegeman, L. (1994). *Introduction to government and binding theory*. Cambridge, MA: Basil Blackwell.

Hickok, G., Canseco-Gonzalez, E., Zurif, E., & Grimshaw, J. (1993). Modularity in locating *wh*-gaps. *Journal of Psycholinguistic Research*, 21, 545–561.

Jackendoff, R. (1990). *Semantic structures*. Cambridge, MA: MIT Press.

Jacobs, B., & Thompson, C.K. (2000). Cross-modal generalization effects of training noncanonical sentence comprehension and production in agrammatic aphasia. *Journal of Speech, Language, and Hearing Sciences*, 43, 5–20.

Jones, E.V. (1986). Building the foundation for sentence production in a nonfluent aphasic. *British Journal of Disorders of Communication*, 21, 63–82.

Kleczewska, M.K., Shapiro, L.P., Steele, R.D., & Weinrich, M. (1987). Design considerations for a computer-based visual communication system for aphasic patients. Seminar presented to the American Speech-Language-Hearing Association, New Orleans.

Levelt, W.J.M. (1999). Producing spoken language: A blueprint of the speaker. In C. Brown & P. Hagoort (Eds.), *The neurocognition of language* (pp. 83–122). New York: Oxford. University Press.

Loverso, F.L., Prescott, T.E., & Selinger, M. (1986). Cueing verbs: A treatment strategy for aphasic adults. *Journal of Rehabilitation Research*, 25, 47–60.

Maas, E., Barlow, J., Robin, D., & Shapiro, L.P. (2002). Treatment of phonological errors in aphasia and apraxia of speech: Effects of phonological complexity. *Aphasiology*, 16, 609–622.

Nicol, J., & Swinney, D. (1989). The role of structure and coreference assignment during sentence comprehension. *Journal of Psycholinguistic Research*, 18, 5–19.

Pustejovsky, J. (1995). *The generative lexicon*. Cambridge, MA: MIT Press.

Radford, A. (1997). *Syntax: A minimalist introduction*. New York: Cambridge University Press.

Radford, A. (2004). *Minimalist syntax: Exploring the structure of English*. New York: Cambridge University Press.

Schmidt, R.A., & Lee, T.D. (1999). *Motor control and learning: A behavioural emphasis*. Champaign, IL: Human Kinetics.

Schwartz, M.F., Linebarger, M., Saffron, E.M., & Pate, D. (1987). Syntactic transparency and sentence interpretation in aphasia. *Language and Cognitive Processes, 2*, 85–113.

Schwartz, M.F., Saffron, E.M., Fink, R.B., Myers, J.L., & Martin, N. (1994). Mapping therapy: A treatment programme for agrammatism. *Aphasiology, 8*, 19–54.

Shapiro, L.P., & Hestvik, A. (1995). On-line comprehension of VP-ellipsis: Syntactic reconstruction and semantic influence. *Journal of Psycholinguistic Research, 24*, 517–532.

Shapiro, L.P., & Thompson, C.K. (1994). The use of linguistic theory as a framework for treatment studies in aphasia. *Clinical Aphasiology, 22*, 291–305.

Shapiro, L.P., & Thompson, C.K. (2005). On-line comprehension of wh-questions in discourse. Unpublished manuscript, San Diego State University, San Diego, CA.

Shapiro, L.P., Nagel, N., & Levine, B.A. (1993). Preferences for a verb's complements and their use in sentence processing. *Journal of Memory and Language, 32*, 96–114.

Shapiro, L.P., Zurif, E., & Grimshaw, J. (1987). Sentence processing and the mental representation of verbs. *Cognition, 27*, 219–246.

Shapiro, L.P., Zurif, E., & Grimshaw, J. (1989). Verb representation and sentence processing: Contextual impenetrability. *Journal of Psycholinguistic Research, 18*, 223–243.

Shapiro, L.P., Brookins, B., Gordon, B., & Nagel, N. (1991). Verb effects during sentence processing. *Journal of Experimental Psychology: Learning, Memory, and Cognition, 17*, 983–996.

Shapiro, L.P., Gordon, B., Hack, N., & Killackey, J. (1993). Verb-argument structure processing in complex sentences in Broca's and Wernicke's aphasia. *Brain and Language, 45*, 423–447.

Shapiro, L.P., Hestvik, A., Lesan, L., & Garcia, A.R. (2003). Charting the time-course of sentence processing: Evidence for an initial and independent structural analysis. *Journal of Memory and Language, 49*, 1–19.

Steele, R.D., Weinrich, M., Wertz, R.T., Kleczewska, M.K., & Carlson, G.S. (1989). Computer-based visual communication in aphasia. *Neuropsychologia, 21*, 409–426.

Swinney, D., Nicol, J., Ford, M., Frauenfelder, U., & Bresnan, J. (1987). The time course of co-indexation during sentence comprehension. Presented at Psychonomic Society Meeting, Seattle.

Thompson, C.K., Fix, S., Gitelman, D.R., Parish, T.B., & Mesulam, M. (submitted). The neurobiology of recovered sentence comprehension in aphasia: Treatment-induced fMRI activation patterns.

Thompson, C.K., Ballard, K.J., & Shapiro, L.P. (1998). The role of complexity in training Wh-movement structures in agrammatic aphasia: Optimal order for promoting generalization. *Journal of the International Neuropsychological Society, 4*, 661–674.

Thompson, C.K., Shapiro, L.P., & Roberts, M. (1993). Treatment of sentence production deficits in aphasia: A linguistic-specific approach to wh-interrogative training and generalization. *Aphasiology, 7*, 111–133.

Thompson, C.K., Shapiro, L.P., Ballard, K.J., Jacobs, B.J., Schneider, S.L., & Tait, M. (1997). Training and generalized production of wh- and NP-movement structures in agrammatic aphasia. *Journal of Speech, Language, and Hearing Research, 40*, 228–244.

Thompson, C.K., Shapiro, L.P., Kiran, S., & Sobecks, J. (2003). The role of syntactic complexity in treatment of sentence deficits in agrammatic aphasia: The complexity account of treatment efficacy (CATE). *Journal of Speech, Language, and Hearing Research, 46*, 591–607.

Thompson, C.K., Shapiro, L.P., Li, L., & Schendel, L. (1995). Analysis of verbs and verb-argument structure: A method for quantification of aphasic language production. *Clinical Aphasiology*, 121–140.

Thompson, C.K., Shapiro, L.P., Tait, M., Jacobs, B.J., & Schneider, S.L. (1996). Training Wh-question productions in agrammatic aphasia: Analysis of argument and adjunct movement. *Brain and Language, 52*, 175–228.

Trueswell, J., & Kim, A. (1998). How to prune a garden-path by nipping it in the bud: Fast priming of verb argument structure. *Journal of Memory and Language, 39*, 102–123.

Wambaugh, J.L., & Thompson, C.K. (1989). Training and generalization of agrammatic aphasic adults' wh-interrogative productions. *Journal of Speech and Hearing Disorders, 54*, 509–525.

Yao, K. (1989). Acquisition of mathematical skills in a learning hierarchy by high and low ability students when instruction is omitted on coordinate and subordinate skills. Unpublished doctoral dissertation, Indiana University.

Zurif, E., Swinney, D., Prather, P., Solomon, J., & Bushell, C. (1993). On-line analysis of syntactic processing in Broca's and Wernicke's aphasia. *Brain and Language, 45*, 448–464.

III

MOTOR ASPECTS AND SIGN LANGUAGE

9

Broca's Region: A Speech Area?

Luciano Fadiga

Laila Craighero

Alice Roy

Since its first description in the nineteenth century, Broca's area, largely coincident with Brodmann areas 44/45 (pars opercularis and pars triangularis of the inferior frontal gyrus (IFG), see Amunts et al. (1999) has represented one of the most challenging areas of the human brain. Its discoverer, the French neurologist Paul Broca (1861), strongly claimed that a normal function of this area is fundamental for the correct functioning of verbal communication. In his view this area, which he considered a motor area, contains a "memory" of the movements necessary to articulate words. Several of Broca's colleagues, however, argued against his interpretation (e.g., Henry C. Bastian, who considered Broca's area a sensory area deputed to tongue proprioception), and perhaps the most famous among them, Paul Flechsig, postulated for Broca's area a role neither motor nor sensory (see Mingazzini, 1913). According to his schema, drawn to explain the paraphasic expression of sensory aphasia, Broca's region is driven by Wernicke's area and, due to its strong connections to the inferior part of the precentral gyrus (*gyrus frontalis ascendens*), it recruits and coordinates the motor elements necessary to produce words articulation. It is important to stress here that the whole set of knowledge on the function of Broca's area possessed by the neurologists of the nineteenth century, derived from the study of the correlation between functional impairment and brain lesions, as assessed post-mortem by neuropathological investigations.

The neurosurgeon Wilder Penfield was the first who experimentally demonstrated the involvement of Broca's region in speech production. By electrically stimulating the frontal lobe in awake patients undergoing brain surgery for intractable epilepsy, he collected dozens of cases and first reported that the stimulation of the inferior frontal gyrus evoked the arrest of ongoing speech, although with some individual variability. The coincidence between the focus of the Penfield effect and the location of the Broca's area was a strongly convincing argument in favor of the motor role of this region (Penfield and Roberts, 1959).

Apart from some pioneeristic investigation of speech-related evoked potentials (Ertl and Schafer, 1967; Lelord et al., 1973), the true scientific revolution in the study of verbal communication was represented by the discovery of brain imaging techniques, such as positron emission tomography (PET), functional magnetic resonance imaging (fMRI), and magnetoencephalography (MEG). This mainly because evoked potential technique, although very fast in detecting neuronal responses, was definitely unable to localize brain activation with enough spatial resolution (the situation has changed now with high-resolution electroencephalography). As soon as PET became available, a series of independent studies on the brain correlates of the verbal function demonstrated the involvement of Broca's region during generation of speech (for a review of early studies, see Liotti et al., 1994). At the same time, however, the finding that Broca's region was activated also during speech perception became increasingly accepted (see Papathanassiou et al., 2000, for review). This finding represents in our view the second revolution in the neuroscience of speech. Data coming from cortical stimulation of collaborating patients undergoing neurosurgery confirmed these observations. According to Schaffler et al. (1993), the electrical stimulation of the Broca's area in, addition to the speech production interference originally shown by Penfield, also produced also comprehension deficits, particularly evident in the case of "complex auditory verbal instructions and visual semantic material." According to the same group, while Broca's region is specifically involved in speech production, Wernicke's and Broca's areas both participate to speech comprehension (Schaffler et al., 1993). This double-faced role of Broca's area is now widely accepted, although with different functional interpretations. The discussion in deep of this debate is, however, outside the scope of the present chapter, but readers will find details on it in other contributions to the present book.

The perceptual involvement of Broca's area seems not to be restricted to speech perception. Since the early 1970s several groups have shown a strict correlation between frontal aphasia and impairment in gestures/pantomimes recognition (Bell, 1994; Daniloff et al., 1982; Duffy and Duffy, 1975, 1981; Gainotti and Lemmo, 1976; Glosser et al., 1986). It is often unclear, however, whether this relationship between aphasia and gestures recognition deficits is due to Broca's area lesion only or if it depends on the involvement of other, possibly parietal, areas. In fact, it is a common observation that aphasic patients are frequently affected by ideomotor apraxia too (see Goldenberg, 1996).

This chapter will present data and theoretical framework supporting a new interpretation of the role played by Broca's area. In a first part, we briefly review a series of recent brain imaging studies that report, among others, the activation of areas 44/45. In consideration of the large variety of experimental paradigms inducing such activation, we will make an interpretative effort by presenting neurophysiological data from the monkey homologue of BA44/BA45. Finally we will report electrophysiological data on humans which connect speech perception to the more general framework of other's action understanding.

DOES ONLY SPEECH ACTIVATE BROCA'S AREA?

In this section we present recent brain imaging experiments reporting Broca's area activation. Experiments will be grouped according to the general cognitive function they explore.

Memory and Attention

Brain imaging studies aiming at identifying the neuronal substrate of the working memory have repeatedly observed activations of Broca's area. However, these results should be taken cautiously as most of the experimental tasks used verbal stimuli and do not allowed to clearly disambiguate the role of BA44 in the memory processes from the well-known one in language processes. Considered as the neuronal substrate of the phonological loop, a component of the working memory system, few memory studies have highlighted the possible contribution of Broca's area in "pure" memory processes. Mecklinger and colleagues (2002) recently reported the activation of BA44 during a delay match-to-sample task in which subjects were required to match the orientation of nonmanipulable objects. When tested with pictures of manipulable objects the activation shifted caudally to the left ventral premotor cortex. While in this study BA44 was mainly associated with the encoding delay, Ranganath and co-workers (2003) failed to demonstrate any preferential activation of Broca's area for the encoding or, conversely, the retrieval phases. Furthermore, the authors found the activation of Broca's area during both a long-term memory task and a working memory task, questioning thus a specific involvement in the working memory system. Interestingly, the stimuli used in this experiment were pictures of face and, as we review later, Broca's area seems particularly responsive to facial stimuli. Moreover, there is a series of papers by Ricarda Schubotz and Yves von Cramon in which they investigate nonmotor and non-language functions of the premotor cortex (for review, see Schubotz and von Cramon, 2003). According to this work, the premotor cortex is also involved in prospective attention to sensory events and in processing serial prediction tasks.

Arithmetics and Calculation

If the role of Broca's area in nonverbal memory remains to be confirmed, its potential participation in calculation tasks is equally confusing. Arithmetic studies face with two problems that could both account for the activation of BA44, the working memory subprocesses and the presence of covert speech (Delazer et al., 2003; Menon et al., 2000; Rickard et al., 2000). To this respect, the study of Gruber et al. (2001) is interesting as they carefully controlled for the covert-speech but still found an activation of Broca's area. Moreover, they compared a simple calculation task with a compound one and once again observed an activation of Broca's area. If the hypothesis of the verbal working memory cannot be ruled out, these authors nevertheless strengthened the potential involvement of Broca's area in processing symbolic meaningful operations and applying calculation rules.

Music

Playing with rules seems to be part of the cognitive attributions of BA44, as repeatedly observed during tasks manipulating syntactic rules. In an elegant study, Maess and colleagues (2001) further extended these observations to musical syntax. Indeed, the predictability of harmonics and the rules underlying music organization has been compared to language syntax (Bharucha and Krumhansl, 1983; Patel et al., 1998). By inserting unexpected harmonics, Maess and co-workers (2001) created a sort of musical syntactic violation. Using MEG, they studied the neuronal counterpart of hearing harmonic incongruity. As expected, based on a previous experiment, they found an early right anterior negativity, a parameter that has already been associated with harmonics violation (Koelsch et al., 2000). The source of the activity pointed out BA44, bilaterally. However, the story is

not that simple, and in addition to a participation in high-order processes, Broca's area takes part in lower-order processes such as tonal frequency discrimination (Muller et al., 2001) or binocular disparity (Negawa et al., 2002).

Motor-Related Functions

Excluding the linguistic field, another important contribution of BA44 is certainly found in the motor domain and motor-related processes. Gerlach et al. (2002) asked subjects to perform a categorization task between natural and man-made objects and found an activation of BA44 extending caudally to BA6 for artefacts only. The authors proposed that categorization might rely on motor-based knowledge, artefacts being more closely linked with hand actions than natural objects. Distinguishing between manipulable and nonmanipulable objects, Kellenbach and colleagues (2003) found a stronger activation of BA44 when subjects were required to answer a question concerning the action evoked by manipulable objects. However, performing a categorization task or answering a question even by the way of a button press is likely to evoked covert speech. Against this criticism are several studies reporting a significant activation of BA44 during execution of distal movements such as grasping (Binkofski et al., 1999ab; Gerardin et al., 2000; Grezes et al., 2003; Hamzei et al., 2003; Lacquaniti et al., 1997; Matsumura et al., 1996; Nishitani and Hari, 2000). Moreover, the activation of BA44 is not restricted to motor execution but spreads over motor imagery (Binkofski et al., 2000; Geradin et al., 2000; Grezes and Decety, 2002).

HOW CAN WE SOLVE THE PUZZLE?

In order to understand how the human brain works, usually neuroscientists try to define which human areas are morphologically closer to electrophysiologically characterized monkey ones. In our case, to navigate through this impressive amount of experimental data, we perform the reversal operation by stepping down the evolutionary scale in order to examine the functional properties of the homologue of BA44 in our "progenitors." From a cytoarchitectonical point of view (Petrides and Pandya, 1997), the monkey's frontal area that closely resembles human Broca's region is an agranular/disgranular premotor area (area

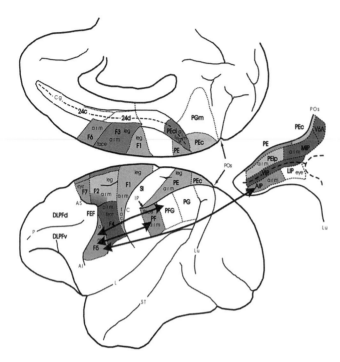

FIGURE 9–1. Lateral view of monkey left hemisphere. Area F5 is buried inside the arcuate sulcus (posterior bank) and emerges onto the convexity immediately posterior to it. Area F5 is bidirectionally connected with the inferior parietal lobule (areas AIP [anterior intraparietal], PF, and PFG) and represents the monkey homologue of human Broca's area (Petrides and Pandya, 1997). Area F5 sends some direct connections also to hand/mouth representations of primary motor cortex (area F1) and to the cervical enlargement of the spinal cord. This last evidence definitely demonstrates its motor nature.

F5 as defined by Matelli et al., 1985) (see Rizzolatti et al., 2002). We therefore examine the functional properties of this area by reporting the results of experiments aiming to find a behavioral correlate to single-neuron responses (Fig. 9–1).

Motor Properties of the Monkey Homologue of Human Broca's Area

Area F5 forms the rostral part of inferior area 6.

Microstimulation (Hepp-Reymond et al., 1994) and single-neuron studies (see Rizzolatti et al., 1988) show that area F5 represents hand and mouth movements. The two representations tend to be spatially segregated: while hand movements are mostly represented in the dorsal part of area F5, mouth movements are mostly located in its ventral part. Although not much is known about the functional properties of "mouth" neurons, the properties of "hand" neurons have been extensively investigated. Rizzolatti et al. (1988) recorded single-neuron activity in monkeys trained to grasp objects of different sizes and shapes. The specificity of the goal seems to be an essential prerequisite in activating these neurons. The same neurons that discharge during grasping, holding, tearing, and manipulating are silent when the monkey performs actions that involve a similar muscular pattern but with a different goal (e.g., grasping to put away, scratching, grooming, etc.). Further evidence in favor of such a goal representation is given by F5 neurons that discharge when the monkey grasps an object with its right hand or with its left hand (Fig. 9–2). This observation suggests that some F5 premotor neurons are capable to generalize the goal, independent of the acting effector. Using the action effective in triggering neuron's discharge as classification criterion, F5 neurons can be subdivided into several classes. Among them, the most common are "grasping," "holding," "tearing," and "manipulating" neurons. Grasping neurons form the most represented class in area F5. Many of them are selective for a particular type of prehension such as precision grip, finger prehension, or whole hand prehension. In addition, some neurons show specificity for different fingers configuration, even within the same grip type. Thus, the prehension of a large spherical object (whole hand prehension, requiring the opposition of all fingers) is coded by neurons different from those coding the prehension of a cylinder (still whole hand prehension but performed with the opposition of the four last fingers and the palm of the hand). The temporal relation between grasping movement and neuron discharge varies from neuron to neuron. Some neurons become active during the initial phase of the

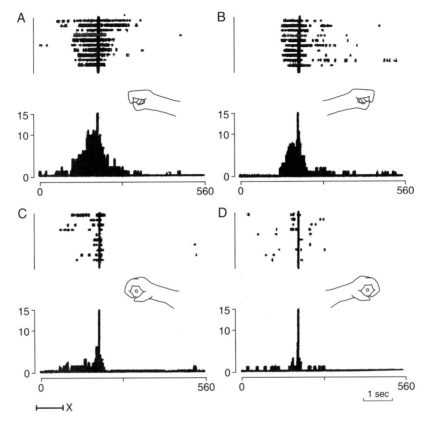

FIGURE 9–2. Example of F5 motor neuron. In each panel, eight trials are represented (rasters in the *top*) together with the sum histogram (*bottom*). Trials are aligned with the moment at which the monkey touches the target (vertical line across rasters and histograms). Ordinates given in spikes per second; abscissae, 20 × millisecond bins. (Modified from Rizzolatti et al., 1988.)

movement (opening of the hand), some discharge during hand closure, and others discharge during the entire grasping movement from the beginning of fingers opening until their contact with the object.

Taken together, the functional properties of F5 neurons suggest that this area stores a set of motor schemata (Arbib, 1997) or, as it was previously proposed (Rizzolatti and Gentilucci, 1988), contains a "vocabulary" of motor acts. The "words" composing this vocabulary are constituted by populations of neurons. Some of them indicate the general category of an action (hold, grasp, tear, manipulate). Others specify the effectors that are appropriate for that action. Finally, a third group is concerned with the temporal segmentation of the actions. What differentiates F5 from the primary motor cortex (M1, BA4) is that while F5 motor schemata code for goal-directed actions (or fragments of specific actions), the primary motor cortex represents movements, which are independent of the action context in which they are used. In comparison with F5, M1 could therefore be defined as a "vocabulary of movements."

Visuomotor Properties of the Monkey Homologue of Human Broca's Area

All F5 neurons share similar motor properties. In addition to their motor discharge, however, several F5 neurons also discharge to the presentation of visual stimuli (visuomotor neurons). Two radically different categories of visuomotor neurons are present in area F5: Neurons of the first category discharge when the monkey observes graspable objects ("canonical" F5 neurons; Rizzolatti et al., 1988; Rizzolatti and Fadiga, 1998). Neurons of the second category discharge when the monkey observes another individual making an action in front of it (di Pellegrino et al., 1992, Gallese et al., 1996; Rizzolatti et al., 1996a). For this peculiar "resonant" properties, neurons belonging to the second category have been named "mirror" neurons (Gallese et al., 1996). The two categories of F5 neurons are located in two different subregions of area F5: canonical neurons are mainly found in that sector of area F5 buried inside the arcuate sulcus, whereas mirror neurons are almost exclusively located in the cortical convexity of F5.

Recently, the visual responses of canonical neurons were reexamined using a formal behavioral paradigm, which allowed separate testing of the response related to object observation, during the waiting phase between object presentation and movements onset, and during movement execution (Murata et al., 1997). The results showed that among the canonical neurons recorded in area F5, two thirds were selective to one or few specific objects. When visual and motor properties of F5 object observation neurons are compared, it becomes clear that there is a strict congruence between the two types of responses. Neurons that become active when the monkey observes small objects also discharge during precision grip. On the contrary, neurons selectively active when the monkey looks at a large object, discharge also during actions directed towards large objects (e.g., whole hand prehension). The most likely interpretation for visual discharge in these visuomotor neurons is that, at least in adult individuals, there is a close link between the most common three-dimensional stimuli and the actions necessary to interact with them. Thus, every time a graspable object is visually presented, the related F5 neurons are addressed and the action is "automatically" evoked. Under certain circumstances, it guides the execution of the movement; under others, it remains an unexecuted representation of it, which might be used also for semantic knowledge.

Mirror neurons, that become active when the monkey acts on an object and when it observes another monkey or the experimenter making a similar goal-directed action, appear to be identical to canonical neurons in terms of motor properties, but they radically differ from them as far as visual properties are concerned (Rizzolatti and Fadiga, 1998). In order to be triggered by visual stimuli, mirror neurons require an interaction between a biological effector (hand or mouth) and an object. The sights of an object alone, of an agent mimicking an action, or of an

individual making intransitive (non–object directed) gestures are all ineffective. The object significance for the monkey has no obvious influence on mirror neuron response. Grasping a piece of food or a geometric solid produces responses of the same intensity.

Mirror neurons show a large degree of generalization. Largely different visual stimuli, but representing the same action, are equally effective. For example, the same grasping mirror neuron that responds to a human hand grasping an object also responds when the grasping hand is that of a monkey. Similarly, the response is, typically, not affected if the action is done near or far from the monkey, despite of the fact that the size of the observed hand is obviously different in the two conditions. It is also of little importance for neuron activation if the observed action is eventually rewarded. The discharge is of the same intensity if the experimenter grasps the food and gives it to the recorded monkey or to another monkey, introduced in the experimental room. The observed actions which most commonly activate mirror neurons are grasping, placing, manipulating, and holding.

Most mirror neurons respond selectively to only one type of action (e.g., grasping). Some are highly specific, coding not only the type of action but also how that action is executed. They fire, for example, during observation of grasping movements but only when the object is grasped with the index finger and the thumb. Typically, mirror neurons show congruence between the observed and executed action. According to the type of congruence they exhibit, mirror neurons have been subdivided into "strictly congruent" and "broadly congruent" neurons (Gallese et al., 1996). Mirror neurons in which the effective observed and effective executed actions correspond in terms of goal (e.g., grasping) and means for reaching the goal (e.g., precision grip) have been classified as "strictly congruent." They represent about one third of F5 mirror neurons. Mirror neurons that, in order to be triggered, do not require the observation of exactly the same action that they code motorically have been classified as "broadly congruent." They represent about two thirds of F5 mirror neurons.

The early studies of mirror neurons concerned essentially the upper sector of F5 where hand actions are mostly represented. Recently, a study was carried on the properties of neurons located in the lateral part of F5 (Ferrari et al., 2003), where, in contrast, most neurons are related to mouth actions. The results showed that about 25% of studied neurons have mirror properties. According to the visual stimuli effective in triggering the neurons, two classes of mouth mirror neurons were distinguished: ingestive and communicative mirror neurons. Ingestive mirror neurons respond to the observation of actions related to ingestive functions, such as grasping food with the mouth, breaking it, or sucking. Neurons of this class form about 80% of the total amount of the recorded mouth mirror neurons. Virtually all ingestive mirror neurons show a good correspondence between the effective observed and the effective executed action. In about one third of them, the effective observed and executed actions are virtually identical (strictly congruent neurons); in the remaining, the effective observed and executed actions are similar or functionally related (broadly congruent neurons). More intriguing are the properties of the communicative mirror neurons. The most effective observed action is for them a communicative gesture such as lip smacking. However, as the ingestive mirror neurons, they strongly discharge when the monkey actively performs an ingestive action.

It seems plausible that the visual response of both canonical and mirror neurons addresses the same motor vocabulary, the words of which constitute the monkey motor repertoire. What is different is the way in which "motor words" are selected: in the case of canonical neurons, they are selected by object observation; in the case of mirror neurons, by the sight of an action. Thus, in the case of canonical neurons, vision of graspable objects activates the motor representations more appropriate to interact with those objects. In the case of mirror neurons, objects alone are no more sufficient to evoke a premotor discharge: what is necessary is a visual stimulus describing a goal-directed hand action in which both an acting hand and a target must be present.

Summarizing the evidence presented here, the monkey precursor of human Broca's area is a premotor area, representing hand and mouth goal-directed actions, provided with strong visual inputs coming from the inferior parietal lobule. These visual inputs originate in distinct parietal areas and convey distinct visual information: (1) object-related information, used by canonical neurons to motorically categorize objects and to organize the hand-object interaction, and (2) action-related information driving the response of mirror neurons during observation of action made by others.

WHICH ARE THE HUMAN AREAS ACTIVATED BY ACTION OBSERVATION?

The existence of a mirror-neuron system in humans has been first demonstrated by electrophysiological experiments. The first pioneer demonstration of a "visuomotor resonance" has been reported by Gastaut and Bert (1954) and Cohen-Seat et al. (1954). These authors showed that the observation of actions made by humans exerts a desynchronizing effect on the electroencephalogram recorded over motor areas, similar to that exerted by actual movements. Recently, more specific evidence in favor of the existence of a human mirror system arose from transcranial magnetic stimulation (TMS) studies of cortical excitability. Fadiga et al. (1995) stimulated the left motor cortex of normal subjects using TMS while they were observing meaningless intransitive arm movements as well as hand grasping movements performed by an experimenter. Motor evoked potentials (MEPs) were recorded from various arm and hand muscles. The rationale of the experiment was the following: If the mere observation of the hand and arm movements facilitates the motor system, this facilitation should determine an increase of MEPs recorded from hand and arm muscles. The results confirmed the hypothesis. A selective increase of MEPs was found in those muscles that the subjects would have used for producing the observed movements. Additionally, this experiment demonstrated that both goal-directed and intransitive arm movements were capable to evoke the motor facilitation. More recently, Strafella and Paus (2000) supported these findings and demonstrated the cortical nature of the facilitation.

The electrophysiological experiments just described, while fundamental in showing that action observation elicits a specific, coherent activation of motor system, do not allow the localization of the areas involved in the phenomenon. The first data on the anatomical localization of the human mirror-neuron system have been therefore obtained using brain-imaging techniques. PET and fMRI experiments, carried out by various groups, demonstrated that when the participants observed actions made by human arms or hands, activations were present in the ventral premotor/inferior frontal cortex (Decety and Chaminade, 2003; Decety et al., 1997; Grafton et al., 1996; Grèzes et al., 1998, 2003; Iacoboni et al., 1999; Rizzolatti et al., 1996b). As already mentioned for TMS experiments by Fadiga et al. (1995), both transitive (goal-directed) and intransitive meaningless gestures activate the mirror-neuron system in humans. Grèzes et al. (1998) investigated whether the same areas became active in the two conditions. Normal human volunteers were instructed to observe meaningful or meaningless actions. The results confirmed that the observation of meaningful hand actions activates the left inferior frontal gyrus (Broca's region), the left inferior parietal lobule plus various occipital and inferotemporal areas. An activation of the left precentral gyrus was also found. During meaningless gesture observation there was no Broca's region activation. Furthermore, in comparison with meaningful action observations, an increase was found in activation of the right posterior parietal lobule. More recently, two further studies have shown that a meaningful hand-object interaction more than pure movement observation is effective in triggering Broca's area activation (Hamzei et al., 2003; Johnson-Frey et al., 2003). Similar conclusions have been reached for mouth movement observation (Campbell et al., 2001).

In all early brain imaging experiments, the participants observed actions made by hands or arms. Recently, experiments were carried out to learn whether mirror system coded actions made by other effectors. Buccino et al. (2001) instructed participants to observe actions made by mouth, foot, and hand. The observed actions were biting an apple, reaching and grasping a ball or a small cup, and kicking a ball or pushing a brake (object-related actions). Similar actions but non–object-related (such as chewing) were also tested. The results showed that (1) During observation of non–object-related mouth actions (chewing), activation was present in areas 6 and in Broca's area on both sides, with a more anterior activation (BA45) in the right hemisphere. During object-related action (biting), the pattern of premotor activation was similar to that found during non–object-related action. In addition, two activation foci were found in the parietal lobe. (2) During the observation of non–object-related hand/arm actions there was a bilateral activation of area 6 that was located dorsally to that found during mouth movement observations. During the observation of object-related arm/hand actions (reaching-to-grasp-movements), there was a bilateral activation of premotor cortex plus an activation site in Broca's area. As in the case of observation of mouth movements, two activation foci were present in the parietal lobe. (3) During the observation of non–object-related foot actions there was an activation of a dorsal sector of area 6. During the observa-

tion of object-related actions, there was, as in the condition without object, an activation of a dorsal sector of area 6. In addition, there was an activation of the posterior part of the parietal lobe. Two are the main conclusions that can be drawn from these data. First, the mirror system is not limited to hand movements, Second, actions performed with different effectors are represented in different regions of the premotor cortex (somatotopy). Third, in agreement with previous data by Grèzes et al. (1998) and Iacoboni et al. (1999), the parietal lobe is part of the human mirror systems and it is strongly involved when an individual observes object-directed actions.

The experiments reviewed in this section tested subjects during action observation only. Therefore, the conclusion that frontal activated areas such as Broca's region have mirror properties was an indirect conclusion based on their premotor nature and, in the case of Broca's area, by its homology with monkey's premotor area F5. However, if one looks at the results of the brain imaging experiments reviewed in the second section of this chapter (*motor-related functions* of Broca's area), it appears clearly that Broca's area is an area becoming active not only during speech generation but also during real and imagined hand movements. If one combines these two observations, it appears that Broca's area might be the highest-order motor region where an observation/execution matching occurs. Direct evidence for an observation/execution matching system was recently provided by two experiments, one using fMRI technique (Iacoboni et al., 1999) and the other using event-related MEG (Nishitani and Hari, 2000).

Iacoboni et al. (1999) instructed normal human volunteers to observe and imitate a finger movement and to perform the same movement after a spatial or a symbolic cue (observation/execution tasks). In another series of trials, the same participants were asked to observe the same stimuli presented in the observation/execution tasks but without giving any response to them (observation tasks). The results showed that activation during imitation was significantly stronger than in the other two observation/execution tasks in three cortical areas: left inferior frontal cortex, right anterior parietal region, and right parietal operculum. The first two areas were active also during observation tasks, while the parietal operculum became active during observation/execution conditions only.

Nishitani and Hari (2000) addressed the same issue using event-related neuromagnetic recordings. In their experiments, normal human participants were requested, under different conditions, to grasp a manipulandum, to observe the same movement performed by an experimenter, and, finally, to observe and simultaneously replicate the observed action. Their results showed that during execution, there was an early activation in the left inferior frontal cortex (Broca's area) with a response peak appearing approximately 250 ms before the touch of the target. This activation was followed within 100 to 200 ms by activation of the left precentral motor area and 150 to 250 ms later by activation of the right one. During observation and during imitation, pattern and sequence of frontal activations were similar to those found during execution, but the frontal activations were preceded by an occipital activation due to visual stimulation occurring in the former conditions.

More recently, two studies of Koski and colleagues (2002, 2003) have made further steps toward the comprehension of imitation mechanism and its relation to Brodmann's area 44. First (Koski et al., 2002), they compared the activity evoked by imitation and observation of finger movements in the presence or conversely the absence of an explicit goal. They found that the presence of goal increases the activity observed in BA44 for the imitation task only. They concluded that imitation may represent a behavior tuned to replicate the goal of an action. Later, the same authors (Koski et al., 2003) investigated the potential difference between anatomical (actor and imitator both move the right hand) and specular imitation (the actor moves the left hand, the imitator moves the right hand as in a mirror). They demonstrated that the activation of Broca's area was present only during specular imitation. In sum, a growing amount of studies established the determinant role of Broca's area in distal and facial motor functions such as movement execution, observation, simulation, and imitation, emphasizing further the fundamental aspect of the goal of the action.

WHAT LINKS HAND ACTIONS WITH SPEECH?

Others' actions do not generate only visually perceivable signals. Action-generated sounds and noises are also very common in nature. One could expect, therefore, that also this sensory information, related to a particular action, could determine a motor activation specific for that same action. A very recent neurophysiological experiment addressed this point. Kohler and colleagues (2002) investigated whether there are neurons in area F5 that discharge when the monkey makes a specific hand action and also when it *hears* the corresponding action-related sounds. The experimental hypothesis started from the remark that a large number of object-related actions (e.g., breaking a peanut) can be recognized by a particular sound. The authors found that 13% of the investigated neurons discharge both when the monkey performed a hand action and when it heard the action-related sound. Moreover, most of these neurons discharge also when the monkey observed the same action demonstrating that these "audiovisual mirror neurons" represent actions independent of whether them are *performed*, *heard*, or *seen*.

The presence of an audio-motor resonance in a region that, in humans, is classically considered a speech-related area evokes the Liberman's hypothesis on the mechanism at the basis of speech perception (motor theory of speech perception, Liberman et al., 1967; Liberman and Mattingly, 1985; Liberman and Wahlen, 2000). The motor theory of speech perception maintains that the ultimate constituents of speech are not sounds but articulatory gestures that have evolved exclusively at the service of language. A cognitive translation into phonology is not necessary because the articulatory gestures are phonological in nature. Furthermore, speech perception and speech production processes use a common repertoire of motor primitives that, during speech production, are at the basis of articulatory gesture generation, while during speech perception, are activated in the listener as the result of an acoustically evoked motor "resonance." Thus, sounds conveying verbal communication are the vehicle of motor representations (articulatory gestures) shared by both the speaker and the listener, on which speech perception could be based upon. In other terms, the listener understands the speaker when his or her articulatory gestures representations are activated by verbal sounds.

Fadiga et al. (2002), in a TMS experiment based on the paradigm used in 1995 (Fadiga et al., 1995), tested for the presence in humans of a system that motorically "resonates" when the individuals listen to verbal stimuli. Normal subjects were requested to attend to an acoustically presented randomized sequence of disyllabic words, disyllabic pseudo-words and bitonal sounds of equivalent intensity and duration. Words and pseudo-words were selected according to a consonant-vowel-consonant-consonant-vowel (CVCCV) scheme. The embedded consonants in the

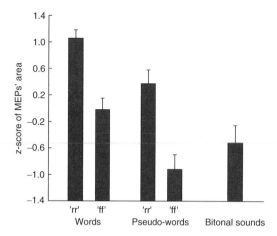

FIGURE 9–3. Average value (+SEM) of intrasubject normalized MEP total areas for each condition. Data from all subjects; 'rr' and 'ff' refer to verbal stimuli containing a double linguapalatal fricative consonant 'r' and containing a double labiodental fricative consonant 'f', respectively. (Modified from Iadija et al., 2002.)

middle of words and of pseudo-words were either a double 'f' (labiodental fricative consonant that, when pronounced, requires slight tongue tip mobilization) or a double 'r' (lingua-palatal fricative consonant that, when pronounced, requires strong tongue tip mobilization). Bitonal sounds, lasting about the same time as verbal stimuli and replicating their intonation pattern, were used as a control. The excitability of motor cortex in correspondence of tongue movements representation was assessed by using single-pulse TMS and by recording MEPs from the anterior tongue muscles. The TMS stimuli were applied synchronously with the double consonant of presented verbal stimuli (words and pseudo-words) and in the middle of the bitonal sounds. Results (see Fig. 9–3) showed that during speech listening there is an increase of motor evoked potentials recorded from the listeners' tongue muscles when the listened word strongly involves tongue movements, indicating that when an individual listens to verbal stimuli his/her speech related motor centers are specifically activated. Moreover, words-related facilitation was significantly larger than pseudo-words–related facilitation.

These results indicate that the passive listening to words that would involve tongue mobilization (when pronounced) induces an automatic facilitation of the listener's motor cortex. Furthermore, the effect is stronger in the case of words than in the case of pseudo-words, suggesting a possible unspecific facilitation of the motor speech center due to recognition that the presented material belongs to an extant word.

The presence of "audio-visual" mirror neurons in the monkey and the presence of "speech-related acoustic motor resonance" in humans indicate that independent of the sensory nature of the perceived stimulus, the mirror-resonant system retrieves from action vocabulary (stored in the frontal cortex) the stimulus-related motor representations. It is, however, unclear if the activation of the motor system during speech listening could be interpreted in terms of an involvement of motor representations in speech processing and, perhaps, perception. Studies of cortical stimulation during neurosurgery and clinical data from frontal aphasics suggest that this is the case (see earlier). However, all of these studies report that comprehension deficits become evident only in the case of complex sentences processing or complex commands accomplishment. Single words (particularly if nouns) are almost always correctly understood. To verify this observation, we applied repetitive TMS (rTMS, that functionally blocks for hundreds of milliseconds the stimulated area) on speech-related premotor centers during single word listening (Fadiga et al., unpublished observation). TMS was delivered on a site 2 cm anterior to the hot spot of the hand motor representation, as assessed during mapping sessions performed on individual subjects. At the end of each trial, participants were required to identify the listened word in a list presented on a computer screen. Data analysis showed that rTMS was ineffective in perturbing subject's performance. As expected, subjects were perfectly able to report the listened word independent of the presence or the absence of the stimulation, from the duration of stimulation itself and from the moment at which the stimulus was delivered with respect to the beginning of the presented word. If one accepts that Broca's region is not concerned with single-word perception but at the same time considers that this area has been classically considered the brain center more involved in phonological processing (at least in production), a possible contradiction emerges. In order to investigate more rigorously the perceptual role of Broca's area, we decided therefore to use an experimental paradigm very sensitive in detecting a possible phonological impairment following Broca's area inactivation. It should be noted, however, that although phonology, among various speech attributes is strictly related to the more motor aspects of speech (phonoarticulatory), this does not mean that other speech attributes, such as lexicon and syntax, are totally unrelated to motor representations. It is well known, in fact, that several Broca's aphasic patients present differential deficits in understanding nouns (less impaired) and verbs (more impaired, particularly in the case of action verbs) (see Bak et al., 2001).

With this aim we applied rTMS on Broca's region during a phoneme discrimination task in order to see if rTMS-induced inhibition was able to produce a specific "deafness" for the phonologic characteristics of the presented stimuli. Subjects were instructed to carefully listen to a sequence of acoustically presented pseudo-words and to categorize the stimuli according to their phonological characteristics by pressing one among four different switches (Craighero, Fadiga, and Haggard, unpublished data). Stimuli consisted of 80 pseudo-words subdivided into four different categories. Categories were formed according to the phonetic sequence of the middle part of the stimulus that could be "dada," "data," "tada," or "tata" (e.g., pipedadali, pelemodatalu, mamipotadame, pimatatape). Subjects had to press as soon as possible the button corresponding to stimulus category. Participants' left hemisphere was magnetically stimulated in three different regions by using rTMS: (a) the focus of the tongue motor representation, (b) a region 2 cm more anterior (ventral premotor/inferior frontal cortex), (c) a region 2 cm more posterior (somatosensory cortex). Repetitive transcranial magnetic stimulation was delivered at a frequency of 20 Hz in correspondence of the second critical formant, in correspondence of the first and of the second critical formants, and also during the whole critical portion of the presented word. The hypothesis was that rTMS delivered in correspondence of the speech-related premotor cortex, by determining the temporary inhibition of the resonance system, should induce slower reaction times and a significant higher amount of errors in the discrimination task with respect to the sessions in which other cortical regions were stimulated. Results, however, showed no difference between the performances obtained during the different experimental conditions (which also included a control without rTMS).

A possible interpretation of the absence of any effect of interference on phonologic perception could be that the discrimination task we used does not, indeed, involve a phonological perception. The task could be considered a mere discrimination task of the serial order of two different (not necessarily phonological) elements: the sound "TA" and the sound "DA." It is possible that the way in which the subjects solve the task is the same he or she would use in the case of two different tones and, possibly, involving structures different from the Broca's area. Another possible interpretation is that the used stimuli (pseudo-words) are treated by the brain as nonspeech stimuli, because they are semantically meaningless.

In order to be sure to investigate subjects with a task necessarily involving phonological perception, we decided to use a paradigm classically considered a phonological one: the "phonological priming" task. Phonological priming effect refers to the fact that a target word is recognized faster when it is preceded by a prime word sharing with it the last syllable (rhyming effect; Emmorey, 1989).

In a single-pulse TMS experiment, we therefore stimulated participants' inferior frontal cortex while they were performing a phonological priming task. Subjects were instructed to carefully listen to a sequence of acoustically presented pairs of verbal stimuli (dysillabic "CVCV" or "CVCCV" words and pseudo-words) in which final phonological overlap was present (rhyme prime) or, conversely, not present. Subjects were requested to make a lexical decision on the second stimulus (target) by pressing with index finger or middle finger one button if the target was a word and another button if the target was a pseudo-word.

The pairs of verbal stimuli could pertain to four categories which differed for presence of lexical content in the prime and in the target:

Prime-word/target-word (W-W)

Prime-word/target-pseudo-word (W-PW)

Prime-pseudo-word/target-word (PW-W)

Prime-pseudo-word/target-pseudo-word (PW-PW).

Each category contained both rhyming and nonrhyming pairs. In some randomly selected trials, we administered single-pulse TMS in correspondence of left BA44 (Broca's region, localized by using "Neurocompass," a frameless stereotactic system built in our laboratory) during the interval (20 ms) between prime and target stimuli.

In trials without TMS, these are the main results: (1) strong and statistically significant facilitation (phonological priming effect) when W-W, W-PW,

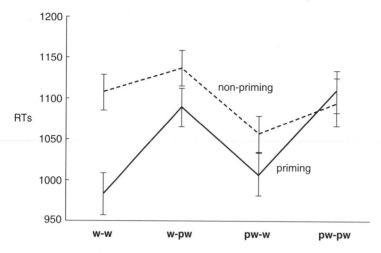

FIGURE 9–4. Reaction time (RTs) in milliseconds (+SEM) relative to the lexical decision during a phonological priming task. *Dotted line*, phonological overlap absent; *solid line*, phonological overlap pre-sent. w-w, prime-word/target-word; w-pw, prime-word/target-pseudo-word; pw-w, prime-pseudo-word/target-word; pw-pw, prime-pseudo-word/target-pseudo-word.

PW-W pairs are presented; (2) no phonological priming effect when the PW-PW pair is presented; and (3) faster responses when the target is a word rather than a pseudo-word (in both W-W and PW-PW) (Fig. 9–4).

An interesting finding emerges from the analysis of these results: the presence or absence of lexical content modulates the presence of the phonological priming effect. When neither the target nor the prime has the access to the lexicon (PW-PW pair), the presence of the rhyme does not facilitate the recognition of the target. In other words, in order to have a phonological effect it is necessary to have the access to the lexicon.

In trials during which TMS was delivered, only W-PW pairs were affected by brain stimulation: the W-PW pair behaving exactly as the PW-PW one. This finding suggests that the stimulation of the Broca's region might have affected the lexical property of the prime. As consequence, the impossibility to have access to the lexicon determines the absence of the phonological effect. According to our interpretation, the TMS-related effect is absent in the W-W and PW-W pairs because of the presence of a meaningful (W) target.

Being aware that a possible criticism to our data is that the task was implying a lexical decision, we replicated the experiment by asking subjects to detect if the final vowel of the target stimulus was A or O. Despite the absence of any lexicon-directed attention, the results were exactly the same as in the case of the lexical decision paradigm. Further experiments are now carried out in order to reinforce this observation. In particular, brain regions other that Broca's area will be stimulated in order to test the specificity of the observed effect.

CONCLUSIONS

The present chapter reviews some literature data and presents some experimental results showing that, in addition to speech-related tasks, Broca's area is also significantly involved during tasks devoid of verbal content. If in some cases one could advance the criticism that internal speech might have been at the origin of this activation, in other cases such possibility is ruled out by appropriate controls. As frequently happens in biology, when too much interpretations are proposed for an anatomic-functional correlate, one should strongly doubt each of them. We started from this skeptical point of view by making an attempt to correlate what was found with brain imaging in humans with what is known in monkeys at single-neuron level. The behavioral conditions triggering the response of neurons recorded in the monkey area that is more closely related to human Broca's (ventral premotor area F5) are (1) grasping with the hand and grasping with the mouth actions, (2) observation of graspable objects, (3) observation of hand/mouth actions performed by other individuals, and (4) hearing sounds produced during manipulative actions. The experimental evidence suggests that, in order to activate F5 neurons, executed/observed/heard actions must be all goal directed. Does the cytoarchitectonical homology, linking monkey area F5 with Broca's area, correspond to some functional homology? Does human Broca's area discharge during hand/mouth action execution/observation/hearing, too? Does make difference, in terms of Broca's activation, if observed actions are meaningful (goal directed) or meaningless? A positive answer to these questions comes from fMRI experiments in which human subjects are requested to execute goal-directed actions and are presented with the same visual stimuli effective in triggering F5 neurons' response (graspable objects or tools and actions performed by other individuals). Results show that in both cases, Broca's area become significantly active. Finally, it is interesting to note that observation of meaningless movements, while strongly activates human area 6 (bilaterally) is definitely less effective in activating Broca's region.

It has been suggested that a motor resonant system, such as that formed by mirror-neurons, might have given a neural substrate to interindividual communication (see Rizzolatti and Arbib, 1998). According to this view, speech may have evolved from a hand/mouth gestural communicative system. A complete theory on the origin of speech is, however, well beyond the scope of this chapter. Our aim in writing was to suggest to the readers some stimulating starting points and to make an attempt to conciliate two streams of research, which start from very different positions: the study of speech representation in humans and the study of hand action representation in monkeys. These two approaches reach a common target: the premotor region of the inferior frontal gyrus where Paul Broca first localized his "frontal speech area." The data presented in the last section of this chapter go in this direction and although they represent only an experimental starting point, we think that they already could allow some preliminary considerations and speculations.

The first important point is that the temporary inactivation of Broca's region during phonological tasks is ineffective in perturbing subjects' performance. This result is definitely against a "pure" phonological role of Broca's region. The interpretation we favor is that it is impossible to dissociate phonology from lex-

icon at Broca's level because there "exist" only words. In other terms, phonologically relevant stimuli are matched on a repertoire of words and not on individually meaningless, "phonemes assembly." Consequently, the motor resonance of tongue representation revealed by TMS during speech listening (Fadiga et al., 2002) is probably a mixed phenomenon that should involve cortical regions others than Broca's area (possibly BA6) being this "acoustically evoked mirror effect" independent of the meaning of the presented stimuli. The motor representation of hand/mouth actions present in Broca's area derives from an ancient execution/observation (hearing) matching system, already present in monkeys. As a consequence, forms of communication other than the verbal one, although expressions of a residual ancient mechanism, should exert a significant effect on Broca's area benefiting of its twofold involvement with motor goals: during execution of own actions and during perception of others' ones. We will investigate this topic in the near future by using brain-imaging techniques.

The intimate *motor* nature of Broca's region cannot be neglected when interpreting the results of experiments testing hypotheses apparently far from pure motor tasks. The hypothesis we suggest here (being aware of its purely speculative nature) is that the original role played by this region in generating/extracting action meanings (by organizing/interpreting motor sequences of individually meaningless movements) might have been generalized during evolution giving to this area a new capability. The capability to deal with meanings (and rules) that share with the motor system similar hierarchical and sequential structures harmonized by a general, supramodal "syntax."

ACKNOWLEDGMENTS   The research presented in this chapter is supported in the framework of the European Science Foundation EUROCORES program "The Origin of Man, Language and Languages", by EC "MIRROR" Contract and by Italian Ministry of Education Grants. The authors deeply thank G. Spidalieri for his fruitful comments on early versions of the manuscript.

This chapter is dedicated to the memory of Massimo Matelli.

References

Amunts, K., Schleicher, A., Burgel, U., Mohlberg, H., Uylings, H.B., & Zilles, K. (1999). Broca's region revisited: Cytoarchitecture and intersubject variability. *Journal of Comparative Neurology, 412,* 319–341.

Arbib, M.A. (1997). From visual affordances in monkey parietal cortex to hippocampo-parietal interactions underlying rat navigation. *Philosophical Transactions of the Royal Society of London B Biology, 352,* 1429–1436.

Bak, T.H., O'Donovan, D.G., Xuereb, J.H., Boniface, S., & Hodges, J.R. (2001). Selective impairment of verb processing associated with pathological changes in Brodmann areas 44 and 45 in the motor neurone disease-dementia-aphasia syndrome. *Brain, 124,* 103–120.

Bell, B.D. (1994). Pantomime recognition impairment in aphasia: An analysis of error types. *Brain and Language, 47,* 269–278.

Bharucha, J., & Krumhansl, C. (1983). The representation of harmonic structure in music: Hierarchies of stability as a function of context. *Cognition, 13,* 63–102.

Binkofski, F., Amunts, K., Stephan, K.M., Posse, S., Schormann, T., Freund, H.J., et al. (2000). Broca's region subserves imagery of motion: A combined cytoarchitectonic and fMRI study. *Human Brain Mapping, 11,* 273–285.

Binkofski, F., Buccino, G., Posse, S., Seitz, R.J., Rizzolatti, G., & Freund, H.-J. (1999a). A fronto-parietal circuit for object manipulation in man: evidence from an fMRI study. *European Journal of Neuroscience, 11,* 3276–3286.

Binkofski, F., Buccino, G., Stephan, K.M., Rizzolatti, G., Seitz, R.J., & Freund, H.-J. (1999b). A parieto-premotor network for object manipulation: evidence from neuroimaging. *Experimental Brain Research, 128,* 21–31.

Broca, P.P. (1861). Loss of speech, chronic softening and partial destruction of the anterior left lobe of the brain. *Bulletin de la Société Anthropologique, 2,* 235–238.

Buccino, G., Binkofski, F., Fink, G.R., Fadiga, L., Fogassi, L., Gallese, V., et al. (2001). Action observation activates premotor and parietal areas in a somatotopic manner: An fMRI study. *European Journal of Neuroscience, 13,* 400–404.

Campbell, R., MacSweeney, M., Surguladze, S., Calvert, G., McGuire, P., Suckling, J., et al. (2001). Cortical substrates for the perception of face actions: An fMRI study of the specificity of activation for seen speech and for meaningless lower-face acts (gurning). *Cognitive Brain Research, 12,* 233–243.

Cohen-Seat, G., Gastaut, H., Faure, J., & Heuyer, G. (1954). Etudes expérimentales de l'activité nerveuse pendant la projection cinématographique. *Revue Internationale de Filmologie, 5,* 7–64.

Daniloff, J.K., Noll, J.D., Fristoe, M., & Lloyd, L.L. (1982). Gesture recognition in patients with aphasia. *Journal of Speech and Hearing Disorders, 47,* 43–49.

Decety, J., & Chaminade, T. (2003). Neural correlates of feeling sympathy. *Neuropsychologia, 41,* 127–138.

Decety, J., Grezes, J., Costes, N., Perani, D., Jeannerod, M., Procyk, E., et al. (1997). Brain activity during observation of actions: Influence of action content and subject's strategy. *Brain, 120,* 1763–1777.

Delazer, M., Domhas, F., Bartha, L., Brenneis, A., Lochy, A., Trieb, T., et al. (2003). Learning complex arithmetic: An fMRI study. *Cognitive Brain Research, 18,* 76–88.

Di Pellegrino, G., Fadiga, L., Fogassi, L., Gallese, V., & Rizzolatti, G. (1992). Understanding motor events: A neurophysiological study. *Experimental Brain Research, 91,* 176–180.

Duffy, R.J., & Duffy, J.R. (1975). Pantomime recognition in aphasics. *Journal of Speech and Hearing Research, 18,* 115–132.

Duffy, R.J., & Duffy, J.R. (1981). Three studies of deficits in pantomimic expression and pantomimic recognition in aphasia. *Journal of Speech and Hearing Research, 24,* 70–84.

Emmorey, K.D. (1989). Auditory morphological priming in the lexicon. *Language and Cognitive Processes, 4,* 73–92.

Ertl, J., & Schafer, E.W. (1967). Cortical activity preceding speech. *Life Sciences, 6,* 473–479.

Fadiga, L., Craighero, L., Buccino, G., & Rizzolatti, G. (2002). Speech listening specifically modulates the excitability of tongue muscles: A TMS study. *European Journal of Neuroscience, 15,* 399–402.

Fadiga, L., Fogassi, L., Pavesi, G., & Rizzolatti, G. (1995). Motor facilitation during action observation: A magnetic stimulation study. *Journal of Neurophysiology, 73,* 2608–2611.

Ferrari, P.F., Gallese, V., Rizzolatti, G., & Fogassi, L. (2003). Mirror neurons responding to the observation of ingestive and communicative mouth actions in the monkey ventral premotor cortex. *European Journal of Neuroscience, 17,* 1703–1714.

Gainotti, G., & Lemmo, M.S. (1976). Comprehension of symbolic gestures in aphasia. *Brain and Language, 3,* 451–460.

Gallese, V., Fadiga, L., Fogassi, L., & Rizzolatti, G. (1996). Action recognition in the premotor cortex. *Brain, 119,* 593–609.

Gastaut, H.J., & Bert, J. (1954). EEG changes during cinematographic presentation. *Electroencephalography and Clinical Neurophysiology, 6,* 433–444.

Gerardin, E., Sirigu, A., Lehéricy, S., Poline, J.-B., Gaymard, B., Marsault, C., et al. (2000). Partially overlapping neural networks for real and imagined hand movements. *Cerebral Cortex, 10,* 1093–1104.

Gerlach, C., Law, I., Gade, A., & Paulson, O.B. (2002). The role of action knowledge in the comprehension of artefacts: A PET study. *Neuroimage, 15,* 143–152.

Glosser, G., Wiener, M., & Kaplan, E. (1986). Communicative gestures in aphasia. *Brain and Language, 27,* 345–359.

Goldenberg, G. (1996). Defective imitation of gestures in patients with damage in the left or right hemispheres. *Journal of Neurology, Neurosurgery and Psychiatry, 61,* 176–180.

Grafton, S.T., Arbib, M.A., Fadiga, L., & Rizzolatti, G. (1996). Localization of grasp representations in humans by PET: 2. Observation compared with imagination. *Experimental Brain Research, 112,* 103–111.

Grezes, J., Armony, J.L., Rowe, J., & Passingham, R.E. (2003). Activations related to "mirror" and "canonical" neurones in the human brain: An fMRI study. *Neuroimage, 18,* 928–937.

Grezes, J., Costes, N., & Decety, J. (1998). Top-down effect of strategy on the perception of human biological motion: A PET investigation. *Cognitive Neuropsychology, 15,* 553–582.

Grezes, J., & Decety, J. (2002). Does visual perception of object afford action? Evidence from a neuroimaging study. *Neuropsychologia, 40,* 212–222.

Gruber, O., Inderfey, P., Steinmeiz, H., & Kleinschmidt, A. (2001). Dissociating neural correlates of cognitive components in mental calculation. *Cerebral Cortex, 11,* 350–359.

Hamzei, F., Rijntjes, M., Dettmers, C., Glauche, V., Weiller, C., & Buchel, C. (2003). The human action recognition system and its relationship to Broca's area: An fMRI study. *Neuroimage, 19,* 637–644.

Hepp-Reymond, M.C., Husler, E.J., Maier, M.A., & Qi, H.X. (1994). Force-related neuronal activity in two regions of the primate ventral premotor cortex. *Canadian Journal of Physiology and Pharmacology, 72,* 571–579.

Iacoboni, M., Woods, R., Brass, M., Bekkering, H., Mazziotta, J.C., & Rizzolatti, G. (1999). Cortical mechanisms of human imitation. *Science, 286,* 2526–2528.

Johnson-Frey, S.H., Maloof, F.R., Newman-Norlund, R., Farrer, C., Inati, S., & Grafton, S.T. (2003). Actions or hand-object interactions? Human inferior frontal cortex and action observation. *Neuron, 39,* 1053–1058.

Kellenbach, M.L., Brett, M., & Patterson, K. (2003). Actions speak louder than functions: the importance of manipulability and action in tool representation. *Journal of Cognitive Neuroscience, 15,* 30–45.

Koelsch, S., Gunter, T., Friederici, A.D., & Schroger, E. (2000). Brain indices of music processing: "Nonmusicians" are musical. *Journal of Cognitive Neuroscience, 12,* 520–541.

Kohler, E., Keysers, C.M., Umiltà, A., Fogassi, L., Gallese, V., & Rizzolatti, G. (2002). Hearing sounds, understanding actions: Action representation in mirror neurons. *Science, 297,* 846–848.

Koski, L., Iacoboni, M., Dubeau, M.-C., Woods, R.P., & Mazziotta, J.C. (2003). Modulation of cortical activity during different imitative behaviors. *Journal of Neurophysiology, 89,* 460–471.

Koski, L., Wohlschlager, A., Bekkering, H., Woods, R.P., Dubeau, M.-C., Mazziotta, J.C., & Iacoboni, M. (2002). Modulation of motor and premotor activity during imitation of target-directed actions. *Cerebral Cortex, 12,* 847–855.

Lacquaniti, F., Perani, D., Guignon, E., Bettinardi, V., Carrozzo, M., Grassi, F., et al. (1997). Visuomotor transformations for reaching to memorized targets: A PET study. *Neuroimage, 5,* 129–146.

Lelord, G., Laffont, F., Sauvage, D., & Jusseaume, P. (1973). Evoked slow activities in man following voluntary movement and articulated speech. *Electroencephalography Clinical Neurophysiology, 35,* 113–124.

Liberman, A.M., & Mattingly, I.G. (1985). The motor theory of speech perception revised. *Cognition, 21,* 1–36.

Liberman, A.M., & Wahlen, D.H. (2000). On the relation of speech to language. *Trends in Cognitive Neuroscience, 4,* 187–196.

Liberman, A.M., Cooper, F.S., Shankweiler, D.P., & Studdert-Kennedy, M. (1967). Perception of the speech code. *Psychological Review, 74,* 431–461.

Liotti, M., Gay, C.T., & Fox, P.T. (1994). Functional imaging and language: Evidence from positron emission tomography. *Journal of Clinical Neurophysiology, 11,* 175–190.

Maess, B., Koelsch, S., Gunter, T.C., & Friederici, A.D. (2001). Musical syntax is processed in Broca's area: An MEG study. *Nature Neuroscience, 4,* 540–545.

Matelli, M., Luppino, G., & Rizzolatti, G. (1985). Patterns of cytochrome oxidase activity in the frontal agranular cortex of macaque monkey. *Behavioral Brain Research, 18,* 125–137.

Matsumura, M., Kawashima, R., Naito, E., Satoh, K., Takahashi, T., Yanagisawa, T., et al. (1996). Changes in rCBF during grasping in humans examined by PET. *NeuroReport, 7,* 749–752.

Mecklinger, A., Gruenewald, C., Besson, M., Magnié, M.-N., & Von Cramon, Y. (2002). Separable neuronal circuitries for manipulable and non-manipulable objects in working memory. *Cerebral Cortex, 12,* 1115–1123.

Menon, V., Rivera, S.M., White, C.D., Glover, G.H., & Reiss, A.L. (2000). Dissociating prefrontal and parietal cortex activation during arithmetic processing. *Neuroimage, 12,* 357–365.

Mingazzini, G. (1908). Lezioni di anatomia clinica dei centri nervosi. Torino: UTET.

Muller, R.-A., Kleinhans, N., & Courchesne, E. (2001). Broca's area and the discrimination of frequency transitions: A functional MRI study. *Brain and Language, 76,* 70–76.

Murata, A., Fadiga, L., Fogassi, L., Gallese, V., Raos, V., & Rizzolatti, G. (1997). Object representation in the ventral premotor cortex (area F5) of the monkey. *Journal of Neurophysiology, 78,* 2226–2230.

Negawa, T., Mizuno, S., Hahashi, T., Kuwata, H., Tomida, M., Hoshi, H., et al. (2002). M pathway and areas 44 and 45 are involved in stereoscopic recognition based on binocular disparity. *Japanese Journal of Physiology, 52,* 191–198.

Nishitani, N., & Hari, R. (2000). Temporal dynamics of cortical representation for action. *Proceedings of the National Academy of Sciences USA, 97,* 913–918.

Papathanassiou, D., Etard, O., Mellet, E., Zago, L., Mazoyer, B., & Tzourio-Mazoyer, N. (2000). A common language network for comprehension and production: A contribution to the definition of language epicenters with PET. *Neuroimage, 11,* 347–357.

Patel, A.D., Gibson, E., Ratner, J., Besson, M., & Holcomg, P. (1998). Processing syntactic relations in language and music: An event-related potential study. *Journal of Cognitive Neuroscience, 10,* 717–733.

Penfield, W., & Roberts, L. (1959). *Speech and brain mechanisms.* Princeton, NJ: Princeton University Press.

Petrides, M., & Pandya, D.N. (1997). Comparative architectonic analysis of the human and the macaque frontal cortex. In *Handbook of neuropsychology* (pp. 17–58), edited by F. Boller & J. Grafman. New York: Elsevier.

Ranganath, C., Johnson, M., & D'esposito, M. (2003). Prefrontal activity associated with working memory and episodic long-term memory. *Neuropsychologia, 41,* 378–389.

Rickard, T.C., Romero, S.G., Basso, G., Wharton, C., Flitman, S., & Grafman, J. (2000). The calculating brain: An fMRI study. *Neuropsychologia, 38,* 325–335.

Rizzolatti, G., & Arbib, M.A. (1998). Language within our grasp. *Trends in Neuroscience, 21,* 188–194.

Rizzolatti, G., & Fadiga, L. (1998). Grasping objects and grasping action meanings: The dual role of monkey rostroventral premotor cortex (area F5). In G.R. Bock & J.A. Goode (Eds.), *Sensory guidance of movement, Novartis Foundation Symposium* (pp. 81–103). Chichester: John Wiley and Sons.

Rizzolatti, G., & Gentilucci, M. (1988). Motor and visual-motor functions of the premotor cortex. In P. Rakic & W. Singer (Eds.), *Neurobiology of Neocortex* (pp. 269–284). Chichester: John Wiley and Sons.

Rizzolatti, G., Camarda, R., Fogassi, L., Gentilucci, M., Luppino, G., & Matelli, M. (1988). Functional organization of inferior area 6 in the macaque monkey: II. Area F5 and the control of distal movements. *Experimental Brain Research, 71,* 491–507.

Rizzolatti, G., Fadiga, L., Gallese, V., & Fogassi, L. (1996a). Premotor cortex and the recognition of motor actions. *Cognitive Brain Research, 3,* 131–141.

Rizzolatti, G., Fadiga, L., Matelli, M., Bettinardi, V., Paulesu, E., Perani, D., et al. (1996b). Localization of grasp representation in humans by PET: 1. Observation versus execution. *Experimental Brain Research, 111,* 246–252.

Rizzolatti, G., Fogassi, L., & Gallese, V. (2003). Motor and cognitive functions of the ventral premotor cortex. *Current Opinion in Neurobiology, 12,* 149–154.

Schaffler, L., Luders, H.O., Dinner, D.S., Lesser, R.P., & Chelune, G.J. (1993). Comprehension deficits elicited by electrical stimulation of Broca's area. *Brain, 116,* 695–715.

Schubotz, R.I., & von Cramon, D.Y. (2003). Functional-anatomical concepts of human premotor cortex: Evidence from fMRI and PET studies. *Neuroimage, 20,* Suppl 1, 120–131.

Strafella, A.P., & Paus, T. (2000). Modulation of cortical excitability during action observation: A transcranial magnetic stimulation study. *NeuroReport, 11,* 2289–2292.

10

Broca's Area in System Perspective: Language in the Context of Action-Oriented Perception

Michael Arbib

The mirror system hypothesis of Rizzolatti and Arbib (1998) gave an evolutionary account of the readiness of the human brain for language, informed by homologies between areas of the human (Fig. 10–1A) and macaque (Fig. 10–1B) brains.[1] The generally accepted view of human cortical areas involved in language gives special prominence to Broca's area and Wernicke's area (although many other areas are also implicated), both lateralized in the left hemisphere for most humans. *Broca's area* is located on the inferior frontal gyrus (pars triangularis and opercularis), and comprises BA (Brodmann area) 44 and BA 45. Some publications use the term Broca's area for BAs 44, 45, and 47; others use it for BA 44 only. *Wernicke's area* is located in the posterior part of the superior temporal gyrus and in the floor of the Sylvian sulcus. It corresponds to the posterior part of BA 22, or area Tpt (temporoparietal) as defined by Galaburda and Sanides (1980). Lesion-based views of Wernicke's area may include not only the posterior part of BA 22

but also (in whole or in part) areas 42, 39, 40, and perhaps 37.

Where Rizzolatti and Arbib (1998) focused on the homology between Broca's area and macaque premotor area F5, the present paper (following Arbib and Bota, 2003) treats other areas as well, placing Broca's area in a systems perspective as part of a network of brain regions whose interactions collectively support language. The account is incomplete, but is informed by lessons learned from computational models of (more or less) homologous areas of the macaque brain.

In my view, a neurolinguistic approach to language is part of a performance approach that explicitly analyzes both perception and production (Fig. 10–2). For production, we have much that we could possibly talk about which might be represented as cognitive structures (cognitive form; schema assemblages [see Schema Theory for more on schemas]) from which some aspects are selected for possible expres-

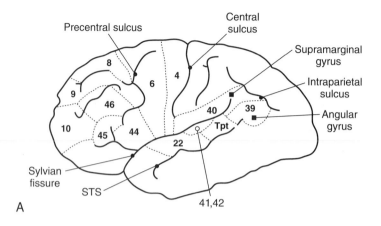

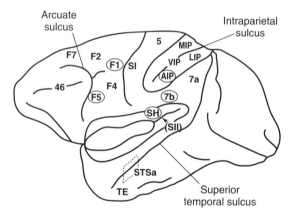

FIGURE 10–1. (A) Lateral view of the left hemisphere of the human brain (after Aboitiz and García, 1997) showing various sulci as well as various cortical areas (numbered according to Brodmann). Tpt, temporoparietal area. (B) A side view of the left hemisphere of the macaque brain (adapted from Jeannerod et al., 1995). Area 7b is also known as area PF. MIP, LIP, VIP, AIP, medial, lateral, ventral, and anterior regions of the intraparietal sulcus; SII, secondary somatosensory cortex; STSa, part of the superior temporal sulcus; TE, the temporal pole.

sion. Further selection and transformation yield semantic structures (hierarchical constituents expressing objects, actions, and relationships) that constitute a semantic form. Finally, the ideas in the semantic form must be expressed in phonological form, that is, as words whose markings and ordering reflect the relationships within semantic form—where, here, I extend phonological form to embrace a wide range of ordered expressive gestures that may include speech, sign, and orofacial expressions. For example, perception of a visual scene may interpret the visual input through an assemblage of perceptual schema instances to reveal "Who is doing what and to whom/which" as part of a nonlinguistic *action-object frame* in cognitive form. By contrast, the *verb-argument structure* is an overt linguistic representation in semantic form—in modern human languages, generally the ac-

tion is named by a verb and the objects are named by nouns or noun phrases (see Arbib, 2005b, Section 7). For perception, the received sentence must be interpreted semantically with the result updating the hearer's cognitive structures.

In many approaches to linguistics, a grammar is viewed as a storehouse of syntactic and other knowledge that can be invoked by mechanisms for both the production and understanding of sentences. However, paralleling the notion of direct and inverse model in motor control, I would argue that this "knowledge" is embedded in two different subsystems. A *production grammar* for a language is then a specific mechanism (whether explicit or implicit) for converting semantic structures into phonological structures—e.g., verb-argument structures into strings of words (and hierarchical compounds of verb-argument structures into

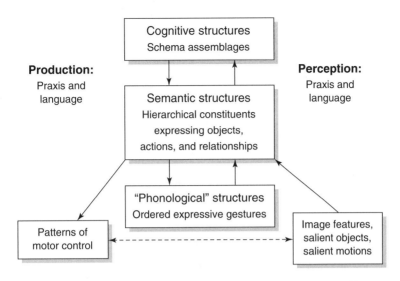

FIGURE 10–2. A performance view of the production and perception of language.

complex sentences)—and vice versa for a *perception grammar*. However, the study of grammars is beyond the scope of this chapter.

SCHEMA THEORY

The workshop on which this volume is based exhibited a tension between a concern with structures (such as Broca's area) and functions (such as those impaired in Broca's aphasia). As such analyses reveal, there is no one-to-one correlation between areas and functions. Arbib (1981; Arbib et al., 1998, Chapter 3) offers a version of *schema theory* to complement neuroscience's terminology for levels of *structural* analysis with a framework for analysis of *function* with no necessary commitment to hypotheses on the localization of each *schema* (unit of functional analysis).

A schema expresses a function that need not be co-extensive with the activity of any single neuronal circuit. Schema-based modeling becomes part of neuroscience when hypotheses on the distribution of schemas across a network of brain regions and neural circuitry is constrained by data provided by, for example, human brain mapping, studies of the effects of brain lesions, or neurophysiology.

Schemas for Perceptual Structures and Distributed Motor Control

A schema is what is learned about some aspect of the world, combining knowledge with the processes for

applying it; a *schema instance* is an active deployment of these processes. Central to my approach is *action-oriented perception*, as the "active organism" seeks from the world the information it needs to pursue its chosen course of action. A *perceptual schema* not only determines whether a given "domain of interaction" (an action-oriented generalization of the notion of object) is present in the environment but can also provide parameters concerning the current relationship of the organism with that domain. *Motor schemas* provide the control systems which can be coordinated to effect the wide variety of movement.

Schema instances may be combined (possibly with those of more abstract schemas, including coordinating schemas) to form *schema assemblages*. For example, an assemblage of perceptual schema instances may combine an estimate of environmental state with a representation of goals and needs. A *coordinated control program* is a schema assemblage which processes input via perceptual schemas and delivers its output via motor schemas, interweaving the activations of these schemas in accordance with the current task and sensory environment to mediate more complex behaviors.

Figure 10–3 shows the original coordinated control program (Arbib, 1981, analyzing data of Jeannerod and Biguer, 1982). As the hand moves to grasp an object, it is *preshaped* so that when it has almost reached the ball, it is of the right shape and orientation to enclose some part of the object prior to gripping it firmly. Moreover (to a first approximation), the movement can be broken into a fast phase and a slow

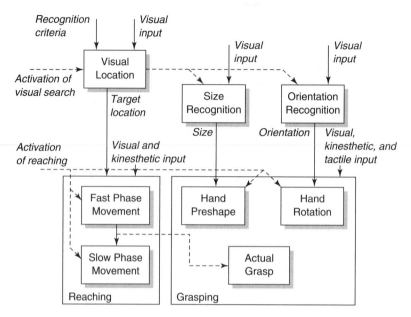

FIGURE 10–3. Hypothetical coordinated control program for reaching and grasping. Note that different perceptual schemas are required for the control of "reaching" (arm transport ≈ hand reaching) and "grasping" (controlling the hand to conform to the object). Note too the timing relations posited here within the "Hand Reaching" motor schema and between the motor schema for "Hand Reaching" and "Grasping." *Dashed lines,* activation signals; *solid lines,* transfer of data. (Adapted from Arbib, 1981.)

phase. The output of three perceptual schemas is available for the control of the hand movement by concurrent activation of two motor schemas, one controlling the arm to transport the hand toward the object and the other preshaping the hand. Once the hand is preshaped, it is only the completion of the fast phase of hand transport that "wakes up" the final stage of the grasping schema to shape the fingers under control of tactile feedback. (This model anticipates the much later discovery of perceptual schemas for grasping in a localized area [AIP] of parietal cortex and motor schemas for grasping in a localized area [F5] of premotor cortex; see below.) Jeannerod (1997) surveys the role of schemas and other constructs in the cognitive neuroscience of action; schemas have also played an important role in the development of behavior-based robots (Arkin, 1998).

VISIONS: Schemas for Visual Scene Understanding

An early example of schema-based interpretation for visual scene analysis in the VISIONS system (Arbib, 1989, Section 5.3; Draper et al., 1989). Low-level processes take an image of an outdoor visual scene and extract an *intermediate representation*—including contours and surfaces tagged with features such as color, texture, shape, size, and location. Perceptual schemas process different features of the intermediate representation to form confidence values for the presence of objects like houses, walls, and trees. The knowledge required for interpretation is stored in LTM (long-term memory) as a network of schemas, while the state of interpretation of the particular scene unfolds in STM (short-term or working memory) as a network of schema instances (Fig. 10–4). Note that this STM is not defined in terms of recency (as in very short term memory) but rather in terms of continuing relevance.

Interpretation of a novel scene starts with the data-driven instantiation of several schemas (e.g., a certain range of color and texture might cue an instance of the foliage schema for a certain region of the image). When a schema instance is activated, it is linked with an associated area of the image and an associated set of local variables. Each schema instance in STM has an associated confidence level that changes on the basis of interactions with other units in STM. The STM

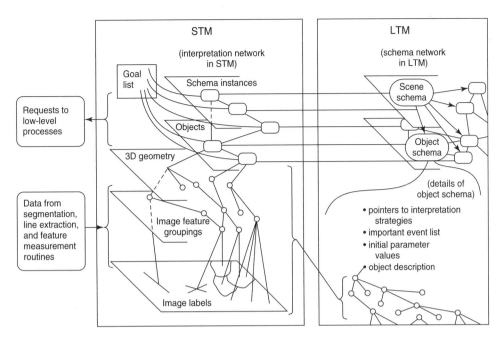

FIGURE 10–4. The VISIONS paradigm for cooperative computation in visual scene analysis. Interpretation strategies are stored in schemas that are linked in a schema network in long-term memory (LTM). Under the guidance of these schemas, the intermediate representation is modified and interpreted by a network of schema instances that label regions of the image and link them to a three-dimensional geometry in short-term memory (STM). (From Arbib, 1989, after Weymouth, 1986.)

network makes context explicit: each object represents a context for further processing. Thus, once several schema instances are active, they may instantiate others in a "hypothesis-driven" way (e.g., recognizing what appears to be a roof will activate an instance of the house schema to seek confirming evidence in the region below that of the putative roof). Ensuing computation is based on the competition and cooperation of concurrently active schema instances. Once a number of schema instances have been activated, the schema network is invoked to formulate hypotheses, set goals, and then iterate the process of adjusting the activity level of schemas linked to the image until a coherent scene interpretation of (part of) the scene is obtained. Cooperation yields a pattern of "strengthened alliances" between mutually consistent schema instances that allows them to achieve high activity levels to constitute the overall solution of a problem. As a result of competition, instances that do not meet the evolving consensus lose activity and thus are not part of this solution (though their continuing subthreshold activity may well affect later behavior). Successful instances of perceptual schemas become part of the current short-term model of the environment.

From Vision to Action and Working Memory

As exemplified in the VISIONS system, schema-based modeling of action-oriented perception views the STM of an organism as an assemblage combining an estimate of environmental state via instances of perceptual schemas. LTM is provided by the stock of schemas from which STM may be assembled. New sensory input as well as internal processes can update STM. Moving beyond visual STM for objects in retinotopic location, note that in action-oriented perception current sensory stimulation is always interpreted within the ongoing state of the organism. Thus, in general, STM is dynamic and task oriented and must include a representation of goals and needs, linking instances of perceptual schemas to motor schemas, providing parameters and changing confidence levels. As their activity levels reach threshold, certain motor schemas create patterns of overt behavior. To see this, consider a driver instructed to "Turn right at the red barn." At first the person drives along looking for something large and red, after which the perceptual schema for barns is brought to bear.

Once a barn is identified, the emphasis shifts to recognition of spatial relations appropriate to executing a right turn "at" the barn but determined rather by the placement of the roadway, etc.

All this is "planning" in a flexible representation strongly conditioned by current goals. Arbib and Liaw (1995) thus suggested extending VISIONS by the inclusion of motor as well as perceptual schemas and the dynamic interaction of working memory with changing sensory input. Activity in inferotemporal cortex accentuates perceptual schemas for the current focus of attention. In this case, only a few intermediate schemas may be active, with STM being updated as new results come in from this focal processing. This leads us to reverse the view of activity/passivity of schemas and instances in the VISIONS system. There, the schema in LTM is the passive code for processes (the program for deciding if a region is a roof, for example), while the schema instance is an active copy of that process (the execution of that program to test a particular region for "roofness"). By contrast, it may be that in the brain, the active circuitry is the *schema*, so that only one or a few instances can apply data-driven updating at a time. Rolls and Arbib (2003) outline how the general schema architecture integrates the "what" system (inferotemporal cortex) and the various "how" systems (posterior parietal cortex), while the MNS model (Oztop and Arbib, 2002) exemplifies this for the special case of grasping an object.

Such considerations offer a different perspective on the neuropsychological view of working memory offered by Baddeley (2003). The initial three-component model of working memory proposed by Baddeley and Hitch (1974) posits a *central executive* (an attentional controller) coordinating two subsidiary systems: the *phonological loop*, capable of holding speech-based information, and the *visuospatial sketchpad*. However, the latter is passive, because the emphasis of Baddeley's work has been on the role of working memory in sentence processing. Baddeley (2003) added an episodic LTM to the Baddeley-Hitch model, with the ability to hold language information complementing the phonological loop and (the idea is less well developed) an LTM for visual semantics complementing the visuospatial sketchpad. He further adds an *episodic buffer*, controlled by the central executive, which is assumed to provide a temporary interface between the phonological loop and the visuospatial sketchpad and LTM. The Arbib-Liaw scheme seems far more general, because it integrates dynamic visual analysis with the ongoing control of action.[2] As such, it seems better suited to encompass Emmorey's notion (this volume) of a visuospatial phonological short-term store. With this, let us see how the above ideas play out in the domain of speech understanding.

HEARSAY: Schemas for Speech Understanding

Jackendoff (2002) makes much use of the AI notion of blackboard in presenting his architecture for language, but does not cite HEARSAY-II (Lesser et al., 1975), perhaps the first AI system to develop a blackboard architecture.[3] While obviously not the state of the art, it is of interest because it foreshadows features of Jackendoff's architecture. Digitized speech data provide input at the *parameter level*; the output at the *phrasal level* interprets the speech signal as a sequence of words with associated syntactic and semantic structure. Because of ambiguities in the spoken input, a variety of hypotheses must be considered. To keep track of all these hypotheses, HEARSAY uses a dynamic global data structure, called the *blackboard*, partitioned into various levels; processes called *knowledge sources* act upon hypotheses at one level to generate hypotheses at another. First, a knowledge source takes data from the *parameter level* to hypothesize a phoneme at the *surface-phonemic level*. Many different phonemes may be posted as possible interpretations of the same speech segment. A lexical knowledge source takes phoneme hypotheses and finds words in its dictionary that are consistent with the phoneme data—thus posting hypotheses at the *lexical level* and allowing certain phoneme hypotheses to be discarded. These hypotheses are akin to the schema instances of the VISIONS system (Fig. 10–4).

To obtain hypotheses at the *phrasal level*, knowledge sources embodying syntax and semantics are brought to bear. Each hypothesis is annotated with a number expressing the current confidence level assigned to it. Each hypothesis is explicitly linked to those it supports at another level. Knowledge sources cooperate and compete to limit ambiguities. In addition to data-driven processing which works upward, HEARSAY also uses hypothesis-driven processing so that when a hypothesis is formed on the basis of partial data, a search may be initiated to find supporting data at lower levels. A hypothesis activated with sufficient confidence will provide context for determination of other hypotheses. However, such an *island of reliability* need not survive into the final interpretation of the sentence. All we can ask is that it forwards the process, which eventually yields this interpretation.

Arbib and Caplan (1979) discussed how the knowledge sources of HEARSAY, which were scheduled serially, might be replaced by schemas distributed across the brain to capture the spirit of "distributed localization" of Luria (e.g., 1973). Today, advances in the understanding of distributed computation and the flood of brain imaging data make the time ripe for a new push at a neurolinguistics informed by the understanding of cooperative computation.

THE MIRROR SYSTEM HYPOTHESIS

Elsewhere in this volume, Fadiga has summarized the neurobiology of macaque canonical and mirror neurons (see Rizzolatti et al., 2002, and Rizzolatti and Craighero, 2004, for further details and references). Here, we briefly present two computational models.

FARS: Modeling the Macaque Canonical System for Grasping

Parietal area AIP, the anterior region of the intraparietal sulcus, and ventral premotor area F5 (Fig. 10–1B) anchor the cortical circuit in macaque that transforms visual information on intrinsic properties of an object into hand movements for grasping it. Discharge in most grasp-related F5 neurons correlates with an action rather than with the individual movements that form it so that one may relate F5 neurons to various *motor schemas* corresponding to the action associated with their discharge:

Fagg and Arbib (1998) developed the FARS (Fagg-Arbib-Rizzolatti-Sakata) model for the control of the *canonical neurons* of F5 (Fig. 10–5). Area cIPS provides visual input to parietal area AIP concerning the position and orientation of the object's surfaces. AIP then extracts the *affordances* the object offers for grasping (i.e., the visually grounded encoding of "motor opportunities" for grasping the object, rather

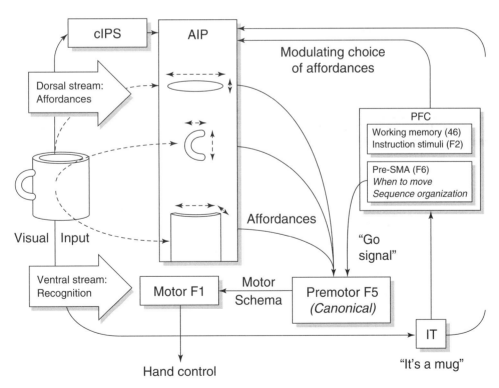

FIGURE 10–5. A reconceptualization of the FARS model in which the primary influence of PFC (prefrontal cortex) on the selection of affordances is on parietal cortex (AIP, anterior intraparietal sulcus) rather than premotor cortex (the hand area F5). cIPS, the caudal area of the intraparietal sulcus.

than its classification). The basic pathway AIP $\rightarrow$ F5$_{canonical}$ $\rightarrow$ F1 (primary motor cortex, also known as M1) of the FARS model then transforms the (neural code for) the affordance to the appropriate motor schema (F5) and thence to the appropriate detailed descending motor control signals (F1).

Going beyond the empirical data then available, Fagg and Arbib (1998) stressed that there may be several ways to grasp an object and thus hypothesized (1) that object recognition (mediated by inferotemporal cortex) can bias the computation of working memory and task constraints and the effect of instruction stimuli in various areas of prefrontal cortex and (2) that strong connections between prefrontal cortex and F5 provide the data for F5 to choose one affordance from the possibilities offered by AIP.

However, following suggestions of Rizzolatti and Luppino (2003), Figure 10–5 shows "FARS Modificato" in which information on object semantics and the goals of the individual directly influence AIP rather than F5. AIP still describes several affordances initially, but only one of these is selected to influence F5. This affordance then establishes in the F5 neurons a command which reaches threshold for the appropriate grip once it receive a "go signal" from F6 (pre-SMA), which (in concert with the basal ganglia) will determine whether external and/or internal contingencies allow the action execution. It is worth noting that this account associates *three* working memory systems with the canonical grasping system:

WM1: Interactions between AIP and F5 keep track of current affordances in the environment.

WM2: Area 46 or other prefrontal cortex regions hold the location and related parameters of unattended or absent objects within the currently relevant environment (see Rolls and Arbib, 2003, for some of the relevant issues in scene perception).

WM3: The basal ganglia works with F6 to keep track of the place of the current action within some overall coordinated control program.

Although it is not part of the FARS model, we should also note the importance of yet another working memory system:

WM4: A working memory that holds information about aspects of the recently executed trajectory. This working memory decays rapidly over time.

MNS: Modeling the Macaque Mirror System for Grasping

As explained at length in Fadiga's chapter, there is a subset of the F5 neurons related to grasping, the *mirror neurons*, which are active not only when the monkey executes a specific hand action but also when it observes a human or other monkey carrying out a similar action. These neurons constitute the "mirror system for grasping" in the monkey and we say that these neurons provide the neural code for matching execution and observation of hand movements. (By contrast, the canonical neurons are active for execution but not observation.)

What is the mirror system "for"? It has often been suggested that the mirror system for grasping first evolved to mediate action recognition as a basis for *social interaction* and *imitation*. However, my counterhypothesis subdivides the emergence of the mirror system into two stages: (1) The mirror system for grasping evolved originally to provide visual feedback for dexterous hand movements requiring attention to object detail. (2) Exaptation then exploited this "self-ability" to map one's own actions onto internal motor representations to recognize other individual's actions and encode them in such a way as to link with similar actions of one's own. Moreover, monkeys have a mirror system for grasping but little or no capacity for imitation. Imitation requires more than action recognition—it requires the ability to recognize that a *novel* action A achieves goal B in context W, and use this as the basis for mastering the skill of performing A, and then using it in future if B is one's goal in a context related to W.

The populations of canonical and mirror neurons appear to be spatially segregated in F5 (Rizzolatti and Luppino, 2001). The region of F5 buried in the dorsal bank of the arcuate sulcus, F5ab, contains the canonical neurons, while the convexity located caudal to the arcuate sulcus, F5c, includes the mirror neurons. Both sectors receive a strong input from the secondary somatosensory area (SII; buried within the Sylvian fissure, Fig. 10–1B) and parietal area PF (shown as 7b in Fig. 10–1B). F5ab is the target of area AIP.

STSa, in the rostral part of STS, has neurons that discharge when the monkey observes such biological actions as walking, turning the head, bending the torso and moving the arms. Of most relevance to us is that a few of these neurons discharged when the monkey

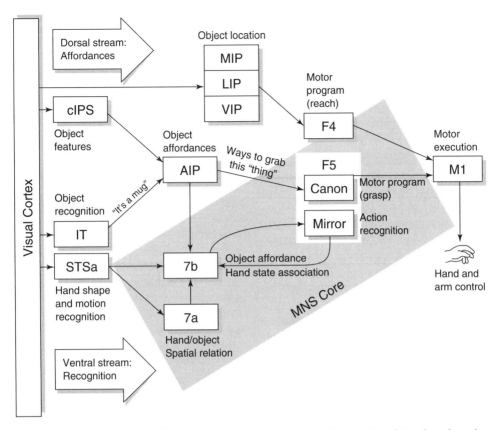

FIGURE 10–6. A schematic view of the mirror neuron system. The mirror neuron system (MNS) model (Oztop and Arbib, 2002) focuses on the circuitry highlighted by the gray diagonal rectangle. (Note that this model omits the functionality of prefrontal cortex (PFC) included in the FARS model in Fig. 10–5.) F4 is the premotor area for control of arm movements. For other abbreviations, see Figure 10-1B and text.

observed goal-directed hand movements, such as grasping objects (Perrett et al., 1990)—although STSa neurons do not seem to discharge during movement execution as distinct from observation. STSa and F5 may be indirectly connected via inferior parietal area PF (BA 7b) (Seltzer and Pandya, 1994).

Just as we have embedded the F5 canonical neurons in a larger system involving both the parietal area AIP and the inferotemporal area, so do we now stress that *the F5 mirror neurons are part of a larger mirror system that includes (at least) parts of the superior temporal gyrus (STS) and area PF of the parietal lobe.* We now discuss a model of this larger system, the MNS model (Fig. 10–6; Oztop and Arbib, 2002). One path in Figure 10–6 corresponds to the basic pathway AIP → F5$_{canonical}$ → M1 of the FARS model (but MNS does not include the material on prefrontal influences). Another pathway completes the "canonical" portion of the MNS model, with intraparietal areas MIP/LIP/VIP providing object location information that enables F4 to instruct F1 to execute a reaching movement which positions the hand appropriately for grasping. The rest of Figure 10–6 presents the core elements for the understanding of the mirror system. The sight of both hand and object—with the hand moving appropriately to grasp the seen (or recently seen) object—is required for the mirror neurons attuned to the given action to fire. This requires schemas for the recognition of both the shape of the hand and analysis of its motion (STSa in the figure), and for analysis of the relation of these hand parameters to the location and affordance of the object (7a and 7b [≈PF] in the figure).

In the MNS model, the *hand state* is defined as a vector whose components represent the movement of the wrist relative to the location of the object and of the hand shape relative to the affordances of the object. Oztop and Arbib (2002) showed that an artificial neural network corresponding to PF and F5$_{mirror}$ could be trained to recognize the grasp type from the *hand state trajectory*, with correct classification often being achieved well before the hand reached the object.

During training, the output of the F5 canonical neurons, acting as a code for the grasp being executed by the monkey at that time, was used as the training signal for the F5 mirror neurons to enable them to learn which hand-object trajectories corresponded to the canonically encoded grasps. As a result of this training, the appropriate mirror neurons come to fire in response to the appropriate trajectories even when the trajectory is not accompanied by F5 canonical firing. What makes the modeling worthwhile is that the trained network not only responded to hand state trajectories from the training set but also exhibited interesting responses to novel hand-object relationships.

This training prepares the F5 mirror neurons to respond to hand-object relational trajectories even when the hand is of the "other" rather than the "self" because the hand state is based on the movement of a hand relative to the object, and thus only *indirectly* on the retinal input of seeing hand and object—the latter can differ greatly between observation of self and other. However, the model only accepts input related to one hand and one object at a time, and so says nothing about the "binding" of the action to the agent of that action.

The MNS model provides an explicit account of how the mirror system may learn to recognize the hand-object relations associated with grasps already in its repertoire. Complementing this, Oztop and colleagues (2004) discuss how the infant may acquire its initial repertoire of grasps. Such learning models, and the data they address, make clear that *neither canonical nor mirror neurons are restricted to recognition of an innate set of actions but can be recruited to recognize and encode an expanding repertoire of novel actions*. Given the debate over innateness with regard to language acquisition, it is worth noting that in the MNS model the focus on hand-object relationships as providing relevant input is "built in"—but not the exact nature of the grasps that will be learned. Similarly, the ILGM model (Oztop et al., 2004) has as its basis that the child reaches for a bright or moving object, executes the grasp reflex if contact is made on the palmar surface, and builds a repertoire of grasps based on those which prove to be stable, which we posit supplies a reinforcement signal. The system thus has certain "innate" hand-related biases but is then able to acquire a range of power grasps and precision pinches through experience without these having to be built in.

Homologies

The notion that a mirror system might exist in humans was tested by PET experiments which showed that grasp observation significantly activated the STS, the inferior parietal lobule, and the inferior frontal gyrus (area 45, part of Broca's area). For further review of related studies using TMS (transcranial magnetic stimulation) as well as PET and fMRI brain imaging, see Fadiga (this volume). F5 in macaque is generally considered to be the homologue of Broca's area in humans.

The relative positions of Broca's area on the inferior part of the frontal cortex and Wernicke's area on the superior part of the temporal lobe suggest that candidates for homologous structures of these language-related areas may be situated in corresponding locations in the macaque cortex. Accordingly, the homologous structures of the human Broca's area may be found on the inferior part of the macaque agranular frontal cortex, in the vicinity of the arcuate sulcus (considered to be the macaque homologue of the human precentral and prefrontal sulci), and the macaque homologues of Wernicke's area may be located at the junction between the temporal and parietal cortices. If the nomenclature proposed by Brodmann is applied to the macaque cortex, one should find corresponding structures of the human areas 44 and 45. Both of these human areas are considered to have their counterparts in the macaque cortex, even though there is no consensus over their exact locations and extensions. The macaque homologue of Wernicke's area appears to include the macaque area Tpt, located on the posterior part of the superior temporal gyrus. For full discussion of this and other relevant homologies see Arbib and Bota (2003) and the chapters by Petrides and Aboitiz et al. in this volume.

Arbib and Bota (2003) hypothesize that the macaque homologues of Broca's area are areas 44 and 45 (as defined in their paper). They also hypothesize that the macaque areas 44 and 45 are *convergence points* of the action recognition information conveyed by the connections with posterior parietal cortices with auditory information from the superior temporal gyrus. Results of Kohler et al. (2002) and Romanski and Goldman-Rakic (2002) indicate a possible functional dissociation between areas 44 and 45, with area

44 involved in processing spatially related auditory information in the context of action recognition, and area 45 possibly involved in nonspatial processing of auditory inputs. In any case, more structural, neurophysiological and functional studies have to be performed in humans, macaques and great apes to more fully explore homologies to human language-related structures across different primate species.

Evolving the Language-Ready Brain

We would all agree that the human genome provides the human child with a brain able to acquire and use language if raised in a community which already has language. Controversy arises over what constitutes this "language readiness". Some would claim that the genome provides a Principles and Parameters style of Universal Grammar[4] (e.g., Chomsky 1981), but Arbib (2002, 2005b) argues that biological evolution only brought hominids to the stage of having protolanguage (an open system of symbolic communication with little or no syntax), whereas the path from protolanguage to language involved a series of historical changes such as those that led to the development of farming, or city dwelling or literacy—changes that define what most of us today would see as part of the essentials of the way we are human, yet which we know to be in the main part "postbiological."

What turns a movement into an action is that it is associated with a goal, so that initiation of the movement is accompanied by the creation of an expectation that the goal will be met. We distinguish "praxic action" in which the hands are used to interact physically with objects or other creatures, from "communicative action" (both manual and vocal). Our assumption is that macaques use hand movements mainly for praxic actions. The mirror system allows other macaques to understand these actions and act on the basis of this understanding. Similarly, the macaque's orofacial gestures register emotional state, and primate vocalizations can also communicate something of the current situation of the macaque. However, seeking to understand why the mirror system for grasping in macaque is the homologue of Broca's area in humans, Rizzolatti and Arbib (1998) developed the following:

The Mirror-System Hypothesis

Language evolved from a basic mechanism *not* originally related to communication: the *mirror system for grasping* with its capacity to generate *and* recognize a set of actions. More specifically, human Broca's area contains a mirror system for grasping which is homologous to the F5 mirror system of macaque, and this provides the evolutionary basis for *language parity*—i.e., an utterance means roughly the same for both speaker and hearer.

This provides a neurobiological "missing link" for the hypothesis that communication based on manual gesture preceded speech in language evolution (e.g., Hewes, 1973; Stokoe, 2001).[5] I view the "openness" or "generativity" that some see as the hallmark of language (i.e., its openness to new constructions, as distinct from having a fixed repertoire like that of monkey vocalizations) as present in manual behavior which can thus supply part of the evolutionary substrate for its appearance in language.

Arbib (2002, 2005b) has amplified the original account of Rizzolatti and Arbib to hypothesize seven stages in the evolution of language, with imitation grounding two of the stages. The first three stages are prehominid:

S1: Grasping

S2: A mirror system for grasping shared with the common ancestor of human and monkey. The mirror neurons can be recruited to recognize and encode an expanding set of novel actions. Stage S2 is subdivided into S2a, providing feedback for dexterous manual control, and S2b, acting with other brain regions to make useful information available for interacting with others.

S3: A simple imitation system for grasping shared with the common ancestor of human and chimpanzee.

The next three stages then distinguish the hominid line from that of the great apes:

S4: A complex imitation system for grasping: This presupposes a capacity for *complex action analysis*, the ability to analyze another's performance as a combination of actions (or approximated by variants of actions) already in the repertoire. This can provide the basis for adding new, complex actions to one's repertoire. The notion is that complex imitation was an evolutionary step of great advantage independent of its implications for communication. However, in modern humans it undergirds the child's ability to acquire language, while complex action analysis is essential for the adult's ability to comprehend the novel compounds of "articulatory gestures" that constitute language.

The next two stages introduces communication intended by the utterer to have a particular effect on the recipient, rather than being involuntary or a side effect of praxis:

S5: *Protosign*, a manual-based communication system, breaking through the fixed repertoire of primate vocalizations to yield an open repertoire. This decomposes into S5a: the ability to engage in pantomime; and S5b: the ability to make conventional gestures to disambiguate pantomime.

S6: *Proto-speech*, resulting from the ability of control mechanisms evolved for protosign to also control the vocal apparatus with increasing flexibility.

It is argued that early protosign provided the scaffolding for early protospeech after which they developed together in an expanding spiral till protospeech became dominant. Recent data on mirror neurons are relevant here. Kohler et al. (2002) show that 15% of mirror neurons in the hand area of macaque F5 can respond to the distinctive sound of an action (breaking peanuts, ripping paper, etc.) as well as viewing the action. Ferrari et al. (2003) find that in the orofacial area of F5, there are "mirror" neurons tuned to communicative gestures such as lip-smacking, although these are *not strictly congruent*—e.g., one "observed" lip protrusion (communicative) but "executed" syringe sucking (ingestive). Some might argue that these results let us apply the mirror system hypothesis to vocalization directly, "cutting out the middleman" of manual gesture. The three papers by Arbib (2005a), MacNeilage and Davis (2005b), and Fogassi and Ferrari (2004) exemplify the current state of the debate.

The final stage is claimed to involve little if any biological evolution, but instead to result from cultural evolution (historical change) in *Homo sapiens*:

S7: *Language*: the change from action-object frames to verb-argument structures to syntax and semantics; the co-evolution of cognitive and linguistic complexity.

Arbib (2005b) offers examples of the discoveries which might have accumulated across tens of millennia to take *Homo sapiens* from protolanguage to language, arguing that the features of language emerged by adding many features as "patches" to a protolanguage, with general "rules" emerging both consciously and unconsciously only as generalizations could be imposed on, or discerned in, a population

of ad hoc mechanisms. Needless to say, this assertion is highly controversial.

Aboitiz and García (1997) offer a somewhat different theory of human brain evolution, also rooted in the study of human–macaque homologies. They propose three stages in the evolution of the capacity of the human brain to support language:

1. The capacity to give names yielded the lexicon that underlies the ability to refer to objects or events in the external world. They associate this with the elaboration of a precursor of Wernicke's area in the superior temporal lobe as a zone for cross-modal associations which include a phonological correlate.
2. The need to combine more and more words to express complex meanings yielded syntax, the expression of regularities in the ways in which different elements are combined to form linguistic utterances. They associate the emergence of syntax with the differentiation of an inferoparietal-frontal (Broca's) area with its connections to the incipient Wernicke's region developing as a phonological rehearsal device that eventually differentiated into the language areas This system they see as yielding a phonological-rehearsal loop (recall the discussion of Baddeley, 2003) that could provide some basic syntactic rules at the levels of phonemes and morphemes.
3. Coordinated operation of networks involving granular frontal cortex and the semantic system represented in the temporoparietal lobes, together with the phonological-rehearsal loop, generated higher levels of syntax and discourse.

Aboitiz et al. (this volume, Chapter 1) provide a fuller exposition of these hypotheses and notes certain modifications they have made in the years since 1997. Arbib and Bota (2003) contrast the two evolutionary theories as follows:

Aboitiz and García assume that the human brain evolved (in part) to support language. They offer an essentially *retrospective* theory working back from a lexicon of spoken words and a syntax that binds them into sentences to suggest how areas of the macaque brain, and their connections, changed (some areas enlarged, some connections are strengthened) to yield a human brain that could support these features of language. By contrast, Rizzolatti and Arbib offer more of a prospective theory. They start from an analysis of the monkey's capabilities, especially the fact that F5, containing a mirror system for hand movements, is homologous to

Broca's area. They then offer hypotheses on how intermediate stages from the mirror system for grasping led via simple and complex imitation and protosign to protospeech. Here I want to place special emphasis on complex imitation and in particular *complex action analysis*, the ability to analyze another's performance in terms of actions already in the repertoire. However, Rizzolatti and Arbib are relatively silent on the phonological loop and other working memory systems whose emphasis is an important feature of the Aboitiz and García analysis. Thus, the relevance of the schema-

theoretic view of memory provided at the end of the Schema Theory section and the range of working memory systems within the FARS model of Figure 10–5.

TOWARD AN ACTION-ORIENTED NEUROLINGUISTICS

Figure 10–7 provides a view of the language-ready brain (Arbib & Bota 2003), informed both by the mir-

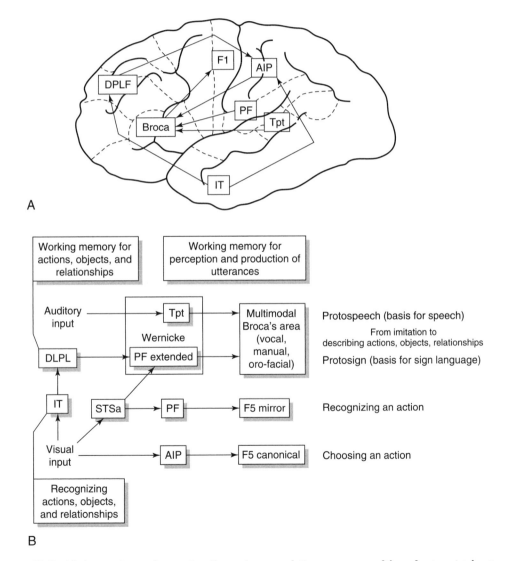

FIGURE 10–7. (A) A recasting and extension (in part) of FARS Modificato (Fig. 10–5) in register with the view of the human brain in Figure 1A, designed for maximal congruence with the schema provided by Aboitiz and García (1997). (B) A high-level view of the cumulative emergence of three frontoparietal systems: choosing an action → recognizing an action → describing an action (in multiple modalities). DLPL, dorsolateral prefrontal cortex. For other abbreviations see Figure 10–1. (Both figures from Arbib and Bota, 2003.)

ror system hypothesis and by the emphasis on working memory of Aboitiz and García. It is a hybrid, mixing macaque and human regions and gives the impression that three frontoparietal systems end in three distinct brain structures. In fact, current research has not really settled the question. In any case, the possibility that one monkey area may be homologous to different human regions implicated in one or more of praxic hand movements, protosign, protospeech, signed language, and speech offers challenge to overly binary views of homology. Much needs to be done to delineate subareas of Broca's area that can be distinguished on this basis and their connections—while noting that differences that are found (and the variations in the pattern of such differences from individual to individual) may reflect the self-organization of the brain as the child grows within a language community rather than any innate "fate map" for these differences. DeRenzi et al. (1966) found that the majority of patients with apraxia of speech had oral apraxia and a high coexistence of oral and limb apraxia while Marquardt and Sussman (1984) found that 12 of their 15 patients with Broca's aphasia had apraxia of speech while 5 had limb apraxia. Double dissociations do occur in some cases. Thus, either separate networks of neurons are engaged in the generation of speech and nonspeech movement of the same muscles, or the same general network underlies speech and nonspeech movements but these have separate control mechanisms which can be differentially damaged (Code, 1998).

Notes

1. Analysis of the macaque brain, and thus of homologies with the human brain, is bedeviled by the fact that different authors use different parcellations to address data acquired since the time of Brodmann. Arbib and Bota (2003) have addressed the issue by developing neuroinformatics tools to create an online knowledge management system, the NeuroHomology Database.

2. See Goldman-Rakic, Ó Scalaidhe, and Chafee, 1999, for the variety of working memories implemented in prefrontal cortex and with links to specific parietal circuitry.

3. The architecture of the VISIONS computer vision system was based on the HEARSAY architecture as well as on neurally inspired schema theory.

4. The concept of universal grammar is protean, and there may be variants for which I would accept a genetic basis. What I do reject is the view that the majority of syntactic rules are preencoded, so that the child's experience simply "sets switches" to select and parameterize those rules appropriate to the language community in which the child is raised. Perhaps the most compelling hypothesis for the evolution of such a universal grammar was advanced by Pinker and Bloom (1990)—but when I read it carefully, I find that the notion of universal grammar is not unequivocally defined, and that many of the stages they posited could have occurred by cultural evolution as easily as by biological evolution.

5. Below, I soften this assertion to the claim that protosign provided scaffolding essential to the evolution of protospeech.

References

Aboitiz, F., & García V.R. (1997). The evolutionary origin of the language areas in the human brain. A neuroanatomical perspective. *Brain Research Reviews*, 25, 381–396.

Arbib, M.A. (1981). Perceptual structures and distributed motor control. In V.B. Brooks (Ed.), *Handbook of Physiology – The Nervous System II. Motor Control* (pp. 1449–1480). Bethesda, MD: American Physiological Society.

Arbib, M.A. (1989). *The metaphorical brain 2: Neural networks and beyond.* New York: Wiley-Interscience.

Arbib, M.A. (2002). The mirror system, imitation, and the evolution of language. In C. Nehaniv & K. Dautenhahn (Eds.), *Imitation in animals and artifacts* (pp. 229–280). Boston: MIT Press.

Arbib, M.A. (2005a). Interweaving protosign and protospeech: Further developments beyond the mirror. *Interaction Studies: Social Behavior and Communication in Biological and Artificial Systems*, 6, 145–171.

Arbib, M.A. (2005). From monkey-like action recognition to human language: An evolutionary framework for neurolinguistics. *Behavioral and Brain Sciences* (in press).

Arbib, M.A., & Bota, M. (2003). Language evolution: Neural homologies and neuroinformatics. *Neural Networks*, 16, 1237–1260.

Arbib, M.A., & Caplan, D. (1979). Neurolinguistics must be computational. *Behavioral and Brain Sciences*, 2, 449–483.

Arbib, M.A., & Liaw, J.-S. (1995). Sensorimotor transformations in the worlds of frogs and robots. *Artificial Intelligence*, 72, 53–79.

Arbib, M.A., Érdi, P., & Szentágothai, J. (1998). *Neural organization: Structure, function, and dynamics.* Cambridge, MA: MIT Press.

Arkin, R.C. (1998). *Behavior-based robotics.* Cambridge, MA: MIT Press.

Baddeley, A. (2003). Working memory: Looking back and looking forward. *Nature Reviews Neuroscience*, 4, 829–839.

Baddeley, A.D., & Hitch, G.J. (1974). Working memory. In G.A. Bower (Ed.), *The psychology of learning and motivation* (pp. 47–89). NY: Academic Press.

Chomsky, N. (1981). *Lectures on government and binding: The Pisa lectures.* Dordrecht: Foris.

Code, C. (1998). Models, theories and heuristics in apraxia of speech. *Clinical Linguistics & Phonetics*, 12, 47–65.

DeRenzi, E., Pieczuro, A., & Vignolo, L.A. (1966). Oral apraxia and aphasia. *Cortex*, 2, 50–73.

Draper, B.A., Collins, R.T., Brolio, J., Hanson, A.R., & Riseman, E.M. (1989). The schema system. *International Journal of Computer Vision*, 2, 209–250.

Fagg, A.H., & Arbib, M.A. (1998). Modeling parietal-premotor interactions in primate control of grasping. *Neural Networks*, 11, 1277–1303.

Ferrari, P.F., Gallese, V., Rizzolatti, G., & Fogassi, L. (2003). Mirror neurons responding to the observation of ingestive and communicative mouth actions in the monkey ventral premotor cortex. *European Journal of Neuroscience*, 17, 1703–1714.

Fogassi, L., & Ferrari, P.F. (2004). Mirror neurons, gestures and language evolution. *Interaction Studies: Social Behavior and Communication in Biological and Artificial Systems*, 5, 345–363.

Galaburda, A.M., & Sanides, F. (1980). Cytoarchitectonic organization of the human auditory cortex. *Journal of Comparative Neurology*, 190, 597–610.

Geschwind, N. (1964). The development of the brain and the evolution of language. *Montreal Series in Language & Linguistics*, 1, 155–169.

Goldman-Rakic, P.S., Ó Scalaidhe, S.P., & Chafee, M.V. (1999). Domain specificity in cognitive systems. In M.S. Gazzaniga (Ed.), *The new cognitive neurosciences* (Chapter 50). Second Edition. Cambridge, MA: MIT Press.

Hewes, G. (1973). Primate communication and the gestural origin of language. *Current Anthropology*, 14, 5–24.

Jackendoff, R. (2002). *Foundations of language: Brain, meaning, grammar, evolution.* Oxford and New York: Oxford University Press.

Jeannerod, M., & Biguer, B. (1982). Visuomotor mechanisms in reaching within extra-personal space. In D.J. Ingle, R.J.W. Mansfield, & M.A. Goodale (Eds.), *Advances in the analysis of visual behavior* (pp. 387–409), Boston: MIT Press.

Jeannerod, M. (1997). *The cognitive neuroscience of action.* Oxford: Blackwell Publishers.

Jeannerod, M., Arbib, M.A., Rizzolatti, G., & Sakata, H. (1995). Grasping objects: The cortical mechanisms

of visuomotor transformation. *Trends in Neurosciences*, 18, 314–320.

Kohler, E., Keysers, C., Umilta, M.A., Fogassi, L., Gallese, V., & Rizzolatti, G. (2002). Hearing sounds, understanding actions: Action representation in mirror neurons. *Science*, 297, 846–848.

Lesser, V.R., Fennel, R.D., Erman, L.D., & Reddy, D.R. (1975). Organization of the HEARSAY-II speech understanding system. *IEEE Transactions on Acoustics, Speech, and Signal Processing*, 23, 11–23.

Luria, A.R. (1973). *The working brain.* Harmondsworth: Penguin Books.

MacNeilage, P.F., & Davis, B. (2005). The frame/content theory of evolution of speech: A comparison with a gestural origins alternative. *Interaction Studies: Social Behavior and Communication in Biological and Artificial Systems*, 6, 173–199.

Marquardt, T.P., & Sussman, H. (1984). The elusive lesion—Apraxia of speech link in Broca's aphasia. In J.C. Rosenbek, M.R. McNeil, & A.E. Aronson (Eds.), *Apraxia of speech: Physiology, acoustics, linguistics, management*, San Diego: College-Hill Press.

Oztop, E., & Arbib, M.A. (2002). Schema design and implementation of the grasp-related mirror neuron system. *Biological Cybernetics*, 87, 116–140.

Oztop, E., Bradley, N., & Arbib, M.A. (2004). Infant grasp learning: A computational model. *Experimental Brain Research*, 158, 480–503.

Perrett, D.I., Mistlin, A.J., Harries, M.H., & Chitty, A.J. (1990). Understanding the visual appearance and consequence of hand actions. In M.A. Goodale (Ed.), *Vision and action: The control of grasping* (pp. 163–342). Norwood, NJ: Ablex.

Pinker, S., & Bloom, A. (1990). Natural language and natural selection. *Behavioural Brain Sciences*, 13, 707–784.

Rizzolatti, G., & Arbib, M.A. (1998). Language within our grasp. *Trends in Neurosciences*, 21, 188–194.

Rizzolatti, G., & Craighero, L. (2004). The mirror-neuron system. *Annual Review of Neuroscience*, 27, 169–192.

Rizzolatti, G., & Luppino, G. (2003). Grasping movements: Visuomotor transformations. In M.A. Arbib (Ed.), *The handbook of brain theory and neural networks* (2nd ed., pp. 501–504). Cambridge, MA: MIT Press.

Rizzolatti, G., Fogassi, L., & Gallese, V. (2002). Motor and cognitive functions of the ventral premotor cortex. *Current Opinions in Neurobiology*, 12, 149–154.

Rolls, E.T., & Arbib, M.A. (2003). Visual scene perception. In M.A. Arbib (Ed.), *The handbook of brain theory and neural networks* (2nd ed., pp. 1210–1251). Cambridge, MA: MIT Press.

Romanski, L.M., & Goldman-Rakic, P.S. (2002). An auditory domain in primate prefrontal cortex. *Nature Neuroscience, 5,* 15–6.

Seltzer, B., & Pandya, D.N. (1994). Parietal, temporal, and occipital projections to cortex of the superior temporal sulcus in the rhesus monkey: A retrograde tracer study. *Journal of Comparative Neurology, 15,* 445–463.

Stokoe, W.C. (2001). *Language in hand: Why sign came before speech.* Washington, DC: Gallaudet University Press.

Weymouth, T.E. (1986). Using object descriptions in a schema network for machine vision, Ph.D. Thesis and COINS Technical Report 86–24, Department of Computer and Information Science, University of Massachusetts at Amherst.

Wilkins, W.K., & Wakefield, J. (1995). Brain evolution and neurolinguistic preconditions. *Behavioral and Brain Sciences, 18,* 161–226.

11

The Role of Broca's Area
in Sign Language

Karen Emmorey

Sign languages provide a powerful tool for investigating the neurobiology and cognitive architecture of human language. Linguistic research has revealed substantial similarities between signed and spoken languages, but this is only a starting point (for reviews, see Emmorey, 2002; Sandler and Lillo-Martin, 2006). The similarities provide a strong basis for comparison and serve to highlight universal properties of human language. In addition, however, sign-speech modality distinctions can be exploited to discover how the input-output systems of language impact the neurocognitive underpinnings of language production and comprehension. In this chapter, we explore whether Broca's area subserves the same behavioral functions for signed and spoken languages and discuss the nature of these functions. First, however, some background on sign language structure needs to be presented.

The discovery that sign languages have a phonology (traditionally defined as the *sound* patterns of language) was ground-breaking and crucial to our understanding of the nature of human language (for reviews, see Brentari, 1998; Corina and Sandler, 1993). In spoken languages, words are constructed out of sounds that in and of themselves have no meaning (duality of patterning). The words "bat" and "pat" differ only in the initial sounds that convey no inherent meanings of their own. Similarly, signs are constructed out of components that are themselves meaningless and are combined to create morphemes and words. Signs can be minimally distinguished by hand configuration, place of articulation, movement, and orientation with respect to the body. Figure 11–1 provides an illustration of four minimal pairs: signs that are identical except for one component, and if you substitute one component for another, it changes the meaning of the sign. Some signs are produced with one hand and some with two hands, but handedness is not distinctive in ASL (American Sign Language) or perhaps in any sign language. There are no ASL signs that differ only on the basis of whether they are made with the right hand or with the left hand. One-

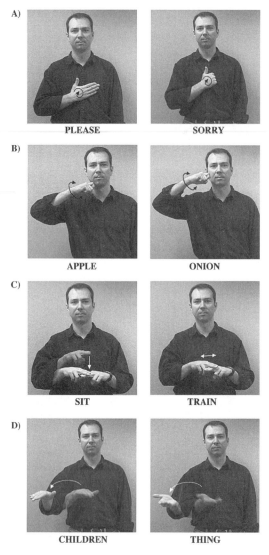

FIGURE 11–1. Examples of minimal pairs in American Sign Language: (A) signs that contrast in hand configuration, (B) signs that contrast in place of articulation, (C) signs that contrast in movement, and (D) signs that contrast in orientation.

handed signs are produced with the signer's dominant hand. Thus, left-handers and right-handers differ in which hand is dominant.

Not all hand configurations nor all places of articulation are distinctive in any given sign language. For example, the T handshape (thumb inserted between index and middle fingers) does not occur in European signed languages. Chinese Sign Language contains a handshape formed with an open hand with all fingers extended expect for the ring finger, which is bent; this hand configuration does not occur in ASL. Although the upper cheek and chin are distinctive places of articulation in ASL (see Fig. 11–1B), the back jaw is not a phonologically contrastive location (e.g., there are no minimal pairs involving this place of articulation).

Spoken languages represent sequential structure in terms of the linear ordering of consonant and vowel segments. Similarly, the linear structure of signs can be represented in terms of sequences of phonological categories akin to consonants and vowels. These are Location and Movement segments within Sandler's phonological model (Sandler, 1989). Other phonological models also propose linear structure, but characterize segments and features somewhat differently (Brentari, 1998; van der Hulst, 1993). Segments in signed languages are characterized by manual features (e.g., selected fingers; body contact) rather than by oral features (e.g., voicing; labial).

There is fairly strong evidence for the existence of syllables in sign languages—the syllable is a unit of structure that is below the level of the word but above the level of the segment. However, there is little evidence for onset-rhyme distinctions within a sign syllable or resyllabification processes. Finally, sign languages exhibit phonological rules such as assimilation, constraints on well-formedness that refer to segmental structure, and form patterns can be accounted for using feature geometry. Thus, both signed and spoken languages exhibit a linguistically significant, yet meaningless, level of structure that can be analyzed as *phonology* for both language types.

Signed and spoken languages are also subject to the same syntactic constraints on form and movement (see Sandler and Lillo-Martin, in press, for review). For example, the basic word order for ASL is SVO (subject-verb-object). The ASL sentence GIRL PUSH BOY[1] unambiguously means "The girl pushes the boy" and BOY PUSH GIRL means "The boy pushes the girl." Topicalization can result in the movement of the object noun phrase to a sentence initial position, as illustrated in example 1 and Figure 11–2.

<u>　　t</u>
(1) BOY, GIRL PUSH _____.
"The boy, the girl pushes him."

This ASL topicalization marker is a combination of a backward head tilt and raised eyebrows, timed to

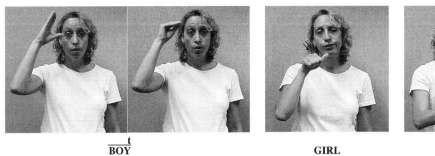

$\overline{\quad\text{t}\quad}$
BOY   **GIRL**   **PUSH**

FIGURE 11–2. Illustration of an American Sign Language sentence with a moved constituent (a topicalized object), corresponding to Example (1) in the text (from Emmorey, 2002).

co-occur with the manual sign(s). The line above BOY in example 1 indicates the scope of the facial expression (i.e., it continues throughout the articulation of BOY), and "t" stands for topic. Topicalization and other movement operations in ASL are subject to the same universal constraints that apply to spoken language (Fischer, 1974; Padden, 1983). For example, in example 2 the subject MOTHER has been topicalized out of an embedded wh-clause, resulting in an ungrammatical sentence (from Lillo-Martin, 1991). Topicalization of a noun phrase from this structural position violates universal constraints on the (structural) distance over which movement can occur.

$$\overline{\qquad\quad\text{t}\qquad\quad}$$
(2) *MOTHER, I DON'T-KNOW WHAT _____ LIKE.
*"Mom, I don't know what _____ likes."

These examples illustrate two points. First, signed languages exhibit embedded structures, movement operations, and follow universal constraints on syntactic form. Second, nonmanual markings (e.g., specific facial expressions) are critical to ASL syntax and mark such structures as topics (Fig. 11–2), relative clauses, conditional clauses, and wh-phrases. Wh-questions in ASL must also be accompanied by a specific facial expression: furrowed brows, squinted eyes, and a slight head shake (Baker and Cokely, 1980). This facial expression must co-occur with the entire wh-phrase, as shown in example 3:

$$\overline{\qquad\qquad\quad\text{wh}\qquad\qquad}$$
(3) a. BOB LIKE WHAT?   "What does Bob like?"
$$\overline{\qquad\qquad\quad\text{wh}\qquad\qquad}$$
   b. WHO LOVE BOB?   "Who loves Bob?"

$$\overline{\qquad\text{wh}\qquad}$$
*c. *WHO LOVE BOB?

The syntactic analysis of WH questions is a topic of current linguistic debate (see Petronio and Lillo-Martin, 1997; Neidle et al., 2000). These accounts disagree on the direction of the WH-movement operation (rightward or leftward) and on the conditions under which the spread of WH marking is obligatory. Nonetheless, it is clear that although emotional facial expressions are universal in humans (Ekman, 1992), the use of facial expressions to mark grammatical structure is unique to signed languages.

Broca's area (Brodmann areas 44/45) and the immediately surrounding cortex have been shown to play a role in several aspects of linguistic, as well as nonlinguistic, processing. Given the similarities between signed and spoken languages outlined above for phonology and syntax (two domains of processing implicated as functions of Broca's area), we examine whether there is any evidence that Broca's area is involved in these aspects of sign language processing and whether this involvement mirrors that found for spoken languages. To the extent that we find parallels between signed and spoken languages, it will indicate that linguistic processing within Broca's area is modality independent and that the perceptual and/or articulatory properties of speech do not drive its organization. To the extent that we find differences between signed and spoken languages, it will indicate that specific properties of the input-output system of a language can affect the behavioral functions subserved by Broca's area. Finally, we explore whether certain modality-dependent aspects of sign language structure modulate activity within this area.

BROCA'S AREA AND SIGN LANGUAGE PRODUCTION

Broca's area area has long been thought to play a role in speech production. Given that Broca's area is anterior to primary motor cortex controlling mouth and lip movements, it is reasonable that an area involved in speech production would be anatomically located near regions involved in control of the speech articulators. Is the same area involved in sign language production? Or is the functional equivalent of Broca's area shifted superiorly so that it is next to the motor representation for the hand and arm? Using cortical stimulation mapping, Corina and colleagues (1999) were able to identify the areas involved in mouth and lip movements in a deaf ASL signer. While the subject produced manual signs in a picture-naming task, they stimulated the posterior aspect of Broca's area (Brodmann's area 44). This site was just anterior to the sites that evoked facial motor responses. Stimulation resulted in signing errors best characterized as phonetic or motor execution errors. Signs were articulated with nonspecific movements and laxed handshape configurations. Semantic naming errors did not occur with stimulation to BA44, nor did phonological errors (e.g., producing an erroneous, but clearly articulated, handshape substitution). In contrast, both phonological substitution errors and semantic errors occurred during sign production when stimulation was applied to the left supramarginal gyrus in the same deaf signer.

The cortical stimulation mapping results with this deaf ASL signer suggest that BA 44 is involved in phonetic aspects of linguistic expression, regardless of the anatomy of the language articulators. This hypothesis is supported by the recent results of Horwitz, Amunts, Bhattacharyya, Patkin, Jeffries, Zilles, and Braun (2003), who used a combination of cytoarchitectonic mapping and PET data to investigate activation of Broca's area during the production of spoken and signed language by hearing ASL-English bilinguals. Subjects were asked to produce autobiographical narratives in either English or ASL, and the baseline comparison tasks were laryngeal and orofacial articulatory movements or bilateral non-routinized hand and arm movements (from Braun et al., 1997, 2001). When contrasted with the baseline articulation conditions, there was little or no activation within BA44 for sign production or for speech production. However, when the articulatory baseline tasks were con-trasted with a rest condition, significant activation was observed in BA44 for both language types (more for orofacial articulation than for manual articulation). Interestingly, activation in BA 44 within the right hemisphere was observed for orofacial articulation compared to rest, but very little activation in right BA 44 was observed for (bimanual) limb articulation.

In contrast to BA 44, Horwitz et al. (2003) found only left hemisphere activation in BA 45 for both signing and speaking. Activation in left BA 45 was only observed when the linguistic tasks (producing an English or an ASL narrative) were contrasted with the articulatory baseline tasks. The contrast between the articulation tasks and rest did not produce activation in BA 45 for either orofacial or manual-limb articulation. Horowitz et al. (2003) concluded that BA45 is the portion of Broca's area that is fundamental to modality-independent aspects of language production.

PET data from prelingually deaf ASL signers naming objects and/or actions also indicate a role for left BA 45 in single sign production, as well as for narrative production (Emmorey et al., 2002, 2003, 2004). Activation maxima were observed in left BA 45 with nearly identical Talairach coordinates when signers named animals (-41, $+28$, $+17$), tools (-42, $+28$, $+18$), tool-based actions (-46, $+26$, $+13$), and actions performed without a tool (-47, $+21$, $+15$). The baseline task required subjects to judge the orientation of unknown faces (overtly responding "yes"/"no" for upright/inverted). A between-subjects ($N = 58$) random effects analysis revealed that BA 45 (peak coordinates: -48, $+27$, $+20$) was equally involved in both speech and sign production (Emmorey & Grabowki, 2004). However, two regions within the parietal lobe were significantly more active during sign production than during word production: the left supramarginal gyrus (peak coordinates: -63, -34, $+25$) and the left superior parietal lobule (two peak coordinates: -29, -46, $+54$; -10, -62, $+59$). We speculate that activation in these regions is linked to modality-specific output parameters of sign language. Specifically, activation within left supramarginal gyrus may reflect aspects of phonological processing in ASL (e.g., selection of hand configuration and place of location features), whereas activation within the superior parietal lobule may reflect proprioceptive monitoring of motoric output.

The neuroimaging data indicate strong left lateralized activation within Broca's area for both covert (McGuire et al., 1997) and overt signing (Braun et al., 2001; Emmorey et al., 2002, 2003, 2004; Petitto et al., 2000). However, in all of these studies, subjects produced signs with their dominant right hand, which is innervated almost exclusively by left primary motor and sensory cortices. In contrast, the speech articulators lie on the midline of the body and are innervated by both hemispheres. Does the fact that the primary articulator for sign language is innervated by left-lateralized sensorimotor cortices influence the laterality of language production systems? Corina and colleagues (2003) recently investigated this question by asking ASL signers to generate verbs with either their left (non-dominate) or right (dominant) hand, while undergoing PET scanning. The verb-generation task (produce a verb that is semantically related to a visually presented ASL noun) was contrasted with a noun repetition task. The data showed no activation in right Broca's area when signers produced verbs with their left hand. In addition, a conjunction analysis with right- and left-hand sign production revealed activation maxima within BA 44/45 ($-54, +18, +16$) and also in BA 46 ($-48, +30, +20$) and BA 47 ($-38, +29, -8$). These findings indicate that lexical-semantic processing in language production relies upon Broca's area (and surrounding cortex) in the left hemisphere, even when the primary language articulator is innervated by the right hemisphere.

In general, the lesion data also support a role for Broca's area in sign language production because left, but not right, frontal damage results in nonfluent, effortful signing (Corina, 1998; Poizner et al., 1987). However, there is only one case study reported thus far in which the location of the cortical damage was clearly restricted to Broca's region (BA 44/45 and immediately surrounding cortex). Hickok and colleagues (1996) report the case of R.S., a congenitally deaf native ASL signer, who suffered an ischemic infarct involving the posterior aspect of the left frontal operculum, inferior motor cortex, and white matter deep to both regions. R.S. exhibited relatively good comprehension of ASL (but see later) and significant deficits in ASL production. Although R.S. had good articulation, she produced frequent phonemic paraphasias and occasional semantic paraphasias. An unusual aspect of R.S.'s phonemic paraphasias was that the errors all occurred with two-handed signs. Specifically, the errors involved bimanual coordination of the two hands. For example, she might incorrectly fail to move one of her hands or incorrectly mirror the movement of one hand with the other when the movement

should be symmetrical. She also tended to shadow one-handed signs with her nondominant (left) hand. Deficits in bimanual coordination were not observed when R.S. produced nonlinguistic bimanual hand and arm movements (e.g., producing alternating windmill movements, finger tapping, tying her shoes, knitting, etc.). R.S.'s deficits in coordinating the two hands may be analogous to the phonetic deficits observed for speakers with nonfluent aphasia who have difficulty coordinating independent speech articulators, e.g., the larynx, tongue, and lips (see Blumstein, 1998).

Another clue to the function of Broca's area (specifically BA 45) in sign language production comes from a recent PET study by Emmorey and colleagues (2005). We contrasted noun production with the production of spatial language (prepositions or locative classifier constructions) in English and ASL by hearing ASL-English bilinguals. Briefly, in ASL the most common way to express the spatial relationship between two objects is to use a classifier construction in which the position of the hands in signing space schematically represents the spatial relation between objects. An illustrative example is provided in Figure 11–3. Within this type of classifier construction, each handshape specifies an object type, such as "long and thin," "cylindrical," or "flat surface." The set of classifier handshape morphemes is closed.

Of interest is the finding that the production of classifier constructions (like the one shown in Fig. 11–3) did not significantly engage Broca's area. In this study, ASL-English bilinguals were asked to describe the spatial relation between two objects in English (with a preposition) or in ASL (with a classifier construction), and on a separate presentation, they named the figure object in either ASL or English (the figure object was colored red). When producing ASL lexical signs (nouns) was contrasted with producing locative classifier constructions, significant activation was observed in left BA 45 for ASL nouns (peak activation coordinates: $-38, +26, +3$). The contrast between spoken English prepositions and English nouns revealed no difference in activation for Broca's area. Furthermore, the interaction analysis indicated that English prepositions engaged left BA 45 ($-41, +29, +9$) to a significantly greater extent than ASL classifier constructions. The PET data from deaf ASL signers also indicated that production of ASL classifier constructions did not engage Broca's area. When the production of classifier constructions was contrasted

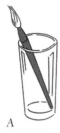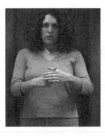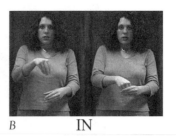

A   B **IN**

FIGURE 11–3. (A) Illustration of an American Sign Language locative classifier construction expression. The signer's right hand (a 1 handshape) represents a long, thin object (the paintbrush), whereas her left hand (a C handshape) represents a cylindrical object (the glass). The spatial relationship between her two hands denotes the spatial relationship between the two objects. (B) Illustration of the lexicalized locative preposition glossed as IN.

with our standard baseline task, no activation was observed within Broca's area; however, when deaf signers viewed the same picture stimuli and named the figure object with an ASL sign, significant activation was observed in Broca's area (BA 45: −49, +24, +15) using the same baseline contrast. Finally, the deaf ASL signers were also asked to name spatial relationships with lexicalized ASL "prepositions" (signs glossed as IN, ON, UNDER, etc.). An example is shown in Figure 11–3. Syntactically, these forms do not function like prepositions in English (McIntire, 1980; Shepard-Kegl, 1985), are not preferred for everyday spatial descriptions, and are usually used for emphasis ("It's *under* the table"). In addition, the handshape of these signs is lexically specified and does not change with the nature of the figure or ground objects, unlike the handshape morphemes within classifier constructions. Also unlike classifier constructions, production of ASL prepositions engaged Broca's area when contrasted with the baseline task (BA 45: −50, +19, +20).

In sum, the production of ASL verbs, nouns, and lexical prepositions activated Broca's area (specifically BA 45), but the production of locative classifier constructions did not. One possible explanation for this somewhat surprising result is that because classifier constructions do not constitute a simple lexical category, their production does not engage the same lexical retrieval processes that have been associated with Broca's area (e.g., Petersen et al., 1988; Thompson-Schill et al., 1997). In our PET studies, signers and speakers were asked to provide a single label for each picture. That is, subjects were required to retrieve a distinct lexical item for each picture stimulus. However, for locative classifier constructions, subjects did not retrieve a specific lexical sign that denoted an object, action, or spatial relationship; rather, they retrieved a handshape morpheme that denoted an object *type* (e.g., long and thin). The same handshape morpheme was appropriate for a number of different objects. For example, the 1 handshape shown in Figure 11–3 could be used for a pencil, a toothbrush, or a spoon. To indicate the spatial relationship between two objects, signers did not retrieve a lexical sign or morpheme. Rather, as illustrated in Figure 11–3, they placed their right hand (representing the figure object) in signing space with respect to their left hand (representing the ground object, which was the same object type for a given stimulus set—either a cylindrical object or a flat surface). In these constructions, the position of the hands in space is not a morphemic, categorical representation (Emmorey and Herzig, 2003). Signing space is schematically mapped in an analogue manner to the physical space shown in the picture stimuli. The finding that the production of these constructions does not significantly engage Broca's area, in contrast to the production of lexical signs, suggests that Broca's area plays a specific role in the selection and/or retrieval of specific lexical items, i.e., *names* of entities, actions, and relationships.

In conclusion, the function of Broca's area is *not* strongly tied to oral-acoustic phonological features of spoken language. Despite the anatomical proximity of Broca's area to the sensorimotor representation of the orofacial articulators and the strong connection between Broca's area and auditory cortices via the arcuate fasciculus, this neural area is nonetheless intimately involved in the production of visual-manual languages. It has been hypothesized that Broca's area is lateralized to the left hemisphere because of the need for unilateral motor control over the bilaterally innervated midline speech articulators (e.g., Cook, 2003). However, the primary articulators for sign language, the hand and arm, are unilaterally innervated, and Broca's area is nonetheless engaged during language production, even when the left hand and arm are the language articulators. Finally, the finding that the production of locative classifier constructions does not engage Broca's area in a picture-naming task (in contrast to nouns, verbs, and lexical prepositions) suggests that Broca's area is engaged in the retrieval and/or selection of stored lexical items that refer to specific entities, actions, or relationships.

BROCA'S AREA AND SIGN LANGUAGE COMPREHENSION

For spoken languages, lesion data indicate that damage to Broca's area results in comprehension deficits that are typically less debilitating than damage to temporal lobe structures, such as Wernicke's area (Goodglass, 1993). Given that Wernicke's area is adjacent to auditory cortex, deficits in comprehension following temporal lobe damage might be expected for spoken language but perhaps not for signed language, which does not depend upon auditory input for perception. However, Hickok, Love-Geffen, and Klima (2002) reported that deaf signers with damage to the left temporal lobe performed significantly worse on tests of ASL comprehension than signers with left frontal and/or parietal damage and worse than signers with right temporal lobe damage. The comprehension deficit associated with left temporal lobe damage was most severe for complex sentences (e.g., multiclausal commands) but was also observed for simple sentences (single clause commands) and single sign comprehension. Hickok et al. (2002) concluded that language comprehension for either spoken or signed language depends upon the integrity of the left temporal lobe.

Functional imaging data support this conclusion. Several studies using a variety of techniques have reported activation within superior temporal cortex during sign language comprehension (Levänen et al., 2001; MacSweeney et al., 2002; Neville et al., 1998; Newman et al, 2004; Petitto et al., 2000; Nishimura et al., 1999; Söderfeldt et al., 1994, 1997). In addition, some studies also reported activation in Broca's area during sign comprehension (Levänen et al.,

2001; MacSweeney et al., 2002; Neville et al., 1998; Newman et al., 2004). Unlike sign production, however, activation in Broca's area was bilateral for sign comprehension in all studies (as was activation in superior temporal cortex). Note, however, that when audio-visual speech is presented to hearing subjects, similar bilateral activation of Broca's area is observed (Capek et al., 2004; MacSweeney et al., 2002). "Audio-visual speech" refers to viewing and listening to a talking person. Sign language comprehension does not appear to recruit more right hemisphere regions than comprehension of audio-visual speech, the most natural way to process spoken language (but see Capek et al., 2004). For both sign and speech, activation within Broca's area is more left-lateralized for language production than for comprehension.

To date, no studies (that I am aware of) have specifically examined the role of Broca's area in the syntactic processing of sign language. However, Hickok, Say, Bellugi, and Klima (1996) investigated the ASL comprehension abilities of the aphasic signer R.S., who had damage restricted primarily to Broca's area. Although her comprehension of single ASL signs and simple sentences was relatively good compared to signers with left temporal lobe damage, R.S. performed poorly on a test assessing the comprehension of signing space to express subject-object distinctions. In this test, the examiner produced a signed description in which two nouns (e.g., CAT, DOG) were associated with two locations in signing space using pointing signs. The examiner then produced a verb (e.g., BITE) with movement between the two spatial locations indicating subject (the first location) and object (the second location). The sentences were reversible, and only the direction of the verb indicated which noun should be understood as the subject or object. R.S. was asked to chose which of two pictures matched the signed sentence (e.g., "The dog bites the cat" or "The cat bites the dog"). R.S. performed significantly worse than control subjects, and her performance was not reliably different from chance.

However, it is not clear whether the source of R.S.'s impairment on this task can be traced to a specific deficit in syntactic processing. For example, Poizner, Klima, and Bellugi (1987) reported that *both* left- and right-hemisphere damaged signers performed poorly on the comprehension test used by Hickok et al. (1996). Furthermore, errors on this test could be due to a number of factors: failures of spatial memory (e.g., forgetting which noun was associated with which location), impairment in the ability to determine verb argument structure, or difficulty with non-canonical structures (in natural discourse, it is rare to find the type of construction tested by Hickok et al. (1996), i.e., two nouns associated with two spatial locations via pointing signs, followed immediately by a directional verb).

Grodzinsky (2000) proposed that Broca's area plays a limited and very specific role in syntactic processing. He hypothesized that Broca's area houses the "receptive mechanisms involved in the computation of the relation between transformationally moved phrasal constituents and their extraction sites" (Grodzinsky, 2000, p. 1). Interestingly, unpublished data from Hickok (1994) indicate that R.S. had particular difficulty comprehending sentences with topicalized objects that involve transformational movement. On a picture-matching task, R.S. scored at chance (7/14) comprehending topicalized object sentences (e.g., BOY, GIRL PUSH; see Fig. 11–2), but performed quite well (13/14) on sentences without movement (e.g., GIRL PUSH BOY). I know of no other lesion or imaging data (published or unpublished) that speak to the neural substrate underlying the comprehension of syntactic movement in sign language.

However, without further investigation, the syntactic specificity of R.S.'s deficit is somewhat suspect. For example, the comprehension deficits observed for R.S. could be due to impairment of working memory. Both the topicalized sentences and the sentences tested by Hickok et al. (1996) require that two potential verb arguments be maintained in working memory until the verb is encountered. Therefore, we next turn to the possible role of Broca's area in working memory for sign language.

BROCA'S AREA AND WORKING MEMORY FOR SIGN LANGUAGE

Models of working memory typically contain two major components, one used for verbal material, the other used for visual spatial material (e.g., Baddeley, 1986; Logie, 1995). Gathercole and Baddeley (1993) characterize these two subcomponents as follows: "The *phonological loop* maintains verbally coded information, whereas the *visuo-spatial sketchpad* is involved in the short-term processing and maintenance of material which has a strong visual or spatial component" (p. 4; italics in the original). Given that sign

languages are both "verbal" (i.e., linguistic) and visual-spatial, they pose a challenge for this characterization of working memory. In a series of studies, Margaret Wilson and I took up this challenge by investigating how language modality might shape the architecture of working memory (Wilson and Emmorey, 1997a, 1997b, 1998, 2000, 2001, 2003).

For hearing speakers, the phonological loop has been argued to consist of a phonological store with an articulatory process that refreshes information within the store. Wilson and Emmorey (1997a) conducted two experiments to discover whether working memory can support an articulatory rehearsal loop in the visuospatial domain (our model is presented in Fig. 11–4). Deaf ASL signers were tested on immediate serial recall. One experiment, using ASL stimuli, provided evidence for manual motoric coding: signers had worse recall under articulatory suppression—repetitive motion of the hands—than under no suppression (hands at rest). This experiment also replicated earlier findings of ASL-based phonological coding (Bellugi et al., 1975; Hanson, 1982). Specifically, signers exhibited worse recall for phonologically similar lists (all signs in a list had the same handshape and the same location, e.g., BROOM, PIE, BOOK) than for phonologically dissimilar lists (signs in a list differed in handshape and movement, e.g., EGG, KEY, SOCKS). The phonological similarity effect and the articulatory suppression effect did not interact, suggesting separate components which both contribute to memory performance. Stimuli in a second experiment were nameable pictures, which must be recoded for ASL-based rehearsal to occur. Under these conditions, articulatory suppression eliminated the phonological similarity effect. Thus, an articulatory process seems to be used in translating pictures

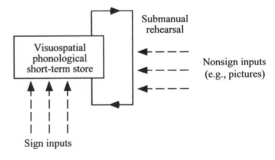

FIGURE 11–4. Illustration of the phonological loop model of sign-based working memory (from Emmorey, 2002).

into a phonological code for memory maintenance (see Fig. 11–4).

In addition, Wilson and Emmorey (1998) found a sign length effect for ASL, analogous to the word length effect for speech. Lists containing long signs (signs which traverse relatively long distances) produced poorer memory performance than lists of short signs (signs that do not change in location). Further, this length effect was eliminated by articulatory suppression, and articulatory suppression produced an overall drop in performance. This pattern of results indicates a configuration of components similar to the phonological loop for speech, suggesting that working memory can develop a language-based rehearsal loop in the visuospatial modality.

However, there is also evidence for modality-dependent processes in working memory. Wilson and Emmorey (2003) found that working memory for ASL is sensitive to irrelevant signed input (and other structured visual input) in a manner similar to the effects of irrelevant auditory input on working memory for speech. Deaf signers were disrupted on serial recall of lists of ASL signs when either pseudosigns or moving shapes were presented during a retention interval. Hearing subjects asked to recall lists of printed English words did not show disruption under the same interference conditions. The results favor models of working memory which hypothesize modality-specific representations, as opposed to amodal representations (e.g., Jones et al., 1996). The results also indicate that working memory for sign language involves visual or quasi-visual representations, suggesting parallels to visuo-spatial working memory. Furthermore, Wilson and Emmorey (2001) found that working memory for ASL may involve a type of spatial coding that is unavailable for spoken languages. This study showed that deaf signers can use signing space as a tool for maintaining serial order information (better performance for lists of signs with a moveable place of articulation (neutral space signs) than lists of signs with a fixed place of articulation on the body). Association of words with locations in space does not improve immediate recall performance for hearing speakers (although a method of loci strategy does enhance long term recall). These findings suggest that working memory for sign and for speech are each at least partially shaped by the sensorimotor modalities in which they are instantiated.

Thus, universal structural properties of language and sensori-motoric processing constraints interact to determine the cognitive architecture of working memory for sign and for speech (for review, see Emmorey, 2002). One question that arises is whether this cognitive architecture is instantiated in the brain in the same way for spoken and signed languages. Does working memory for sign language engage brain regions known to be involved in working memory for speech? Or does language modality influence the neural circuitry recruited during verbal working memory? For spoken language, working memory has been argued to involve inferior parietal regions subserving storage processes and left prefrontal regions subserving rehearsal and executive control processes (e.g., Smith and Jonides, 1997; Wagner, 2002). Specifically, Broca's area has been implicated as a potential substrate for rehearsal processes within the phonological loop of verbal working memory (Paulesu et al., 1993; Smith et al., 1998; Wagner et al., 2001).

Unfortunately, there has been little research investigating the neural circuitry for sign-based working memory. A recent fMRI study by Buchsbaum and colleagues (2005) suggests that both modality-independent and modality-dependent regions are engaged during working memory for sign language. In that study, deaf signers viewed ASL nonsense signs (phonologically possible, but nonexistent signs) and then silently rehearsed them. Buchsbaum et al. (2005) reported that Broca's area was active both while viewing the ASL stimuli and during silent (submanual) rehearsal. In a parallel study with hearing English speakers, Buchsbaum et al. (2001) found similar activation in Broca's area when subjects listened to nonsense words and when they rehearsed subvocally. Signers and speakers differed, however, with respect to the site of posterior parietal activation during rehearsal and encoding of linguistic stimuli. Signers showed activation in a site along the intraparietal sulcus, whereas the most dominant response for speakers was more ventral, along the posterior superior temporal gyrus at the parietal junction. Similarly, in a working memory study using PET, Rönnberg et al. (2004) found more parietal activation during an overt serial recall task with Swedish Sign Language compared to (spoken) Swedish, but no difference in activation within Broca's area for the two languages.

Buchsbaum et al. (2005), following Hickok and Poeppel (2000), argue that parietal activation during working memory tasks does not reflect the activation of the phonological storage buffer per se, rather this activation is due to a sensorimotor integration system that mediates between frontal articulatory systems and posterior sensory systems in which phonological information is represented. Therefore, they argue that the more dorsal parietal activation observed during sign-based working memory reflects visual-motor integration required for sign language and the more ventral and temporal activation during speech-based working memory reflects auditory-motor integration.

In sum, behavioral data indicate the cognitive architecture for verbal working memory is parallel for sign and for speech (see Fig. 11–4). However, effects of the different perceptual-motor systems of sign and speech can be found in the nature of phonological representations that must be stored and rehearsed (e.g., unlike speech-based working memory, sign-based working memory is affected by irrelevant visual input and can take advantage of spatial coding). The left frontal-parietal system that subserves the rehearsal and storage components of working memory for speech may also subserve these same components for sign-based working memory. However, there is some evidence that the specific neural sites within parietal (storage-relevant) cortex may be influenced by modality-specific properties of sign and speech.

BROCA'S AREA AND MANUAL ACTIONS

Recently, primate studies have identified mirror neurons within area F5 (inferior ventral premotor cortex) that respond both when a monkey manipulates an object and when the monkey observes another individual grasping or manipulating an object (Gallese et al., 1996; Rizzolatti et al., 1988, 1996). It has been hypothesized that the human homologue of area F5 in monkey is Broca's area (Iacoboni et al., 1999; Rizzolati and Arbib, 1998). Given that the articulators required for signing are the same as those involved in non-linguistic reaching and grasping, one might expect Broca's area to play an important role in both signing and in nonlinguistic action production.

However, unlike reaching and grasping, sign articulations are structured within a phonological system of contrasts. For grasping tasks, hand configuration is determined by the nature of the object to be held or manipulated. For sign production, hand configuration is determined by the phonological specification stored in the lexicon. For example, as shown in Figure 11–1, the hand configuration for the ASL

sign PLEASE is a B handshape, and this hand configuration contrasts with that for SORRY (an A handshape). As noted in the introduction, there is a limited inventory of contrasting hand configurations in ASL, and this inventory differs from other signed languages. The hand configuration used to grasp objects is generally functionally determined, but the hand configuration for signs is dependent on the lexicon and phonology of a particular sign language (e.g., the sign for PLEASE in British Sign Language is formationally distinct from ASL).

However, ASL contains some signs that appear to mimic grasping motions and the hand configuration in these signs represents how the human hand holds or manipulates an instrument or the hand represents the instrument itself. Specifically, ASL handling classifier verbs denote actions performed with an implement. For example, the sign BRUSH-HAIR is produced with a grasping handshape and a brushing motion at the head (see Fig. 11–5). Such verbs are referred to as *classifier* verbs because the handshape is morphemic and refers to a property of the referent object (e.g., the handle of a brush); see papers in Emmorey (2003) for a discussion of classifier constructions in signed languages). As can be seen in Figure 11–5A, the form of handling classifier verbs is quite iconic, depicting the hand configuration used to grasp and manipulate an object and the movement that is typically associated with the object's manipulation.

In addition, ASL nouns denoting tools or manipulable objects are often derived from instrument classifier verbs. For instrument classifier verbs, the object itself is represented by the articulator, and the movement of the sign reflects the stylized movement of the tool or implement. For example, the sign SCREW-DRIVER shown in Figure 11–5B is made with a twisting a motion, and the H handshape (fist with index and middle fingers extended) depicts the screwdriver itself, rather than how the hand would hold a screwdriver. In general, the movement of a noun in ASL reduplicates and shortens the movement of the related verb (Supalla and Newport, 1978). Thus, the twisting motion of the sign SCREWDRIVER is repeated and relatively short.

Given the motoric iconicity of handling classifier verbs and of many ASL nouns referring to manipulable objects, Emmorey et al. (2004) investigated whether such iconicity impacts the neural systems that underlie tool and action naming for deaf ASL

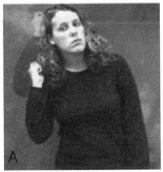 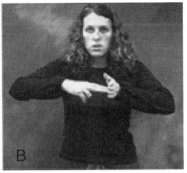 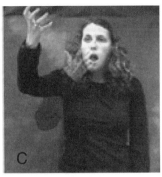

| BRUSH-HAIR | SCREWDRIVER | YELL |

FIGURE 11–5. Illustration of an American Sign Language verb and noun that resemble pantomime (A and B) and a verb that does not exhibit such sensory-motor iconicity (C). (A) BRUSH-HAIR; (B) SCREWDRIVER; (C) YELL.

signers. In this PET study, signers were asked to name actions performed with an implement (producing handling classifier verbs), actions performed without a tool (e.g., YELL in Figure 11–5C), and manipulable objects (nouns referring to tools or utensils). The results showed that the sensory-motoric iconicity of ASL signs denoting tools (e.g., SCREWDRIVER) and of handling classifier verbs denoting actions performed with a tool (e.g., BRUSH-HAIR) does not alter the neural systems that underlie lexical retrieval or sign production.

Specifically, naming tools or tool-based actions engages a left premotor-parietal cortical network for both signers and speakers. The neural activation maximum observed within left premotor cortex for ASL handling classifier verbs (−39, +1, +41) was similar to the premotor activation observed when English speakers named the function or use of tools (−39, −6, +51; Grafton et al., 1997). Naming tools with iconic ASL signs also engaged left premotor cortex (−40, 0, +35), and this activation maximum was similar to that found when English speakers named tools: −52, +11, +29 (Grabowski et al., 1998); −50, +3, +25 (Chao and Martin, 2000). These premotor sites are generally superior to Broca's area. Activation maxima within the left inferoparietal cortex when naming tools or tool-based actions were also similar for signers and speakers. When signers or speakers named actions that did not involve tools (e.g., yelling, sleeping) or nonmanipulable objects (e.g., animals that are not pets) activation within this left premotor-parietal network was not observed (Damasio et al., 1996, 2001; Emmorey

et al., 2004, 2003). Thus, activation within this network may represent retrieval of knowledge about the sensory- and motor-based attributes of grasping movements associated with tools and commonly manipulated objects.

In addition, Broca's area was activated when signers named tools (−42, +28, +18), tool-based actions (−46, +26, +13), and actions without tools (−47, +21, +15) (Emmorey et al., 2004). As suggested earlier, this activation may reflect lexical retrieval and/or selection processes during naming. Activation in Broca's area is not reported when subjects are asked to pantomime tool use (Choi et al., 2001; Moll et al., 2000). The fact that the production of ASL verbs resembling pantomime (e.g., BRUSH-HAIR) and non-pantomimic verbs (e.g., YELL) both engaged Broca's area suggests that handling classifier verbs are lexical forms, rather than nonlinguistic gestures. This result is complemented by two case studies of aphasic signers who exhibit a dissociation between the ability to sign and to pantomime (Corina et al., 1992; Marshall et al., 2004). Corina et al. (1992) describe the case of WL who had a large frontotemporoparietal lesion in the left hemisphere. The lesion included Broca's area, the arcuate fasciculus, a small portion of inferoparietal lobule (Brodmann's area 40) and considerable damage to the white matter deep to the inferoparietal lobule. WL exhibited poor sign comprehension, and his signing was characterized by phonological and semantic errors with reduced grammatical structure. An example of a phonological error by WL was his production of the sign SCREWDRIVER. He substituted an A-bar handshape (fist with thumb extended, touching the palm of the non-dominant hand) for the required H handshape (see Fig. 11–1B). In contrast to his sign production, WL was unimpaired in his ability to produce pantomime. For example, instead of signing DRINK (a C handshape (fingers extended and curved as if holding a cup) moves toward the mouth, with wrist rotation—as if drinking), WL cupped his hands together to form a small bowl. WL was able to produce stretches of pantomime and tended to substitute pantomimes for signs, even when pantomime required more complex movements. Such pantomimes were not evident before his brain injury.

Marshall et al. (2004) report a second case of a deaf aphasic signer who also demonstrated a striking dissociation between gesture and sign (in this case, British Sign Language). "Charles" had a left temporoparietal lesion and exhibited sign anomia that was parallel to speech anomia. For example, his sign finding difficulties were sensitive to sign frequency and to cueing, and he produced both semantic and phonological errors. However, his gesture production was intact and superior to his sign production even when the forms of the signs and gestures were similar. Furthermore, this dissociation was impervious to the iconicity of signs. His production of iconic signs was as impaired as his production of non-iconic signs. Thus, the lesion data support the neuroimaging results. The neural systems supporting sign language production and pantomimic expression are non-identical. Specifically, Broca's area is engaged during the lexical retrieval of signs denoting tools and tool-based actions, but not during tool-use pantomime (Choi et al., 2001; Moll et al., 2000).

Although Broca's area (specifically, BA 44) is activated when subjects imitate non-linguistic finger movements (Iacoboni et al., 1999; Tanaka and Inui, 2002), activation in Broca's area has not been found when signers imitate (repeat) visually presented signs, in contrast to visual fixation (Petitto et al., 2000; supplemental material). Activation in the posterior inferior frontal gyrus (including Broca's area) is rarely reported when speakers repeat (i.e., imitate) spoken words (Indefrey and Levelt, 2000). Repetition of manual signs (or oral words) does not require lexical retrieval/selection and is cognitively quite distinct from imitating novel manual movements because mental representations specifying form exist only for lexical items, not for finger/hand movements. Thus,

although Broca's area may be engaged during the imitation of manual actions, it appears to play a different role in sign language production.

CONCLUSIONS

Overall, the functions associated with Broca's area for spoken language parallel those for signed language. With respect to language production, the imaging data indicate a critical role for Broca's area (particularly BA 45) in lexical retrieval and/or selection. More posterior cortex (BA 44) appears to be involved in the coordination of linguistic articulation, regardless of whether the articulators are manual-brachial or orofacial (Horowitz et al., 2003). The precise role of Broca's area in sign language comprehension is less clear. Imaging studies that presented signed sentences for comprehension reported activation in Broca's area (MacSweeney et al., 2001; Neville et al., 1998; Newman et al., 2004), but Petitto et al. (2000; supporting material) reported no such activation for viewing single signs compared to fixation (but see Levänen et al., 2001). Data from a deaf aphasic signer with specific damage to Broca's area suggested impairment in comprehension of sentences with moved constituents (object topicalization), but much more detailed studies of the effects of anterior and posterior damage on the syntactic abilities of aphasic signers are needed.

Broca's area has also been identified as critical to rehearsal processes for spoken language materials. Behavioral data from signers indicates that sign-based working memory exhibits a cognitive architecture that is similar to speech-based working memory (see Fig. 11–4). Much more research is needed to determine whether the neural systems that instantiate working memory are parallel for signed language. The few existing imaging studies suggest that Broca's area is also engaged during rehearsal of signs (Buchsbaum et al., 2005; Rönnberg et al., 2004).

Finally, Broca's area (specifically BA 44) has been hypothesized to house mirror neurons in humans. Although Broca's area has been found to be engaged during human action perception (e.g., observing a person drink from a cup) and during verb generation, the peak activation sites for action observation and verb production were distinct for individual subjects (Hamzei et al., 2003). Data from signed languages suggest that action production (e.g., pantomime) and sign production are distinct and subserved by non-identical neural systems. However, imaging studies that directly compare sign and gesture production or compare action observation and sign/gesture comprehension have not yet been conducted. Such studies will help determine whether mirror neurons (or the human functional equivalent) are specific to non-linguistic action production/observation or respond during the production/observation of linguistic actions as well.

ACKNOWLEDGMENTS   Preparation of this chapter was supported by NIH grants RO1 HD13249 and RO1 DC00146.

Note

1. By convention, ASL signs are written in capital letters representing English glosses (the nearest equivalent translation).

References

Baddeley, A. (1986). *Working memory.* Oxford: Clarendon Press.

Baker, C., & Cokely, D. (1980). *ASL: A teacher's resource text on grammar and culture.* Silver Spring, MD: TJ Publishers.

Bellugi, U., Klima, E. S., & Siple, P. (1974). Remembering in signs. *Cognition, 3,* 93–125.

Blumstein, S. (1998). Phonological aspects of aphasia. In M.T. Sarno (Ed.), *Acquired aphasia* (pp. 157–185), third edition. San Diego: Academic Press.

Braun, A.R., Varga, M., Stager, S., Shulz, G., Selbie, S., Maisog, J.M., et al. (1997). Altered patterns of cerebral activity during speech and language production in developmental stuttering. An H2O-15 positron emission tomography study. *Brain, 120,* 761–784.

Braun, A.R., Guillemin, A., Hosey, L., & Varga, V. (2001). The neural organization of discourse: An $H_2^{15}O$ PET study of narrative production in English and American Sign Language. *Brain, 124,* 2028–2044.

Brentari, D. (1998). *A prosodic model of sign language phonology.* Cambridge, MA: MIT Press.

Buchsbaum, B., Hickok, G., & Humphries, C. (2001). Role of left posterior superior temporal gyrus in phonological processing for speech perception and production. *Cognitive Science, 15,* 663–678.

Buchsbaum, B., Pickell, P., Love, T., Hatrak, M., Bellugi, U., & Hickok, G. (2005). Neural substrates for verbal working memory in deaf signers: fMRI study and lesion case report. *Brain and Language, 95,* 265–272.

Capek, C.M., Bavelier, D., Corina, D., Newman, A.J., Jezzard, P., & Neville, H.J. (2004). The cortical organization of audio-visual sentence comprehension: An fMRI study at 4 Tesla. *Cognitive Brain Research, 20,* 111–119.

Chao, L., & Martin, A. (2000). Representation of manipulable man-made objects in the dorsal stream. *NeuroImage, 12,* 478–484.

Choi, S.H., Na, D.L., Kang, E., Lee, K.M., Lee, S.W., & Na, D.G. (2001). Functional magnetic resonance imaging during pantomiming tool-use gestures. *Experimental Brain Research, 139,* 311–317.

Cook, N.D. (2003). Hemispheric dominance has its origins in the control of the midline organs of speech. *Behavioral and Brain Sciences, 26,* 216–217.

Corina, D.P., & Sandler, W. (1993). On the nature of phonological structure in sign language. *Phonology, 10,* 165–207.

Corina, D.P. (1998). Aphasia in users of signed languages. In P. Coppens, Y. Lebrun, & A. Basso (Eds.), *Aphasia in atypical populations* (pp. 261–310). Mahwah, NJ: Lawrence Erlbaum Associates.

Corina, D.P., McBurney, S.L., Dodrill, C., Hinshaw, K., Brinkley, J., & Ojemann, G. (1999). Functional roles of Broca's area and supramarginal gyrus: Evidence from cortical stimulation mapping in a deaf signer. *NeuroImage, 10,* 570–581.

Corina, D.P., Poizner, H., Bellugi, U., Feinberg, T., Dowd, D., & O'Grady-Batch, L. (1992). Dissociation between linguistic and non-linguistic gestural systems: A case for compositionality. *Brain and Language, 43,* 414–447.

Corina, D.P., San Jose-Robertson, L., Guillemin, A., High, J., & Braun, A. (2003). Language lateralization in a bimanual language. *Journal of Cognitive Neuroscience, 15,* 718–730.

Damasio, H., Grabowski, T.J., Tranel, D., Hichwa, R., & Damasio, A.R. (1996). A neural basis for lexical retrieval. *Nature, 380,* 499–505.

Damasio, H., Grabowski, T.J., Tranel, D., Ponto, L.L.B., Hichwa, R.D., & Damasio, A.R. (2001). Neural correlates of naming actions and of naming spatial relations. *NeuroImage, 13,* 1053–1064.

Ekman, P. (1992). Facial expression of emotion: An old controversy and new findings. In V. Bruce (Ed.), *Processing the facial image* (pp. 63–69). Oxford: Clarendon Press.

Emmorey, K., & Grabowki, T. (2004). Neural organization for sign versus speech production. *Journal of Cognitive Neuroscience Supplement, F69,* 205.

Emmorey, K., & Herzig, M. (2003). Categorical versus gradient properties of classifier constructions in ASL. In K. Emmorey (Ed)., *Perspectives on classifier constructions in signed languages* (pp. 222–246). Mahwah, NJ: Lawrence Erlbaum Associates.

Emmorey, K. (Ed.) (2003). *Perspectives on classifier constructions in signed languages*. Mahwah, NJ: Lawrence Erlbaum and Associates.

Emmorey, K. (2002). *Language, cognition, and the brain: Insights from sign language research*. Mahwah, NJ: Lawrence Erlbaum and Associates.

Emmorey, K., Damasio, H., McCullough, S., Grabowski, T., Ponto, L., Hichwa, R., et al. (2002). Neural systems underlying spatial language in American Sign Language. *NeuroImage, 17,* 812–824.

Emmorey, K., Grabowski, T., McCullough, S., Damasio, H., Ponto, L., Hichwa, R., et al. (2003). Neural systems underlying lexical retrieval for sign language. *Neuropsychologia, 41,* 85–95.

Emmorey, K., Grabowski, T., McCullough, S., Damasio, H., Ponto, L., Hichwa, R., et al. (2004). Motor-iconicity of sign language does not alter the neural systems underlying tool and action naming. *Brain and Language, 89,* 27–37.

Emmorey, K., Grabowski, T., McCullough, S., Ponto, L., Hichwa, R., & Damasio, H. (submitted). The neural correlates of spatial language in English and American Sign Language: A PET study with hearing bilinguals.

Fischer, S. (1974). Sign language and linguistic universals. In C. Rohrer & N. Ruwet (Eds)., *Actes du Colloque Franco-Allemand de Grammaire Transformationelle, Band II: Etudes de Sémantique et Autres* (pp. 187–204). Tübingen: Max Neimery Verlag.

Gallese, V., Fadiga, L., Fogassi, L., & Rizzolatti, G. (1996). Action recognition in the premotor cortex. *Brain, 119,* 593–609.

Gathercole, S., & Baddeley, A. (1993). *Working memory and language*. Hove, UK: Lawrence Erlbaum Associates.

Goodglass, H. (1993). *Understanding aphasia*. San Diego, CA: Academic Press.

Grabowski, T.J., Damasio, H., & Damasio, A. (1998). Premotor and prefrontal correlates of category-related lexical retrieval. *NeuroImage, 7,* 232–243.

Grafton, S., Fadiga, L., Arbib, M., & Rizzolatti, G. (1997). Premotor cortex activation during observation and naming of familiar tools. *NeuroImage, 6,* 231–236.

Grodzinsky, Y. (2000). The neurology of syntax: Language use without Broca's area. *Brain and Behavior Sciences, 23,* 1–71.

Hamzei, F., Rijntjes, M., Dettmers, C., Glauche, V., Weiller, C., & Büchel, C., (2003). The human ation recognition system and its relationship to Broca's area: An fMRI study. *NeuroImage, 19,* 637–644.

Hanson, V.L. (1982). Short-term recall by deaf signers of American Sign Language: Implications of encoding strategy for order recall. *Journal of Experimental Psychology, 8,* 572–583.

Hickok, G., & Poeppel, D. (2000). Towards a functional neuroanatomy of speech perception. *Trends in Cognitive Sciences, 4,* 131–138.

Hickok, G., Kritchevsky, M., Bellugi, U., & Klima, E.S. (1996). The role of the left frontal operculum in sign language aphasia. *Neurocase, 2,* 373–380.

Hickok, G., Love-Geffen, T., & Klima, E.S. (2002). Role of the left hemisphere in sign language comprehension. *Brain and Language, 82,* 167–178.

Hickok, G., Say, K., Bellugi, U., & Klma, E.S. (1996). The basis of hemispheric asymmetries for language and spatial cognition: Clues from focal brain damage in two deaf native signers. *Aphasiology, 10,* 577–591.

Horwitz, B., Amunts, K., Bhattacharyya, R., Patkin, D., Jeffries, K., Zilles, K., et al. (2003). Activation of Broca's area during the production of spoken and signed language: A combined cytoarchitectonic mapping and PET analysis. *Neuropsychologia, 41,* 1868–1876.

Iacoboni, M., Woods, R.P., Brass, M., Bekkering, H., Mazziotta, J.C., & Rizzolatti, G. (1999). Cortical mechanisms of human imitation. *Science 286,* 2526–2528.

Indefrey, P., & Levelt, W. (2000) The neural correlates of language production. In M. Gazzaniga (Ed.), *The new cognitive neurosciences* (pp. 845–865). Cambridge, MA: MIT Press.

Jones, D.M., Beaman, P., & Macken, W.J. (1996). The object-oriented episodic record model. In S. Gathercole (Ed.), *Models of short-term memory* (pp. 209–237). Hove, UK: Psychology Press.

Levänen, S., Uutela, K., Salenius, S., & Hari, R. (2001). Cortical representation of sign language: Comparison of deaf signers and hearing non-signers. *Cerebral Cortex, 11,* 506–512.

Lillo-Martin, D. (1991). *Universal grammar and American sign language: Setting the null argument parameters*. Dordrecht, the Netherlands: Kluwer Academic Publishers.

Logie, R.H. (1995). *Visuo-spatial working memory*. Hillsdale, NJ: Lawrence Erlbaum and Associates.

MacSweeney, M., Woll, B., Campbell, R., McGuire, P.K., David, A.S., Williams, S.C.R., et al. (2002). Neural systems underlying British Sign Language and audio-visual English processing in native users. *Brain, 125,* 1583–1593.

Marshall, J., Atkinson, J., Smulovitch, E., Thacker, A., & Woll, B. (2004). Aphasia in a user of British Sign

Language: Dissociation between sign and gesture. *Cognitive Neuropsychology, 21(5)*, 537–554.

McGuire, P., Robertson, D., Thacker, A., David, A.S., Kitson, N., Frackovwiak, R.S.J., & Frith, C.D. (1997). Neural correlates of thinking in sign language. *NeuroReport, 8*, 695–697.

McIntire, M. 1980. *Locatives in American Sign Language*. Unpublished Ph.D. dissertation, University of California, Los Angeles.

Moll, J., de Oliveira-Souza, R., Passman, L.J., Cimini Cunha, F., Souza-Lima, F., & Andreiuolo, P.A. (2000). Functional MRI correlates of real and imagined tool-use pantomimes. *Neurology, 54*, 1331–1336.

Neidle, C., Kegl, J., MacLaughlin, D., Bahan, B., & Lee, R.G. (2000). *The syntax of American Sign Language: Functional categories and hierarchical structure*. Cambridge, MA: MIT Press.

Neville, H., Bavelier, D., Corina, D., Rauschecker, J., Karni, A., Lalwani, A., et al. (1998). Cerebral organization for language in deaf and hearing subjects: Biological constraints and effects of experience. *Proceedings of the National Academy of Science USA, 95*, 922–929.

Newman, A., Supalla, T., Hauser, P., Newport, E., & Bavelier, D. (2004). Brain organization for morphosyntactic and narrative structure in American Sign Language: An fMRI study. *Journal of Cognitive Neuroscience Supplement, E91*, 175.

Nishimura, H., Hashikawa, K., Doi, D., Iwaki, T., Watanabe, Y., Kusuoka, H., et al. (1999). Sign language 'heard' in the auditory cortex. *Nature, 397*, 116.

Padden, C. (1983). *Interaction of morphology and syntax in American Sign Language*. Doctoral dissertation, published in 1988 in Outstanding Dissertations in Linguistics, Series IV, New York: Garland.

Paulesu, E., Frith, C.D., & Frackowiak, R.S. (1993). The neural correlates of the verbal component of working memory. *Nature, 362*, 342–345.

Petersen, S.E., Fox, P.T., Posner, M.I., Mintun, M.A., & Raichle, M.E. (1988). Positron emission tomographic studies of the cortical anatomy of single-word processing. *Nature, 331*, 585–589.

Petitto, L.A., Zatorre, R.J., Gauna, K., Nikelski, E.J., Dostie, D., & Evans, A. (2000). Speech-like cerebral activity in profoundly deaf people processing signed languages: Implications for the neural basis of human language. *Proceedings of the National Academy of Sciences USA, 97*, 13961–13966.

Petronio, K., & Lillo-Martin, D. (1997). WH-movement and the position of spec-CP: Evidence from American Sign Language. *Language, 73*, 18–57.

Poizner, H., Klima, E.S., & Bellugi, U. (1987). *What the hands reveal about the brain*. Cambridge, MA: MIT Press.

Rizzolati, G., & Arbib, M. (1998). Language within our grasp. *Trends in Neuroscience, 21*, 188–194.

Rizzolatti, G., Carmarda, R., Fogassi, L., Gentilucci, M., Luppino, G., & Matelli, M. (1988). Functional organization of inferior area 6 in the macaque monkey. II. Area F5 and the control of distal movements. *Experimental Brain Research, 71*, 491–507.

Rizzolatti, G., Fadiga, L, Gallese, V., & Fogassi, L. (1996). Premotor cortex and the recognition of motor actions. *Cognitive Brain Research, 3*, 131–141.

Rönnberg, J., Rudner, M., & Ingvar, M. (2004). Neural correlates of working memory for sign language. *Cognitive Brain Research, 20*, 165–182.

Sandler, W., & Lillo-Martin, D. (2006). *Sign language and linguistic universals*. Cambridge University Press.

Sandler, W. (1989). *Phonological representation of the sign: Linearity and nonlinearity in American Sign Language*. Dordrecht, Holland: Foris Publications.

Shepard-Kegl, J. (1985). *Locative relations in American Sign Language word formation, syntax, and discourse*. Ph.D. Dissertation, MIT, Cambridge, MA.

Smith, E.E., & Jonides, J. (1997). Working memory: A view from neuroimaging. *Cognitive Psychology, 33*, 5–42.

Smith, E.E., Jonides, J., Marshuetz, C., & Koeppe, R.A. (1998). Components of verbal working memory: Evidence from neuroimaging. *Proceedings of the National Academy of Sciences USA, 95*, 876–882.

Söderfeldt, B., Ingvar, M., Rönnberg, J., Eriksson, L., Serrander, M., & Stone-Elander, S. (1997). Signed and spoken language perception studied by positron emission tomography. *Neurology, 49*, 82–87.

Söderfeldt, B., Rönnberg, J., & Risberg, J. (1994). Regional cerebral blood flow in sign language users. *Brain and Language, 46*, 59–68.

Supalla, T., & Newport, E. (1978). How many seats in a chair? The derivation of nouns and verbs in American Sign Language. In P. Siple (Ed.), *Understanding language through sign language research*. New York: Academic Press.

Tanaka, S., & Inui, T. (2002). Cortical involvement for action imitation of hand/arm versus finger configurations: An fMRI study. *NeuroReport, 13*, 1599–1602.

Thompson-Schill, S.L., D'Esposito, M., Aguirre, G.K., & Farah, M.J. (1997). Role of left inferior prefrontal cortex in retrieval of semantic knowledge: A reevaluation. *Proceedings of the National Academy of Sciences USA, 94*, 1472–14797.

Van der Hulst, H. (1993). Units in the analysis of signs. *Phonology, 10*, 209–241.

Wagner, A.D. (2002). Cognitive control and episodic memory: Contributions from prefrontal cortex. In

L. Squire & D. Schachter (Eds)., *Neuropychology of memory* (pp. 174–192). New York: The Guilford Press.

Wagner, A.D., Maril, A., Bjork, R., & Schachter, D. (2001). Prefrontal contributions to executive control: fMRI evidence for functional distinctions within lateral prefrontal cortex. *NeuroImage, 14,* 1337–1347.

Wilson, M., & Emmorey, K. (1997a). A visual-spatial "phonological loop" in working memory: Evidence from American Sign Language. *Memory and Cognition, 25,* 313–320.

Wilson, M., & Emmorey, K. (1997b). Working memory for sign language: A window into the architecture of working memory. *Journal of Deaf Studies and Deaf Education, 2,* 123–132.

Wilson, M., & Emmorey, K. (1998). A "word length effect" for sign language: Further evidence on the role of language in structuring working memory. *Memory and Cognition, 26,* 584–590.

Wilson, M., & Emmorey, K. (2000). When does modality matter? Evidence from ASL on the nature of working memory. In K. Emmorey & H. Lane (Eds.), *The signs of language revisited: An anthology to honor Ursula Bellugi and Edward Klima* (pp. 135–142). Mahwah, NJ: Lawrence Erlbaum and Associates.

Wilson, M., & Emmorey, K. (2001). Functional consequences of modality: Spatial coding in working memory for signs. In V. Dively, M. Metzger, S. Taub, & A.M. Baer (Eds.), *Sign languages: Discoveries from international research* (pp. 91–99). Washington, DC: Gallaudet University Press.

Wilson, M., & Emmorey, K. (2003). The effect of irrelevant visual input on working memory for sign language. *Journal of Deaf Studies and Deaf Education, 8,* 97–103.

IV

PSYCHOLINGUISTIC INVESTIGATIONS

12

Broca's Area and
Lexical-Semantic Processing

Stefano F. Cappa
Daniela Perani

Every neurologist gets acquainted early in her training with the syndrome of Broca's aphasia. It is a fairly common consequence of an acute lesion, usually a left-sided infarction in the territory of the anterior branches of the middle cerebral artery, and the clinical presentation is relatively straightforward. The patients' speech is impaired, which is what would be expected in a condition bearing the rather pessimistic name of aphasia. The articulation is affected, resulting in speech production, which is often hard to understand; what the listener often grasps are a few isolated words, which do not appear to be integrated in proper sentences. On the other hand, the patient appears to understand what is said, at least in the limited context of a neurological examination: simple commands, such as close your eyes, raise your arms, etc. During our neurology training, which took place in sophisticated aphasiological environments, we soon became aware that the idea of "articulated language" sitting in a small chunk of brain tissue, namely the foot of the left third frontal convolution, was fairly simplistic. As a possible consequence of this, we were hooked up to the relationship between language and the brain for the rest of our life. It was not a bad time to get into this area. In the late seventies, the availability of computerized axial tomography (CAT scan) was revamping the rather stale field of clinicoanatomical correlations in neurology. Aphasia, the traditional battlefield of localizer and antilocalizer, was of course immediately invested by the new developments.

In the present chapter our arbitrary choice, due to reasons of space, is to focus the review on the relationship between Broca's area and lexical-semantic processing starting from that period. In the first section, we will briefly review the aphasiological evidence for lexical and/or semantic impairment in the syndrome of Broca's aphasia. In the second, we will consider the relationship between damage to Broca's area and neighboring structures and specific aspects of linguistic impairment in the syndrome, including disorders of lexical/semantic processing. Finally, we will review the contribution of functional imaging to the issue of the role of Broca's area in lexical/semantic processing.

LEXICAL DISORDERS IN BROCA'S APHASIA

The classic description of the syndrome of Broca's aphasia is centered on a cluster of symptoms of speech and language impairment. Goodglass and Kaplan (1972) provide a concise description: "its essential characteristics are awkward articulation, restricted vocabulary, restriction of grammar to the simplest, more over-learned forms, and relative preservation of auditory comprehension." A lexical disorder was thus considered to be an integral part of the syndrome of Broca's aphasia. Actually, Goodglass and Kaplan observe that, in the case of good recovery, Broca's aphasia loses its distinctive features, leaving a residual picture of word-finding difficulties, which makes it "barely distinguishable" from anomic aphasia. A more precise description of naming difficulties in Broca's aphasia can be found in an earlier, classic paper about "semantic word categories in aphasia" (Goodglass et al., 1966). Here, Broca's aphasics are shown to be defective in naming all categories of stimuli (objects, action words, colors, numbers and letters), with an overall performance level which is not different from fluent aphasics. As for error types, Kohn and Goodglass (1985) found that the production of semantic and phonological errors in picture naming was comparable for all diagnostic categories. In other words, Broca's aphasics were as likely to produce semantic and phonemic paraphasias as Wernicke's. However, Goodglass and coworkers clearly formulated the concept that a similar level of performance can be associated to different mechanisms of impairment. The finding that Broca's aphasics, but not Wernicke's, are facilitated by phonemic cueing, and show the TOT phenomenon was taken to indicate that the naming disorder in BA reflects a "difficulty in the programming of phonological information for articulation."

The clinical observation that the production of patients with Broca's aphasia might be characterized by a difficulty with verbs, both at the single word and at the sentence level, has opened an active field of psycholinguistic investigation. The representation of lexical items includes syntactic and semantic information. In the case of verbs, crucial aspects are subcategorization frame, argument structure and thematic roles (see Shapiro and Nagel, 1995). Since agrammatism is one of the crucial aspects of Broca's aphasia, it has been hypothesized that defective verb retrieval may reflect an impairment in dealing with lexical items associated with complex argument structure (Thompson et al., 1997; see also Collina et al., 2001). The situation however appears to be more complex. Shapiro and Levine (1990) found that, during sentence comprehension, agrammatic Broca's aphasics activate complex argument structures at the same level as normal subjects, suggesting a preservation of this information in real-time verb processing. Further, there is evidence from production indicating the role of morphological impairment. The verbs, which are produced by agrammatic subjects, are often lacking in inflection (Miceli et al., 1989). Grodzinsky (1984) observed that in the case of languages in which the production of inflectional morphology is required for lexical or lexical/phonological well formedness (such as Italian and Hebrew), the most frequent errors are morphological substitutions, usually towards a default form (typically the infinitive).

It is noteworthy that most of the case reports of patients with selective, or relatively selective, disorders in the processing of nouns and verbs have capitalized on the results of tasks at the single word level (typically, picture naming and word-picture matching; Miceli et al., 1988). In general, these case studies were not aimed at the definition of the anatomical correlates of the observed dissociation. However, an analysis of the reported lesion sites, assessed with computerized brain tomography, indicated that, while patients with selective disorders of noun processing had lesions centered on the left temporal lobe, verb impairment was associated to damage involving, or limited, to the left prefrontal cortex. The first careful anatomical study of a patient with selective action naming impairment was reported by Damasio and Tranel in 1993. The MRI lesion involved the left premotor frontal cortex. In a recent study, Tranel et al. (2001) have shown that damage to a region involving the left frontal operculum, the inferior sector of the pre-central and post-central gyri and the anterior part of the insula is associated with severe action-naming impairment. However, patients with lesions involving this area were often impaired also in object naming, and damage to other posterior areas (mesial occipital cortex, white matter underlying the posterior temporoparietal region) was also associated with action naming impairment. A striking disorder of action naming and comprehension has also been reported in motor neuron disease patients with pathologically verified involvement of Ba 44 and 45 (Bak et al., 2001). More recently, several case reports have indicated the presence of a severe, selective disorder of action naming in patients with nonfluent progressive aphasia, the variant of fronto-temporal dementia associated with prevalent atrophy in the Broca's region (Gorno-Tempini et al., 2004; Hillis et al., 2004).

Other case reports further indicate that action naming impairment can be associated with lesions sparing Broca's area. Lesions centered in the left parietal lobe were observed in several patients with a disproportionate deficit in verb processing (see, for example, Silveri and Di Betta, 1997).

These findings indicate that patients with a selective difficulty in action naming and, maybe, also of other aspects of language processing involving the grammatical category of verbs are as a rule affected by lesions which involve the frontal and parietal part of the left perisylvian language areas. The temporal lobe, and in particular its anterior part, are usually spared in these patients. It is noteworthy that, within the category of nouns, an interesting pattern of anatomical correlation has been derived from the investigation of patients with category-specific semantic disorders. Patients with defective naming of animals and persons usually have lesions affecting the temporal lobe, in particular its anterior part, while tool naming impairments are associated with perisylvian damage in the temporo-parietal and frontal areas (Damasio et al., 1996; Saffran and Schwartz, 1994).

Taken together, these findings support the hypothesis of a crucial role of areas in the left hemispheric convexity, including Broca's area, in the retrieval of lexical items related to action. These include verbs, but also nouns referring to tools. This issue will be discussed in more detail in the section on functional imaging studies.

BROCA'S APHASIA AND BROCA'S AREA

As indicated in the introduction, we will neglect many years of active research and hot debate about the language function of Broca's area, leaving out of the story important contributors such as Marie, Moutier, and Niessl von Mayendorf. A landmark of "modern" investigation of the role of Broca's area in language is the study of surgical lesions of "F3" by Hecaen and Consoli (1973). The sample of 19 patients was very heterogeneous from the point of view of the etiology (mostly tumor ablations) and of time post surgery (from 12 days to 17 years!). However, lesion localization appears to have been exceptionally careful, and a relatively detailed neurolinguistic examination was available for all patients. All the patients showed some aspect of language impairment, with the exception of the two angioma cases (the latter finding suggests that some reorganization of the language areas can be expected to take place in the case of congenital lesions). It is noteworthy that disorders of lexical retrieval in spontaneous production were observed in some of the patients. Impaired picture naming was found in five patients, in which it was associated with defective auditory comprehension. None of the patients with right-sided lesions had a similar pattern of impairment.

Only a few years later, several investigators started to apply the new technology of CT brain scanning to the investigation of the lesion correlates of aphasia syndromes. These were defined according to traditional classification schemes, based on the patient's performance on a cluster of language task. For example, in the Milan study (Mazzocchi and Vignolo, 1979), Broca's aphasia was defined on the basis of the results of a standardized examination. The Boston series was based on the results of the BDAE (Naeser and Hayward, 1978). The main result of these early investigations was that the syndrome of Broca's aphasia is associated with lesions, which extend beyond Broca's area proper, extending to other regions of the left hemisphere (motor cortex, insula, subcortical white matter, basal ganglia). No attempt was made at this time to fractionate the components of Broca's aphasia, with a remarkable exception. Jay P. Mohr and his colleagues (1978) published a remarkable paper, which was based on a personal series of 22 cases of Broca's aphasia, in which lesion information was available on the basis of "autopsy, CT scan, radionuclide brain scan or angiography" and included a review of cases published "from 1820 onward." The main result of this study, which expanded earlier reports by the same author, was that lesion limited to Broca's area proper were only associated with "mild, transient anomia." The authors' conclusion is that the multiple aspects of language function that are affected in the full-fledged syndrome reflect the synergistic function of the entire opercular and insular region. Within this area, there is no strict localization of function, but a sort of "team action," with ample possibility for vicariation due to neural plasticity. The authors underline that this rejection of a specific role for

Broca's area does not imply a complete denial of language localization. The deficit in Broca's aphasia is not the same as in Wernicke's aphasia, and it "involves grammar in particular."

In the following years, the Boston VA group, in particular, attempted an anatomical fractionation of the components of the syndrome. Tonkonogy and Goodglass (1981) provided important evidence, based on two pathologically verified cases, for the fractionation of articulatory impairment, due to damage to the rolandic operculum, and lexical impairment, associated with lesion of Broca's area proper. Naeser et al. (1989) correlated severe nonfluency to damage to specific white matter tracts. A crucial role of insular damage in the production of apraxia of speech was indicated by the lesion study of Dronkers (1996).

BROCA'S AREA AND LEXICAL PROCESSING: FUNCTIONAL IMAGING

Given the association of Broca's areas with multiple aspects of language processing indicated by clinical studies, the engagement of the same regions in normal subjects in tasks going beyond "speech production" should not have came as much surprise. An early language activation study with positron emission tomography clearly established, for example, that a purely input task, such as phoneme discrimination, resulted in activation of Broca's area (Zatorre et al., 1992). Many different tasks have been applied to the investigation of the brain correlates of lexical selection and retrieval. A very widely used task has been single word production according to a cue. The first published PET study of language activation (Petersen et al., 1988) showed that, in comparison to repetition, generating a "use" for a presented word resulted in an activation of several areas in left dorsolateral prefrontal cortex, as well as in anterior cingulate. The latter activation was attributed to the non-language-specific requirement for response selection, while the prefrontal activity was suggested to reflect, "some computation related to semantic processing or association between words" (Petersen and Fiez, 1993).[1] It is noteworthy that the foci of activation included areas 45 and 47, but not area 44. This finding opened a lively discussion about the convergence of imaging and lesion data. The reaction from the aphasiological community was that semantic dysfunction is not typically observed in Broca's aphasia. On the other hand, prefrontal lesions are associated with defective performance in "fluency" tasks, in which the patient is asked to generate as many items as possible belonging to a given category. Frith et al. (1991a) reported that generation of words (following semantic—names of jobs—or orthographic—beginning with a—cues) resulted in activation in area 46, i.e., in the same region activated by random movements generation (Frith et al., 1991b). This was interpreted as reflecting a non-linguistic ("intrinsic generation") rather than a semantic role of the prefrontal activity. No activation in Broca's area and surrounding region was observed during lexical decision, which extensively activated superior temporal areas (including BA 22) bilaterally. The conclusion was compatible with traditional views of language representation in the brain: the superior temporal regions were suggested to be "the store of word representations" (Wortschatz). We have summarized this debate, which now may seem outdated (even if it was only 12 years ago!), in some detail, because it includes all the crucial issues presently under investigation. First, is there a specific role of Broca's area in lexical-semantic processing, or are we observing in activation data a reflection of nonspecific aspects, such as selection among competitors, retrieval effort, working memory, etc.? Second, the classical question: what are we talking about, in terms of anatomy of Broca's area? Let us now consider analytically other imaging studies, subdivided according to the task involved.

Word Generation

Phonological vs. Semantic Cues

There is considerable evidence that retrieving a word following a phonological or semantic cue results in a differential pattern of activity within Broca's area. Mummery et al. (1996) found a selective activation of BA 44/6 during phonological fluency. Using fMRI, we found an engagement of area 44 only in the case of phonological cues, while both engaged Ba 45 (Paulesu et al., 1997).

Semantic Category Effects

Martin et al. (1995) were the first to show that the semantic content of the word to be retrieved mattered. In particular, generating action words (action associated with an achromatic object picture) activated Broca's area (BA 44) more extensively than generating the color of the object. A similarly located activation was found by Warburton et al. (1996) in the comparison between generating multiple actions appropriate to a heard concrete noun, and generating nouns belonging to a heard superordinate noun. The contrast between generating natural kinds versus objects, and vice versa, did not result in prefrontal differences in the PET study by Mummery et al. (1996). Recently, we have performed a functional magnetic resonance study of semantic fluency for animal and tool names (Vitali et al., 2005). A similar network of left prefrontal and premotor, parietal, and occipital regions was active for both conditions, but the direct comparisons revealed areas selectively engaged by the retrieval of tool names. An effective connectivity analysis indicated the existence of two partially segregated systems of functional integration. During the tool condition, there was an enhancement of the effective connectivity between left hemispheric regions including the inferior prefrontal, and premotor cortex, the inferoparietal lobule and the lateral fusiform gyrus/inferotemporal cortex; during the animal condition, there was an enhanced pattern of connectivity in the left visual associative regions. Noteworthy, the left inferofrontal gyrus (Brodmann's area 45) was more connected with the lateral part of the fusiform gyrus during tool production and with its medial part during animal production. Taken together, these studies indicate a relationship between retrieval of names of action and tools, and Broca's area activation.

Picture Naming

The brain activations observed when subjects retrieve the name of a visually presented stimulus reflects complex cognitive performance involving visual perceptual processes, semantic identification, lexical retrieval, and speech production. A careful consideration of the experimental conditions is thus necessary in order to interpret the possible contribution of Broca's area. A particularly relevant investigation in this respect is the PET study of (Murtha et al., 1999), which clearly indicated the presence of activation in BA 44, 45, and 46 during semantic judgment and picture naming.

A number of studies suggest that, as in the case of word generation, semantic category, and/or grammatical class play an important role in recruiting pre-

frontal regions during picture naming. Martin et al. (1996) found an extensive activation of BA 44/6 when comparing tool naming with animal naming. It is noteworthy that a close area of activation (BA 45/46) had been reported a few months before by our group in a picture-matching task, contrasting animals with man-made tools (Perani et al., 1995). Martin et al. (1995) found that the comparison between color naming and action naming indicated selective activations related to action naming in the left frontoparietal cortex, the middle temporal gyrus, and the cerebellum. Another investigation of the cerebral correlates of action naming has been recently reported by Damasio et al. (2001). Naming actions, compared to a perceptual baseline (verbal judgment of the orientation of unknown faces), resulted in left frontal, temporal, and parietal activations. A comparison of naming actions performed with an implement, with naming tools and implements resulted in bilateral activations in area MT in the temporal lobe, a region associated with motion processing. We have recently compared the cerebral activations associated with naming pictures of manipulation and nonmanipulation actions, with those associated with naming tools and objects which cannot be manipulated (Saccuman et al., submitted). The items related to manipulation, independent from their noun-verb status, selectively activated Broca's area, suggesting that semantic reference, independent of grammatical class, plays a crucial role in the recruitment of this area.

Lexical Decision

In a PET experiment with lexical decision, Perani et al. (1999) compared respectively, nouns referring to tools and psychological states, and manipulation and psychological verbs. The results indicated the existence of incompletely overlapping neurological substrates for verb and noun processing. There was no double dissociation between frontal and temporal cortex, but only the presence of "verb-specific" areas (Broca's, left middle temporal gyrus). Noun and verb processing equally activated the other areas, associated with the lexical task. No significant interactions between grammatical class and semantic content were observed, suggesting that the observed difference is verb specific. A similar study has been recently reported by Tyler et al. (2001), with negative results. No differences were found between closely matched nouns and verbs, both in a lexical decision and in a semantic judgment task. The reason for this discrepancy is unclear, and deserves further investigation.

Passive Listening to Single Words

Mazoyer et al. (1993) reported activation in Broca's area while subjects were listening to words in their mother language, in comparison to stories in a language they could not understand. This is evidence for a role of lexical processing independent from speech production.

"Semantic Encoding"

This heading includes a number of tasks, characterized by the presentation (visual or auditory) of word lists, on which the subjects are asked to perform semantic decisions. Monitoring a list of words for the names of dangerous animals resulted in a left prefrontal activation (Petersen et al., 1989). Similar tasks are often used as the "encoding" phase of an episodic memory test. In comparison to "shallow" encoding of visual words (to decide if there was a letter "a"), a living-nonliving decision resulted in extensive activation in BA 45, 46, 47, and 10 (Kapur et al., 1994). Demb et al. (1995) showed that this activation could not be explained by "task difficulty," as it was observed in the comparison with both an easy and a difficult shallow encoding task. A contrast between form-based and semantic judgment resulted in a fractionation of activity within LIPC similar to that observed for word generation (Mummery et al., 1996; Paulesu et al., 1997), indicating a prevalent role of the posterior part of Broca's area in phonological processing, and of BA 45/47 for semantic processing (Poldrack et al., 1999).

We can conclude from this that, while the fractionation of semantic and grammatical factor has not been conclusively shown, there is strong evidence for separate activations in Broca's area associated with phonological and semantic aspects of lexical retrieval.

Selection Demands and Other Task Manipulations

Other important evidence for the involvement of Broca's area in semantic processing comes for studies, which have attempted to manipulate task requirements, using one of the paradigms described above. Murtha et al. (1999) contrasted word generation, semantic classification and comparison in different conditions. In the first task, the subjects had to generate a verb when confronted with a noun. The baseline was word reading. In the high selection (HS) condition, the noun had many possible associates, without a dominant response. In low selection (LS), the associates were few, or there was a clearly dominant response. For classification of pictures, the baseline was an identity judgment. HS involved pictures had to be classified according to a single feature, LS required an analysis of the entire representation. Comparison involved visual words: the HS required a judgment on a single feature (for example, color), LS, a global analysis. The HS-LS comparison yielded a significant activation in left BA 44, suggesting that the prefrontal activation is driven by the selection requirements of the task, rather than by semantic processing per se. This conclusion was supported by a lesion study in which patients with lesions affecting BAs 44/45 were impaired in producing actions associated to objects only in the HS condition (Thompson-Schill et al., 1998).

Task repetition can be expected to reduce retrieval demands (i.e., make the task "easier"). Raichle et al. (1994) found a decrease in activation of a network of areas (anterior cingulate-left prefrontal-left temporal and right cerebellum) during repetition of the generation of verbs to the same list of nouns. A decrease was also observed with repetition of a semantic encoding task (Demb et al., 1995). Thompson-Schill et al. (1999) attempted to contrast in the same experiment the effects of repetition and selection demands. The reasoning is as follows: if a subject is asked to generate an action word associated with an object name, and the task is repeated, the repetition priming effect is expected to reduce both retrieval demands and selection demands. If the repetition however requires the generation of a different word (a color) to the same stimulus, the reduction of retrieval demand is associated with an increase in selection demands. The fMRI findings indicated a decrease of LIFG activity with repetition, but an increase in the "different" task. It is noteworthy that behavioral priming (reaction time decrease) was present for both the repetition "same" and "different" conditions.

Sentence Processing

There is ample evidence for the contribution of Broca's area to morphological and syntactic level processing, thus confirming aphasiological evidence. A general conclusion we can draw from our own studies

TABLE 12–1. Talairach Coordinates of Broca's Area Activation in Four Different Experiments

Lexical-Semantic

Lexical decision on verbs (Perani et al., 1999)

BA 46/9	−28	28	28
BA 45/46	−36	30	20

Listening to action-related sentences (Tettamanti et al., 2005)

BA 44	−52	10	16

Morpho-Syntactic

Detection of morphosyntactic anomalies (Moro et al., 2001)

BA 45	−28	34	8

Learning of possible rules (Musso et al., 2003)

BA 45	−45	21	6

of Broca's area activation during "lexical-semantic" versus morphosyntactic tasks is that the activations which we consider to be related to the processing of action-related language do not seem to coincide with those observed in the case of tasks which emphasize morphological and syntactic processing (see Table 12–1). The evidence on which this finding is based is too limited in its anatomical precision to allow further speculation about the precise correlates of each aspect of language processing. The presently available improvements in the anatomical localization of functional activations, however, will probably allow a more precise answer in the near future.

CONCLUSIONS

The convergence of findings derived from both lesion and functional imaging studies provides firm indication that Broca's area plays a necessary role in lexical retrieval (Friston and Price, 2003). The semantic dimension of action (in particular manipulative action), interacting with the grammatical distinction between noun and verb, appears to be a crucial determinant of Broca's area involvement. Whether these two aspects are independent in the anatomical sense, i.e. reflected in an anatomical segregation, or interactive is a question that cannot be answered with confidence at the present time. There is however some evidence supporting the hypothesis that the activations associated with "action words" involve the same component

(pars opercularis, BA 44) of Broca's area that are activated by motor imagery (Binkofski et al., 1999). It has been proposed that this area represents the human homologue of monkey area F5, containing mirror neurons, i.e. an observation/execution matching system (Rizzolatti et al., 2001).

What are the implications of these findings for lexical theories? While the brain system underlying somatosensory and motor functions is well known, very little is known about the format assumed by the conceptual level representations accessed by language. Two main theories have been proposed. The first claims that the meaning of an action, when verbally presented, is accessed using abstract and amodal units (Fodor, 2001; Pylyshyn, 1984). An alternative hypothesis suggests that understanding words semantically related to actions depends upon the motor structures involved in the execution of the very same actions (Lakoff and Johnson, 1999; Pulvermueller, 2002). The findings reviewed in this chapter appear to support the latter theory. A possible criticism is that the activation shown by functional imaging may represent a form of mental imagery (visual or motor), which is associated with tasks such as naming, controlled associations, etc., but is not necessary to perform the task. The data from patient studies, however, appear to support the hypothesis of a functional role of dorsal prefrontal (as well as of parietal) areas in the processing of action-related language.

While Broca's area appears to be part of this network, there is ample evidence that its role is not limited to it. The evidence for its participation in a variety of tasks involving word form has also been briefly discussed here. Its involvement in morphological and syntactic processing has been mentioned in this chapter only in relationship with the lexicon, and is dealt with extensively in other chapters. This multifunctional role leads to the issue of the anatomical fractionation of the Broca's region (including neighboring structures, such as the rolandic operculum, the insula, the basal ganglia) according to the linguistic distinctions between phonology, lexical-semantics, and morpho-syntax. Lesion data and functional imaging results support the idea of subcomponents, but the precise assignment of specific roles to definite areas may be premature. A more advanced understanding of the cortical anatomy of functional activations and of anatomical and functional connectivity is required to allow a more precise definition of the networks involved in specific aspects of linguistic processing.

Note

1. The same authors later modified this interpretation. In a subsequent study with the same task (in which the focus of prefrontal activation was actually in area 46), they conclude for a role in using internalized knowledge to guide behavior, when the response is not based on strong association with the presented stimuli (Raichle et al., 1994)

References

Bak, T.H., O'Donovan, D.G., Xuereb, J.H., Boniface, S., & Hodges, J.R. (2001). Selective impairment of verb processing associated with pathological changes in Brodmann areas 44 and 45 in the motor neurone disease-dementia-aphasia syndrome. *Brain*, *124*, 103–120.

Binkofski, F., Buccino, G., Posse, S., Seitz, R.J., Rizzolatti, G., & Freund, H. (1999). A fronto-parietal circuit for object manipulation in man: evidence from an fMRI-study. *European Journal of Neuroscience*, *11*, 3276–3286.

Collina, S., Marangolo, P., & Tabossi, P. (2001). The role of argument structure in the production of nouns and verbs. *Neuropsychologia*, *39*, 1125–1137.

Damasio, A.R., & Tranel, D. (1993). Nouns and verbs are retrieved with differently distributed neural systems. *Proceedings of the National Academy of Science USA*, *90*, 4957–4960.

Damasio, H., Grabowski, T.J., Tranel, D., Hichwa, R.D., & Damasio, A.R. (1996). A neural basis for lexical retrieval. *Nature*, *380*, 499–505.

Damasio, H., Grabowski, T.J., Tranel, D., Ponto, L.L.B., Hichwa, R.D., & Damasio, A.R. (2001). Neural correlates of naming actions and of naming spatial relations. *Neuroimage*, *13*, 1053–1064.

Demb, J.B., Desmond, J.E., Wagner, A.D., Vaidya, C.J., Glover, G.H., & Gabrieli, J.D.E. (1995). Semantic encoding and retrieval in the left inferior prefrontal cortex: A functional MRI study of task difficulty and process specificity. *Journal of Neuroscience*, *15*, 5870–5878.

Dronkers, N.F. (1996). A new brain region for coordinating speech articulation. *Nature*, *384*, 159–161.

Frith, C.D., Friston, K.J., Liddle, P.F., & Frackowiak, R.S.J. (1991a). A PET study of word finding. *Neuropsychologia*, *29*, 1137–1148.

Frith, C.D., Friston, K.J., Liddle, P.F., & Frackowiak, R.S.J. (1991b). Willed action and the prefrontal cortex in man: A study with PET. *Proceedings of the Royal Society of London B*, *244*, 241–246.

Gorno-Tempini, M.L., Dronkers, N.F., Rankin, K.P., Ogar, J.M., Phengrasamy, L., Rosen, H.J., et al. (2004). Cognition and anatomy in three variants of primary progressive aphasia. *Annals of Neurology*, *55*, 335–346.

Grodzinsky, Y. (1984). The syntactic characterization of agrammatism. *Cognition*, *16*, 99–120.

Hecaen, H., & Consoli, S. (1973). Analyse des troubles du langage au cours des lésions de l'aire de Broca. *Neuropsychologia*, *11*, 377–388.

Hillis, A., Oh, S., & Ken, L. (2004). Deterioration of naming nouns vs. verbs in primary progressive aphasia. *Annals of Neurology*, *55*, 268–275.

Kapur, S., Craik, F.I.M., Tulving, E., Wilson, A.A., Houle, S., & Brown, G.M. (1994). Neuroanatomical correlates of encoding in episodic memory: Levels of processing effect. *Proceedings of the National Academy of Science USA*, *91*, 2008–2011.

Kohn, S.E., & Goodglass, H. (1985). Picture-naming in aphasia. *Brain Language*, *24*, 266–283.

Lakoff, G., & Johnson, M. (1999). *The flesh: The embodied mind and its challenge to western thought*. New York: Basic Books.

Martin, A., Haxby, J.V., Lalonde, F.M., Wiggs, C.L., & Ungerleider, L.G. (1995). Discrete cortical regions associated with knowledge of color and knowledge of action. *Science*, *270*, 102–105.

Martin, A., Wiggs, C.L., Ungerleider, L.G., & Haxby, J.V. (1996). Neural correlates of category-specific knowledge. *Nature*, *379*, 649–652.

Mazoyer, B.M., Tzourio, N., Frank, V., Syrota, A., Murayama, N., Levrier, O., et al. 1993. The cortical representation of speech. *Journal of Cognitive Neuroscience*, *5*, 467–479.

Mazzocchi, F., & Vignolo, L.A. (1979). Localisation of lesions in aphasia: Clinical-CT scan correlations in stroke patients. *Cortex*, *15*, 627–654.

Miceli, G., Silveri, M.C., Nocentini, U., & Caramazza, A. (1988). Patterns of dissociation in comprehension and production of nouns and verbs. *Aphasiology*, *2*, 251–258.

Miceli, G., Silveri, M.C., Romani, C., & Caramazza, A. (1989). Variations in the pattern of omissions and substitutions of grammatical morphemes in the spontaneous speech of so-called agrammatic patients. *Brain and Language*, *36*, 447–492.

Mohr, J.P., Pessin, M.S., Finkelstein, S., Funkestein, H.H., Duncan, G.W., & Davis, K.R. (1978). Broca aphasia. Pathologic and clinical. *Neurology*, *28*, 311–324.

Moro, A., Tettamanti, M., Perani, D., Donati, C., Cappa, S.F., & Fazio, F. (2001). Syntax and the brain: Disentangling grammar by selective anomalies. *Neuroimage*, *13*, 110–118.

Mummery, C.J., Patterson, K., Hodges, J.R., & Wise, R.S.J. (1996). Generating "tiger" as an animal name or a word beginning with T: Differences in brain activation. *Proceedings of the Royal Society of London B, 263*, 989–995.

Murtha, S., Chertkow, H., Beauregard, M., & Evans, A. (1999). The neural substrate of picture naming. *Journal of Cognitive Neuroscience, 11*, 399–423.

Musso, M., Moro, A., Glauche, V., Rijntjes, M., Reichenbach, J., Buchel, C., et al. (2003). Broca's area and the language instinct. *Nature Neuroscience, 6*, 774–781.

Naeser, M.A., & Hayward, R.W. (1978). Lesion localization in aphasia with cranial computed tomography and the Boston Diagnostic Aphasia exam. *Neurology, 28*, 545–551.

Naeser, M.A., Palumbo, C.L., Helm-Eastabrooks, N., Stiassny-Eder, D., & Albert, M.L. (1989). Severe nonfluency in aphasia. Role of the medial subcallosal fasciculus and other white matter pathways in the recovery of sponataneous speech. *Brain, 112*, 1–38.

Paulesu, E., Goldacre, B., Scifo, P., Perani, D., Cappa, S.F., Gilardi, M.C., et al. (1997). Differential activation of left frontal cortex during phonemic and semantic word fluency. An EPI-fMRI activation study. *Neuroreport, 8*, 2011–2016.

Perani, D., Cappa, S.F., Bettinardi, V., Bressi, S., Gorno Tempini, M.L., Matarrese, M., et al. (1995). Different neural networks for the recognition of biological and man-made entities. *Neuroreport, 6*, 1637–1641.

Perani, D., Cappa, S.F., Schnur, T., Tettamanti, M., Collina, S., Rosa, M.M., et al. (1999). The neural correlates of verb and noun processing: A PET study. *Brain, 122*, 2337–2344.

Petersen, S.E., & Fiez, J.A. (1993). The processing of single words studied with positron emission tomography. *Annual Review of Neuoscience, 160*, 509–530.

Petersen, S.E., Fox, P.T., Posner, M.I., Mintun, M., & Raichle, M.E. (1988). Positron emission tomography studies of the cortical anatomy of single-word processing. *Nature, 331*, 585–589.

Petersen, S.E., Fox, P.T., Posner, M.I., Mintun, M., & Raichle, M.E. (1989). Positron emission tomographic studies of the processing of single words. *Journal of Cognitive Neuroscience, 1*, 153–170.

Pylyshyn Z.W. (1984). Computation and cognition: Towards a foundation for cognitive science. Cambridge, MA: MIT Press.

Raichle, M.E., Fiez, J.A., Videen, T.O., MacLeod, A.M.K., Pardo, J.V., Fox, P.T., et al. (1994). Practice-related changes in human brain functional anatomy during non-motor learning. *Cerebral Cortex, 4*, 8–26.

Saffran, E.M., & Schwartz, M.F. (1994). Of cabbages and things: Semantic memory from a neuropsychological perspective—a tutorial review. In C. Umiltà & M. Moscovitch (Eds.), *Attention and performance. XV: conscious and unconscious processes*. Cambridge, MA: MIT Press.

Shapiro, L., & Levine, B. (1990). Verb processing during sentence comprehension in aphasia. *Brain and Language, 38*, 21–47.

Shapiro, L.P., & Nagel, H.N. (1995). Lexical properties, prosody, and syntax: Implications for normal and disordered language. *Brain and Language, 50*, 240–257.

Silveri, M.C., & Di Betta, A.M. (1997). Noun-verb dissociations in brain-damaged patients: Further evidence. *Neurocase, 3*, 477–488.

Tettamanti, M., Danna, M., Scifo, P., Fazio, F., Saccuman, C., Buccino, G., et al. (2005). Understanding action-related sentences activates fronto-parietal motor circuits. *Journal of Cognitive Neuroscience, 17*, 273–281.

Thompson, C.K., Lange, K.L., Schneider, S.L., & Shapiro, L.P. (1997). Agrammatic and non-brain-damaged subjects' verb and verb argument structure production. *Aphasiology, 11*, 473–490.

Thompson-Schill, S.L., D'Esposito, M., & Kan, I.P. (1999). Effects of repetition and competititon on activity in left prefrontal cortex during word generation. *Neuron, 23*, 513–522.

Tonkonogy, J., & Goodglass, H. (1981). Language function, foot of the third frontal gyrus and rolandic operculum. *Archives of Neurology, 38*, 486–490.

Tranel, D., Adolphs, R., Damasio, H., & Damasio, A.R. (2001). A neural basis for the retrieval of words for actions. *Cognitive Neuropsychology, 18*, 655–670.

Tyler, L.K., Russell, R., Fadili, J., & Moss, H.E. (2001). The neural representation of nouns and verbs: PET studies. *Brain, 124*, 1619–1634.

Vitali, P., Abutalebi, J., Tettamanti, M., Rowe, J., Scifo, P., Fazio, F., Cappa, S.F., & Perani, D. (2005). Generating animal and tool names: An FMRI study of effective connectivity. *Brain and Language, 93*, 32–45.

Warburton, E., Wise, R.S.J., Price, C.J., Weiller, C., Hadar, U., Ramsay, S., et al. (1996). Noun and verb retrieval by normal subjects. Studies with PET. *Brain, 119*, 159–179.

Zatorre, R.J., Evans, A.C., Meyer, E., & Gjedde, A. (1992). Lateralization of phonetic and pitch discrimination in spech processing. *Science, 256*, 846–849.

13

The Neural Basis of Sentence Processing: Inferior Frontal and Temporal Contributions

Angela D. Friederici

Sentence comprehension consists of a number of sub-processes bridging the way from auditory (or visual) input to the ultimate representation of the sentence's meaning.

Psycholinguistic models of sentence comprehension agree that different subprocesses underlie the comprehension process. They disagree, however, with respect to the issue, whether there are different components responsible for the different subprocesses, and if so, to what extent these subprocesses interact in time (see Frauenfelder and Tyler, 1987 for a review). Two extreme positions can be identified with respect to the current models. On the one hand there are the so-called serial or syntax-first models (e.g., De Vincenzi, 1991; Frazier, 1978, 1987a, 1987b; Gorrell, 1995), which claim that the language processing system, called the parser, initially builds up a syntactic structure independent of lexical-semantic or sentential-semantic information and that semantic aspects only come into play during a second processing stage. These models assume that syntactic and semantic processes are supported by different components in the language comprehension system and that these may be implemented at the neuronal level by distinct brain regions. The so-called interactive models (e.g., Marslen-Wilson and Tyler, 1980) and models within the constraint-satisfaction framework (MacDonald, Pearlmutter and Seidenberg, 1994a, 1994b; McClelland et al., 1989; Trueswell and Tanenhaus, 1994) on the other hand assume that the parser uses multiple sources of information, including semantic and world knowledge at the same time. Interactive approaches are either neutral with respect to the assumption of different components in the processing systems, as for example proposed by MacDonald et al. (1992) who in versions of constraint based models assume such subcomponents but allow them to interact directly, or they deny separate components for syntactic and semantic processes (Marslen-Wilsen and Tyler, 1980). The latter approach can be taken as an example of a model of non-component processes.

Overviews concerning the behavioral evidence for each of these views are given in Mitchell (1994), Tanenhaus and Trueswell (1995), Frazier and Clifton (1996), and different articles published in the readers edited by Garfield (1987), Carlson and Tanenhaus (1989), Altmann (1990), Balota et al. (1990), Simpson (1991), Clifton et al. (1994), and Hemforth and Konieczny (2000). Each of the different type of models is supported by empirical data from behavioral experiments, thus disallowing to draw a final conclusion with respect to the ultimate cognitive architecture of sentence processing.

The present paper will not reiterate the empirical behavioral data that have been collected over the last two decades providing support for each of these models of sentence processing, but it will rather provide neurocognitive evidence critical to this discussion. Given the fact that the difference between the models crucially depends on the separability of different

linguistic subdomains, such as syntax and semantics as well as the temporal relation between these, an adequate description of the neural basis of sentence processing will have to specify not only the brain areas involved, but also the temporal aspects of language-related brain activation.

NEUROCOGNITIVE MODEL OF SENTENCE PROCESSING

The neurocognitive model proposed here emerges from the temporal and neurotopological parameters as gathered by electrophysiological (EEG), magneto-physiological (MEG), and functional magnetic resonance imaging (fMRI) or position emission tomography (PET) studies presented in the following sections (see Fig. 13–1).

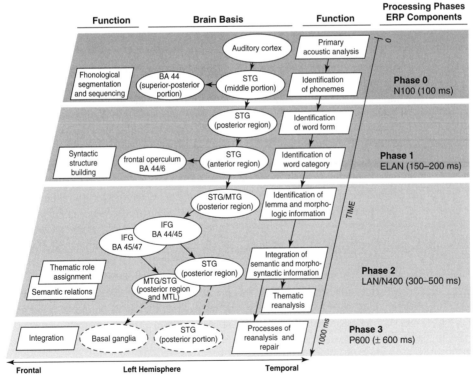

FIGURE 13–1. Schematic neurocognitive model of sentence processing. BA, Brodmann areas; STG, superior temporal gyri; MTG, middle temporal gyri; MTL, middle temporal lobe; IFG, inferior frontal gyri. For further explanations of their functional significance, see the text. The different components of the event-related brain potential, that is, N100, ELAN (early left anterior negativity), LAN (left anterior negativity), N400, and P600, are described with respect to the shape and function in the text.

The *temporal aspects* of the diagram (Phase 0–Phase 3) are modeled on the basis of EEG and MEG data, indicated by the relevant event-related brain potential (ERP) components: the ELAN, an early anterior negativity with a maximum over the left hemisphere occuring between 150 and 200 ms, the LAN, a left anterior negativity occuring between 300 and 500 ms, the N400, a negative centroparietally distributed component occuring around 400 ms, and the P600, a positive component with a centroparietal distribution occuring after 600 ms. The *spatial aspects* of the diagram are modeled on the basis of either fMRI and PET data (indicated by Brodmann areas and descriptions of the relevant brain regions), or on the basis of MEG dipole localization or EEG/MEG distributional effects (indicated by distributional descriptions). The former is true for semantic on-line processes whereas the latter holds for the description of the syntactic processes. Note, that the diagram reflects a schematic representation of the state of the art. It must be considered to be preliminary, as not all aspects have been investigated so far. It is meant to provide a structured view on our present knowledge concerning the processing of sentences during language comprehension.

The present model primarily concentrates on language processes located in the left hemisphere. But, note that there are a number of behavioral studies, lesion studies, and recent imaging studies suggesting that the right hemisphere is also involved in several stages of language processing, in particular in the processing of prosodic information (for a recent review on this issue, see Friederici and Alter, 2004).

In the following the model graphed in Figure 13–1 will be sketched briefly before the available evidence is discussed in more detail.[1]

On-line processes during language comprehension, depicted in Figure 13–1, are modeled to occur in an incremental serial order. Phonological processes precede three phases of sentence processing. Phase 1 represents structure building, which precedes Phase 2 during which semantic processes and processes of thematic role assignment take place and which in turn precede Phase 3 reflecting processes of integration and reanalysis. The temporal course of theses Phases is indicated by the vertical line at the outer left of Figure 13–1. Phases 1 and 2 are assumed to involve temporal as well as inferior frontal brain structures. Phase 3 seems to be supported by the temporal regions and

the basal ganglia (BG). The spatial dimensions are indicated by the lower horizontal line in Figure 13–1. Temporal brain structures of the left hemisphere are taken to support the identification of a given element and whereas frontal structures rather seem to be recruited by phonological sequencing, structure building processes, and the build up and judgment of semantic relations.

The available brain imaging data discussed in detail in Neuroimaging suggest that identification of a particular type of information in the input is supported by the superotemporal region (superior temporal gyrus [STG]/superior temporal sulcus [STS]) and the middle temporal gyrus (MTG) with different subparts being responsible for different information types. Within the temporal lobe, the identification of phonemes (speech sounds) appears to be supported by regions adjacent to the primary auditory cortex. In an anterolateral regions (possibly comprising belt and parabelt regions in primates) the spectrotemporal structure of sounds are processed, whereas the region lateral and anterior to this is involved in the identification of phonetic features relevant for the recognition of phonemes. The identification of word form is supported by the posterior portion of the STG. The identification of word category (e.g., noun versus verb) seems to involve the anterior portion of the STG, that is the planum polare, which together with the inferior portion of BA 44 is responsible for on-line local phrase structure building. The identification of the information encoded in the lemma (part of the lexical entry in the lexicon), that is, meaning information, verb argument information, syntactic gender information, is assumed to be subserved by the posterior region of the MTG/STG. Phonological sequencing, as well as the build up of syntactic and semantic relations are taken to be supported by the inferior frontal gyrus (IFG). Within this gyrus, phonological segmentation and sequencing appears to involve the superior-posterior portion of BA 44. Local syntactic structure building seem to involve the frontal operculum, whereas processing of complex structures rather involve BA 44/45. Executive processes in the semantic domain rather recruit BA 45/47.

Finally, processes of reanalysis, which become necessary when the different types of representations cannot be integrated successfully may be differentiated into processes of thematic reanalysis (revision of thematic role assignment) and those of structural re-

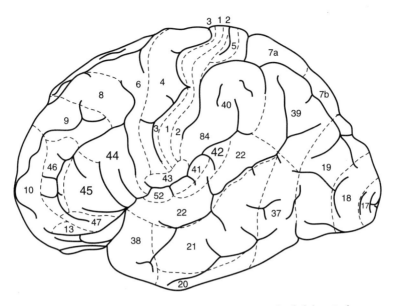

FIGURE 13–2. Specification of Brodmann areas in the left hemisphere.

analysis (recomputation of the syntactic structure). Neurophysiologically, the two aspects are reflected in an early (345 ms) and a late (600 ms) centroparietally distributed ERP effect. As a supporting system of the latter processes, the BG has been discussed as a possible neural correlate. However, the neural anatomy of these processes as well as those of thematic revision has not yet been specified.

The data justifying this model will be presented as follows. We first discuss the electrophysiological data relevant to the temporal structure of sentence processing. We then turn to a description of the neuroanatomic parameters based on results from PET studies and from fMRI studies. Given the limited temporal resolution of these techniques we will use results from dipole modeling studies to map the different processing phases onto its neural substrates whenever possible.

NEUROPHYSIOLOGICAL DATA: THE TEMPORAL ASPECTS OF SENTENCE PROCESSING

The data informing the on-line processes Phase 1 to Phase 3 in the present neurocognitive model will be presented following the proposed time course of the language comprehension process.[2]

Phase 1

Function

Phase 1 is the stage that could be termed first-pass parsing. During this phase the parser is assumed to build up the initial syntactic structure on the basis of word category information (Friederici, 1995; Frazier, 1987a, 1987b; Gorrell, 1995). Each incoming element is integrated into the current structure following the specific principles of the grammar under investigation and following the general principle of simplicity (Gorrell, 1995). If an incoming element's word category does not fit the rules of the grammar, it cannot be integrated into the current structure.

Temporal Parameters

The brain reacts immediately whenever the word category of the incoming element does not match the expectations based on the rules of the grammar. A number of ERP studies have observed an early left anterior negativity between 150 and 200 ms, when the brain is confronted with such a situation (Friederici et al., 1993; Hahne and Friederici, 1999; Hahne and Jescheniak, 2001; Hahne, 2001; Kubota et al., 2003; Neville et al., 1991). This component has been labeled ELAN (Friederici, 1995). Other studies investigating word category violation reported a left anterior negativity peaked somewhat later (Friederici et al., 1996; Münte et al., 1993). The latency difference appears to be a function of when the relevant word category information is available to the parser and, moreover, as a function of the mode of presentation. The ELAN's latency is early when word category information is available early. This could be due to the fact that the word category information can be accessed rapidly, as in example 1, in a short function word (Kubota et al., 2003; Neville et al., 1991) or as in example 2, in a prefix of the main verb (Hahne and Friederici, 1999) (critical elements are underlined).[3]

(1a) *Max's _of_ proof the theorem.
(1b) Max's proof of the theorem.
(2a) *Das Bild wurde im _gemalt_.
     The picture was in the painted.
(2b) Das Bild wurde im Atelier gemalt.
     The picture was in the studio painted.

The latency of the ELAN is prolonged when the ERP is time-locked to the word onset, although the relevant word category information only becomes available late in the critical word, e.g., in the suffix of the main verb as in example 3 (Friederici et al., 1996)[4] or only after accessing the lexical entry fully as in example 4 (Münte et al., 1993).

(3a) *Das Metall wurde zur veredel_t_ . . .
     The metal was by the refined . . .
(3b) Das Metall wurde zur Veredel_ung_ . . .
     The metal was by the refinement . . .
(4a) *your _write_
(4b) your letter

Moreover, it has been shown that the latency of the left anterior negativity depends on optimal input conditions: the left anterior negativity is early when the sentence is presented as normal connected speech or rapid, high contrast reading conditions (Friederici et al., 1993; Hahne and Friederici, 1999; Neville et al., 1991). This component appears somewhat later when presented visually either in a slow word-by-word fashion or with a poor visual contrast (Gunter et al., 1999).

Thus, it seems that all studies investigating word category violations discussed thus far found a left anterior negativity either between 150 and 200 ms or between 200 and 400 ms. The latency difference was explained by two factors: first, by differences in the word category decision point and second, by the input conditions. Reading a sentence word-by-word with a slow presentation time (pauses up to 300 ms or more between each word) or poor visual contrast conditions appear to slow down the fast and high automatic first-pass parsing processes. The notion that local phrase structure building is indeed highly automatic is supported by a recent ERP experiment varying the proportion of grammatical and ungrammatical sentences (Hahne and Friederici, 1999). The ELAN component was unaffected by this variation indicating this component reflects highly automatic processes.[5]

Temporospatial Parameters

The spatial parameters for the early syntactic processes as reflected in the (E)LAN component are hard to specify as this component is usually part of a biphasic ERP pattern with a P600 as its second part. The interpretation of the P600 as a component reflecting late processes of syntactic reanalysis and integration clearly separates it form the ELAN functionally. The particular question of which brain areas support the early phrase structure building processes reflected by the ELAN was approached by using different dipole modeling techniques applied to MEG data (Gross et al., 1998; Friederici et al., 2000; Knösche et al., 1999). The study by Friederici et al. (2000) applied fMRI constraints for the dipole location and found two dipoles in the left hemisphere, a larger dipole in the anterior left temporal brain region and a smaller in the left inferior frontal brain region in the time window reflecting the ELAN. This suggests an involvement of the anterior portion of the left temporal cortex as well as in the inferior frontal cortex during early structure building processes. This localization nicely conicides with data from a functional imaging study using the same material (Friederici et al., 2003c). Syntactic processes were shown to involve the frontal operculum and the anterior portion of the STG (for a detailed discussion of these data see Neuroimaging).

At this point, the question arises what the function of these two brain areas may be. One hypothesis is that the temporal area provides information about the different words' categories, whereas the inferior frontal area builds the structure of the incoming elements on the basis of this information. Further research must show whether this hypothesis holds true.

Summary Phase 1

Local phrase structure processes are early as indicated by the ELAN component.[6] The available data suggest that local structure building proceeds incrementally as soon as word category information is available. This process is fast and automatic.

Phase 2

Function

During Phase 2 of sentence processing lexically based information becomes available and thematic and relational properties are determined. After the word category information is accessed and used for initial local structure building, the full information encoded in the lexical entry is retrieved. Beside word category information the lexical entry contains at least two different types of information: meaning information of content words as well as idiosyncratic syntactic information, i.e., syntactic gender of nouns and verb argument structure information of verbs. During this phase the available morpho-syntactic information determining the relation between different words is also processed. Here it is proposed that these semantic and syntactic processing domains work in parallel (but independent of each other) to achieve a meaning representation.

Temporal Parameters

Processes attributed to Phase 2 are correlated with two components in the ERP the N400 and the LAN.

N400 as a Marker of Semantic Processes   The N400 is a negativity with a centro-parietal maximum generally observed between 300 and 500 ms post-stimulus onset. The N400 has been shown to occur in response to words that cannot be integrated semantically into the preceding sentential context (Kutas and Hillyard, 1980, 1983). Furthermore, it is also elicited by words that are possible, but semantically unexpected in the context in which they appear (Kutas and Hillyard, 1984). I will not review the rich literature on the N400 here, the reader is referred to comprehensive overviews by Kutas and Van Petten (1994) and Kutas and Federmeier (2000). There has

been some discussion as to whether the N400 reflects processes of lexical access and/or lexical integration. On the psycholinguistic assumption that the former process is automatic whereas the latter is controlled, Chwilla et al. (1995) argued that the N400 reflects processes of lexical integration. They had demonstrated that the N400 to a target word varied as a function of the task demands (semantic judgment versus physical task).

LAN as a Marker of Morphosyntactic Processes   The LAN is a left anterior negativity observed between 300 and 500 ms poststimulus outset. The LAN was found in response to agreement violations in a number of different languages: for subject-verb-agreement violations in English (Kutas and Hillyard, 1983; Osterhout and Mobley, 1995; but see Osterhout and Nicol, 1999), in Dutch (Gunter et al., 1997), in German (Penke et al., 1997; but see Münte et al., 1997) and in Italian (Angrilli et al., 2002) for article-noun gender agreement in German (Gunter et al., 2000) as well as for noun-verb gender agreement in Hebrew (Deutsch and Bentin, 2001). As a large number of studies across different languages consistently show an LAN in response to subject-verb agreement violations.

N400/LAN in Verb-Argument Processsing   There is a long-standing discussion to what extend verb-argument structure must be considered to fall into the domain of syntax or semantics. Interestingly, violations of verb-argument-structure elicit a LAN under some conditions and an N400 under others. An LAN, for example, was observed in English for a noun phrase (*we*) whose case marking indicated an argument position (i.e., subject), which was already occupied by another noun phrase (*the plan*) (Coulson et al., 1998) as in example 8.

(8a) *The plane took we to paradise.*
(8b) *The plane took us to paradise.*

A study in German focusing explicitly on two different aspects of verb-argument structure information using the fact that in German subordinate clauses the verb is in clause final position (Friederici and Frisch, 2000). A LAN was found in German when the sentence-final critical element violating the verb-argument-structure with respect to the type of arguments (marked by case) was the verb as in example 9.

(9a) *Anna weiß, dass der Kommissar den Banker bei-stand.
Anna knows, that the commissar the (ACC) banker helped.

(9b) Anna weiß, dass der Kommissar dem Banker beis-tand.
Anna knows, that the commissar the (DAT) banker helped.

In contrast, an N400 was observed for the sentence final verb when of thematic role assignment was implausible as in example 10 in which the number of arguments associated with the verb was incorrect thus, disallowing an interpretation (Friederici and Frisch, 2000).

(10) *Anna weiß, dass der Kommissar den Banker abreiste.
Anna knows that the inspector (NOM) the banker (ACC) left town.

The two violation types tap different aspects of verb-argument structure information. While the verb in example 9 is a two-place-argument verb with a preceding incorrect morpho-syntactically marked NP, the verb in example 10 a one-place-argument verb with two preceding arguments both asking for thematic implementation. These two different aspects morpho-syntactic versus thematic are reflected in two ERP component, the LAN and the N400, respectively.

N400 as a Marker of Thematic Processes   In more recent studies an N400 component was observed systematically in German sentences with case marking errors that signal incorrect thematic role assignment (Bornkessel et al., 2002; Frisch and Schlesewsky, 2001). Note, that in languages that mark case thematic roles can be derived directly from the case itself. Bornkessel (2002) proposed that the German parser must implement two parallel processing routes: one route that considers case when marked unambiguously and maps thematic roles directly and one route which is used for ambiguously marked noun phrase and which considers other morphosyntactic information (e.g., subject-verb agreement) similar to parsers of languages without case marking.

Temporospatial Parameters

The issue of which brain areas support semantic processes and thematic processes has only been investigated partially. So far, this issue has been approached mainly for semantic processes by using intracranial ERP recording and by dipole modeling based on MEG data for the N400 component.

Most recently, however, the processing of subject-verb-agreement was investigated in studies using a standard oddball mismatch paradigm (Pulvermüller and Shtyrov, 2003; Shtyrov et al., 2003). In the EEG and MEG experiments, pronouns were combined with verbs which matched or did not match the pronoun in their inflectional form. For syntactic violations, a left lateralized effect was found about 100 ms after the divergence point at the end of the verb (e.g., we come vs *we comes). While EEG findings revealed a left anterior negativity (Pulvermüller and Shtyrov, 2004), an MEG study reported a significant temporal source (Shtyrov et al., 2003). This apparent difference in localization may be due to the different methodologies and their differential sensitivity to the spatial orientation of the source.

With respect to N400, it has been proposed that this component arises from a number of functionally and spatially distinct generators (Nobre and Mc-Carthy, 1995). This suggestion is largely based on data from intracranial depth recordings during word reading. These data specify medial temporal structures close to the hippocampus and the amygdala as possible locations for the N400 generators. Data from a study with intracranial recordings from less deep structures, however, suggest that the superior temporal sulcus is also involved in the generation of the N400 (Halgren et al., 1994).

Helenius et al. (1998) used the approach of whole-head MEG recording to identify the generators of the N400 during sentence reading. They reported structures in the "immediate vicinity of the left auditory cortex" (p. 1133) to be implicated most consistently with the N400 in reading comprehension.

Summary Phase 2

The combined findings show that during the Phase 2 lexical-semantic, morpho-syntactic and argument structure information is retrieved and thematic role assignment takes place. Different subsystems seem to be responsible for lexical-semantic and thematic processes on the one hand (N400) and morpho-syntactic processes (LAN) on the other. The processing of verb argument structure information appears to fall in one of the two processing domains dependent on whether the critical feature has direct consequences for thematic assignment or whether it has consequences for the syntactic structure. Future research must show whether the N400 observed in response to semantic anomalies and the N400 elicited by thematic processing difficulties are of the same kind.[7]

Functional Relation of Phase 1 and Phase 2

The temporal parameters of Phase 1 and Phase 2 suggest a relative seriality between the two phases. A number of studies have been devoted to the issue of the temporal and functional relation of the phrase structure building processes of Phase 1 and the processes of Phase 2.

A crucial test with respect to the functional relation between the processes of Phase 1 and Phase 2 are sentences in which the crucial violations are realized within the same critical element. If phrase structure building processes of Phase 1 indeed functionally precede processes of Phase 2 the following prediction should hold: processes of Phase 1 may influence processes of Phase 2, but not vice versa. A number of experiments conducted in German demonstrate that this prediction holds true.

In these experiments phrase structure violations were crossed either with semantic violations (Friederici et al., 1999; Hahne and Friederici, 2002) or with verb argument structure violations (Frisch et al., 2004) on the critical target element. The general pattern of results from these experiments was as follows. All single violation conditions showed the expected components: namely an ELAN for the syntactic violation condition, and an N400 for the semantic violation condition as well as for the verb argument violation condition. Critically for all double violation conditions only an ELAN, but no N400 effect was observed. This ERP pattern indicates that once the word category of an item does not fit the preceding syntactic structure, the parser abandons further lexical processing, leading to an absence of the N400. This finding, which was replicated in three studies, is in direct agreement with models assuming a primacy of syntactic processes.

A relevant question, however, is whether this relation between Phase 1 and Phase 2 is due to the relative timing of the availability of the relevant information to a parser or due to some functional aspects of parsing itself. In the experiment by Hahne and Friederici (2002), stimulus material was used in which the violating word category information was available from the verb prefix *ge-* of the critical element *gefüttert*/fed as in example 13a, whereas the violating semantic information was available from the verb stem *-füttert* (Hahne and Friederici, 2002). For a semantically and syntactically correct sentence see example 13b.

(13a) *Die Burg wurde im gefüttert.*
      The castle was in the fed.
(13b) Die Gans wurde gefüttert.
      The goose was fed.

An additional experiment has investigated a double violation of phrase structure and semantics in sentences with target words that contained word category information in the suffix, i.e., after the semantic information encoded in the verb stem was processed as in example 14 (Friederici et al., 2004). The word stem *verpflanz-*/repott in the verb *verpflanz-t*/repotted is identical to the word stem in the noun *Verpflanzung*/repottment. Thus, word category identification is only possible after the stem, i.e., in the suffix. In example 14a, an example of a double violation is given, whereas example 14b provides a correct example.

(14a) *Das Buch wurde trotz verpflanzt . . .*
      The book was despite repotted . . .
(14b) Der Busch wurde trotz Verpflanzung . . .
      The bush was despite repottment . . .

Even in this situation we observed an ELAN but no N400. This suggests that the target word was not integrated semantically in the double violation condition even when the word category information was available after the semantic information.

This finding is clear evidence for the functional seriality of phrase structure building processes and semantic processes, thus, for the functional seriality of Phase 1 and Phase 2 as predicted by syntax-first models. Moreover, with respect to the temporal ordering within Phase 2, De Vincenzi et al. (2003) most recently argued on the basis of ERP results in Italian for an inherent serialty of morpho-syntactic and semantic processes.

Phase 3

Function

During Phase 3 the structural representation, the semantic representation and thematic representation are mapped onto each other. When these different representation can be mapped successfully *integration*, i.e., comprehension, has taken place. When these representations cannot be mapped the parser diagnoses this mismatch and *reanalyzes* the initial structure that was built. When no structural or thematic reanalysis[8] is possible based on the input, the parsing system has to consider processes of *repair.*

From this functional description the question arises as to whether there are certain neurophysiological parameters that reflect processes of *structural reanalysis* and *thematic reanalysis*, and if so, whether these can provide evidence for different subprocesses during the reanalysis phase.

Temporal Parameters

Reanalysis   There is a particular ERP component that is taken to reflect processes of syntactic recomputation: The so-called *P600*. This component is a centro-parietally distributed positivity between 600 and 900 ms that is elicited by the element that disambiguates a structurally ambiguous sentence, i.e., a garden-path sentence, first reported by Osterhout and Holcomb (1992, 1993). The positivity around 600 ms elicited by the processing of nonpreferred sentence structures was shown to vary in amplitude as a function of the "cost of reprocessing" (Osterhout et al., 1994). The P600 observed in correlation with garden-path sentences may be considered to reflect processes of *structural reanalysis.*

Friederici and Mecklinger (1996) formulated the assumption that the latency of the positivity may vary as a function of difficulty to recover from a garden-path. They found a very early positivity (P345) in correlation with the processing of nonpreferred object relatives compared to subject relatives in German, but a later positivity (P600) for difficult-to-revise object-first complement compared to subject-first complement sentences. The revision of a subject relative clause into an object relative clause interpretation is a relatively easy process, achieved simply by recoindexing subject and object NP and its thematic roles,

but requiring no alteration of the underlying structure. The revision of a subject-first complement clause towards an object-first complement clause, in contrast, requires an alteration of the underlying structural hierarchy and could be predicted to require more effort (Mecklinger et al., 1995).

An alternative interpretation for the early positivity (P345) and the late positivity (P600) on the basis of more recent data, however, is given by Bornkessel et al. (2002). As they found a P345 to be present in sentences, which call for a thematic reanalysis, they interpret the P345 to reflect *thematic reanalysis* and the P600 to reflect structural reanalysis. This latter interpretation of the P345 also explains the Mecklinger et al. (1995) data under the assumption that in case ambiguous sentences thematic roles of the NPs are assigned on the basis of word order, and that the underlying process of reanalysis is similar to case marked sentences in which thematic roles are assigned on the basis of case information.

Repair   There are a number of ERP studies in different languages investigating the processing of syntactic violations and thus, processes of syntactic repair. Most of these report a biphasic pattern with a P600 following a preceding left anterior negativity. The P600 has been found to covary with a variety of syntactic anomalies such as garden-path sentences and other syntactically nonpreferred structures (Friederici et al., 1996, 1993; Hagoort et al., 1993; Mecklinger et al., 1995; Osterhout et al., 1994; Osterhout and Holcomb, 1992;), outright phrase structure violations (Friederici et al., 1996; Neville et al., 1991; Osterhout et al., 1992, 1993), subjacency violations (McKinnon and Osterhout, 1996; Neville et al., 1991), and agreement violations (Coulson et al., 1998; Friederici et al., 1993; Gunter et al., 1997; Hagoort et al., 1993; Osterhout and Mobley, 1995).

Integration   There is one study that investigated the issue of whether the P600 reflects the brain's response to a syntactic violation or a preference violation. Kaan et al. (2000) constructed correct sentences, which varied in the difficulty of integration while keeping all other aspects constant. They found a P600 for the difficult-to-integrate element and argued that the P600 is a marker for syntactic integration difficulty. This notion may describe the P600 in most general terms.

However, the finding that the syntax related positivity varies systematically in amplitude, latency and distribution across a number of studies may indicate that different aspects of integration problems find their different signatures in the "late positivity."

Temporospatial Parameters of P600

Our current knowledge concerning the neural generators, syntactic integration, reanalysis, and repair processes is limited. This is due to a number of facts. First, so far no study focusing on syntactic *integration* has systematically varied the difficulty of integration in accord with any type of parsing theory. Second, dipole modeling for EEG or MEG so far has not successfully been applied to late components such as the P600. Third, due to the low temporal resolution of PET and fMRI imaging, studies investigating the processing of syntactic violations cannot distinguish between early processes (detection of error as reflected in the (E)LAN) and the late processes (as reflected in the P600). Therefore, the only indication with respect to spatial parameters of the different processing aspects during Phase 3 come from scalp recorded ERPs and from ERP studies in brain-lesioned patients.

Given that scalp distributions are difficult to interpret relative to the underlying neural generators only some topographic differences of the P600 will be mentioned. Reviewing the literature, Hagoort, Brown and Osterhout (1999) proposed that the topography of the P600 may vary as a function of whether it reflects processes of reanalysis and repair. Friederici, Hahne and Saddy (2002) directly compared processes correlated with syntactic complexity and processes of repair and observed a distributional difference. They found the P600 elicited by syntactic violations had a centro-parietal focus, whereas the P600 observed with the processing of syntactic complexity had a centro-frontal focus. This difference in the distributional pattern suggests that the two P600s partly involve different brain systems.

Two recent ERP studies with patients with deficient functioning of the BG suggest an involvement of this structure in the generation of the P600 (Kotz et al., 2003). In one study investigating patients with lesions in the BG, the P600 was found to be attenuated (Friederici et al., 1999), in another study testing patients which suffered from Parkinson's disease affecting the BG, the P600 was found to be absent (Friederici et al., 2003).

In order to evaluate whether the effects of BG lesions on the P600 were specific to the ERP component, a study was conducted in which patients with lesions in the BG were tested with sentence material usually eliciting a P600 and stimulus material known to elicit a domain unspecific P300 (Frisch et al., 2003). This study indicated that the BG are specifically involved in syntactic repair processes as no P600 was observed, although a P300 was found.

Summary Phase 3

Phase 3 can be best-described neurocognitively on the basis of the available ERP data. Difficulty of syntactic *integration* induced by complexity and syntactic *repair* induced by syntactic violation can be distinguished on the basis of neurotopographic parameters with the latter showing a centro-parietal distributed P600 and the former demonstrating a centro-frontal distributed P600. Processes of different domains of *reanalysis* may be distinguishable on the basis of the latency of the positivity, namely an early positivity reflecting thematic reanalysis (P345) and a late positivity reflecting syntactic reanalysis/repair and integration (P600). The data at hand suggest that at least processes of syntactic repair are partly supported by the BG. Further studies, however, are necessary before a more detailed description of the neural basis of those processes reflected by the P600 and the P345 can be given.

The question as to what extent the different processes reflected by the P600 are dependent on memory resources can be approached by considering those ERP studies that specifically examine participants with different general working memory capacities. This literature indicates an interesting difference between the P600 and the P345: the P600 varies systematically as a function of memory capacity, whereas the P345 does not (Vos et al., 2001). This suggests that the P600 reflects processes, which are not part of the parsing system per se, but may lay outside the linguistic system and are, therefore, subject to general working memory resources.[9] The P345, on the other hand, may reflect processes that are part of the linguistic system proper.

Implication for Psycholinguistic Models

The empirical neurophysiological data lead to a model which assumes three processing phases (Friederici, 1995, 2002): a first phase during which local phrase structure is build on the basis of word category information, a second phase (which may incrementally have a temporal overlap with Phase 1) during which lexical-semantic, morpho-syntactic and thematic information is considered in parallel and a third phase during which integration and if necessary syntactic reanalysis takes place. Interestingly, the ELAN component is present whenever there is a word category violation, its presence is not affected either by variation in semantic or thematic information, nor by strategic manipulations. Semantic processes as reflected by the N400 can be blocked by processes of Phase 1, e.g., by syntactic incongruency at the word category level. When processing morpho-syntactic information (Phase 2) and semantic or thematic information (Phase 2) these two information types do not seem to interact. These two types of information, however, seem to interact during a later processing stage.

Gunter et al. (2000) used sentences in which gender agreement violation between the noun and its determiner was crossed with a variation in cloze probability. The results revealed the LAN effect to be present independent of the cloze probability manipulation and the N400 to be present independent of the agreement violation, again suggesting the LAN and the N400 to be independent. Interestingly, the factor of gender agreement and semantic cloze probability were found to interact, however, in the P600 time window: The P600 varied as a function of both information types. For a similar result see Gunter et al. (1997).

Thus, the neurophysiological findings available thus far, suggest that different subprocesses do not interact unconstraintly during the first two processing phases. It appears that a failure to build up a correct structure can block lexical integration processes. Morpho-syntactic and semantic systems appear to work in parallel and independently during Phase 2. The different types of information, however, do interact during Phase 3. It appears that the fine-grained temporal resolution of the ERP, which allows monitoring the brain's activity from the onset of the stimulus presentation millisecond-by-millisecond can provide data relevant for the discussion of different psycholinguistic models. The data partly support syntax-first models, but they clearly indicate an interaction between different information types during a late processing phase thus also supporting interactive models, but only those that do not assume immediate interaction of semantic and syntactic information.

NEUROIMAGING DATA: THE NEUROANATOMY OF SENTENCE PROCESSING

A consideration of the neural structures underlying the different subprocesses involved in language comprehension is clearly limited given by the relatively poor temporal resolution of the PET and fMRI method, which are tied to the hemodynamic response of the brain. Thus, a description of the early versus late syntactic processes can only be achieved indirectly.

Syntactic Processes

Neurophysiological studies over the last 30 years suggest that Broca's area plays a crucial role in the processing of syntactic information (for a recent review, see Grodzinsky, 2000). The actual role of this brain region during sentence processing may be describable in more detail in reference to those functional neuroimaging studies that investigated sentence processing, with a special focus on syntactic processes. Earlier studies compared the brain activation during the comprehension of sentences or short passages to resting baselines or non-language control conditions (e.g., Bavelier et al., 1997; Bottini et al., 1994; Lechevalier et al., 1989; Mazoyer et al., 1993; Müller et al., 1997) and found a broadly distributed network of areas in the peri-Sylvian region active. One of these studies, however, compared sentence processing and the processing of random word lists (including function words and content words) and found the left IFG and the left STG to be active in the word list condition and the left temporal pole together with the left STG to be active in the sentence condition (Mazoyer et al., 1993). This finding was taken to suggest a special involvement of the temporal pole in syntactic processing. More recent studies focusing on syntactic processes do not support this notion. Moreover, however, these studies do not provide a unified picture either. This may partly be due to the different types of language material used and/ or to the task required in the different experimental settings.

In the following the various studies will be discussed with respect to different aspects of syntactic processing that is (1) the processing of syntactic violations and the processing of syntactic structure in the absence of lexical-semantics and (2) the processing of syntactically complex sentences.

Syntactic Violations/Syntax in Focus

Syntactic violations were investigated in a number of fMRI and PET experiments. Meyer, Friederici, and von Cramon (2000) presented syntactically correct and syntactically incorrect sentences auditorily and observed stronger activation in the left temporal regions (i.e., planum polare, Heschl's gyrus and planum temporale) for incorrect than for correct sentences compared to baseline, the activation in the IFG was present though weak, but not influenced by the presence of syntactic violations (i.e., word category or agreement).

In a different approach, Friederici, Meyer, and von Cramon (2000) studied syntactic processes in an auditory fMRI study by systematically varying the presence of semantic and syntactic information in the input. Participants listened to normal sentences in active and passive voice (i.e., syntax and semantics), to lists of semantically unrelated words (no syntax, but semantics), to lists of pseudowords (no syntax, no semantics) and, most critically, to so-called syntactic prose sentences in which all content words were replaced by pseudowords but in which all function words and inflectional morphology were present (syntax, but no semantics). They were requested to judge whether the stimulus contained a syntactic structure and/or content words. Normal and syntactic prose sentences, i.e., the two conditions in which syntax was present, activated the anterior portion of the STG (planum polare) selectively (in addition to activation in the planum temporale and the Heschl's gyrus). Activation in the deep frontal operculum, maximal in the left hemisphere, was observed only in the syntactic prose condition, i.e., the condition in which only syntactic information was available. Thus no clear activation of the Broca's area (BA 44/45) proper, but rather an activation of the deep frontal operculum was found as a function of stimulus types.

In a more recent study, syntactic violations in the auditory domain were investigated in an event-related fMRI experiment in German (Friederici et al., 2003c). The study used sentences identical to those used in the ERP experiments Hahne and Friederici (2002) and similar to the previous ERP studies a grammaticality judgment task was used. Syntactic phrase structure violations during auditory sentence comprehension revealed an increased involvement of the anterior portion of the left STG and the frontal operculum as well as the putamen in the BG, when considering the activation of the syntactically incorrect sentences (versus baseline) compared to those of the correct sentences (versus baseline). Thus from these studies it appears that a syntactic violation in a sentence does not selectively increase activation in BA 44/45, the classic Broca's region.

Quite a number of studies have investigated syntactic processes during reading. Moro et al. (2001) report a PET study on processing syntactic violations during visual sentence comprehension. They found activation in the anterior portion of the left insula and the right homologue of Broca's area (BA 44/45), which was selectively increased for the violation conditions (i.e., word order violation and subject-verb agreement violation) compared to the correct condition. Ni et al. (2000) investigated syntactic and semantic violations during visual sentence processing and observed a number of brain areas similarly active in both conditions. These included bilateral activation of the inferior frontal gyri (BA 44, 45, and 47), the middle frontal gyri (BA 46/49) and the superior and middle temporal gyri. No region specific for the processing of syntactic violations could be identified. Kuperberg et al. (2000) contrasting syntactic, semantic, and pragmatic violations during reading also found no area specifically activated by syntactic violations.

A clear involvement of Broca's area (BA 44/45), however, is reported in studies as a function of task. Dapretto and Bookheimer (1999) report an fMRI study in which the activation of different brain areas was investigated as a function of whether participants directed their attention towards syntactic or semantic aspects of a sentence. This study uses a paradigm in which two sentences were presented visually one after the other and participants were required to make a same/different decision. The processing of syntactic information,, was correlated with a bilateral activation in the pars opercularis (BA 44), but with maximal activations in the left hemisphere.

Embick et al. (2000) used an error detection paradigm in which subjects had to detect misspelled words or a syntactic error in visually presented sentence. They reported a larger activation in the grammar than in the spelling task for Broca's area as compared to Wernicke's area or the angular and supramarginal gyrus. They claim that this result suggests a selective involvement of Broca's area in syntactic processing.

In a PET study Indefrey and colleagues (Indefrey et al., 2001) also investigated the processing of syntactic errors in meaningless sentences using different syntactic and nonsyntactic tasks. Stimuli were presented visually in a whole sentence format. Their findings reveal that an area of the left dorso-lateral prefrontal cortex, "dorsally adjacent to BA 45 or Broca's area" is specifically involved in the detection of syntactic errors. More anterior prefrontal areas were activated bilaterally for all tasks including those requiring non-syntactic error detection.

Suzuki and Sakai (2003) varied the task demands in a sentence processing study in Japanese and found the left IFG (BA 44/45) to be specifically increased during explicit syntactic processing compared to implicit processing.

These studies, in which syntax was put into focus by particular task demands, Broca's area (BA 44/45) appears to be activated.

Thus, from the combined studies we may conclude that syntactic violations during on-line processing do not automatically give rise to a specific activation pattern in Broca's area, but rather in the left deep frontal operculum. When syntactic processes are in focus due to task demands the left pars opercularis and the pars triangularis are selectively activated.

Syntactic Complexity/Syntactic Memory

A number of PET and fMRI studies which have attempted to specify those brain areas that vary systematically as a function of syntactic complexity. By comparing syntactically complex to syntactically less complex sentences, and keeping the lexical elements identical, these studies aimed to substract out lexical-semantic processes and to look at pure syntactic processes. The majority of these studies were carried out in English, used language in which the variation of syntactic complexity was directly confounded with working memory demands. Caplan and collaborators (Caplan et al., 1998, 2000; Stromswold et al., 1996) for example, compared the processing of visually presented right-branching subject relative clauses (11a) and center-embedded object relative clauses (11b). The "i" in sentences (11a/11b) indexes the *filler* and the _____ indexes the *gap* or *trace* the filler leaves behind when moved out of its original position.

(11a) *The child spilled the juice that$_i$ _____$_i$ stained the rug.*
      (subject-first)
(11b) *The juice that$_i$ the child spilled _____$_i$ stained the rug.*
      (object-first, center embedded)

Sentences of this structural type were presented which were either semantically plausible or semantically implausible. Participants had to perform a plausibility judgment task. In a first PET study the authors reported a focal activation in the left pars opercularis (BA 44) for object relative clauses compared to subject relative clauses for male subjects (Stromswold et al., 1996). Similar studies using cleft subjects and cleft object sentences with female participants and in the auditory domain (Caplan et al., 1998) also reported activation in "Broca's area." However, the precise location of the activation varies considerably between these studies (including BA 44, 45, and 47 and regions beyond these areas).

Just et al. (1996) conducted an fMRI study using three types of sentences with different syntactic complexity: sentences in which two simple clauses were conjoined by "and," sentences with center-embedded subject relative clauses and sentences with center-embedded object relative clauses. They reported increased activation as a function of syntactic complexity in left "Broca's area" and left "Wernicke's area" and to a lesser degree their right hemisphere homologues. As, however, no coordinates of the activation are provided in their report, results from this study cannot be directly compared to those of others. The authors attributed the increased activation to the amount of cognitive resources necessary to perform the task, without, however, specifying what these "cognitive resources" are.

In an investigation of the processing of simple and center-embedded sentences in Japanese, Inui et al. (1998), using fMRI, found left inferior frontal regions (BA 44 and 45) as well as the premotor area to be active. In a Dutch study, Stowe et al. (1998) investigated the processing of simple, complex and ambiguous sentences as well as word lists using PET. When comparing all sentence conditions to the word list condition they found increased activation in the left anterior STG. The combined findings suggest that syntactic processes are supported by the anterior portion of the left STG (i.e., the planum polare), in addition to the left IFG. A German study also comparing activations to simple and those to more complex sentences reported the left IFG and the left STG and MTG to show an increase as a function of complexity (Roeder et al., 2002).

Fiebach, Schlesewsky, and Friederici (2001) also used German as the test language as this language allows varying aspects of syntactic complexity (subject-initial versus object-initial structures) independent of working memory required to bridge the distance between filler and gap (short distance vs long distance). Applying an event-related fMRI technique activation in the left IFG was found to increase as a function of the filler-gap distance. Interestingly, two foci in the IFG could be separated by cluster analysis: inferior portion of BA 44 and the superior portion of BA 44 extending to BA 45. Functionally, the latter region may be correlated with syntactic working memory processes whereas the inferior portion of BA 44 may support structure-building processes.

A very similar finding was reported for English when comparing filler-gap dependencies of different length in subject and object relative clause sentences (Cooke et al., 2001). Significant activation in BA 44/45 was observed when the distance of the filler and its gap was long. Thus, the combined data suggest that activation in the superior portion of BA 44/45 is due to processes of syntactic working memory rather than processes of structure building perse.

Using Hebrew, Ben-Shachar et al. (2003) investigated syntactic transformations and found the left IFG (Broca's area) and the posterior STS bilaterally to support syntactic transformations, which they consider to be the core of syntax. As the left posterior STS was also activated as a function of verb complexity, the left IFG activation is taken to be selectively involved in the processing of syntactic transformations.

Recently, Fiebach, Schlesewsky, and Friederici (2001) conducted a study in which the processing of transformations was directly compared to the processing of syntactic violations. The results indicate that the processing of transformations is supported by left BA 44/45, whereas the processing of syntactic violations does not recruit this area, but rather a region in the left ventral premotor cortex (inferior BA 44/6) in the direct vicinity to the frontal operculum.

On the basis of the combined studies, the notion was put forward that local syntactic violations are correlated with an increase of the frontal operculum (and the adjacent premotor cortex, i.e., inferior BA 44/6), whereas processing of sentences involving syntactic movement and long distance dependencies are correlated with activation in Broca's areas, i.e., BA 44/45 (Friederici, 2004). It is argued that the proposed functional neuroanatomical segregation may be related to the phylogenetic differentiation between older and younger brain structures. Under such a view, the left frontal operculum which according to Sanides (1962) is most likely older evolutionary territory derived from insular proisocortex may be differentiated from adjacent cortex structures which are phylogenetically younger, that is Broca's area.

Summary Syntactic Processes

The reviewed findings suggest that the left IFG as well as the anterior portion of the left STG (planum polare) constitute a network that is specifically involved in syntactic processes. The left planum polare appears to support on-line structure-building processes. Within the left IFG two brain areas may be functionally separable: the frontal operculum appears to come into play when local syntactic structure building is in focus and the superior-anterior portion of BA 44/45 seems to support more demanding syntactic processes, e.g., those involving syntactic movement and non-local dependencies.

Semantic Processes

Semantics has been in the focus of PET and fMRI research from the beginning. It is, however, only very recent that sentence level studies have been. Earlier studies have focused on word level processes and on semantic memory.

There are quite a number of imaging studies, which tried to specify the neural correlate of semantic processes at the word level (e.g., Demonet et al., 1992; Fiez, 1997; Gabrieli et al., 1998; Paulesu et al., 1993; Price et al., 1997; Shaywitz et al., 1995; Thompson-Schill et al., 1997; Vandenberghe et al., 1996; Wise et al., 1991). Overviews of the relevant literature on word level semantic processes suggest a systematical involvement of the posterior portion of the STG and the MTG in semantic processes as indicated across different tasks in reading or listening. Inferior frontal activation (BA 45/47), however, is observed only under particular task demands (Fiez, 1997; Thompson-Schill et al., 1997). This has lead to the notion that the IFG only comes into play when strategic or executive aspects of semantic processes are at order.

Only those few studies that examined semantic processes at the sentence level will be reviewed in somewhat for detail here. In general fMRI sentence studies reported a variety of loci of activation in correlation with semantic processes including the left inferior frontal gyrus (BA 47) (Dapretto and Bookheimer, 1999), the right superior and left middle temporal gyrus (Kuperberg et al., 2000) and the posterior temporal region (Ni et al., 2000). While the latter two studies used a task in which subjects were required to judge after each sentence whether it "made sense," the first study presented two sentences visually at the same time and subjects had to judge whether they "mean the same."

Friederici et al. (2003c) used a grammaticality judgment task in a study investigating the processing of semantic and syntactic violations. For semantic violations the event-related fMRI revealed activation in the mid portion of the STG and the insular cortex bilaterally. For both types of violation, semantic and syntactic, additional activation was observed in the superoposterior portion of the STG. This latter activation may thus, be correlated with general processes of sentential integration, rather than with semantic processes in particular.

Summary Semantic Processes

Overall, the combined findings from these studies together with results from semantic studies at the word level suggest that semantic processes are supported by the left MTG, whereas the left IFG is recruited whenever strategic processes (Thompson-Schill et al., 1997) or, more generally, executive processes (Poldrack et al., 1999) come into play.

The neural substrate can currently only be specified with respect to lexical-semantic but not with respect to thematic aspects of processing. Lexical-semantic access and semantic integration processes at the sentence level are supported by temporal structures, in particular, the MTG and possibly the posterior temporal region. Strategic processes in the semantic domain as well as processes of semantic memory are located in the IFG, in particular, BA 45 and 47.

In addition to what has been sketched so far, it is assumed that the system must represent the output from the phase of thematic role assignment in some form, possibly in a representation specifying the thematic structure hierarchy of the sentence (Schlesewsky, 2001). The locus of such a representation in memory is not yet identified, as there is no single study

investigating this issue. It is not unlikely that frontal memory systems are involved when it comes to hold such a thematic representation in memory.

CONCLUSION

It is not easy to draw a final conclusion from these studies as they used different languages, sentence types, tasks and different functional imaging methodologies. Nonetheless, the empirical data reviewed here lead to the formulation of the model presented at the outset of the chapter. As a general principle of functional organization the model proposes a temporofrontal network for sentence processing. The model suggests that temporal areas analyze and identify the elements at each processing phase with respect to their specific characteristics while the inferofrontal areas are responsible for aspects of sequencing and building of dependency relations.

The semantic network, more specifically, is assumed to consist of the posterior portion of the STG and the MTG together with the more ventral portion of the IFG (BA 45/47). The network subserving online syntactic processes, in contrast, seems to consist of the anterior portion of the STG and the Broca's area (BA 44/45), i.e., pars triangularis/pars opercularis and the frontal operculum. Processes of late integration and reanalyis may partly be supported by the posterior portion of the STG and the BG, respectively.

It appears that in the language evidence (provided here) as well as in a nonlanguage domain (Binkofski et al., 2000; Rizzolatti et al., 1988; Schubotz and von Cramon, 2002) temporal and parieto-temporal areas, including Broca's area, in concert with frontal areas are active during perception. A crucial question that arises, given these findings, clearly is: Due to what extent one can claim a functional specificity to Broca's area? The notion promoted here is that Broca's area receives its specificity as part of a specialized network (which should vary between domains). Within the syntax-specific network, Broca's area's special function is to support the processing of sentences involving syntactic movements and of nonlocal syntactic dependencies.

ACKNOWLEDGMENTS The author would like to thank Kai Alter, Christian Fiebach, Anja Hahne, Christoph Herrmann, Martin Meyer, David Swinney, and three anonymous reviewers for helpful comments on an earlier version of the manuscript.

This work was supported by the Leibniz-Prize awarded to Angela Friederici by the Deutsche Forschungsgemeinschaft (German Research Foundation).

Notes

1. Note that the model only displays the initial processing step for the auditory domain. Reading sentences additionally involves occipital and parietal brain structures paving the way from primary visual processes, to letter recognition, to word form recognition and to lexical access (for a review and recent findings on word reading see Cohen et al., 2000; Fiebach et al., 2002). We will not consider these processes or those involved in grapheme-to-phoneme conversion in this paper, but rather describe the processes of sentence comprehension beyond those specific to reading.

2. Phase 0 will not be discussed here. For recent reviews on the neural basis of processes from auditory input to speech recognition see Hickok and Poeppel (2000), Griffiths (2002), and Scott and Johnsrude (2003).

3. Note that in (2) the sentence final position of the verb is correct as German is a verb final language, but that (2a) is incorrect as the preposition 'im' requires a noun or an adjective-noun combination to follow; thus the main verb following the preposition is syntactically incorrect.

4. A more valuable time locking in cases (3) would require to the ERP component to be time-locked not to the word onset, but to the word category decision point when the ERP component is time-locked to the word category decision point which is the third syllable of the critical word 'veredelt' in (3a). The time-locked to this point, the latency of the left anterior negativity is again early.

5. It should be noted at this point that there are some studies, which report no left anterior negativity in correlation with presumed word category violations. In these studies stimulus material are such that their targets do not actually violate local syntactic word category related rules (e.g., Ainsworth-Darnell et al., 1998, Exp. 1). A similar argument holds for the study by Hagoort et al. (1993) in Dutch for the condition they labelled their 'phrase structure violation' condition, but which rather represents, as they admit, a "less frequent, more complex, but syntactically legal structure in Dutch."

6. There is some recent discussion as to whether the ELAN component that reflects the detection of a phrase structure violation can be separate from the so-called mismatch negativity (MMN) observed for auditory stimuli that mismatch prior context with respect to physical parameters such as frequency, duration and location.

This issue was investigated in a recent study in which the target item in a sentence like (2) was not only violating the preceding context in the syntactic domain, but also in location of the auditory stimulus (left vs. right) (Hahne et al., 2002). The observed additivity of these factors suggest's a relative independence of the ELAN form the physical MMN.

7. The question whether the N400 is a component specific for language processing has been discussed in the literature. Recent studies investigating the domain-specificity of the N400 with respect to language report an N400 for the processing of pictures in sentence context (for a review see Kutas and Federmeier, 2000). An N400 was also observed in the domain of gesture comprehension for a violation of meaningful gestures in the play "Paper, Scissors, Rock" (Gunter et al., 2002). These studies suggest that an N400 can be elicited by a processing difficulty of an anomaly of meaning even when not encoded in words.

8. Recently the idea has been put forward that case marking languages in which the grammatical, and thereby the thematic, role of an NP can be assigned solely on the basis of case information may not enter processes of structural reanalysis, but may rather enter directly into processes of *thematic reanalysis* as soon as the relevant disambiguating case information is available (Bornkessel, 2002; Schlesewsky, 2001).

9. As with the other language related ERP components the issue about the domain-generality versus domain specificity of the P600 has been raised. Within the language domain several studies have investigated the P600's modulation as a function of proportion variation since the domain general P300 context-up-dating component varies its amplitude systematically as a function of proportion (Donchin and Coles, 1988; Osterhout et al., 1996) used a proportion of 40%:60% correct versus incorrect sentences and found no variation of the P600 and suggested its domain specificity. Hahne and Friederici (1999) had a 20%:80% proportion and observed a variation of the P600 that was present when 80% of the sentences were incorrect but not when 20% were incorrect. Studies focusing on nonlanguage domain report a P600 for the processing of anomalies in musical sequences (Patel et al., 1998), and a P600 for the processing of anomalies in gestural sequences (Gunter et al., 2000). These findings suggest that the P600 may be less domain specific than the early syntactic component (E/LAN) (for a similar argument, see Münte et al., 1997). It may be interesting to note the sequential violation in the music domain elicited an early negativity with a right hemispheric maximum (Koelsch et al., 2000; Patel et al., 1998), and the sequential violation the gestural domain an early negativity over the occipital sites know to cover visual processing areas (Gunter et al., 2002).

References

Ainsworth-Darnell, K., Shulman, H.G., & Boland, J.E. (1998). Dissociating brain responses to syntactic and semantic anomalies: Evidence from event-related brain potentials. *Journal of Memory and Language, 38,* 112–130.

Altmann, G.T.M. (Ed.) (1990). *Cognitive models of speech processing.* Cambridge, MA: MIT Press.

Angrilli, A., Penolazzi, B., Vespignani, F., De Vincenzi, M., Job, R., Ciccarelli, L., et al. (2002). Cortical brain responses to semantic incongruity and syntactic violation in Italien language: An event-related potential study. *Neuroscience Letters, 322,* 5–8.

Balota, D.A., Flores d'Arcais, G.B., & Rayner, K. (Eds.) (1990). *Comprehension processes in reading.* Hillsdale, NJ: Lawrence Erlbaum.

Bavelier, D., Corina, D., Jezzard, P., Padmanabhan, S., Clark, V.P., Karni, A., et al. (1997). Sentence reading: A functional MRI study at 4 Tesla. *Journal of Cognitive Neuroscience, 9,* 664–686.

Ben-Shachar, M., Hendler, T., Kahn, I., Ben-Bashat, D., & Grodzinsky, Y. (2003). The neural reality of syntactic transformations: Evidence from fMRI. *Psychological Science, 14,* 433–440.

Binkofsi, F., Amunts, K., Stephan, K.M., Posse, S., Schormann, T., Freund, H.-J., et al. (2000). Broca's region subserves imagery of motion: A combined cytoarchitectonic and fMRI study. *Human Brain Mapping, 11,* 273–285.

Bornkessel, I. (2002). *The argument dependency model: A neurocognitive approach to incremental interpretation.* In Max Planck Institute of Cognitive Neuroscience (Ed.), *MPI Series in Cognitive Neuroscience, vol. 28,* Leipzig.

Bornkessel, I., Schlesewsky, M., & Friederici, A.D. (2002). Language-related positivities reflect the revision of hierarchies. *Neuroreport, 13,* 361–364.

Bottini, G., Corcoran, R., Sterzi, R., Paulesu, E., Schenone, P., Scarpa, P., et al. (1994). The role of right hemisphere in interpretation of figurative aspects of language. A positron emission tomography activation study. *Brain, 117,* 1241–1253.

Caplan, D., Alpert, N., & Waters, G. (1998). Effects of syntactic structure and propositional number on patterns of regional cerebral blood flow. *Journal of Cognitive Neuroscience, 10,* 541–552.

Caplan, D., Alpert, N., Waters, G., & Olivieri, A. (2000). Activation of Broca's area by syntactic processing under conditions of concurrent articulation. *Human Brain Mapping, 9,* 65–71.

Carlson, G.N., & Tanenhaus, M.K. (Eds.) (1989). *Linguistic structure in language processing.* Dordrecht: Kluwer Academic Publishers.

Caplan, D., & Waters, G.S. (1999). Verbal working memory and sentence comprehension. *Behavioral Brain Sciences, 22,* 114–126.

Chwilla, D.J., Brown, C., & Hagoort, P. (1995). The N400 as a function of the level of processing. *Psychophysiology, 32,* 274–285.

Clifton, C., Frazier, L., & Rayner, K. (Eds.) (1994). *Perspectives on sentence processing.* Hillsdale, NJ: Lawrence Erlbaum.

Cohen, L., Dehaene, S., Naccache, L., Lehéricy, S., Dehaene-Lambertz, G., Hénaff, M.-A., et al. (2000). Spatial and temporal characterization of an initial stage of reading in normal subjects and posterior split-brain patients. *Brain, 123,* 291–307.

Cooke, A., Zurif, E.B., DeVita, C., Alsop, D., Koenig, P., Detre, J., et al. (2001). Neural basis for sentence comprehension: Grammatical and short-term memory components. *Human Brain Mapping, 15,* 80–94.

Coulson, S., King, J., & Kutas, M. (1998). Expect the unexpected: Event-related brain responses of morpho-syntactic violations. *Language and Cognitive Processes, 13,* 21–58.

Dapretto, M., & Bookheimer, S. Y. (1999). Form and content: Dissociating syntax and semantics in sentence comprehension. *Neuron, 24,* 427–432.

Demonet, J.F., Chollet, F., Ramsay, S., Cardebat, D., Nespoulous, J.L., Wise, R., et al. (1992). The anatomy of phonological and semantic processing in normal subjects. *Brain, 115,* 1753–1768.

De Vincenzi, M. (1991). *Syntactic parsing strategies in Italian: The minimal chain principle* (Studies in theoretical psycholinguistics, Vol. 12). Dordrecht: Kluwer Academic Publishers.

De Vincenzi, M., Job, R., Di Matteo, R., Angrilli, A., Penolazzi, B., Ciccarelli, L., et al. (2003). Differences in the perception and time course of syntactic and semantic violations. *Brain and Language, 85,* 280–296.

Deutsch, A., & Bentin S. (2001). Syntactic and semantic factors in processing gender agreement in Hebrew: Evidence form ERPs and eye movements. *Journal of Memory and Language, 45,* 200–224.

Donchin, E., & Coles, M. (1988). Is the P300 component a manifestation of context updating? *Behavioral and Brain Sciences, 11,* 357–374.

Embick, D., Marantz, A., Miyashita, Y., O'Neil, W., & Sakai, K.L. (2000). A syntactic specialization for Broca's area. *Proceedings of the National Academy of Sciences of the USA, 97,* 6150–6154.

Fiebach, C.J., Friederici, A.D., Müller, K., & von Cramon, D.Y. (2002). fMRI evidence for dual routes to the mental lexicon in visual word recognition. *Journal of Cognitive Neuroscience, 14,* 11–23.

Fiebach, C.J., Schlesewsky, M., & Friederici, A.D. (2001). Syntactic working memory and the establishment of filler-gap dependencies: Insights from ERPs and fMRI. *Journal of Psycholinguistic Research, 30,* 321–338.

Fiez, J.A. (1997). Phonology, semantics, and the role of the left inferior prefrontal cortex. *Human Brain Mapping, 5,* 79–83.

Fodor, J.D., & Inoue, A. (1994). The diagnosis and cure of garden path. *Journal of Psycholinguistic Research, 23,* 407–434.

Frauenfelder, U.H., & Tyler, L.K. (1987). The process of spoken word recognition: An introduction. *Cognition, 25,* 1–20.

Frazier, L. (1978). *On comprehension sentences: Syntactic parsing strategies.* Doctoral Dissertation, University of Connecticut.

Frazier, L. (1987a). Sentence processing: A tutorial review. In M. Coltheart (Ed.), *Attention and performance XII: The psychology of reading.* London: Lawrence Erlbaum.

Frazier, L. (1987b). Theories of sentence processing. In J. Garfield (Ed.), *Modularity in knowledge representation and natural-language processing.* Cambridge, MA: MIT Press.

Frazier, L., & Clifton, C., Jr. (1996). *Construal.* Cambridge, MA: MIT Press.

Frazier, L., & Flores d'Arcais, G.B. (1989). Filler driven parsing: A study of gap filling in Dutch. *Journal of Memory and Language, 28,* 331–344.

Frazier, L., & Rayner, K. (1982). Making and correcting errors during sentence comprehension: Eye movements in the analysis of structurally ambiguous sentences. *Cognitive Psychology, 14,* 178–210.

Friederici, A.D. (1995). The time course of syntactic activation during language processing: A model based on neuropsychological and neurophysiological data. *Brain and Language, 50,* 259–281.

Friederici, A.D. (2002). Towards a neural basis of auditory sentence processing. *Trends in Cognitive Sciences, 6,* 78–84.

Friederici, A.D. (2004). Processing local transitions versus long-distance syntactic hierarchies. *Trends in Cognitive Sciences, 8,* 245–247.

Friederici, A.D., & Alter, K. (2004). Lateralization of auditory language functions: A dynamic dual pathway view. *Brain and Language, 89,* 267–276.

Friederici, A.D., & Frisch, S. (2000). Verb-argument structure processing: The role of verb-specific and argument-specific information. *Journal of Memory and Language, 43,* 476–507.

Friederici, A.D., Gunter, T.C., Hahne, A., & Mauth, K. (2004). The relative timing of syntactic and semantic processes in sentence comprehension. *NeuroReport, 15,* 165–169.

Friederici, A.D., Hahne, A., & Mecklinger, A. (1996). The temporal structure of syntactic parsing: Early and late event-related brain potential effects elicited by syntactic anomalies. *Journal of Experimental Psychology: Learning, Memory, and Cognition, 22,* 1219–1248.

Friederici, A.D., Hahne, A., & Saddy, D. (2002). Distinct neurophysiological patterns for aspects of syntactic complexity and syntactic repair. *Journal of Psycholinguistic Research, 31,* 45–63.

Friederici, A.D., Kotz, S.A., Steinhauer, K., & von Cramon, D.Y. (2003a). The neural basis of the prosody-syntax interplay: The role of the corpus callosum. *Brain and Language, 87,* 133–134.

Friederici, A.D., Kotz, S.A., Werheid, K., Hein, G., & von Cramon, D.Y. (2003b). Syntactic comprehension in Parkinson's desease: Investigating early automatic and late integrational processes using event-related brain potentials. *Neuropsychology, 17,* 133–142.

Friederici, A.D., & Mecklinger, A. (1996). Syntactic parsing as revealed by brain responses: First-pass and second-pass parsing processes. *Journal of Psycholinguistic Research, 25,* 157–176.

Friederici, A.D., Meyer, M., & von Cramon, D.Y. (2000). Auditory language comprehension: An event-related fMRI study on the processing of syntactic and lexical information. *Brain and Language, 74,* 289–300.

Friederici, A.D., Pfeifer, E., & Hahne, A. (1993). Event-related brain potentials during natural speech processing: Effects of semantic, morphological and syntactic violations. *Cognitive Brain Research, 1,* 183–192.

Friederici, A.D., Rüschemeyer, S.-A., Hahne, A., & Fiebach, C.J. (2003c). The role of left inferior frontal and superior temporal cortex in sentence comprehension: Localizing syntactic and semantic processes. *Cerebral Cortex, 13,* 170–177.

Friederici, A.D., Steinhauer, K., & Frisch, S. (1999). Lexical integration: Sequential effects of syntactic and semantic information. *Memory and Cognition, 27,* 438–453.

Friederici, A.D., von Cramon, D.Y., & Kotz, S.A. (1999). Language-related brain potentials in patients with cortical and subcortical left hemisphere lesions. *Brain, 122,* 1033–1047.

Friederici, A.D., Wang, Y., Herrmann, C.S., Maess, B., & Oertel, U. (2000). Localization of early syntactic processes in frontal and temporal cortical areas: A magnetoencephalographic study. *Human Brain Mapping, 11,* 1–11.

Frisch, S., Hahne, A., & Friederici, A.D. (2004). Word category and verb-argument structure information in the dynamics of parsing. *Cognition, 91,* 191–219.

Frisch, S., Kotz, S.A., von Cramon, D.Y., & Friederici, A.D. (2003). Why the P600 is not just a P300: The role of the basal ganglia. *Clinical Neurophysiology, 114,* 336–340.

Frisch, S., & Schlesewsky, M. (2001). The N400 reflects problems of thematic hierarchizing. *Neuroreport, 12,* 3391–3394.

Gabrieli, J.D.E., Poldrack, R.A., & Desmond, J.E. (1998). The role of left prefrontal cortex in langauge and memory. *Proceedings of the National Academy of Sciences USA, 95,* 906–913.

Garfield, J.L. (Ed.) (1987). *Modularity in knowledge representation and natural-language understanding.* Cambridge, MA: MIT Press.

Gibson, E. (1991). *A computational theory of human linguistic processing: Memory limitations and processing breakdown.* Unpublished Ph.D. dissertation. Carnegie Mellon University.

Gorrell, P. (1995). *Syntax and parsing.* Cambridge, UK: Cambridge University Press.

Gorrell, P. (1996). Parsing theory and phrase-order variation in german V2 clauses. *Journal of Psycholinguistic Research, 25,* 135–156.

Griffiths, T.D. (2002). The planum temporale as a computational hub. *Trends in Neurosciences, 25,* 348–353.

Grodzinsky, Y. (2000). The neurology of syntax: Language use without Broca's area. *Behavioral and Brain Sciences, 23,* 1–21.

Gross, J., Ioannides, A.A., Dammers, J., Maess, B., Friederici, A.D., & Müller-Gärtner, H.-W. (1998). Magnetic field tomography analysis of continious speech. *Brain Topography, 10,* 273–281.

Gunter, T.C., Friederici, A.D., & Hahne, A. (1999). Brain responses during sentence reading: Visual input affects central processes. *NeuroReport, 10,* 3175–3178.

Gunter, T.C., Friederici, A.D., & Schriefers, H. (2000). Syntactic gender and semantic expectancy: ERPs reveal early autonomy and late interaction. *Journal of Cognitive Neuroscience, 12,* 556–568.

Gunter, T.C., Knoblich, G, Bach, P., Prinz, W., & Friederici, A.D. (2002). Meaning and structure in action comprehension: electrophysiological evidence. *Journal of Cognitive Neuroscience, Supplement,* S80.

Gunter, T.C., Stowe, L.A., & Mulder, G. (1997). When syntax meets semantics. *Psychophysiology, 34,* 660–676.

Hagoort, P., Brown, C., & Groothusen, J. (1993). The syntactic positive shift as an ERP measure of syntactic processing. *Language and Cognitive Processes, 8,* 439–483.

Hagoort, P., Brown, C.M., & Osterhout, L. (1999). The neurocognition of syntactic processing. In C.M. Brown & P. Hagoort (Eds.). *The neurocognition of language* (pp. 273–316). Oxford/New York: Oxford University Press.

Hahne, A. (2001). What's different in second language processing? Evidence from event-related brain potentials. *Journal of Psycholinguistic Research, 30,* 251–266.

Hahne, A., & Friederici, A.D. (1999). Electrophysiological evidence for two steps in syntactic analysis: Early automatic and late controlled processes. *Journal of Cognitive Neuroscience, 11,* 194–205.

Hahne, A., & Friederici, A.D. (2002). Differential task effects on semantic and syntactic processes as revealed by ERPs. *Cognitive Brain Research, 13,* 339–356.

Hahne, A., & Jescheniak, J.D. (2001). What's left if the Jabberwocky gets the semantics? An ERP investigation into semantic and syntactic processes during auditory sentence comprehension. *Cognitive Brain Research, 11,* 199–212.

Hahne, A., Schröger, E., & Friederici, A.D. (2002). Segregating early physical and syntactic processes in auditory sentence comprehension. *Neuroreport, 13,* 305–309.

Halgren, E., Baudena, P., Heit, P., Clarke, J.M., Marinkovic, K., & Clarke, M. (1994). Spatio-temporal stages in face and word processing. 1. Depth-recorded potentials in the human occipital, temporal and parietal lobes [corrected] [published erratum appears in *Journal de Physiologie Paris,* 1994, 88, following ISI]. *Journal de Physiologie, 88,* 1–50.

Helenius, P., Salmelin, R., Service, E., & Connolly, J.F. (1998). Distinct time courses of word and context comprehension in the left temporal cortex. *Brain, 121,* 1133–1142.

Hemforth, B., & Konieczny, L. (Eds.) (2000). *German sentence processing.* Dordrecht/Boston/London: Kluwer Academic Publishers.

Hickok, G. (1993). Parallel parsing: Evidence from reactivation in garden-path sentences. *Journal of Psycholinguistic Research, 22,* 239–250.

Hickok, G., & Poeppel, D. (2000). Towards a functional neuroanatomy of speech perception *Trends in Cognitive Sciences, 4,* 131–138.

Indefrey, P., Hagoort, P., Herzog, H., Seitz, R.J., & Brown, C.M. (2001). Syntactic processing in left prefrontal cortex is independent of lexical meaning. *NeuroImage, 14,* 546–555.

Inoue, A., & Fodor, J.D. (1995). Information-paced parsing of Japanese. In R. Mazuka & N. Nagai (Eds.), *Japanese sentence processing* (pp. 9–63). Hillsdale, NJ: Lawrence Erlbaum.

Inui, T., Otsu, Y., Tanaka, S., Okada, T., Nishizawa, S., & Konishi, J. (1998). A functional MRI analysis of comprehension processes of Japanese sentences. *NeuroReport*, 9, 3325–3328.

Just, M.A., & Carpenter, P. (1992). A capacity theory of comprehension: Individual differences in working memory. *Psychological Review*, 99, 122–149.

Just, M.A., Carpenter, P.A., Keller, T.A., Eddy, W.F., & Thulborn, K.R. (1996). Brain activation modulated by sentence comprehension. *Science*, 274, 114–116.

Kaan, E., Harris, A., Gibson, E., & Holcomb, P.J. (2000). The P600 as an index of syntactic integration difficulty. *Language and Cognitive Processes*, 15, 159–201.

Knösche, T., Maess, B., & Friederici, A.D. (1999). Processing of syntactic information monitored by brain surface current density mapping based on MEG. *Brain Topography*, 12, 75–87.

Koelsch, S., Gunter, T.C., Friederici, A.D., & Schröger, E. (2000). Brain indices of music processing: Non-musicians are musical. *Journal of Cognitive Neuroscience*, 12, 520–541.

Kotz, S.A., Frisch, S., von Cramon D.Y., & Friederici, A.D. (2003). Syntactic language processing: ERP lesion data on the role of the basal ganglia. *Journal of the International Neuropsychological Society*, 9, 1053–1060.

Kubota, M., Ferrari, P., & Roberts, T.P.L. (2003). Magnetoencephalography detection of early syntactic processing in humans: Comparison between L1 speakers and L2 learners of English. *Neuroscience Letters*, 353, 107–110.

Kuperberg, G.R., McGuire, P.K., Bullmore, E.T., Brammer, M.J., Rabe-Hesketh, S., Wright, I.C., et al. (2000). Common and distinct neural substrates for pragmatic, semantic, and syntactic processing of spoken sentences: An fMRI study. *Journal of Cognitive Neuroscience*, 12, 321–341.

Kutas, M., & Federmeier, K.D. (2000). Electrophysiology reveals semantic memory use in language comprehension. *Trends in Cognitive Sciences*, 4, 463–470.

Kutas, M., & Hillyard, S.A. (1980). Reading senseless sentences: Brain potentials reflect semantic incongruity. *Science*, 207, 203–205.

Kutas, M., & Hillyard, S.A. (1983). Event-related potentials to grammatical errors and semantic anomalies. *Memory and Cognition*, 11, 539–550.

Kutas, M., & Hillyard, S. A. (1984). Brain potentials during reading reflect word expectancy and semantic association, *Nature*, 307, 161–163.

Kutas, M., & Van Petten, C. (1994). Psycholinguistics electrified: Event-related brain potential investigations. In M.A. Gernsbacher (Ed.). *Handbook of psycholinguistics* (pp. 83–143). San Diego: Academic Press.

Lechevalier, B., Petit, M., Eustache, F., Lambert, J., Chapon, F., & Viader, F. (1989). Regional cerebral blood flow during comprehension and speech (in cerebrally healthy subjects). *Brain and Language*, 37, 1–11.

MacDonald, M.C., Just, M.A., & Carpenter, P.A. (1992). Working memory constraints on the processing of syntactic ambiguity. *Cognitive Psychology*, 24, 56–98.

MacDonald, M.C., Pearlmutter, N.J., & Seidenberg, M.S. (1994a). The lexical nature of syntactic ambiguity resolution. *Psychological Review*, 101, 676–703.

MacDonald, M.C., Pearlmutter, N.J., & Seidenberg, M.S. (1994b). *Syntactic ambiguity resolution as lexical ambiguity resolution*. In C. Clifton, Jr., L. Frazier and K. Rayner (Eds.), *Perspectives on sentence processing* (pp. 123–154). Hillsdale, NJ: Lawrence Erlbaum.

Marslen-Wilson, W.D., & Tyler, L.K. (1980). The temporal structure of spoken language understanding. *Cognition*, 8, 1–71.

Mazoyer, B.M., Tzourio, N., Frak, V., Syrota, A., Murayama, N., Levrier, O., et al. (1993). The cortical representation of speech. *Journal of Cognitive Neuroscience*, 5, 467–479.

McClelland, J.L., St.John, M., & Taraban, R. (1989). An interaction model of context effects in letter perception: Part I: An account of basic findings. *Language and Cognitive Processes*, 4, 287–336.

McKinnon, R., & Osterhout, L. (1996). Constraints on movement phenomena in sentence processing: Evidence from event-related brain potentials. *Language and Cognitive Processes*, 11, 495–523.

Mecklinger, A., Schriefers, H., Steinhauer, K., & Friederici, A.D. (1995). Processing relative clauses varying on syntactic and semantic dimensions: An analysis with event-related potentials. *Memory and Cognition*, 23, 477–494.

Meyer, M., Alter, K., Friederici, A.D., Lohmann, G., & von Cramon, D.Y. (2002). FMRI reveals brain regions mediating slow prosodic modulations in spoken sentences. *Human Brain Mapping*, 17, 73–88.

Meyer, M., Friederici, A.D., & von Cramon, D.Y. (2000). Neurocognition of auditory sentence comprehension: Event-related fMRI reveals sensitivity to syntactic violations and task demands. *Cognitive Brain Research*, 9, 19–33.

Mitchell, D.C. (1994). Sentence parsing. In M.A. Gernsbacher (Ed.), *Handbook of Psycholinguistics*. San Diego: Academic Press.

Moro, A., Tettamanti, M., Perani, D., Donati, C., Cappa, S.F., & Fazio, F. (2001). Syntax and the brain: Disentangling grammar by selective anomalies. *NeuroImage*, 13, 110–118.

Müller, R.-A., Rothermel, R.D., Behen, M.E., Muzik, O., Mangner, T.J., & Chugani, H.T. (1997). Receptive and expressive language activations for sentences: A PET study. *NeuroReport*, 8, 3767–3770.

Münte, T.F., Heinze, H.J., & Mangun, G.R. (1993). Dissociation of brain activity related to syntactic and semantic aspects of language. *Journal of Cognitive Neuroscience*, 5, 335–344.

Münte, T.F., Szentkui, A., Wieringa, B.M., Matzke, M., & Johannes, S. (1997). Human brain potentials to reading syntactic errors in sentences of different complexity. *Neuroscience Letters*, 235, 105–108.

Neville, H.J., Nicol, J., Barss, A., Forster, K.I., & Garrett, M.F. (1991). Syntactically based sentence processing classes: Evidence from event-related brain potentials. *Journal of Cognitive Neuroscience*, 3, 151–165.

Ni, W., Constable, R.T., Mencl, W.E., Pugh, K.R., Fulbright, R.K., Shaywitz, S.E., et al. (2000). An event-related neuroimaging study distinguishing form and content in sentence processing. *Journal of Cognitive Neuroscience*, 12, 120–133.

Nobre, A.C., & McCarthy, G. (1995). Language-related field potentials in the anterior-medial temporal lobe: II. Effects of the word type and semantic priming. *The Journal of Neuroscience*, 15, 1090–1098.

Osterhout, L., & Holcomb, P.J. (1992). Event-related potentials and syntactic anomaly. *Journal of Memory and Language*, 31, 785–804.

Osterhout, L., & Holcomb, P.J. (1993). Event-related potentials and syntactic anomaly: Evidence of anomaly detection during the perception of continuous speech. *Language and Cognitive Processes*, 8, 413–437.

Osterhout, L., Holcomb, P.J., & Swinney, D. (1994). Brain potentials elicited by garden-path sentences: Evidence of the application of verb information during parsing. *Journal of Experimental Psychology: Learning, Memory, and Cognition*, 20, 786–803.

Osterhout, L., McKinnon, R., Bersick, M., & Corey, V. (1996). On the language-specificity of the brain response to syntactic anomalies: Is the syntactic positive shift a member of the P300 family? *Journal of Cognitive Neuroscience*, 8, 507–526.

Osterhout, L., & Mobley, L.A. (1995). Event-related brain potentials elicited by failure to agree. *Journal of Memory and Language*, 34, 739–773.

Osterhout, L., & Nicol, J. (1999). On the distinctiveness, independence, and time course of the brain responses to syntactic and semantic anomalies. *Language and Cognitive Processes*, 14, 283–317.

Patel, A., Gibson, E., Ratner, J., Besson, M., & Holcomb, P. (1998). Processing syntactic relations in language and music: An event-related potential study. *Journal of Cognitive Neuroscience*, 10, 717–733.

Paulesu, E., Frith, C.D., & Frackowiak, R.S.J. (1993). The neural correlates of the verbal component of working memory. *Nature*, 362, 342–345.

Penke, M., Weyerts, H., Gross, M., Zander, E., Münte, T.F., & Clahsen, H. (1997). How the brain processes complex words: An ERP-study of German verb inflections. *Cognitive Brain Research*, 6, 37–52.

Poldrack, R.A., Wagner, A.D., Prull, M.W., Desmond, J.E., Glover, G.H., & Gabrieli, J.D.E. (1999). Functional specialization for semantic and phonological processing in the left inferior prefrontal cortex. *NeuroImage*, 10, 15–35.

Price, C.J., Moore, C.J., Humphreys, G.W., & Wise, R.J.S. (1997). Segregating semantic from phonological processes during reading. *Journal of Cognitive Neuroscience*, 9, 727–733.

Pulvermüller, F., & Shtyrov, Y. (2003). Automatic processing of grammar in the human brain as revealed by the mismatch negativity. *NeuroImage*, 20, 159–172.

Rizzolatti, G., Camarda, R., Fogassi, L., & Gentillucci, M. (1988). Functional organization of inferior area 6 in the macaque monkey. II. Area F5 and the control of distal movements. *Experimental Brain Research*, 71, 491–507.

Roeder, B., Stock, O., Neville, H., Bien, S., & Roesler, F. (2002). Brain activation modulated by the comprehension of normal and pseudo-word sentences of different processing demands: A functional magnetic resonance imaging study. *NeuroImage*, 15, 1003–1014.

Sanides, F. (1962). Die Architektonik des menschlichen Stirnhirns. In M. Müller, H. Spatz, & P. Vogel (Eds.), *Monographien der Gesamtgebieten der Neurologie und Psychiatrie* (Vol. 98). Berlin: Springer.

Schlesewsky, M. (2001). Die thematische Natur morphologischer Kasus: Beobachtungen und Konsequenzen. Habilitation thesis, University of Potsdam.

Schubotz, R.I., & von Cramon, D.Y. (2002). A blueprint for target motion: fMRI reveals perceived sequential complexity to modulate premotor cortex. *NeuroImage*, 16, 920–935.

Scott, S.K., & Johnsrude, I.S. (2003). The neuroanatomical and functional organization of speech perception. *Trends in Neurosciences*, 26, 100–107.

Shaywitz, B.A., Pugh, K.R., Constable, R.T., Shaywitz, S.E., Bronen, R.A., Fulbright, R.K., et al. (1995). Localization of semantic processing using functional resonance imaging. *Human Brain Mapping*, 2, 149–158.

Shtyrov, Y., Pulvermüller, F., Näätänen, R., & Ilmoniemi, R.J. (2003). Grammar processing outside the focus of attention: An MEG study. *Journal of Cognitive Neuroscience*, 15, 1195–1206.

Simpson, G.B. (Ed.) (1991). *Understanding word and sentence*. Amsterdam: North-Holland.

Steinhauer, K., Alter, K., & Friederici, A.D. (1999). Brain potentials indicate immediate use of prosodic cues in natural speech processing. *Nature Neuroscience*, 2, 191–196.

Stowe, L.A., Broere, C.A.J., Paans, A.M.J., Wijers, A.A., Mulder, G., Vaalburg, W., et al. (1998). Localization components of a complex task: Sentence processing and working memory. *NeuroReport*, 9, 2995–2999.

Stromswold, K., Caplan, D., Alpert, N., & Rauch, S. (1996). Localization of syntactic comprehension by positron emission tomography. *Brain and Language*, 10, 132–144.

Suzuki, K., & Sakai, K.L. (2003). An event-related fMRI study of explicit syntactic processing of normal/anomalous sentences in contrast to implicit syntactic processing. *Cerebral Cortex*, 13, 517–526.

Tanenhaus, M.K., & Trueswell, J.C. (1995). Sentence comprehension. In J.L. Miller & P.D. Eimas (Eds.), *Speech, language and communication*. San Diego: Academic Press.

Thompson-Schill, S.L., D'Esposito, M., Aguirre, G.K., & Farah, M.J. (1997). Role of left inferior prefrontal cortex in retrieval of semantic knowledge: A reevaluation. *Proceedings of the National Academy of Sciences USA*, 94, 14792–14797.

Trueswell, J.C., & Tanenhaus, M.K. (1994). Toward a lexicalist framework of constraint-based syntactic ambiguity resolution. In C. Clifton Jr., L. Frazier, & K. Rayner (Eds.), *Perspectives on sentence processing* (pp. 155–180). Hillsdale, NJ: Lawrence Erlbaum.

Vandenberghe, R., Price, C., Wise, R., Josephs, O., & Frackowiak, R.S. (1996). Functional anatomy of a common semantic system for words and pictures. *Nature*, 383, 254–256.

Vos, S.H., Gunter, T.C., Schriefers, H., & Friederici, A.D. (2001). Syntactic parsing and working memory: The effects of syntactic complexity, reading span, and concurrent load. *Language and Cognitive Processes*, 16, 65–103.

Wise, R., Chollet, F., Hadar, U., Friston, K., Hoffner, E., & Frackowiak, R. (1991). Distribution of cortical neural networks involved in word comprehension and word retrieval. *Brain*, 114, 1803–1817.

14

Involvement of the Left and Right Frontal Operculum in Speech and Nonspeech Perception and Production

Martin E. Meyer

Lutz Jäncke

For a future understanding of the neural underpinnings of auditory functions it is essential to elucidate how the brain processes distinctive acoustic cues available in spoken utterances, nonspeech sounds, and music. Recent review articles agree in emphasizing the role the superior temporal lobes play in speech and nonspeech processing (Friederici, this volume, Chapter 13; Indefrey and Cutler, 2004; Scott and Wise, 2004). In particular, the auditory cortices that stretch along the entire supratemporal plane including the planum polare and the planum temporale support a multitude of auditory functions even when complex linguistic stimuli have to be processed. With respect to the latter the majority of brain imaging studies support the notion of left hemisphere dominance in speech function while the precise contribution of the right superior temporal cortex still remains somewhat clouded. Notably, recent studies provided some evidence for the importance of the superior temporal sulcus during speech and nonspeech comprehension

(Belin and Zatorre, 2003; Boemio et al., 2005; von Kriegstein and Giraud, 2004).

Aside from the temporal lobes it has been known for a long time that the left inferior frontal gyrus is also indispensibly involved in speech and articulatory functions. According to the seminal reports by Paul Broca a disturbance in articulation was associated with a lesion within the posterior part of the third frontal convolution in the left hemisphere and was characterized by deficient speech production but not by difficulty in language comprehension (Broca, 1861, 1863). From this time on the foot of the third left frontal convolution was called Broca's area. In the early 1960s the notion of a distinct brain region in the left hemisphere accounting for expressive speech functions had been replaced by a revised view. Due to clinical observations it has been demonstrated that patients suffering from damage to Broca's area indeed display particular deficits in producing function words and appropriate inflections, as well as a limited range of syntactic structures (Goodglass, 1976). Additionally, careful tests also evidenced that Broca's aphasia has frequently been accompanied by deficient sentence comprehension. These observations made an increasing number of aphasiologists and neurolinguists believe that Broca's area can be considered the locus of syntactic functions until a case study by Mohr et al. (1978) substantiated that the relation between Broca's aphasia and lesion in Broca's area was not as consistent as once believed. It became highly apparent that damage which is not exclusively confined to Broca's area but also affects the surrounding frontal operculum and may even extend to the anterior insula accounts for the majority of observed serious disturbances in speech functions. With the advent of brain imaging a decade ago a pile of evidence has been collected which corroborates the fundamental role of the frontal operculum in general auditory processing. The frontal operculum covers the lateral convexity of the posterior inferior frontal gyrus (IFG) encompassing Broca's area[1] and its immediate environment, which is the deeply buried portion of the frontal operculum and the adjacent anterior insula.

In this review, we concentrate on sublexical and prelexical modes of speech processing, all types of nonspeech and music processing and speech and nonspeech production. We have explicitly refrained from incorporating and discussing higher levels language comprehension, i.e., semantics and syntax. With respect to semantics a review of the current literature clearly demonstrates that the orbital part of the IFG (corresponding to BA 47) (Bookheimer, 2002) mediate complex semantic executive processes while simple processing of lexical information is subserved by the temporal lobes (Giraud et al., 2001). A review by Cappa and Perani (this volume, Chapter 12) concludes that there is considerable evidence supporting a necessary role of Broca's area in aspects of lexical retrieval. According to Cappa and Perani both grammatical and semantic factors, as well as task requirements, appear to modulate the engagement of Broca's area during lexical-semantic processing. Even though the orbital part seems to differ in cytoarchitecture from the triangular and the opercular part of the IFG it is considered part of Broca's area by some authors (Amunts and Zilles, this volume, Chapter 2). With respect to sentence-level syntactic processing we refer to recently published overview article that conclusively discusses the potential functional-structural re-

lationship between differential aspects of syntactic processing and distinct subportions of the frontal operculum (Friederici, 2004). Several other review papers comprehensively discuss and delineate the potential role the temporal lobes play during auditory sentence perception (Friederici, 2002; Friederici and Alter, 2004; Friederici, this volume, Chapter 13; Indefrey and Cutler, 2004; Hickok and Pöppel, 2004; Scott and Wise, 2004). In the context of this synopsis we completely ignore studies which researched the involvement of the frontal operculum in written language processing. Readers with potential interest in this matter may address the review papers by Burton (2001), Gernsbacher and Kaschak (2003), Martin (2003), and the eloquent position paper by Stowe et al. (2005). A comprehensive review on the role Broca's area plays in sign language production and comprehension has been composed by Emmorey (this volume, Chapter 11).

The multitude of linguistic and paralinguistic functions that could be associated with Broca's area and its contralateral analogue imply that this region cannot be considered a unifunctional area. It is plausible to assume that Broca's area supports nonspecific processing devices which are modality independent. The traditional notion of Broca's area as a core centre for language in the brain has been discarded since a plethora of neuroimaging studies has revealed an engagement of this area in a multitude of cognitive and perceptuomotor functions, i.e., visually prompted digit sequence learning (Müller et al., 2002), perception of the rhythm of motion (Schubotz and von Cramon, 2001), imagery of motion (Binkofski et al., 2000; Binkofski and Buccino, 2004; Fadigo et al., this volume, Chapter 9; Jäncke et al., 1999) subvocal rhythm encoding and maintenance (Gruber et al., 2000), mapping of nonlinguistic structural information (Hoen et al., in press), visual pattern matching (Fink, this volume, Chapter 16), etc. Evidence in favor of an essential involvement of Broca's area in the "articulatory loop," the subvocal rehearsal system, stems from a positron emission tomography study by Paulesu et al. (1993). Furthermore, a review article by Pöppel (1996) provided additional evidence for the close relation between Broca's area and verbal working memory. Aboitiz and colleagues provide a complementary hypothesis proposing that language networks emerged as a specialization of frontoparietal-prefrontal circuits involved in cognitive processes such as working memory (Aboitiz et al., this volume,

Chapter 1). Of particular interest in this context is the notion of "mirror neurons" in the frontal lobe, which have been reported to activate during observation, recognition, and imitation of nonverbal actions (Buccino et al., 2004; Rizzolatti and Luppino, 2001). To date there is still an ongoing debate on the potential neuroanatomical correspondence of monkey area F5 and Broca's area in humans. Notably the proponents of this correspondence advance the idea that the principle of mirror neurons may have shaped the basis for the emergence of spoken communication (Rizzolatti and Arbib, 1999).

Due to the heterogenity and variety of cognitive and perceptuomotor functions outlined earlier, it is almost impossible to draw a unifying picture that plausibly delineates the functional determination of the frontal operculum. One recently published innovative account of research provides an attempt to bridge at least the gap between nonlinguistic processes subserved by Broca's area and its preference to support linguistic functions (Müller and Basho, 2004). Adopting an ontogenetic perspective, the authors conclude that elementary perceptuomotor functions, i.e., audiomotor and visuomotor imitation can be considered indispensable principles of language acquisition. Once the crucial steps of language acquisition have been completed, Broca's area may serve general nonlinguistic processes of sequencing or segmenting visual and auditory language input for which precise linguistic relevance has to be determined in the future.

This review subsumes various relevant auditory functions that have been attributed to multiple anatomical locations and attempts to illustrate the commonalities between them. For this (admittedly arbitrary approach), we used classic terms and expressions that are associated with auditory perception in neuroscience studies of auditory functions (tone perception, speech perception, perception of speech complexity, perception of degraded speech, music perception, perception of sound, perception of phonology, perception of affective auditory information, speech and music production, dichotic listening, and processing of auditory mismatch information). These auditory functions have been explored in the reviewed neuroimaging studies by statistically contrasting an operationalized function of interest against an appropriate control condition. Based on a comprehensive synopsis of these contrasts, we are able to address some important and hotly debated issues in current neuroscience of speech and audition as outlined below.

Primarily, the current review aims at publishing a comprehensive synopsis of recent brain imaging studies that observed a recruitment of the frontal operculum including Broca's area in auditory functions. The vast majority of studies investigated perceptive issues while merely a few investigations examined expressive aspects. A systematic comparison between the mean MNI (Montreal Neurological Institute; http://www. mni.mcgill.ca) coordinates would allow speculation upon potential differences or overlaps of auditory domains based on precise localization. It is conceivable that domains primarily deal with linguistic information (phonology, lexical tone) cover an area of the frontal operculum that is clearly distinct from domains which are primarily related to melodic modulations (music perception, affective prosody). By means of a hierarchical cluster analysis based on the Euclidian distance between MNI coordinates, we identified clusters including up to four auditory domains in at least three distinct subregions of the left frontal operculum.

Besides the cardinal relevance the left frontal operculum has in the context of cognitive and perceptuomotor task, it has become more and more obvious that the contralateral region is also involved in a variety of functions, even though its precise role is poorly understood. Activity in the right frontal operculum has been observed in studies investigating cognitive and perceptuomotor processing in the visual and auditory domain. In particular, in the realm of auditory studies on speech, intonation and music production the right frontal operculum seems to play an important role (Meyer et al., 2004; Perry et al., 1999; Riecker et al., 2000). Interestingly, it has been observed that the right frontal operculum preferentially coactivates with the left frontal operculum (Friederici et al., 2000; Meyer et al., 2004; Plante et al., 2002; Zatorre et al., 1994) that has opened the court for speculations on neurofunctional connectivity between left and right frontoopercular areas. However, this potential connectivity has not yet been proved. In the context of the current review we take a careful look on the present evidence which may help elucidate the functional role the right frontal operculum plays in auditory and speech processing.

A few recent fMRI studies observed functional responses in the deep frontal operculum extending into the anterior insula while participants listened to speech signals that had been physically manipulated in that normal speech signals had been turned into acoustically degraded percepts (Davis and Johnsrude, 2003; Giraud et al., 2004; Meyer et al., 2002). We go into this issue by reviewing brain imaging studies that investigated the processing of distorted speech signal and compare the location of hemodynamic responses.

PROCEDURES

This review includes 56 brain imaging studies using either the positron emission tomography (n = 21) or the fMRI technique (n = 33). All studies were published in peer-reviewed journals in the years 1992 through 2004. All studies investigated right-handed participants, which prohibits a discussion on variable lateralization of speech functions in the brain of left-handed persons. All studies report activity either in the left or right frontal operculum, which encompasses the lateral convexity of the posterior IFG (Broca's region and Broca's analog in the right hemisphere) and the deeply buried opercular part adjacent to the anterior insula.[2] The studies assembled here investigated production or perception of speech and nonspeech at different levels. We structured this heterogeneous bulk of studies by nominating 12 processing domains under which we classified the 56 brain imaging studies. There are a few among this array of studies that provided contrasts for not only one but two domains. All studies assigned to a particular main are listed in one table. We should mention that the studies included in this review considerably differed in terms of the tasks that the volunteers performed.

Tables 14–1 through 14–12 list the particular contrasts that entered the review in that each table represents one particular expressive or perceptive mode. Activation foci reported in Talairach coordinates were converted into the MNI space using the nonlinear algorithm of Brett (2002; http://www.mrc-cbu.cam.ac.uk/Imaging/Common/mnispace.shtml). Each table lists coordinates of fronto-opercular foci for the left and right hemisphere separately. For reasons of intermode comparability we calculated mean values and standard deviations for x, y, and z coordinates.

Figures 14–1 through 14–12 (see color insert) show the averaged spherical distribution of mode-dependent

coordinates superimposed on the normalized single T1-weighted anatomical scan that is implemented in SPM99 (http://www.fil.ion.ucl.ac.uk/spm). Horizontal brain scans are plotted in natural convention, which means the left side of the scan corresponds to the left side of the brain. The center of the sphere corresponds to the mean x, y, and z coordinates (cf. Results section). The radius of the sphere corresponds to the standard deviation of x coordinates. Spheres encompassing left hemisphere coordinates are plotted in white. Spheres encompassing right hemisphere coordinates are plotted in green. We assigned neuroanatomical labels to center of spheres by using the digital version of macroscopic anatomical parcellation of the MNI magnetic resonance imaging single-subject brain (Tzourio-Mazoyer et al., 2002) as implemented in the MRICRO software (http://www.sph.sc.edu/comd/rorden/mricro.html).

We performed a hierarchical cluster analysis for each hemisphere separately based on the Euclidian distance between MNI coordinates to elucidate to what extent single auditory domains might be grouped together (Fig. 14–13).

RESULTS

Phonology

Table 14–1 and Figure 14–1 show an overview of imaging studies that examined "phonological processing." As recently pointed out by Indefrey and Cutler (2004) neuroimaging studies have failed to provide a substantial basis for a dissociation between phonetic and phonological processing. Therefore, we follow their suggestion and use the notion "phonology" as an umbrella term in a loose sense in that we included studies that researched the processing of discrete speech categories (syllables, phonemes, rhymes, consonants, etc.). The current analysis includes 10 neuroimaging studies (6 positron emission tomography, 4 fMRI) that incorporate 17 conditional contrasts yielding 28 activational clusters associated with phonological processing. Of 28 activational clusters, 25 (89%) are localized in the left hemisphere, while 3 of 28 clusters (11%) are situated in the right hemisphere, which speaks of a clear prevalence of the left frontal regions in phonological processing. The mean left hemisphere coordinate "−46 17 20" corresponds to

TABLE 14-1. MNI Coordinates in Neuroimaging Studies of Phonological Speech Processing

Study	Phonological Processing Contrast	Left Hemisphere			Right Hemisphere		
		x	y	z	x	y	z
Zatorre et al. (1992)	Syllable perception—noise	−51	22	13	—	—	—
	Phonetic perception—syllable perception	−48	2	26	—	—	—
Zatorre et al. (1996)	Phonetic discrimination—passive words	−35	20	24	—	—	—
	Phonetic monitoring—passive words	−44	7	30	—	—	—
	Phonetic discrimination—pitch discrimination	−57	5	32	—	—	—
	Phonetic discrimination—noise	−43	4	30	—	—	—
Poldrack et al. (2001)	Rhyme judgment	−48	34	12	—	—	—
		−52	16	0	—	—	—
Burton et al. (2000)	Segmentation in phonological processing	−47	16	27	—	—	—
Demonet et al. (1992)	Sequential phoneme monitoring—tones	−51	18	23	—	—	—
Demonet et al. (1994)	Sequential phoneme monitoring—tones	−40	3	31	—	—	—
	Sequential phoneme monitoring—simple phoneme monitoring	−42	5	31	—	—	—
Fiez et al. (1995)	Phon. target detection	−40	16	10	41	22	6
	Phon. discrimination	−37	16	10	41	22	6
Hsieh et al. (2001)	Consonant discrimination versus passive listening	−54	13	20	—	—	—
		−52	9	28	—	—	—
		−42	38	6	—	—	—
	Vowel discrimination versus passive listening	−44	4	30	—	—	—
		−35	30	17	—	—	—
		−39	38	4	—	—	—
Noesselt et al. (2003)	Indirect phonological processing	−60	20	28	—	—	—
		−48	28	16	—	—	—
		−56	32	24	—	—	—
Golestani and Zatorre (2004)	Phonemes versus noise subtraction	−34	18	5[a]	31	21	5[a]
		−45	19	25[a]	—	—	—
Mean		−46	17	20	38	22	6
Standard deviation		7	11	10	6	1	1

[a]Averaged data.

TABLE 14-2. MNI Coordinates in Neuroimaging Studies of Processing Lexical Tones and Sublexical Intonation

Study	Lexical Tones/ Sublexical Intonation Contrast	Left Hemisphere			Right Hemisphere		
		x	y	z	x	y	z
Gandour et al. (2000)	Lexical tone—pitch	−39	13	20	—	—	—
Gandour et al.(2002)	Lexical tone—pitch	−46	15	41	—	—	—
	Duration nonspeech—passive nonspeech	−44	13	28	49	16	26
Gandour et al. (2003)	Intonation perception	−41	4	39	43	21	35
	Lexical tone perception	−41	4	36	—	—	—
	Intonation versus lexical tone	—	—	—	46	16	36
Hsieh et al. (2001)	Lexical tone versus passive listening	−48	9	28	—	—	—
Mean		−43	10	32	46	18	32
Standard deviation		3	5	8	3	3	6

TABLE 14–3. MNI Coordinates in Neuroimaging Studies of Nonlexical Tone and Pitch Perception

Study	Tone and Pitch Perception — Contrast	Left Hemisphere			Right Hemisphere		
		x	y	z	x	y	z
Klein et al. (2001)	Tone discrimination—silent baseline	−36	18	4	35	20	13
Müller et al. (2001)	Tonal discrimination versus white noise perception	−45	14	24	42	21	14
		−48	−2	36	—	—	—
		−42	2	29	—	—	—
Ackermann et al. (2001)	Hearing trains of click stimuli (high-pass)	−33	15	−3	—	—	—
	Hearing trains of click simuli (low-pass)	—	—	—	42	15	3
Gandour et al. (2003)	Pitch perception versus listening-to-hums	−41	6	34	—	—	—
Pöppel et al. (2004)	FM sweeps—categorial perception	—	—	—	42	−6	−5
Gaab et al. (2003)	Pitch memory versus motor control	−52	6	25	—	—	—
Zatorre et al. (1994)	Pitch memory versus passive melodies	−31	22	10	38	20	7
Zatorre et al. (1992)	Pitch judgment—syllable perception	—	—	—	46	32	12
Mean		−41	10	20	41	17	7
Standard deviation		7	8	14	4	13	7

TABLE 14–4. MNI Coordinates in Neuroimaging Studies of Processing Degraded Speech

Study	Degraded Speech — Contrast	Left Hemisphere			Right Hemisphere		
		x	y	z	x	y	z
Golestani and Zatorre (2004)	Nonnative phonemes versus noise subtraction	−34	16	5	—	—	—
Kotz et al.(2003)	Sentence melody versus normal speech	−32	23	1	31	23	7
Meyer et al. (2002)	Sentence melody versus normal speech	−34	17	9	27	20	4
Meyer et al. (2004)	Sentence melody versus normal speech	−39	13	10	26	16	8
	Sentence melody versus flattened speech	−43	13	9	26	16	8
Wong et al. (2002)	Reversed sentences versus silent baseline	−35	24	1	39	19	3
Plante et al. (2002)	Pure sentence melody	−31	24	8	31	28	4
Davis and Johnsrude (2003)	Disorted speech versus normal speech	−48	14	−6	—	—	—
Giraud et al. (2004)	Temporal complexity (broad–narrow)	−40	20	−10	40	26	−16
Joanisse and Gati (2003)	Nonspeech > speech	−39	−7	1	28	24	8
	Nonspeech > speech	—	—	—	40	7	10
Poldrack et al. (2001)	Compression-related increase	—	—	—	34	26	−4
	Convex compression-related increase	−34	14	20	36	26	8
		−38	34	8	—	—	—
Gelfand and Bookheimer (2003)	Hums > syllables	—	—	—	48	9	31
		—	—	—	46	7	18
Mean		−37	17	5	35	19	7
Standard deviation		5	10	8	7	8	11

TABLE 14–5. MNI Coordinates in Neuroimaging Studies of Processing Speech Complexity

Study	Speech Complexity Contrast	Left Hemisphere			Right Hemisphere		
		x	y	z	x	y	z
Vouloumanos et al. (2001)	Speech versus complex nonspeech	—	—	—	40	24	19
	Speech versus simple tones	—	—	—	48	15	27
		—	—	—	32	24	14
Benson et al. (2001)	Speech complexity	—	—	—	23	19	−5
	Speech × complexity interaction	—	—	—	27	21	1
Mean		—	—	—	34	21	11
Standard deviation		—	—	—	10	4	13

TABLE 14–6. MNI Coordinates in Neuroimaging Studies of Covert and Overt Speech Production

Study	Speech Production Contrast	Left Hemisphere			Right Hemisphere		
		x	y	z	x	y	z
Müller et al. (1997)	Generating sentences versus repetition	−35	21	5	—	—	—
Riecker et al. (2000)	Overt speech versus covert speech	−69	−9	17	66	−4	18
		−35	19	−4	—	—	—
	Covert speech versus overt speech	−66	5	20	—	—	—
Riecker et al. (2002)	Isochronous syllable repetition	−27	18	3	24	18	3
	Rhythmic syllable repetition	−30	18	3	33	20	3
Blank et al. (2002)	Overt speech versus nonspeech perception	−60	10	8	—	—	—
		−36	10	8	—	—	—
Fox et al. (2000)	Syllable production	−43	−13	−21	—	—	—
Ingham et al. (2004)	Stuttering	—	—	—	44	11	3
		—	—	—	36	8	−2
Mean		−45	9	9	41	11	5
Standard deviation		16	12	9	16	10	8

TABLE 14–7. MNI Coordinates in Neuroimaging Studies of Covert and Overt Music Production

Study	Music Production Contrast	Left Hemisphere			Right Hemisphere		
		x	y	z	x	y	z
Perry et al. (1999)	Singing versus complex pitch perception	—	—	—	44	1	11
Riecker et al. (2000)	Overt singing versus covert singing	−69	−9	19	66	−4	20
		—	—	—	32	17	−6
	Covert singing versus overt singing	—	—	—	69	−6	18
Brown et al. (2004)	Monotonic vocalization	−42	25	6	44	8	11
	Melody repetition	−48	6	11	40	14	12
	Harmonization	−42	24	8	40	16	10
		—	—	—	44	10	12
Mean		−50	12	11	47	7	11
Standard deviation		13	17	6	13	9	8

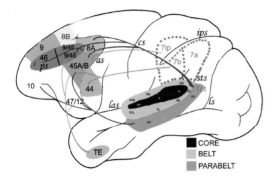

FIGURE 1–1. Diagram indicating some connections between the parietotemporal and the inferior prefrontal areas in the monkey. The auditory region in the superior temporal lobe is subdivided into core, belt, and parabelt regions, and has two main processing streams: the rostral belt and parabelt (the "what" pathway, RTL and RP), which projects to the inferior convexity of the prefrontal lobe; and the caudal belt and parabelt (the "where" pathway, CM, CL, and CP), which projects to more dorsolateral areas. The intraparietal and inferior parietal regions (7ip, 7b) project to the inferior convexity. Numbers indicate Brodmann's areas. Data from Hackett et al. (1998), Romanski et al. (1999a, 1999b), and Petrides and Pandya (2001, 1999). as, arcuate sulcus; cs, central sulcus; ips, intraparietal sulcus; las, lateral sulcus; ls, lunate sulcus; ps, principal sulcus; sts, superior temporal sulcus.

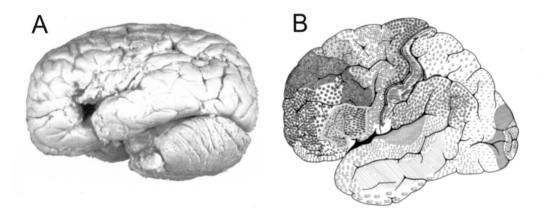

FIGURE 2–1. (A) Lateral view of the brain of Leborgne with lesion in the left frontal lobe. It was the first brain region to which a circumscribed function, overt speech, had been related. This speech region was called Broca's area (or region) and the syndrome that results from its damage was called Broca's aphasia. The lesion included the posterior portion of the left inferior frontal gyrus as seen on the photograph but also parts of subcortical white matter, temporal lobe, and inferior parietal lobe (Signoret et al., 1984). (B) Lateral view of Brodmann' map (1909). Areas 44 and 45 (marked by a bold line) occupy the posterior inferior frontal gyrus and, thus, have been assumed to constitute the microstructural correlates of Broca's region.

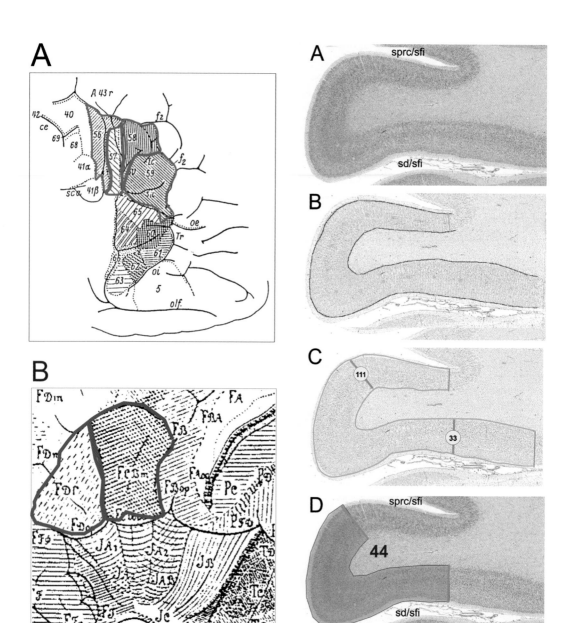

FIGURE 2–2. (A) Adopted cytoarchitectonic maps of an individual brain (right hemisphere) of Riegele (1931; see the historical part of this volume) and (B) von Economo and Koskinas (left hemisphere; 1925). Riegele defined a Broca region comprising areas 56 to 66 as well as 41 (nomenclature of Vogt), corresponding roughly to Brodmann's areas 44, 45, and 47 (1909). Areas 57, 58, and 59 constitute the Pars triangularis (area FDΓ of von Economo and Koskinas), whereas 56 constitutes the Pars opercularis (FCB$_m$ of von Economo and Koskinas). Note the different parcellation schemes of the different authors with respect to Broca's region.

FIGURE 2–3. Algorithm-based definition of areal borders in the inferior frontal cortex of a left hemisphere. (A) Regions of interest are defined in cell body stained histological sections. (B) The GLI (Schleicher and Zilles, 1990) as a measure of the volume fraction of cell bodies is defined, and GLI (grey level index) images are obtained in which each pixel corresponds to a certain value grey value, that is, the *volume* fraction. The cortex is covered by consecutive traverses, reaching from the layer I–layer II border to the cortex–white matter border. Profiles are obtained along these traverses that quantify laminar changes in the GLI. (C) Multivariate statistical analysis is applied in order to define the positions of those profiles (here at positions 111 and 33) at which the shape of the profiles, that is, the cytoarchitecture, changes abruptly. (D) These positions indicate areal borders—in this section, the borders of BA 44. sprc/sfi, junction of the precentral and the inferior frontal sulcus; sd/sfi, junction of the diagonal and the inferior frontal sulcus.

FIGURE 2–4. Cytoarchitectonic dissimilarities between Brodmann's areas (BA) 44, 45, and 6 and areas V1 and V2 for left and right hemispheres. Data are based on the analysis of 10 human postmortem brains. Euclidean distances were calculated as multivariate measures of dissimilarity between profiles of different cortical areas (=interareal differences). They are calculated using features that characterize the shape of the profiles of an area. Multidimensional scaling was applied for visualization of interareal differences and for data reduction to a two-dimensional plane defined by dimension 1 and dimension 2 (Schleicher et al., 2000). The greater the dissimilarity in cytoarchitecture between two areas, the larger is the distance between them in the graph. Although left hemispheric areas 44 and 45 were found to be very similar in cytoarchitecture, both areas differed from area 6 and even more from visual areas V1 and V2. Differences in cytoarchitecture between areas 6 on the one hand and areas 44 and 45 on the other were less pronounced in the right hemisphere. Area 44 seems to take an intermediate position between areas 45 and 6 with respect to its cytoarchitecture, the location in rostrocaudal direction, and in receptorarchitecture (see Fig. 2–5). The two visual areas (V1 and V2) can clearly be distinguished on the basis of their cytoarchitecture from the three frontal ones (6, 44, and 45).

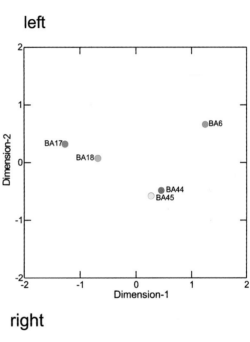

left

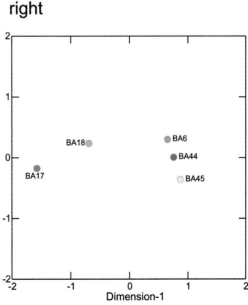

right

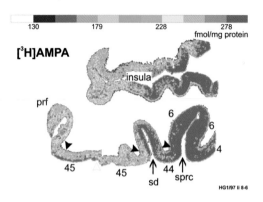

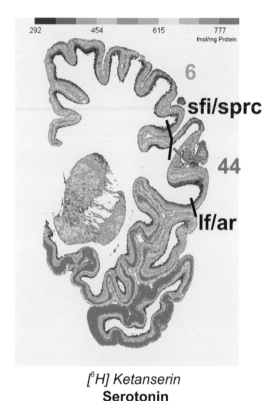

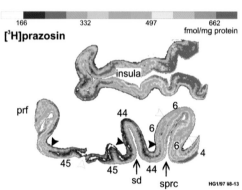

[³H] Ketanserin
Serotonin

FIGURE 2–5. Regional distributions of glutamatergic AMPA and noradrenergic α_1 receptors (demonstrated with [³H]AMPA and [³H]prazosin) in horizontal sections through the human frontal lobe (Amunts, Palomero-Gallagher, and Zilles; unpublished observation). Grey value images were scaled, enhanced in contrast, and color coded (Zilles, 2003). The color scales indicate the total binding in fmol/mg protein. The receptors are heterogeneously distributed and, therefore, allow mapping of cortical areas including 4, 6, 44, and 45 (*arrowheads*). In addition to these cortical areas, subdivisions have been identified on the basis of receptorarchitectonic mapping (*open arrowheads*). Borders obtained by receptor architectonic mapping were compared with borders revealed by cytoarchitectonic mapping. Note the decrease in receptor density from caudal to rostral positions. The different architectonic techniques supplement each other and are the basis of multimodal architectonic mapping. sprc, precentral sulcus; sd, diagonal sulcus; prf, prefrontal cortex (*arrows*).

FIGURE 2–6. Regional distributions of serotonergic 5-HT$_2$ receptors (demonstrated with [³H]ketanserin) in a coronal section through the human frontal lobe (Amunts, Palomero-Gallagher, and Zilles; unpublished observation). Designation of areas as in Figure 2–5. lf/ar, ascending branch of the lateral fissure. sfi, inferior frontal sulcus.

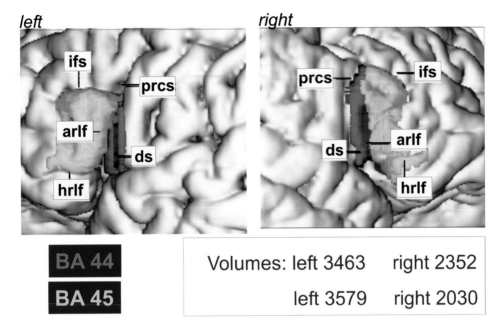

BA 44

BA 45

Volumes: left 3463 right 2352

left 3579 right 2030

FIGURE 2–7. Surface rendering of Brodmann's area (BA) 44 (red) and BA 45 (yellow) in a postmortem brain of the left and the right hemispheres based on cell body stained histological sections and observer-independent definition of cytoarchitectonic borders in serial histological sections (Amunts et al., 1999). The volumes (in mm^3) of the areas have been calculated using Cavalieri's principle. Note that the different extents of the areas on the free surface do not reflect their volumes. For example, BA 45 occupies a considerably larger portion of the free surface than BA 44, but the volumes show very similar values. In addition, BA 44 seems to be slightly larger on the right side as judged by its extent on the free surface, but the volume is greater on the left side by a factor of 1.5. arlf, ascending branch of the lateral fissure; ds, diagonal sulcus; hrlf, horizontal branch of the lateral fissure; ifs, inferior frontal sulcus; prcs, precentral sulcus.

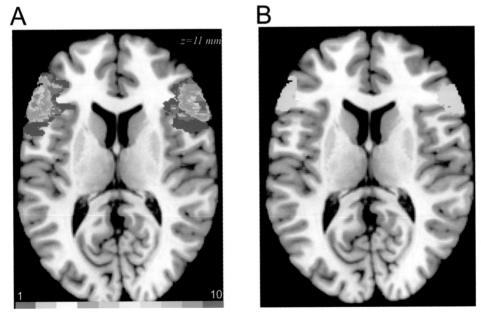

FIGURE 2–8. Probabilistic map of Brodmann's area 45 in standard stereotaxic space (T1-weighted single-subject brain of the MNI; Evans et al., 1993). (A) Complete probabilistic map showing the frequency with which Brodmann's area 45 was present in a particular voxel of the standard reference space. Frequencies are color-coded, whereby red means maximal overlap of all 10 brains, dark orange corresponds to an overlap of 9 brains, etc. (B) 50% map of the area. All of the voxels are part of the 50% map that overlapped in at least 5 of 10 brains.

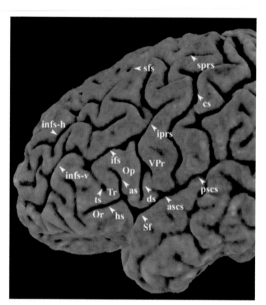

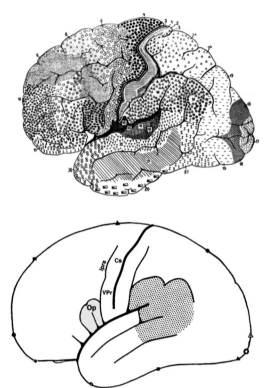

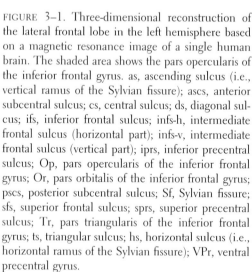

FIGURE 3–1. Three-dimensional reconstruction of
the lateral frontal lobe in the left hemisphere based
on a magnetic resonance image of a single human
brain. The shaded area shows the pars opercularis of
the inferior frontal gyrus. as, ascending sulcus (i.e.,
vertical ramus of the Sylvian fissure); ascs, anterior
subcentral sulcus; cs, central sulcus; ds, diagonal sulcus; ifs, inferior frontal sulcus; infs-h, intermediate
frontal sulcus (horizontal part); infs-v, intermediate
frontal sulcus (vertical part); iprs, inferior precentral
sulcus; Op, pars opercularis of the inferior frontal
gyrus; Or, pars orbitalis of the inferior frontal gyrus;
pscs, posterior subcentral sulcus; Sf, Sylvian fissure;
sfs, superior frontal sulcus; sprs, superior precentral
sulcus; Tr, pars triangularis of the inferior frontal
gyrus; ts, triangular sulcus; hs, horizontal sulcus (i.e.,
horizontal ramus of the Sylvian fissure); VPr, ventral
precentral gyrus.

FIGURE 3–2. (*Top*) Cytoarchitectonic map of Brodmann (1909) with the pars opercularis (area 44)
marked in yellow. (*Bottom*) Summary of electrical
stimulation studies causing aphasic arrest of speech
(adapted from Rasmussen and Milner, 1975). In the
lateral frontal cortex, aphasic arrest of speech is obtained from stimulation of the pars opercularis
(marked in yellow). Cs, central sulcus; Iprs, inferior
precentral sulcus; Op, pars opercularis of the inferior
frontal gyrus; VPr, ventral precentral gyrus.

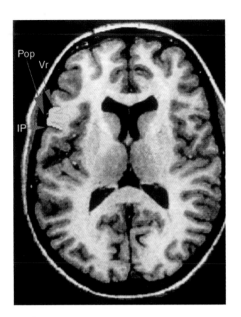
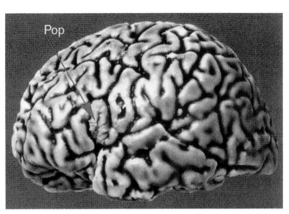

FIGURE 3–3. Three-dimensional reconstruction of the lateral surface of the left hemisphere based on a magnetic resonance image of a single human brain (*right*). A horizontal section through the pars opercularis is shown (*left*). The pars opercularis of the inferior frontal gyrus (Pop) is marked in yellow. Note that it is formed by two vertically oriented convolutions separated by the diagonal sulcus. IP, inferior precentral sulcus; Pop, pars opercularis of the inferior frontal gyrus; Vr, vertical ramus (ascending sulcus) of the Sylvian fissure.

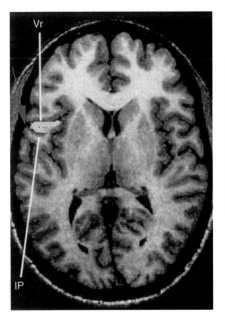
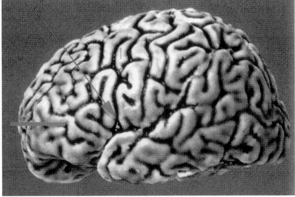

FIGURE 3–4. Three-dimensional reconstruction of the lateral surface of the left hemisphere based on a magnetic resonance image of a single human brain (*right*). A horizontal section taken at the level marked by the blue line is shown (*left*). The pars opercularis of the inferior frontal gyrus is marked in yellow. Note that it is mostly hidden within the inferior precentral sulcus. IP, inferior precentral sulcus; vr, vertical ramus (ascending sulcus) of the Sylvian fissure.

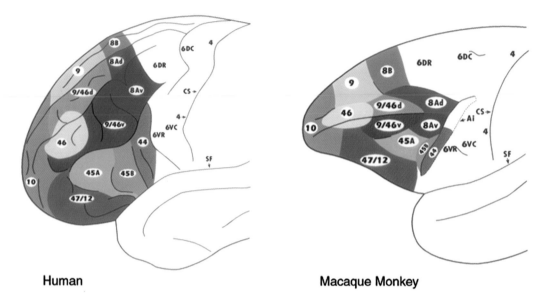

Human   **Macaque Monkey**

FIGURE 3–6. Comparative cytoarchitectonic maps of the lateral frontal lobe of the human and the macaque monkey brain by Petrides and Pandya (1994). Ai, inferior ramus of the arcuate sulcus; CS, central sulcus; SF, Sylvian fissure.

FIGURE 3–8 (see insert for enlarged Figure 3–8).Photomicrographs of cortical areas 6VR, 44, and 45 of the macaque monkey frontal lobe. The axial section perpendicular to the direction of the inferior ramus of the arcuate sulcus shows the location of the photomicrographs. Area 6VR is the anterior part of the ventral agranular premotor cortex and lacks layer IV. This area lies along the inferior ramus of the arcuate sulcus and continues for a variable distance within the upper part of the posterior bank of the sulcus. The dysgranular area 44 succeeds area 6VR within the caudal bank of the inferior ramus of the arcuate sulcus and continues within the fundus of the sulcus. Granular area 45 replaces area 44 at the lower part of the anterior bank of the inferior ramus of the arcuate sulcus. The Roman numerals indicate the cortical layers. Note the absence of layer IV in area 6VR (agranular), the emergence of a layer IV in area 44 (dysgranular), and the well-developed layer IV in area 45 (granular). Note also that in area 45 the granular layer IV happens to be inclined downward at this particular part of the section. Ai, inferior ramus of the arcuate sulcus; Ipd, infraprincipalis dimple. Directions: C, caudal; L, lateral; M, medial; R, rostral. The horizontal calibration bar placed in layer I in the photomicrograph of area 45 is 200 μm, and the calibration bar in the lower left side of the axial section indicates 1 mm.

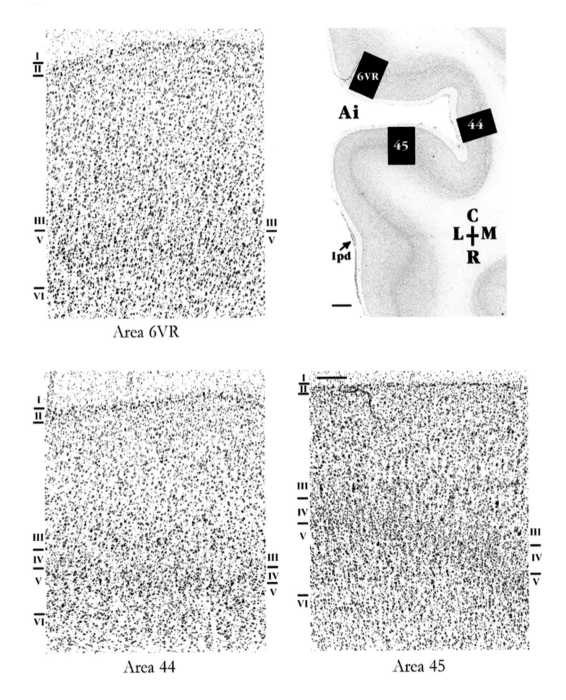

Area 6VR

Area 44

Area 45

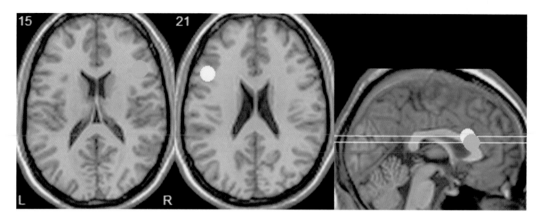

FIGURE 14–1. Sublexical phonological perception of speech.

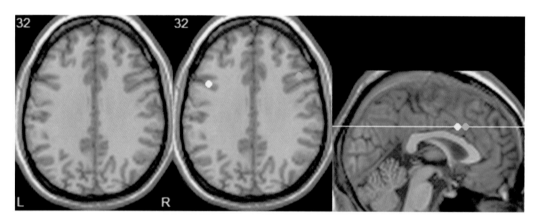

FIGURE 14–2. Perception of lexical tones and sublexical intonation.

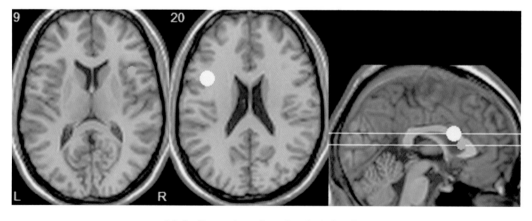

FIGURE 14–3. Perception of tonal and pitch information.

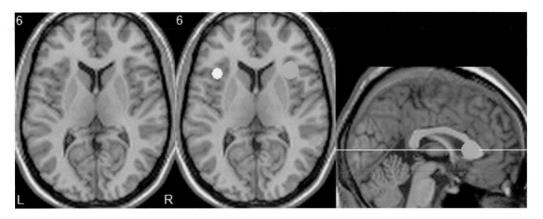

FIGURE 14–4. Perception of degraded speech.

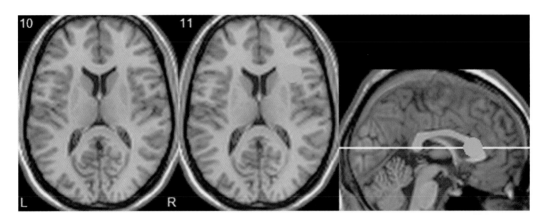

FIGURE 14–5. Perception of speech complexity.

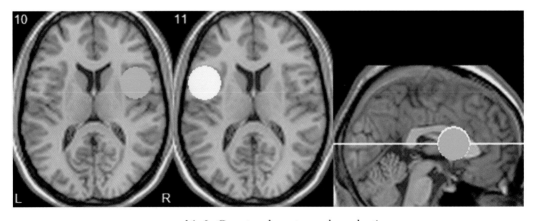

FIGURE 14–6. Covert and overt speech production.

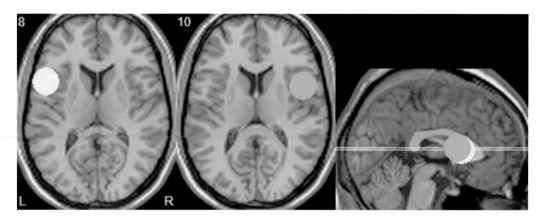

FIGURE 14–7. Covert and overt music production.

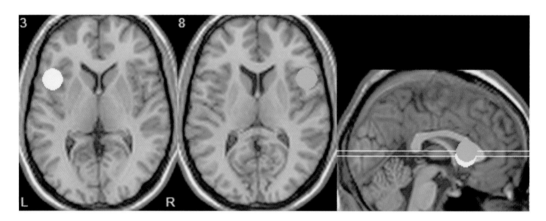

FIGURE 14–8. Perception of music.

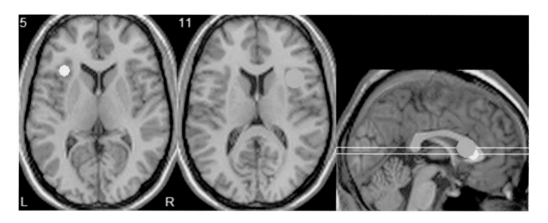

FIGURE 14–9. Perception of sounds.

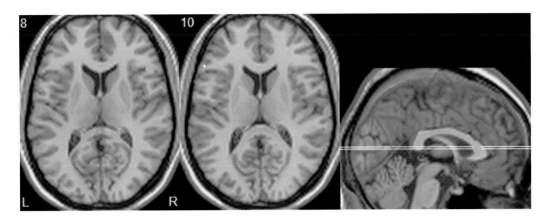

FIGURE 14–10. Perception of affective prosody.

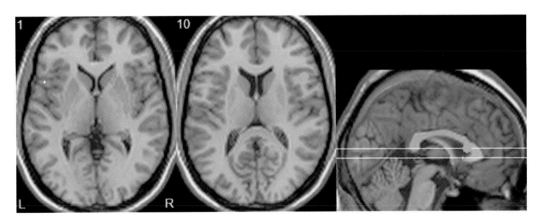

FIGURE 14–11. Perception of auditory deviants in a train of tonal stimuli.

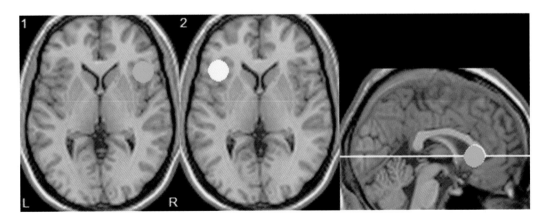

FIGURE 14–12. Dichotic listening.

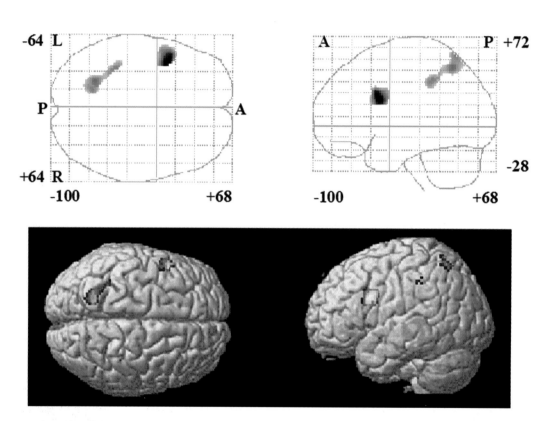

FIGURE 16–2. Main effect of task (EFT versus CT) as reported by Manjaly et al. (2003), random effects analysis (16 subjects). All activations from the EFT versus CT contrast (masked inclusively by the CT versus baseline contrast), significant at a cluster-level corrected threshold of $P < 0.05$, are shown. *Top row:* Maximum intensity projections (glass brains). A, anterior; P, posterior; L, left; R, right. *Bottom row:* Activations overlaid on a rendered template brain.

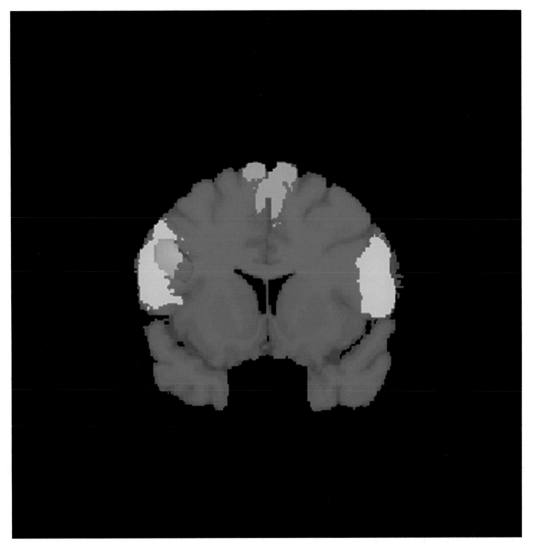

FIGURE 16–3. Overlay of the functional activation of pIFG during EFT (red) with a cytoarchitectonically defined probability map of Brodmann area 44 (light gray).

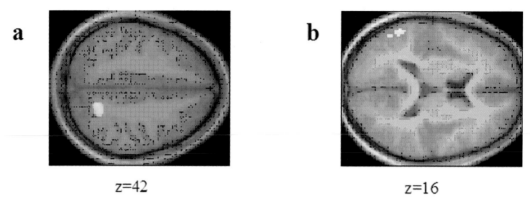

a

z=42

b

z=16

FIGURE 16–5. Results of the PPI analysis for left IPS, random effects analysis (16 subjects). As in Figures 16–2 through 16–4, results are shown at a cluster-level threshold of $P < 0.05$, corrected for multiple comparisons across the whole brain (voxel-level threshold of $P < 0.001$). (*a*) The only area to receive an increased contribution from left IPS during EFT compared with the control task was the right posterior parietal cortex (18, −62, 42; $t_{max} = 6.69$; $P < 0.001$). (*b*) Similar to the PPI results for the left pIFG (compare with Fig. 16–4), the left temporoparietal cortex (−58, −50, 16; $t_{max} = 4.57$; $P < 0.001$) was found to receive a decreased contribution from the left IPS during EFT relative to the control task.

TABLE 14–8. MNI Coordinates in Neuroimaging Studies of Musical Perception

Study	Music Perception Contrast	Left Hemisphere x	y	z	Right Hemisphere x	y	z
Janata et al. (2002)	Music perception	—	—	—	56	19	5
		—	—	—	60	22	20
Tillmann et al. (2003b)	Dissonant—consonant	—	—	—	45	−4	15
	Unrelated consonant—related consonant	−52	8	0	49	15	0
		−38	19	5	34	22	0
Mean		−45	14	3	49	15	8
Standard deviation		10	8	4	10	11	9

TABLE 14–9. MNI Coordinates in Neuroimaging Studies of Sound Perception Production

Study	Sounds Contrast	Left Hemisphere x	y	z	Right Hemisphere x	y	z
Engelien et al. (1995)	Environmental sound perception versus rest	—	—	—	34	26	14
	Environmental sound categorization versus rest	—	—	—	24	19	−8
		−42	20	18	—	—	—
Maeder et al. (2001)	Sound recognition > sound localization	—	—	—	36	−14	21
	Sound localization > sound recognition	−28	17	−6	—	—	—
Alain et al. (2001)	Sound recognition > sound localization	—	—	—	45	25	12
		—	—	—	52	18	14
Mean		−35	19	6	39	15	11
Standard deviation		10	2	17	11	16	11

TABLE 14–10. MNI Coordinates in Neuroimaging Studies of Processing Affective Prosody

Study	Affective Prosody Contrast	Left Hemisphere x	y	z	Right Hemisphere x	y	z
Buchanan et al. (2000)	Emotion versus verbal	—	—	—	44	20	16
Kotz et al. (2003)	Positive > neutral	−51	13	2	53	13	5
		−54	19	5	44	21	15
	Negative > neutral	−44	21	15	—	—	—
		−53	21	4	—	—	—
Mean		−51	19	7	47	18	12
Standard deviation		5	4	6	5	4	6

TABLE 14–11. MNI Coordinates in Neuroimaging Studies of Mismatch Responses Obtained from Auditory Oddball Paradigms

	Mismatch Response	Left Hemisphere			Right Hemisphere		
Study	Contrast	x	y	z	x	y	z
Opitz et al. (2002)	Mismatch response (medium deviant versus standard)	—	—	—	46	20	8
Doeller et al. (2003)	Mismatch response (small deviant versus medium deviant)	—	—	—	54	24	6
	Mismatch response (large deviant versus medium deviant)	−54	26	8	50	24	6
Mean		−54	26	8	50	23	7
Standard deviation		—	—	—	4	2	1

the rostrodorsal part of the lateral pars opercularis. The mean right hemisphere coordinate "38 22 6" matches the anterior insula.

Lexical Tones/Sublexical Intonation

Table 14–2 and Figure 14–2 depict an overview of imaging studies that examined two related processing domains that play a cardinal role in "prosodic processing." As comprehensively described by Gandour and colleagues (2000, 2002, 2003), native speakers of tonal languages (like Chinese and Thai) are more amenable to pick up pitch contours that span shorter temporal integration windows since these fine-grained acoustic cues help decode the lexical meaning of a spoken word. In contrast, speakers of intonational lan-

TABLE 14–12. MNI Coordinates in Neuroimaging Studies of Dichotic Listening

	Dichotic Listening	Left Hemisphere			Right Hemisphere		
Study	Contrast	x	y	z	x	y	z
Jäncke et al. (2003)	Dichotic tone listening > rest	—	—	—	48	12	20
		—	—	—	44	16	−8
	Divided > focussed attention	−36	24	−4	—	—	—
Jäncke and Shah (2002)	Divided > binaural	−60	12	8	56	24	−16
		−44	24	−8	—	—	—
	FL > binaural	—	—	—	48	28	8
	FR > binaural	−48	28	8	—	—	—
Jäncke et al. (2001)	Dichotic versus rest	−56	16	12	51	17	16
Pollmann et al. (2004)	CV-syllable (left ear) versus null event	−43	13	20	—	—	—
Hugdahl et al. (1999)	CV versus tones (dichotic)	−38	24	4	32	22	2
Hugdahl et al. (2000)	CV versus music (dichotic divided)	−53	19	3[a]	—	—	—
	FL versus FR	—	—	—	62	16	4
Thomsen et al. (2004b)	FL	−32	22	−5	32	23	−5
		—	—	—	48	13	21
		−40	32	9	—	—	—
Thomsen et al. (2004a)	Dichotic versus binaural	−30	25	−5	32	25	−8
	Divided versus forced	−34	19	−9	36	23	−13
	FR versus FR binaural	−30	25	−5	32	25	−6
	FL versus FL binaural	−30	25	−6	34	25	−6
Mean		−41	22	2	43	21	1
Standard deviation		10	6	9	10	5	12

[a]Averaged data.

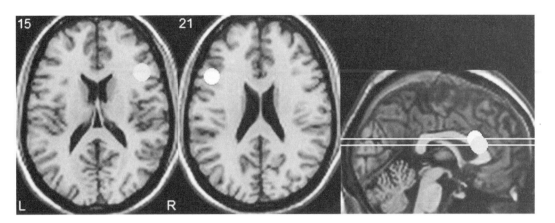

FIGURE 14–1. Sublexical phonological perception of speech.

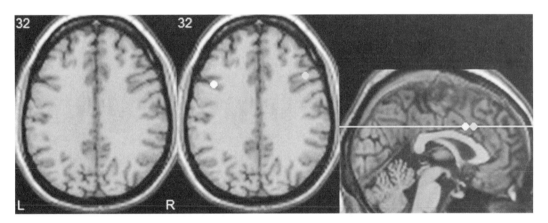

FIGURE 14–2. Perception of lexical tones and sublexical intonation.

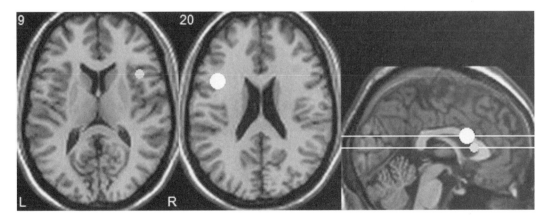

FIGURE 14–3. Perception of tonal and pitch information.

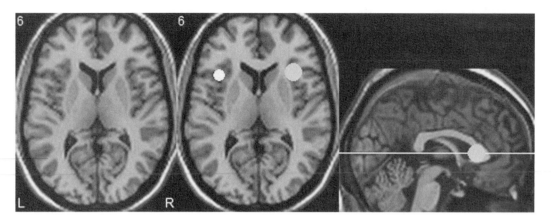

FIGURE 14–4. Perception of degraded speech.

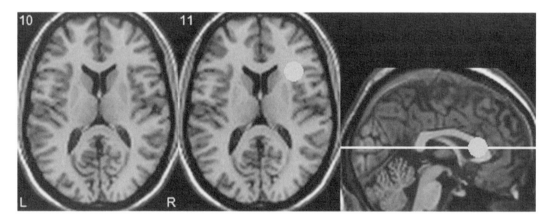

FIGURE 14–5. Perception of speech complexity.

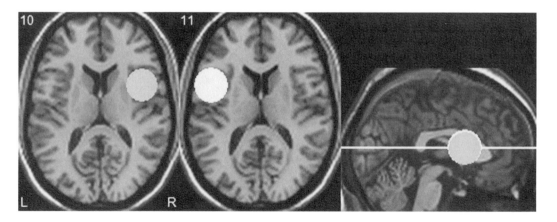

FIGURE 14–6. Covert and overt speech production.

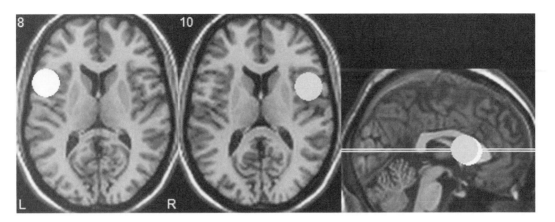

FIGURE 14–7. Covert and overt music production.

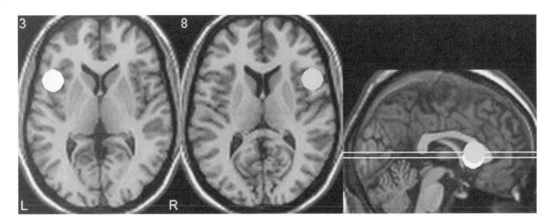

FIGURE 14–8. Perception of music.

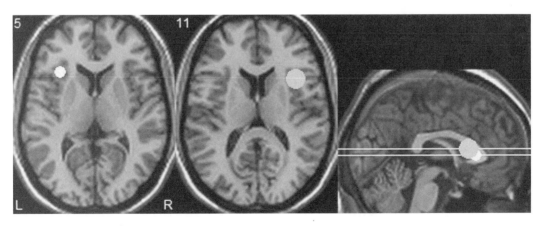

FIGURE 14–9. Perception of sounds.

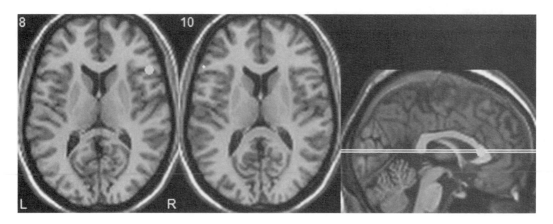

FIGURE 14–10. Perception of affective prosody.

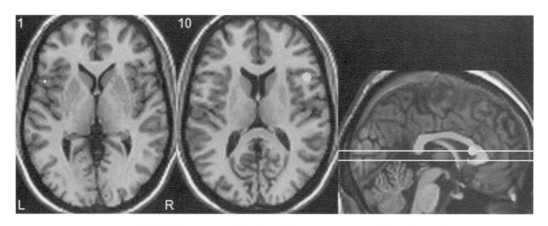

FIGURE 14–11. Perception of auditory deviants in a train of tonal stimuli.

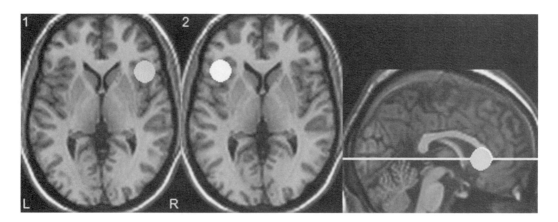

FIGURE 14–12. Dichotic listening.

Dendogram Left Hemisphere

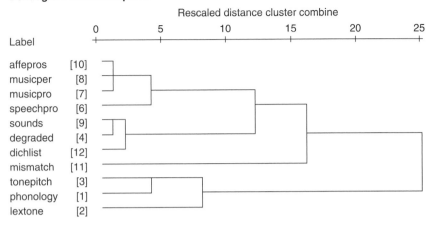

Dendogram Right Hemisphere

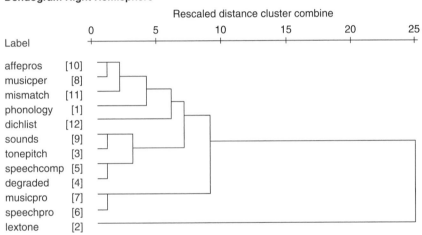

FIGURE 14–13. Results of hierarchical cluster analysis based on Euclidian distance. (*Top*) The extent to which auditory domains cluster in the left hemisphere (LH). (*Bottom*) The extent to which auditory domains cluster in the right hemisphere (RH). Short code labels correspond to single auditory domains listed in Tables 1 through 12. Numbers in parentheses refer to the numbering of Tables 1 through 12. There is no LH cluster for speech complexity which results in uneven number of domains for LH (n = 11) and RH (n = 12).

guages (like English or German) are more sensitive to slow prosodic modulations that may convey linguistically relevant information, i.e. sentence modus. The current analysis includes four neuroimaging studies (two positron emission tomography, two fMRI) that incorporate seven conditional contrasts yielding nine activational clusters associated with either processing of lexical tones or sublexical intonation. Of nine activational clusters, six (67%) are localized in the left hemisphere, while three out of nine clusters (33%) are situated in the right hemisphere. The mean left hemisphere coordinate "−43 10 32" corresponds to the ventral border of the precentral gyrus adjoining the dorsal part of the pars opercularis. The mean right hemisphere coordinate "46 18 32" can be precisely localized in the pars opercularis. Four of seven contrasts were derived from analyses testing the processing of lexical tones and exclusively revealed activational increases in the left hemisphere. The remaining three contrasts focused on perception of intonational cues and exposed bilateral and rightward activity patterns.

Tone and Pitch Perception

Table 14–3 and Figure 14–3 sketch an overview of imaging studies focusing primarily on basic auditory functions which are supposed to be essential in speech and musical processing (Zatorre et al., 2002). The current analysis comprises eight neuroimaging studies (four positron emission tomography, four fMRI) that incorporate nine conditional contrasts yielding 14 activational clusters associated with either processing of tonal and pitch information. Of 14 activational clusters, 8 (57%) are localized in the left hemisphere while 6 of 14 clusters (43%) are situated in the right hemisphere. Both the mean left hemisphere coordinate "−41 10 20" and the mean right hemisphere coordinate "41 17 7" correspond to the dorsomedial part of the pars opercularis with the latter being close to the insular cortex. Based on this analysis, it appears that neither the left nor the right frontal operculum displays a dominating preference for tone and pitch perception in a nonlinguistic context.

Degraded Speech

Table 14–4 and Figure 14–4 compile a number of imaging studies that triggered frontal operculum activity by exposing participants to speech that had been artificially or naturally manipulated. More specifically, intelligibility was reduced or even canceled out by applying filtering techniques that (partly) removed segmental information or recorded human humming was presented which also lacked any segmentable linguistic information. The current analysis is made up of 11 neuroimaging studies (1 positron emission tomography, 10 fMRI) that comprise 14 conditional contrasts resulting in 25 activational clusters that supported the processing of unintelligible speech. Precisely, 12 of 25 activational clusters (48%) are localized in the left hemisphere and 13 of 25 clusters (52%) are identified in the right hemisphere. Both the mean left hemisphere coordinate "−37 17 5" and the mean right hemisphere coordinate "35 19 7" correspond to the anterior portion of the insular cortex bordering the medial wall of the Rolandic operculum. Based on this analysis, it seems plausible that processing a degraded acousticc percept like unintelligible speech necessi-

tates both the left and right intra-Sylvian regions. Notably, the mean left and right hemisphere coordinates are outside the frontal operculum and refer to a locus in the phylogenetically distinct anterior insula.

Speech Complexity

Table 14–5 and Figure 14–5 list two fMRI studies that identified the neural substrates underlying speech complexity. Benson and co-workers (2001) used multivariate multiple regression of fMRI responses to stimuli that systematically contrasted along speech/nonspeech, acoustic, or phonetic complexity and natural/synthetic dimensions. In an oddball detection task, Vouloumanos and colleagues (2001) contrasted speech with nonspeech analogues that were matched along key temporal and spectral dimensions. The two studies provide four conditional contrasts yielding five activational clusters corresponding to the processing of speech complexity. Notably, all clusters were consistently localized in the right hemisphere. The mean right hemisphere coordinate "34 21 11" refers to the most anterior tip of the right insular cortex directly adjacent to the deeply buried compartment of the frontal operculum. The analysis suggests that the processing of speech complexity preferentially drives the right hemisphere.

Speech Production

Table 14–6 and Figure 14–6 summarize imaging studies that examined overt and covert speech production and stuttering. The current analysis comprises six neuroimaging studies (four positron emission tomography, two fMRI) that include eight conditional contrasts yielding 14 activational clusters generated by a variety of speech production tasks. Of 14 activational clusters, 9 (65%) are localized in the left hemisphere, while 5 of 14 clusters (35%) are situated in the right hemisphere. The mean left hemisphere coordinate "−45 9 9" is medially situated near the border between the caudal part of the pars opercularis and the rostral part of the Rolandic operculum. The mean right hemisphere coordinate "41 11 5" refers to a voxel in the insular cortex in the vicinity of the medial wall of the pars opercularis and the Rolandic operculum. However, standard deviations for these samples are relatively large, so that the picture drawn by this analysis may be inconclusive. Large differences between expressive modes, i.e., overt versus covert production, simple repetition versus sentence generation, may account for these inconsistencies. Even though two thirds of the contrasts point to an involvement of the left hemisphere fronto-opercular cortex in expressive functions, at least one third of contrasts indicate an engagement of the right intra-Sylvian cortex, in particular, when the neural underpinnings of stuttering are imaged.

Music Production

Table 14–7 and Figure 14–7 depict an overview of imaging studies that addressed the role the frontal operculum plays in music production. The present analysis includes three neuroimaging studies (two positron emission tomography, one fMRI) that comprise six conditional contrasts resulting in 12 activational clusters associated with either overt or covert singing. Of 12 activational clusters, 4 (33%) are localized in the left hemisphere, while 8 of 12 clusters (67%) are situated in the right hemisphere. The mean left hemisphere coordinate "−50 12 11" corresponds to the ventral part of the pars opercularis. The mean right hemisphere coordinate "47 7 11" could be localized at the junction of the Rolandic operculum, the pars opercularis, and the insular cortex. Interestingly, the right mean coordinate observed for music production is almost identical to the right mean coordinate observed for speech production. The two modes additionally share relatively large standard deviation scores, which belies the considerable variance between contrasts entered in this analysis. In sum, the analysis implies that music production accompanies an activational rightward asymmetry in the intra-Sylvian cortex. Furthermore, it is reasoned that this particular area can be considered to play a fundamental role in both speech and music production.

Music Perception

Table 14–8 and Figure 14–8 present two fMRI studies that image the frontal operculum while participants heard musical melodies. The review on music perception comprises three conditional contrasts resulting in seven activational clusters that accompany the perception of music. Of seven activational clusters, two (29%) are localized in the left hemisphere and five of seven clusters (61%) are identified in the

right hemisphere. Both the mean left hemisphere coordinate "−45 14 3" and the mean right hemisphere coordinate "49 15 8" correspond to the ventromedial strip of the pars opercularis, with the first bordering the insular cortex. Even though Tillmann and colleagues (2003a) observed clusters in the left frontal cortex, this analysis implicates a general right frontal superiority in music perception. The specific demands imposed by the task in the study by Tillmann and colleagues apparently addressed aspects of sequence expectancies that may account for the recruitment of Broca's region.

Sounds

Table 14–9 and Figure 14–9 show an overview of three imaging studies (one positron emission tomography, two fMRI) that examined sound processing and incorporates five conditional contrasts yielding seven activational clusters associated with sound processing. Of seven activational clusters, two (29%) are localized in the left hemisphere and five of seven clusters (61%) are identified in the right hemisphere, which displays a clear prevalence of the right frontal regions in sound processing. Both the mean left hemisphere coordinate "−35 19 6" and the mean right hemisphere coordinate "39 15 11" correspond to the anterior insula with the latter adjoining to the medial wall of the pars opercularis. Notably, tasks that explicitly focused on sound recognition activated the right frontal cortex, while sound localization and categorization excited the left frontal cortex.

Affective Prosody

Table 14–10 and Figure 14–10 depict an overview of two fMRI studies that addressed the role the frontal operculum plays in affective prosody. This analysis comprises three conditional contrasts resulting in seven activational clusters associated with processing affective spoken utterances. Of seven activational clusters, four (57%) are localized in the left hemisphere while three of seven clusters (43%) are situated in the right hemisphere. The left hemisphere coordinate "−51 19 7" corresponds to the most posterior part of the pars triangularis. The mean right hemisphere coordinate "47 18 12" could also be localized in the lateral pars opercularis close to the small ascending branch of the anterior segment of the Sylvian fissure.

Mismatch Response

Table 14–11 and Figure 14–11 compile two fMRI studies that elicited frontal operculum activity during participant's performance of a preattentive auditory oddball task. More specifically, volunteers heard continuous trains of identical tones that comprised a small proportion of deviant tones differing in acoustic parameters (e.g., intensity, frequency). The current analysis contains three conditional contrasts resulting in four activational clusters more strongly activated by deviant relative to standard tones. Of four activational clusters, one (25%) is localized in the left hemisphere and three of four clusters (75%) are identified in the right hemisphere. Both the mean left hemisphere coordinate "−54 26 8" and the mean right hemisphere coordinate "50 23 7" correspond to the triangular part of the IFG. Based on this analysis, it seems plausible that the right IFG more prevalently subserves the neurofunctional mechanism underlying deviancy detection.

Dichotic Listening

Table 14–12 and Figure 14–12 show evidence from eight studies (two positron emission tomography, six fMRI) that induces activity within the frontal operculum while participants performed a dichotic listening test. This analysis comprises 15 conditional contrasts resulting in 27 activational clusters. Of 27 activational clusters, 14 (52%) are localized in the left hemisphere and 13 of 27 clusters (48%) are identified in the right hemisphere. Both the mean left hemisphere coordinate "−41 22 2" and the mean right hemisphere coordinate "43 21 1" correspond to the ventromedial strip of the pars triangularis bordering the anterior insular cortex. In the context of this overview, it is evident that lateralization of activational cluster varies as a function of monaural and binaural presentation.

Cluster Analysis

Figure 14–13 presents the results of hierarchical cluster analysis based on the Euclidian distance between MNI coordinates, implicating a differential pattern in the left relative to the right hemisphere. In the left hemisphere, we identify three clusters that include up to four functional domains. The first cluster (mean "−48 14 8", ventral part of pars opercularis) subsumes "affective prosody," "music perception," "music pro-

duction," and "speech production." The second cluster (mean "−38 19 4", anterior insula) groups "sounds," "degraded speech," and "dichotic listening." The third cluster (mean "−43 12 24", dorsal part of pars opercularis) includes "tone and pitch perception," "phonology," and "lexical tones/sublexical intonation." The domain "mismatch response" reveals a large distance to the other clusters. A different picture can be drawn for the right hemisphere. The analysis yields four clusters showing "close" distances. Analogous to the left hemisphere the first cluster (mean "49 19 9", anterior ventral part of pars opercularis) subsumes "affective prosody," "music perception," and in moderate distance "mismatch response." Also similar to the left hemisphere, a second cluster (mean "44 9 8", border zone between pars opercularis, insula, and Rolandic operculum) configures "music production" and "speech production." A third cluster (mean "40 16 9", junction at pars opercularis and anterior insula) groups "sounds" and "tone and pitch perception." A fourth cluster (mean "35 20 9", anterior insula) includes "speech complexity" and "degraded speech." According to the analysis, the latter cluster is in a close distance to the third cluster, while both the third and the fourth cluster are remotely distant from the first and the second cluster. "Phonology," "dichotic listening," and "lexical tones/sublexical intonation" reveal a large distance to the other clusters.

DISCUSSION

A comprehensive discussion of all studies or contrasts we have included is beyond the potentialities of this review. We therefore concentrate on the discussion of clustered domains and attempt to illustrate the commonalities between them. Generally, the results obtained from this review demonstrate that a multitude of heterogeneous tasks and processes illuminate the role of the frontal operculum in both the left and the right hemisphere with the first primarily involved in phonological processing and the latter preferentially driven by paralinguistic and nonlinguistic domains, i.e., speech complexity, music perception and production, and sound perception. We discuss results for left and right hemisphere separately in turn.

Interestingly, the mean coordinates for "phonology" are located in the most dorsal part of the pars opercularis, while all other spots we subsumed are situated in more ventral parts of the pars opercularis. In the left hemisphere, "phonology" clusters with "tone and pitch perception" and "lexical tones." It holds in particular for the latter domain that linguistically relevant stimuli were tested. The majority of phonological contrasts reviewed here and the perception of pitch contours associated with lexical tones have in common that rapidly changing acoustic cues play a decisive role. Therefore, it is possible that the dorsal part of the left pars opercularis belongs to the neural circuit that contributes to the processing of rapidly changing acoustic information. The second cluster integrates domains that particularly deal with musical and intonational information. One might note that both music and affective prosody comprise emotional information. However, this does not hold for the kind of speech investigated in the speech production paradigms reviewed here. Therefore, it is more likely to assume that more general aspects involved in expressive and receptive functions related to (speech) melody account for this observation. Both perception of sounds and degraded speech activated the anterior insula. Like sounds, degraded speech does not comprise any lexical information but only speech melody. In the studies we reviewed, volunteers had to either recognize, categorize, or localize sounds, which is a demanding task. This assertion also holds for the perception of degraded speech and addresses our introductory reasoning on the potential functional role of this area as a provider of extracomputational resources. We will get back to this issue later. Even though the cluster analysis grouped "dichotic listening" together with sounds and degraded speech, we believe that we should consider the latter as not being part of former duo as the spot corresponding to dichotic listening seems to be located in the pars triangularis.

Traditionally, the right hemisphere has been considered to be more amenable to musical processing (Zatorre et al., 2002) even though more recent views indicate that particular acoustic features, that is, slowly changing acoustic cues, account for the right hemisphere preference for music and melodic contours rather than music per se. Our review cannot fully corroborate this view as music perception was found to activate both left and right hemisphere sites. Analogous to the left hemisphere, "affective prosody" and "music perception" clustered closely together in the ventral pars opercularis in the vicinity of the "mismatch response." Based on this finding we are not

able to detect any commonality between these functions. At least this finding speaks to a general responsiveness of the right pars opercularis to auditory stimuli. Also similar to the left hemisphere is the finding that mean coordinates for "speech production" and "music production" are nearby. However, in the right hemisphere, this duo is situated in the Rolandic operculum, which corresponds to the ventral premotor cortex. Since this brain region represents supralaryngeal articulators (lips, tongue), which play a role in (sub)articulation (Kolb and Whishaw, 1995), its engagement in speech and music production is compelling. Obviously both speaking and singing consistently recruit the right Rolandic operculum. Interestingly, two recent fMRI studies that investigated the perception of intonation contour in sentences also observed an engagement of the right Rolandic operculum, which makes this region a candidate for functions of auditory-motor integration (Meyer et al., 2002, 2004). There are two additional clusters in the right hemisphere. The first spot is situated more deeply in the medial part of the pars opercularis close to the anterior insula (recognition and perception of sounds as well as perception of simple tones and pitch). The second spot can be directly localized in the anterior insula ("degraded speech" and "speech complexity"). Considering the variance between methods, experiments, subjects, etc. across all reviewed studies, we do not think it is beneficial to discuss a difference between these two clusters. We rather state that the right (and partly left) deep frontal operculum and the anterior insula are part of the neural network processing multiple elementary aspects provided by auditory stimuli. Neuroanatomically the anterior insula cannot be considered part of the frontal operculum. The anterior insula has been attributed to a variety of vascular, vestibular, olfactory, gustatory, visual, somatosensory, motor, and even auditory modulation (Bamiou et al., 2003; Flynn et al., 1999; Türe et al., 1999; Wise et al., 1999). Due to the poor spatial resolution of positron emission tomography and fMRI studies, it is hard to decide to what extent an activational cluster covering both the anterior insula and the deep frontal operculum originates from the first or the latter (or even from both the first and the latter). Little is known about the cytoarchitectonic structure of the deep portion of the frontal operculum so far. Thus, the precise border between the most anterior tip of the anterior insula and the deep frontal operculum cannot be exactly determined, which leaves researchers insecure about the origin and potential functional implication of activational clusters situated in this brain region. Notably, activity in the "borderland" between (left and right) anterior insula and the deep frontal operculum has primarily been reported by brain imaging studies that examined the perception of degraded auditory percepts (Davis and Johnsrude, 2003; Giraud et al., 2004; Meyer et al., 2004; Plante et al., 2002; Wong et al., 2002). One recent statement that attempts to provide an interpretation proposes that bilateral activity in this region during the perception of degraded speech might reflect the effort to achieve a meaningful segmentation of the inflowing auditory input (Meyer et al., 2003). This view is affirmed by results obtained from a positron emission tomography study that demonstrated a bilateral activational increase in the deeply buried frontopercular cortex reflecting an increase in processing effort while participants performed a demanding pitch memory task (Zatorre et al., 1994). Thus, we think it is plausible to assume the existence of two distinct processing systems in the frontal operculum. While the dorsolateral part of the pars opercularis and triangularis are preferentially adept at processing sequential information as required by phonological and working memory tasks, the deep frontal operculum (and eventually the anterior insula) activates when the perception of auditory information interacts with the application of additional effort required to extract all relevant auditory information from the acoustic signal. With respect to functional lateralization, we would like to emphasize that our review reveals a considerable proportion of right hemisphere clusters involved in a variety of auditory functions. Based on our review, it is not possible to determine differential functional roles for the left and the right frontal operculum. It rather seems that the proper performance of receptive and expressive auditory tasks necessitates either a consistent or even a cooperative functioning of both the left and the right frontal opercula with a clear leftward asymmetry only observed for phonological processing. In sum, we conclude that neither the left nor the right frontal operculum is selective for a particular function during auditory perception and production. The review rather provides compelling evidence that multiple heterogeneous tasks and experimental contrasts recruit a relatively small territory in the human inferior frontal cortex.

The purpose of this review was to summarize the different auditory functions processed by the frontoopercular region including the so-called Broca's area

and the right-sided homotopic area. The 56 studies we reviewed here have used a variety of experimental auditory tasks tapping multiple auditory functions that (partly) engaged Broca's area. We arbitrarily have tried to find a plausible way to classify and distinguish these functions on the basis of current psycholinguistic and/or perception theories of auditory functions. In fact, we revealed several subregions either completely or partly within the "classic" Broca's area that are associated with different auditory functions. Thus, one might conclude we may have identified several distinct cortical sites that accommodate neural assemblies responsible for very specific auditory functions. However, that is not the aim of this review. We rather would like to emphasize the importance of being very careful in interpreting the collected data for several reasons: First, we have to be aware that the majority of the studies included here used fMRI to localize hemodynamic responses. However, the relationship between neural excitement and the BOLD response measured by fMRI has not been fully clarified so far. Although most current authorities speculate that BOLD responses are mainly triggered by synaptic activity (Logothetis, 2003; Logothetis et al., 2001), more recent papers discuss the possible influence of electric activity of the neurons on the measured BOLD response (Xiong et al., 2003). In addition, it is an open question to what extent peak activation or the spatial extension of activation is based on the same neural underpinnings (Marcar and Loenneker, 2004). Furthermore, fMRI and, to a greater degree, positron emission tomograph are neuroimaging methods with a relatively crude temporal resolution ranging from 4 seconds to 2 minutes, which adds to the list of methodological limitations associated with neuroimaging techniques. Taken together, the hemodynamic response is a composite signal modulated by several neurophysiological processes that are hardly to dissociate and it is subject to a relatively sparse temporal resolution. Obviously, these constraints constrict the suitability of these methods to research auditory functions that occur in a range of milliseconds.

A second concern that is even more important in our view addresses an objection that is often raised against the basic idea that the neuroimaging approach relies on. Present neuroimagers (and even the authors of this review) are often (at least implicitly) misguided to interpret the circumscribed activation spots in a more or less phrenological way. For example, the confined sphere including MNI coordinates we report for phonological processing must not be considered to cover the particular region solely processing phonological functions. We rather need to reconcile these neuroimaging findings with insights obtained from classic lesion and human neurophysiological studies using MEG or EEG methods. From the latter, we know that psychologically relevant information is coded in terms of the neural firing rate (firing over time) and the correlated activity of neural oscillation (periodical neural activation patterns). Thus, as some researchers pointed out, "time is the essence" when we are attempting to understand what the brain is really doing (Ringo et al., 1994). Principally, due to the temporal constraints, neuroimaging research presently is not able to implement a closer analysis of the temporal aspects of the brain function. Currently and in the face of the outstanding popularity of neuroimaging, more and more studies using traditional neurophysiological methods (EEG, MEG) have nicely demonstrated that a particular sensory or cognitive process corresponds to the coupled firing of a focal or even largely distributed neural network. Thus, as a general rule, a particular and circumscribed brain region does not control a psychological function; it is more plausible to assume that the particular manner of neural coupling within a neurofunctional network and not the intensity of its activation is the main parameter determining the quality of psychological functions (Engel et al., 2001). Recently developed electrical imaging methods, such as LORETA (Pascual-Marqui et al., 1994; Pascual-Marqui, 1999), even allow for decent estimation of the neural sources of EEG signals recorded from scalp electrodes and can therefore compete with conventional brain imaging. We believe this development has two implications for the neuroimaging community. First, it becomes more and more imperative to carefully cross-check hemodynamic data obtained from fMRI and positron emission tomography with neurophysiological data derived from EEG and MEG to optimize our knowledge on both temporal and spatial aspects of sensory, motor, and cognitive processes. Second, there is a compelling need to strictly pursue model-driven neuroimaging research rather than using neuroimaging in a more explorative manner, which can lead to neuroimaging suffering from the detrimental and undeserved reputation of "neophrenology."

ACKNOWLEDGMENTS   The authors wish to thank Katrin Amunts, Yosef Grodzinsky, Adam McNamara, and Natalia Estévez for helpful comments on the manuscript. During the preparation of this manuscript, Martin Meyer was supported by Schweizer National Fonds (Swiss National Foundation) SNF 46234101, "Short-term and long-term plasticity in the auditory system."

Notes

1. Since the exact size, borders, subportions, and location of Broca's area are still matters of debate (Amunts et al., 1999, 2004; Amunts and Zilles, Chapter 2; Foundas et al., 1998; Petrides, Chapter 3; Uylings et al., 1999; Tomaiuolo et al., 1999), we do not aim to functionally and anatomically dissociate between Brodmann areas 44 and 45. In the context of the present review, the commonly used notions "Broca's region" and "Broca's area" are used exchangeably.

2. Besides activity in the frontal operculum, the majority of studies reviewed here also illuminated the role of temporal and even extra-Sylvian areas. However, the latter are not subject to the present paper and are therefore not considered.

3. The latter studies tested the perception of pure sentence melody, which can also be considered a degraded percept as proper sentence constitutes sentence melody as well as lexical and syntactic in formation.

References

Ackermann, H., Riecker, A., Mathiak, K., Erb, M., Grodd, W., & Wildgruber, D. (2001). Rate-dependent activation of a prefrontal-insular-cerebellar network during passive listening to trains of click stimuli: an fMRI study. *NeuroReport, 12*, 4087–4092.

Alain, C., Arnott, S.R., Hevenor, S., Graham, S., & Grady, C.L. (2001). 'What' and 'where' in the human auditory system. *Proceedings of the National Academy of Science USA, 98*, 12301–12306.

Amunts, K., Schleicher, A., Bürgel, U., Mohlberg, H., Uylings, H.B.M., & Zilles, K. (1999). Broca's region revisited: cytoarchitecture and intersubject variability. *Journal of Comparative Neurology, 412*, 319–341.

Amunts, K., Schleicher, A., & Zilles, K. (2004). Outstanding language competence and cytoarchitecture in broca's speech region. *Brain and Language, 89*, 346–353.

Bamiou, D.-E., Musiek, F.E., & Luxon, L.M. (2003). The insula (Island of Reil) and its role in auditory processing. *Behavioural Brain Research, 42*, 143–154.

Belin, P., & Zatorre, R.J. (2003). Adaptation to speaker's voice in right anterior temporal lobe. *NeuroReport, 14*, 2105–2109.

Benson, R.R., Whalen, D.H., Richardson, M., Swainson, B., Clark, V.P., Lai, S., et al. (2001). Parametrically dissociating speech and nonspeech perception in the brain using fMRI. *Brain and Language, 78*, 364–396.

Binkofski, F., Amunts, K., Stephan, K.M., Posse, S., Schormann, T., Freund, H.J., et al. (2000). Broca's region subserves imagery of motion: A combined cytoarchitectonic and fMRI study. *Human Brain Mapping, 11,* 273–285.

Binkofski, F., & Buccino, G. (2004). Motor functions of Broca's region. *Brain and Language, 89,* 362–369.

Blank, S.C., Scott, S.K., Murphy, K., Warburton, E., & Wise, R.J.S. (2002). Speech production: Wernicke, Broca and beyond. *Brain, 125,* 1829–1838.

Boemio, A., Fromm, S., Braun, A., & Pöppel, D. (2005). Hierarchical and asymmetric temporal sensitivity in human auditory cortices. *Nature Neuroscience, 8,* 389–395.

Bookheimer, S. (2002). Functional MRI of language: New approaches to understanding the cortical organization of semantic processing. *Annual Reviews of Neuroscience, 25,* 151–188.

Brett, M., Johnsrude, I.S., & Owen, A.M. (2002). The problem of functional localization in the human brain. *Nature Neuroscience Review, 3,* 243–249.

Broca, P. (1861). Remarques sur la siège de la faculté de langage suivies d'une observation d'aphemie. *Bulletin de la Société d'Anatomie, 6,* 330–357.

Broca, P. (1863). Localisation des fonctions cérébrales: Siége de langage articulé. *Bulletin de la Société d'Anthropologie de Paris, 4,* 200–208.

Brown, S., Martinez, M.J., Hodges, D.A., Fox, P.T., & Parsons, L.M. (2004). The song system of the human brain. *Brain Research Cognitive Brain Research, 20,* 363–375.

Buccino, G., Binkofski, F., & Riggio, L. (2004). The mirror neuron system and action recognition. *Brain and Language, 89,* 370–376.

Buchanan, T.W., Lutz, K., Mirzazade, S., Specht, K., Shah, N.J., Zilles, K., et al. (2000). Recognition of emotional prosody and verbal components of spoken language: An fMRI study. *Brain Research & Cognitive Brain Research, 9,* 227–238.

Burton, M.W. (2001). The role of inferior frontal cortex in phonological processing. *Cognitive Science, 25,* 695–709.

Burton, M.W., Small, S.L., & Blumstein, S.E. (2000). The role of segmentation in phonological processing: an fMRI investigation. *Journal of Cognitive Neuroscience, 12,* 679–690.

Davis, M.H., & Johnsrude, I.S. (2003). Hierarchical processing in spoken language comprehension. *Journal of Neuroscience, 23,* 3423–3431.

Demonet, J.-F., Chollet, F., Ramsay, S., Cardebat, D., Nespoulous, J., Wise, R., et al. (1992). The anatomy of phonological and semantic processing in normal subjects. *Brain, 115,* 1753–1768.

Demonet, J.-F., Price, C.J., Wise, R., & Frackowiak, R.S.J. (1994). A PET study of cognitive strategies in normal subjects during language tasks: Influence of phonetic ambiguity and sequence processing on phoneme monitoring. *Brain, 117,* 671–682.

Doeller, C.F., Opitz, B., Mecklinger, A., Krick, C., Reith, W., & Schröger, E. (2003). Prefrontal cortex involvement in preattentive auditory deviance detection: Neuroimaging and electrophysiological evidence. *NeuroImage, 20,* 1270–1282.

Engel, A.K., Fries, P., & Singer, W. (2001). Dynamic predictions: Oscillations and synchrony in top-down processing. *Nature Neuroscience Review, 2,* 704–716.

Engelien, A., Silbersweig, D., Stern, E., Huber, W., Döring, W., Frith, C., et al. (1995). The functional anatomy of recovery from auditory agnosia. A PET study of sound categorization in a neurological patient and normal controls. *Brain, 118,* 1395–1409.

Fiez, J.A., Raichle, M.E., Miezin, F.M., Petersen, S.E., Tallal, P., & Katz, W.F. (1995). PET studies of auditory and phonological processing: Effects of stimulus characteristics and task demands. *Journal of Cognitive Neuroscience, 7,* 357–375.

Flynn, F.G., Benson, D.F., & Ardila, A. (1999). Anatomy of the insula—functional and clinical correlates. *Aphasiology, 13,* 55–78.

Foundas, A.L., Eure, K.F., Luevano, L.F., & Weinberger, D.R. (1998). MRI asymmetries of Broca's area: The pars triangularis and pars opercularis. *Brain and Language, 64,* 282–296.

Fox, P.T., Ingham, R.J., Ingham, J.C., Zamarripa, F., Xiong, J.H., & Lancaster, J.L. (2000). Brain correlates of stuttering and syllable production. A PET performance-correlation analysis. *Brain, 123,* 1985–2004.

Friederici, A.D. (2002). Towards a neural basis of auditory sentence processing. *Trends in Cognitive Sciences, 6,* 78–84.

Friederici, A.D. (2004). Processing local transitions versus long-distance syntactic hierarchies. *Trends in Cognitive Sciences, 8,* 245–247.

Friederici, A.D., & Alter, K. (2004). Lateralization of auditory language functions: A dynamic dual pathway model. *Brain and Language, 89,* 267–276.

Friederici, A.D., Meyer, M., & von Cramon, D.Y. (2000). Auditory language comprehension: An event-related fMRI study on the processing of syntactic and lexical information. *Brain and Language, 75,* 465–477.

Gaab, N., Gaser, C., Zaehle, T., Jäncke, L., & Schlaug, G. (2003). Functional anatomy of pitch memory—An fMRI study with sparse temporal sampling. *NeuroImage, 19,* 1417–1426.

Gandour, J., Dzemidzic, M., Wong, D., Lowe, M., Tong, Y., Hsieh, L., et al. (2003). Temporal integration of speech prosody is shaped by language experience: An fMRI study. *Brain and Language, 84*, 318–336.

Gandour, J., Wong, D., Hsieh, L., Weinzapfel, B., Van Lancker, D., & Hutchins, G.D. (2000). A crosslinguistic PET study of tone perception. *Journal of Cognitive Neuroscience, 12*, 207–222.

Gandour, J., Wong, D., Lowe, M., Dzemidzic, M., Satthamnuwong, N., Tong, Y., et al. (2002). A crosslinguistic fMRI study of spectral and temporal cues underlying phonological processing. *Journal of Cognitive Neuroscience, 14*, 1076–1087.

Gelfand, J.R., & Bookheimer, S.Y. (2003). Dissociating neural mechanisms of temporal sequencing and processing phonemes. *Neuron, 38*, 831–842.

Gernsbacher, M.A., & Kaschak, M.P. (2003). Neuroimaging studies on language production and comprehension. *Annual Review of Psychology, 54*, 91–114.

Giraud, A.L., Kell, C., Thierfelder, C., Sterzer, P., Russ, M.O., Preibisch, C., et al. (2004). Contributions of sensory input, auditory search and verbal comprehension to cortical activity during speech processing. *Cerebral Cortex, 14*, 247–255.

Giraud, A.L., Price, C.J., Graham, J.M., Truy, E., & Frackowiak, R.S.J. (2001). Cross-modal plasticity underpins language recovery after cochlear implantation. *Neuron, 30*, 657–663.

Golestani, N., & Zatorre, R.J. (2004). Learning new sounds of speech: Reallocation of neural substrates. *NeuroImage, 21*, 494–506.

Goodglass, H. (1976). Agrammatism. In H. Whitacker & H.A. Whitacker (Eds.), *Studies in neurolinguistics.* Vol. 1 New York: Academic Press.

Gruber, O., Kleinschmidt, A., Binkofski, F., Steinmetz, H., & von Cramon, D.Y. (2000). Cerebral correlates of working memory for temporal information. *NeuroReport, 11*, 1689–1693.

Hickok, G., & Pöppel, D. (2004). Dorsal and ventral streams: A framework for understanding aspects of the functional anatomy of language. *Cognition, 92*, 67–99.

Hoen, M., Pachot-Clouard, M., Segebarth, C., & Dominey, P.F. (in press). When Broca experiences the Janus syndrome. An er-fMRI study comparing sentence comprehension and cognitive sequence processing. *Cortex.*

Hsieh, L., Gandour, J., Wong, D., & Hutchins, G.D. (2001). Functional heterogeneity of inferior frontal gyrus is shaped by linguistic experience. *Brain and Language, 76*, 227–252.

Hugdahl, K., Bronnick, K., Kyllingsbaek, S., Law, I., Gade, A., & Paulson, O.B. (1999). Brain activation during dichotic presentations of consonant-vowel and musical instrument stimuli: A ^{15}O-PETstudy. *Neuropsychologia, 37*, 431–440.

Hugdahl, K., Law, I., Kyllingsbaek, S., Bronnick, K., Gade, A., & Paulson, O.B. (2000). Effects of attention on dichotic listening: A ^{15}O-PET study. *Human Brain Mapping, 10*, 87–97.

Indefrey, P., & Cutler, A. (2004). Prelexical and lexical processing in listening. In M.A. Gazzaniga (Ed.), *The new cognitive neuroscience* (pp. 759–774). Cambridge, MA: MIT Press.

Ingham, R.J., Fox, P.T., Ingham, J.C., Xiong, J., Zamarripa, F., Hardies, L.J., et al. (2004). Brain correlates of stuttering and syllable production: Gender comparison and replication. *Journal of Speech, Language, and Hearing Research, 14*, 321–341.

Janata, P., Birk, J.L., Van Horn, J.D., Leman, M., Tillmann, B., & Bharucha, J.J. (2002). The cortical topography of tonal structures underlying Western music. *Science, 298*, 2167–2170.

Jäncke, L., Buchanan, T., Lutz, K., & Shah, N.J.S. (2001). Focused and non-focused attention in verbal and emotional dichotic listening: an fMRI study. *Brain and Language, 78*, 349–363.

Jäncke, L., Kleinschmidt, A., Mirzazade, S., & Freund, H.-J. (1999). The sensorimotor role of parietal cortex in linking the perception and creation of object shapes: An fMRI study. *Cerebral Cortex, 11*, 114–121.

Jäncke, L., & Shah, N.J. (2002). Does dichotic listening probe temporal lobe functions? *Neurology, 58*, 736–743.

Jäncke, L., Specht, K., Shah, N.J., & Hugdahl, K. (2003). Focused attention in a simple dichotic listening task: An fMRI experiment. *Brain Research Cognitive Brain Research, 16*, 257–266.

Joanisse, M.F., & Gati, J.S. (2003). Overlapping neural regions for processing rapid temporal cues in speech and nonspeech signals. *NeuroImage, 19*, 64–79.

Klein, D., Zatorre, R.J., Milner, B., & Zhao. V. (2001). A cross-linguistic PET study of tone perception in Mandarin Chinese and English speakers. *NeuroImage, 13*, 646–653.

Kolb, B., & Whishaw, I.Q. (1995). *Fundamentals of human neuropsychology.* New York: Freeman.

Kotz, S.A., Meyer, M., Alter, K., Besson, M., von Cramon, D.Y., & Friederici, A.D. (2003). On the lateralization of emotional prosody: An event-related functional MR investigation. *Brain and Language, 86*, 366–376.

Logothetis, N.K. (2003). The underpinnings of the BOLD functional magnetic resonance imaging signal. *Journal of Neuroscience, 23*, 3963–3971.

Logothetis, N.K., Pauls, J., Augath, M., Trinath, T., & Oeltermann, A. (2001). Neurophysiological investigation of the basis of the fMRI signal. *Nature, 412,* 150–157.

Maeder, P.P., Meuli, R.A., Adriani, M., Bellmann, A., Fornari, E., Thiran, J.-P., et al. (2001). Distinct pathways involved in sound recognition and localization: A human fMRI study. *NeuroImage, 14,* 802–816.

Marcar, V.L., & Loenneker, T. (2004). The BOLD response: A new look at an old riddle. *NeuroReport, 15,* 1997–2000.

Martin, R.C. (2003). Language processing: Functional organization and neuroanatomical basis. *Annual Review of Psychology, 54,* 55–89.

Meyer, M., Alter, K., & Friederici, A.D. (2003). Functional MR imaging exposes differential brain responses to syntax and prosody during auditory sentence comprehension. *Journal of Neurolinguistics, 16,* 277–300.

Meyer, M., Alter, K., Friederici, A.D., Lohmann, G., & von Cramon, D.Y. (2002). Functional MRI reveals brain regions mediating slow prosodic modulations in spoken sentences. *Human Brain Mapping, 17,* 73–88.

Meyer, M., Steinhauer, K., Alter, K., Friederici, A.D., & von Cramon, D.Y. (2004). Brain activity varies with modulation of dynamic pitch variance in sentence melody. *Brain and Language, 89,* 277–289.

Mohr, J.P., Pessin, M.S., Finkelstein, S., Funkenstein, H.H., Duncan, G.W., & Davis, M.D. (1978). Broca aphasia: Pathologic and clinical. *Neurology, 28,* 311–324.

Müller, R.-A., & Basho, S. (2004). Are nonlinguistic functions in "Broca's area" prerequisites for language acquisition? fMRI findings from an ontogenetic viewpoint. *Brain and Language, 89,* 329–336.

Müller, R.-A., Kleinhans, N., & Courchesne, E. (2001). Broca's area and the discrimination of frequency transitions: A functional MRI study. *Brain and Language, 76,* 70–76.

Müller, R.-A., Kleinhans, N., Pierce, K., Kemmotsu, N., & Courchesne, E. (2002). Functional MRI of motor sequence acquisition: Effects of learning stage and performance. *Brain Research Cognitive Brain Research, 14,* 277–293.

Müller, R.-A., Rothermel, R.D., Behen, M.E., Muzik, O., Mangner, T.J., & Chugani, H.T. (1997). Receptive and expressive language activations for sentences: A PET study. *NeuroReport, 8,* 3767–3770.

Noesselt, T., Shah, N.J., & Jäncke, L. (2003). Top-down and bottom-up modulation of language related areas—An fMRI study. *BMC Neuroscience, 4.*

Opitz, B., Rinne, T., Mecklinger, A., von Cramon, D.Y., & Schröger, E. (2002). Differential contribution of frontal and temporal cortices to auditory change detection: fMRI and ERP results. *NeuroImage, 15,* 167–174.

Pascual-Marqui, R.D. (1999). Reviews of methods for solving the EEG inverse problem. *International Journal of Bioelectromagnetism, 1,* 75–86.

Pascual-Marqui, R.D., Michel, C.M., & Lehmann, D. (1994). Low resolution electromagnetic tomography: A new method for localizing electrical activitiy in the brain. *International Journal of Psychophysiology, 18,* 49–65.

Paulesu, E., Frith, C.D., & Frackowiak, R.S.J. (1993). The neural correlates of the verbal components of working memory. *Nature, 362,* 342–345.

Perry, D.W., Zatorre, R.J., Petrides, M., Alivisatos, B., Meyer, E., & Evans, A.C. (1999). Localization of cerebral activity during simple singing. *NeuroReport, 10,* 3979–3984.

Plante, E., Creusere, M., & Sabin, C. (2002). Dissociating sentential prosody from sentence processing: activation interacts with task demands. *NeuroImage, 17,* 401–410.

Pöppel, D. (1996). A critical review of PET studies of phonological processing. *Brain and Language, 55,* 317–351.

Pöppel, D., Guillemin, A., Thompson, J., Fritz, J., Bavelier, D., & Braun, A.R. (2004). Auditory lexical decision, categorical perception, and FM direction discrimination differentially engage left and right auditory cortex. *Neuropsychologia, 42,* 183–200.

Poldrack, R.A., Temple, E., Protopapas, A., Nagarajan, S., Tallal, P., Merzenich, M., et al. (2001). Relations between the neural bases of dynamic auditory processing and phonological processing: Evidence from fMRI. *Journal of Cognitive Neuroscience, 13,* 687–697.

Pollmann, S., Lepsien, J., Hugdahl, K., & von Cramon, D.Y. (2004). Auditory target detection in dichotic listening involves the orbitofrontal and hippocampal paralimbic belts. *Cerebral Cortex, 14,* 903–913.

Riecker, A., Ackermann, H., Wildgruber, D., Dogil, G., & Grodd, W. (2000). Opposite hemispheric lateralization effects during speaking and singing at motor cortex, insula and cerebellum. *NeuroReport, 11,* 1997–2000.

Riecker, A., Wildgruber, D., Dogil, G., Grodd, W., & Ackermann, H. (2002). Hemispheric lateralization effects of rhythm implementation during syllable repetitions: An fMRI study. *NeuroImage, 16,* 169–176.

Ringo, J.L., Doty, R.W., Demeter, S., & Simard, P.Y. (1994). Time is of the essence: A conjecture that hemispheric specialization arises from interhemispheric conduction delay. *Cerebral Cortex, 4,* 331–343.

Rizzolatti, G., & Arbib, M.A. (1999). Language within our grasp. *Trends in Neurosciences, 21,* 188–196.

Rizzolatti, G., & Luppino, G. (2001). The cortical motor system. *Neuron, 31,* 889–901.

Schubotz, R.I., & von Cramon, D.Y. (2001). Interval and ordinal properties of sequences are associated with distinct premotor areas. *Cerebral Cortex, 11,* 210–222.

Scott, S.K., & Wise, R.J.S. (2004). The functional neuroanatomy of prelexical processing in speech perception. *Cognition, 92,* 13–45.

Stowe, L.A., Haverkort, M., & Zwarts, F. (2005). Rethinking the neurological basis of language. *Lingua, 115,* 997–1045.

Thomsen, T., Rimol, L.M., Ersland, L., & Hugdahl, K. (2004a). Dichotic listening reveals functional specificity in prefrontal cortex: An fMRI study. *NeuroImage, 21,* 211–218.

Thomsen, T., Specht, K., Hammar, A., Nyttingnes, J., Ersland, L., & Hugdahl, K. (2004b). Brain localization of attentional control in different age groups by combining functional and structural MRI. *NeuroImage, 22,* 912–919.

Tillmann, B., Janata, P., & Bharucha, J.J. (2003a). Activation of the inferior frontal cortex in musical priming. *Annals of New York Academy of Science, 999,* 209–211.

Tillmann, B., Janata, P., & Bharucha, J.J. (2003b). Activation of the inferior frontal cortex in musical priming. *Brain Research Cognitive Brain Research, 16,* 145–161.

Tomaiuolo, F., McDonald, J., Caramanos, Z., Posner, G., Chiavaras, M., Evans, A.C., et al. (1999). Morphology, morphometry and probability mapping of the pars opercularis of the inferior fontal gyrus: An in vivo MRI analysis. *European Journal of Neuroscience, 11,* 3033–3046.

Tzourio-Mazoyer, N., Landeau, B., Papathanassiou, D., Crivello, F., Etard, O., Delcroix, N., et al. (2002). Automated anatomical labeling of activations in SPM using a macroscopic anatomical parcellation of the MNI MRI single-subject brain. *NeuroImage, 15,* 273–289.

Türe, U., Yasargil, D.C.H., Al-Mefty, O., & Yasargil, M.G. (1999). Topographic anatomy of the insular region. *Journal of Neurosurgery, 90,* 720–733.

Uylings, H.B.M., Malofeeva, L.I., Bogolepova, I.N., Amunts, K., & Zilles, K. (1999). Broca's language area from a neuroanatomical and developmental perspective. In P. Hagoort & C. Brown (Eds.), *The neurocognition of language* (pp. 319–336) New York: Oxford University Press.

Von Kriegstein, K., & Giraud, A.L. (2004). Distinct functional substrates along the right superior temporal sulcus for the processing of voices. *NeuroImage, 22,* 948–955.

Vouloumanos, A., Kiehl, K., Werker, J.F., & Liddle, P.F. (2001). Detection of sounds in the auditory stream: Event-related fMRI evidence for differential activation to speech and nonspeech. *Journal of Cognitive Neuroscience, 13,* 994–1005.

Wise, R.J.S., Greene, J., Buchel, C., & Scott, S.K. (1999). Brain regions involved in articulation. *Lancet, 353,* 1057–1061.

Wong, D., Pisoni, D.B., Learn, J., Gandour, J.T., Miyamoto, R.T., & Hutchins, G.D. (2002). PET imaging of differential cortical activation by monoaural speech and nonspeech stimuli. *Hearing Research, 166,* 9–23.

Xiong, J., Fox, P.T., & Gao, J. (2003). Directly mapping of magnetic field effects of neuronal activity by magnetic resonance imaging. *Human Brain Mapping, 20,* 41–49.

Zatorre, R.J., Belin, P., & Penhune, V.B. (2002). Structure and function of auditory cortex: Music and speech. *Trends in Cognitive Sciences, 6,* 37–46.

Zatorre, R.J., Evans, A.C., & Meyer, E. (1994). Neural mechanisms underlying melodic perception and memory for pitch. *Journal of Neuroscience, 14,* 1908–1919.

Zatorre, R.J., Evans, A.C., Meyer, E., & Gjedde, A. (1992). Lateralization of phonetic and pitch discrimination in speech processing. *Science, 256,* 846–849.

Zatorre, R.J., Meyer, E., Gjedde, A., & Evans, A.C. (1996). PET studies of phonetic processing of speech: Review, replication, and reanalysis. *Cerebral Cortex, 6,* 21–30.

15

On Broca, Brain, and Binding

Peter Hagoort

Not all brain areas are equal. Some have triggered the attention and fascination of mankind more than others. Few have even seen books devoted to them or entered the domain of general awareness. Broca's area is one of these areas. No doubt, one of the main reasons is that this area is often seen as distinctly human. After all, isn't it Broca's area that is connected to the faculty that makes us uniquely human, the faculty of language? However, sometimes fascination breeds confusion. In this case, our fascination makes us believe that "Broca's area" is a coherent notion. Closer inspection reveals that it stands for a family of concepts that are loosely connected at best. We thus need to begin by deconstructing the concept of Broca's area. Only then we can see it more clearly.

Broca's area has different interpretations across different domains of research. We should at least distinguish between Broca's area in neuroanatomical, neuropsychological, and functional terms. At all these levels one can ask the question: Is Broca's area a natural kind? That is, does it carve brain and mind at its

joints? We discuss these issues in the first part of this chapter. The second part presents a proposal about the role of the left inferior frontal cortex, which contains Broca's area as classically defined.

DECONSTRUCTING BROCA'S AREA

The Neuroanatomical Perspective

Despite some disagreement in the literature (see Uylings et al., 1999), most authors agree that Broca's area comprises Brodmann's areas 44 and 45 of the left hemisphere. In the classic textbooks, these areas coincide at the macroscopic level with the pars opercularis (BA 44) and the pars triangularis (BA 45) of the third frontal convolution. However, given anatomical variability, in many brains these two parts are not easy to identify (Uylings et al., 1999), and clear microanatomical differences (see Amunts and Zilles, this volume, Chapter 2) have been missed when macro-anatomical landmarks are used (Tomaiuolo et al., 1999). Furthermore, cytoarchitectonic analysis (Amunts et al., 2003) shows that areas 44 and 45 do not neatly coincide with the sulci that have been assumed to form their boundaries in gross anatomical terms. More fundamentally, one has to question the justification for subsuming these two cytoarchitectonic areas under the overarching heading of Broca, rather than, say, areas 45 and 47. Areas 44 and 45 show a number of clear cytoarchitectonic differences, one of which is that 45 has a granular layer IV, whereas 44 is dysgranular. In contrast, like area 45, area 47 is part of the heteromodal component of the frontal lobe, known as the granular cortex (see Fig. 15–1) (Mesulam, 2002). In addition, areas 44 and 45 have clearly distinct postnatal developmental trajectories and show a difference in their patterns of lateral asymmetry (Uylings et al., 1999). Using an observer-independent method for delineating cortical areas, Amunts et al. (1999) analyzed histological sections of 10 human brains. They found a significant left-over-right asymmetry in cell density for area 44, whereas no significant left-right differences were observed for area 45. However, areas 44 and 45 are cytoarchitectonically more similar to each other than 44 and 6 or than 45 and 6 (Amunts and Zilles, 2001).

Studies on corresponding regions in the macaque brain (Petrides and Pandya, 2002) have shown that area 44 receives projections from mainly somatosensory and motor-related regions like SII, the rostral inferior parietal lobule, supplementary, and cingulate motor areas. There is input from portions of the ventral prefrontal cortex but only sparse projections from inferotemporal cortex (Pandya and Yeterian, 1996). Conversely, area 45 receives massive projections from most parts of prefrontal cortex, from auditory areas of the superotemporal gyrus, and visually related areas in the posterior superior temporal sulcus. In other words, the connectivity patterns of macaque BA 44 and 45 suggest clear functional differences between these areas.

Finally, studies on the receptorarchitecture of left inferofrontal areas indicate that functionally relevant subdivisions within BA 44 and 45 might be necessary (for more details, see Amunts and Zilles, this volume, Chapter 2). For instance, there is a difference within BA 44 of the receptor densities, for example, of the 5-HT$_2$ receptor for serotonin, with relatively low density in dorsal BA 44 and relatively high density in ventral BA 44.

In short, from a cytoarchitectonic and receptorarchitectonic point of view, Broca's area, comprising BA 44 and BA 45, is a heterogeneous patch of cortex and not a uniform cortical entity. However, the degree of uniformity required for an inference of functional unity is not known.

With respect to language areas in prefrontal cortex, it has become clear that, in addition to BA 44 and 45, at least BA 47 and the ventral part of BA 6 should be included in the left frontal language network. Recent neuroimaging studies indicate that the pars orbitalis of the third frontal convolution (roughly corresponding to BA47) is involved in language processing (e.g., Devlin et al., 2003; Hagoort et al., 2004).

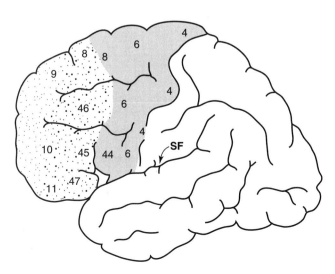

FIGURE 15–1. Lateral view of the frontal lobes. The numbers refer to Brodmann areas. *Dark grey markings*, motor-premotor cortex; *dotted markings*, heteromodal association cortex. SF, Sylvian fissure. (After Mesulam, 2002. Used by permission of Oxford University Press.)

From a functional anatomical perspective, it thus makes sense to use the term *Broca's complex* for this set of areas. Broca's complex is used here to distinguish it from Broca's area as classically defined. The latter definition of Broca's area is both too broad, because it comprises anatomically and functionally distinct areas, and too narrow, because it leaves out adjacent areas that are shown to be crucial for language processing. Broca's complex as here defined is the set of anatomical areas in left inferior frontal cortex that are known to play a crucial, but by no means exclusive, role in language processing.

The Neuropsychological Perspective

The name and fame of Broca's area can be traced back to 1861, when Paul Broca presented a detailed case history of a patient with a restricted brain lesion and a language disorder, which he referred to as aphemia (see Schiller, 1992). In fact, the autopsy of this patient (Leborgne, better known as Tan, since the syllable "tan" was the only utterance the patient could produce) demonstrated an extensive lesion in the left hemisphere encompassing the frontal, parietal, and temporal cortex. Broca's conclusion that the third inferior frontal part of the lesion caused the aphemia was inferred from the degree of necrosis and an analysis of the patient's medical history (Whitaker, 1998). What Broca referred to as aphemia is now known as aphasia, a term introduced by Trousseau in 1864 to refer to brain-related language disorders (Ryalls, 1984). In the decades following Broca's influential papers, other types of aphasia were described as well, pointing out that disorders might involve not only speech production but also comprehension. The publication by Carl Wernicke of "Der Aphasische Symptomencomplex" (1874) was a further hallmark in this initial era of aphasia research.

The history of neuropsychological research since Broca has resulted in the description of a series of aphasic syndromes, including Broca's aphasia and Wernicke's aphasia. Although these aphasias were described in terms of their symptoms, they were also associated with particular lesions, with their focus in what we now refer to as Broca's area and Wernicke's area, respectively. Although it is certainly true that the field of aphasiology has contributed enormously to our current understanding of the relation between brain and language, certainly the implicit link between functional symptom complexes of Broca's and Wernicke's aphasia and particular brain areas has also resulted in some confusion. I focus here particularly on the problematic relationship between Broca's aphasia and Broca's area. To do so, I first have to clarify what is commonly referred to as Broca's aphasia (e.g., Caplan, 1992).

Despite substantial individual variation in severity, characteristic features of Broca's aphasia are the nonfluent speech and the reduced syntactic complexity of the utterances, sometimes resulting in telegraphic speech in which function words and grammatical morphemes are omitted (agrammatism). In contrast to what is often used as a defining characteristic of Broca's aphasia, this type of aphasia is not restricted to language production but also comprises syntactic and other deficits in comprehension (Caramazza and Zurif, 1976; Kolk and Friederici, 1985; Zurif et al., 1972). Only in very rare cases does one find an impairment of language production with an intact language comprehension (Kolk and Friederici, 1985; Miceli et al., 1983; Nespoulous et al., 1988). On the basis of the neurolinguistic studies in the 1970s, Broca's area came to be seen as crucially involved in both grammatical encoding and parsing operations. Modality-independent grammatical knowledge was also thought to be represented in this area (Zurif, 1998). However, since then the pivotal role of Broca's area in syntactic processing has faced a number of serious challenges. Studies that correlated aphasic syndromes with site of lesion led to the conclusion that the relation between Broca's area and Broca's aphasia is not as straightforward as once believed, for a number of reasons.

First, lesions restricted to Broca's area often do not seem to result in lasting aphasic (including agrammatic) symptoms (Mohr et al., 1978). In other words, a lesion in Broca's area is not a sufficient condition for a Broca's aphasia.

Second, large-scale correlational studies have found a substantial number of exceptions to the general rule that left frontal lesions go together with Broca's aphasia (Basso et al., 1985; Willmes and Poeck, 1993). Basso et al. (1985) correlated cortical lesions as revealed by computed tomography scans with aphasiological symptomatology for a group of 207 patients. They reported a substantial number of exceptions (17%) to the classic associations between lesion site and aphasia syndromes. Among these exceptions were patients with lesions restricted to left anterior areas, but with a fluent aphasia of the Wernicke type (seven cases), as well as nonfluent Broca's aphasics with posterior lesions and sparing of Broca's area (six cases). Willmes and Poeck (1993) investigated the computed tomography lesion localization for a group of 221 aphasic patients with a vascular lesion in the territory of the middle cerebral artery. Their results were even more dramatic. The conditional probability of an anterior lesion given a Broca's aphasia was no higher than 59%, whereas the probability that an anterior lesion resulted in a Broca's aphasia was only 35%.

In addition, later studies indicate that the syntactic deficit in Broca's aphasics is probably more limited than was believed in the 1970s. Many agrammatic patients with Broca's aphasia show a relatively high sensitivity to syntactic structure in tasks such as judging the grammaticality of sentences (Linebarger et al., 1983). With respect to language output, other analyses indicate that the telegraphic style of agrammatic aphasics follows the syntactic regularities of elliptic utterances, and therefore these patients show syntactic competence at least to some degree (Kolk and Heeschen, 1992).

In summary, the view that a central syntactic deficit is the distinguishing feature of Broca's aphasia, and therefore that Broca's area is crucial for grammatical encoding and parsing, is difficult to maintain in the light of more recent neurolinguistic studies and lesion studies correlating Broca's aphasia with the concomitant lesion sites.

However, there are good reasons to consider all this evidence as not really decisive with respect to the role of Broca's area in syntactic processing. One major reason is that the characterization of the language disorder in lesion studies usually is based on clinical impressions (Mohr et al., 1978) or clinical aphasia test batteries (Basso et al., 1985; Willmes and Poeck, 1993), which are often insufficient to determine the degree and specificity of the syntactic impairment. The classification of aphasic patients in terms of a limited set of syndromes does not guarantee that core language operations are singled out according to articulated cognitive architectures for speaking, listening, or reading (cf. Shallice, 1988). Willmes and Poeck (1993) therefore rightly conclude that "localization studies along the traditional lines will not yield results that lend themselves to a meaningful interpretation of

impaired psychological processes such as aphasia. Small-scale in-depth studies lend themselves better to characterizing the functional impairment in an information-processing model" (pp. 1538–1539).

In one of these in-depth studies, Caplan et al. (1996) tested patients on a series of sentence types that required them to process a range of syntactic structures. These studies showed that the task performance for the different sentence types did not differ between patients with anterior (Broca's area) lesions and those with posterior lesions. The size of the lesion within the peri-Sylvian area also did not correlate with the syntactic task performance. Caplan et al. (1996) gave two possible explanations for these results. One is that syntactic processing is fairly strictly localized, but the exact site can vary quite substantially between individuals within the borders of the left peri-Sylvian area including the insula (Caplan, 1987; Vanier and Caplan, 1990). The other possibility is that the syntactic machinery is organized as a distributed neural network in which several regions of the left peri-Sylvian cortex are critically involved.

Grodzinsky (2000) acknowledges the problems of the classic view of the relation between the syntactic deficit in Broca's aphasia and the role of Broca's area. He proposes a much more restricted role of Broca's area. In his view, "Broca's area and its vicinity (operculum, insula, and adjacent white matter) support receptive language mechanisms that implement some, but not all aspects of syntax, namely those pertaining to syntactic movement rules in comprehension (as well as limited aspects of tree building in speech production)" (Grodzinsky, 2000, p. 7). However, one has to realize that BA 44 and 45, operculum, and insula together constitute a substantial amount of cortex. It would be surprising if no further functional subdivisions were to be found within this large area.

Finally, a more general problem of the lesion approach is that for some cognitive functions, alternative brain systems might be available. This is referred to as degeneracy (Price and Friston, 2002). In addition, one area within association cortex might be a node in different functional networks (Mesulam, 1998). This implies, on the one hand, that the absence of a cognitive deficit after a lesion to a specific site does not necessarily imply that the lesioned area is not involved in the spared function and, on the other hand, that a lesion to one particular area will often not result in a deficit that conforms to the idea that deficits can be easily parcellated into different cognitive domains.

In conclusion, our view on Broca's area from a neuropsychological perspective has suffered from the assumption that the symptoms of a Broca's aphasia are related in a straightforward way to a lesion of Broca's area. In fact, the contribution of Broca's area cannot be easily inferred from the symptoms of patients with a Broca's aphasia. The functional lesion of patients with Broca's aphasia thus cannot be directly mapped onto Broca's area.

Broca's Area From a Cognitive Neuroscience Perspective

In this chapter, I will not be able to review the rapidly increasing number of neuroimaging studies on different aspect of language processing and on the role of the left inferior frontal cortex in this context. However, what I will do is highlight several lessons to be learnt from this recent body of evidence that cognitive neuroscience has provided.

A first important lesson is that it would be a serious mistake to assume that Broca's area is a language-specific area and that within the language domain it only subserves one very specific function. As Mesulam has argued in a series of classic papers (1990, 1998), "Many cortical nodes are likely to participate in the function of more than one network. Conceivably, top-down connections from transmodal areas could differentially recruit such a cortical node into the service of one network or another" (1998, p. 1040). In this conception, a particular cognitive function is most likely served by a distributed network of areas, rather than by one local area alone. In addition, a local area participates in more than one function. A one-to-one mapping between Broca's area and a specific functional component of the language system would thus be a highly unlikely outcome. Even for the visual system, it is claimed that the representations of, for example, objects and faces in ventral temporal cortex are widely distributed and overlapping (Haxby et al., 2001). It would indeed be highly surprising if the different representational domains in the language network would behave according to a principle of localization that is less distributed than for the visual system. Moreover, Broca's area has been found activated in imaging studies on nonlanguage functions. For instance, Fink et al. (Chapter 16) found activation in Broca's area when subjects had to search for

a target hidden within a complex geometric pattern. Broca's area is also activated in action recognition (Decety et al., 1997; Hamzei et al., 2003) and movement preparation (Thoenissen et al., 2002). Of course, all of this does not mean that cognitive functions are not localized and that the brain shows equipotentiality. It only means that the one-area–one-function principle is in many cases not an adequate account of how cognitive functions are neuronally instantiated.

The second lesson to be learnt is that, within Broca's complex, there might be functionally defined subregions. By now, there is some indication that this complex shows an anterior-to-posterior gradient (Bookheimer, 2002). Roughly speaking, BA 47 and BA 45 are involved in semantic processing, while BA 45, 44, and 46 contribute to syntactic processing. Finally BA 44 and BA 6 have a role in phonological processing. Broca's complex is thus involved in at least three different domains of language processing (semantic, syntactic, phonological), with a certain level of relative specialization within different subregions of Broca's complex. However, the overlap of activations for these three different types of processing is substantial. For this reason, subregional specificity within Broca's complex cannot (yet) be concluded.

Based on the neuroanatomical, neuropsychological, and cognitive neuroscience perspectives, it is evident that Broca's area is not a natural kind at the level of either brain structure or cognitive function. Instead, within the left inferior prefrontal cortex, it refers to a grouping of related but cytoarchitectonically distinct areas with a responsivity to distinct information types within the domains of language comprehension and production. Most likely, the conglomerate contributes to other cognitive functions as well. In the remainder of this chapter, I propose a role for Broca's complex in what I refer to as binding or unification of information retrieved from the mental lexicon.

BROCA'S COMPLEX AS PART OF THE UNIFICATION SPACE

The proposed role for Broca's complex is based on (1) an embedding of this complex in the overall functional architecture of prefrontal cortex and (2) a general distinction between memory retrieval of linguistic information and combinatorial operations on information retrieved from the mental lexicon. These

Phonological structure

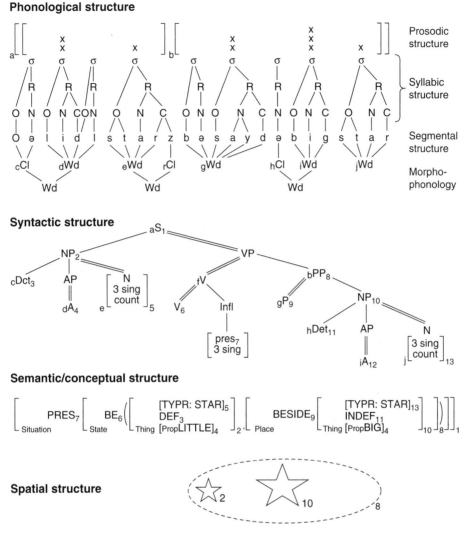

Syntactic structure

Semantic/conceptual structure

Spatial structure

FIGURE 15–2. The phonological, syntactic, and semantic/conceptual structures for the sentence "The little star's beside the big star." (Jackendoff, 2002. Used by permission of Oxford University Press.) The unification operations involved are suggested to require the contribution of Broca's complex.

operations are referred to as unification or binding. The notion of binding is inspired by the visual neurosciences, where one of the fundamental questions is: How do we get from the processing of different visual features (color, form, motion) by neurons that are far apart in brain space to a unified visual percept? This is known as the *binding problem*. In the context of the language system, the binding problem refers to an analogous situation but now transferred to the time domain: How is information that is incrementally retrieved from the mental lexicon unified into a coherent overall interpretation of a multiword utterance?

Most likely, unification needs to take place at the conceptual, syntactic, and phonological levels, as well as between these levels (see Fig. 15–2) (Jackendoff, 2002). Binding in this context refers to a problem that the brain has to solve, not to a concept from a particular linguistic theory.

Broca's Complex as Part of Prefrontal Cortex

Integration is an important part of the function of the prefrontal cortex. This holds especially for integration of information in the time domain (Fuster, 1995). To fulfill this role, prefrontal cortex needs to be able to hold information on-line (Mesulam, 2002) and to select among competing alternatives (Thompson-Schill et al., 1999). Electrophysiological recordings in the macaque monkey have shown that this area is important for sustaining information triggered by a transient event for many seconds (Miller, 2000). This allows prefrontal cortex to establish unifications between pieces of information that are perceived or retrieved from memory at different moments in time Fuster (1995).

Recent neuroimaging studies indicate that Broca's complex contributes to the unification operations required for binding single-word information into larger structures. In psycholinguistics, integration and unification refer to what is usually called postlexical processing. These are the operations on information that is retrieved from the mental lexicon. It seems that prefrontal cortex is especially well suited to contribute to postlexical processing, because this includes selection among competing unification possibilities, so that one unified representation spanning the whole utterance remains.

In short, the properties of neurons in the prefrontal cortex of macaques suggest that this part of the brain is suitable for integrating pieces of information that are made available sequentially, that is spread out over time, regardless of the nature of the material to be handled (Owen et al., 1998). Clearly, there are interspecies differences in terms of the complexity of the information binding operations (Fitch and Hauser, 2004), possibly supported by a corresponding increase in the amount of frontal neural tissue from monkey to humans (Passingham, 2002). With respect to language processing in humans, different complex binding operations take place. Hereafter, I will propose that subregions in the Broca complex contribute to the different unification operations that are required for binding single-word information into larger structures.

Broca's Complex as the Unification Space for Language

Accounts of the human language system (Jackendoff, 1999, 2002; Levelt, 1999) generally assume a cognitive architecture, which consists of separate processing levels for conceptual/semantic information, orthographic/phonological information, and syntactic

information. Based on this architecture, most current models of language processing agree that, in on-line sentence processing, different types of constraints are very quickly taken into consideration during speaking and listening/reading. Constraints on how words can be structurally combined operate alongside qualitatively distinct constraints on the combination of word meanings, on the grouping of words into phonological phrases, and on their referential binding into a discourse model (see Fig. 15–2).

Moreover, in recent linguistic theories, the distinction between lexical items and traditional rules of grammar is vanishing. For instance, Jackendoff (2002) proposes that the only remaining rule of grammar is UNIFY PIECES, "and all the pieces are stored in a common format that permits unification" (p. 180). The unification operation clips together lexicalized patterns with one or more variables in it. The operation MERGE in Chomsky's Minimalist Program (Chomsky, 1995) has a similar flavor. Thus, phonological, syntactic, and semantic/pragmatic constraints determine how lexically available structures are glued together. In Jackendoff's (2002) recent account, for all three levels of representation (phonological, syntactic, semantic/conceptual), information retrieved from the mental lexicon has to be unified into larger structures. In addition, interface operation link these three levels of analysis. The gradient observed in Broca's complex can be specified in terms of the unification operations at these three levels. In short, the left inferior frontal cortex recruits lexical information, mainly stored in temporal lobe structures, and unifies them into overall representations that span multiword utterances. Hereafter I will show in more detail how this could work for the syntactic level of analysis (see Hagoort, 2003). The challenge for the future is to specify computational models with similar detail for the unification of conceptual and phonological information.

According to the Unification Model for parsing (see Vosse and Kempen, 2000), each word form in the mental lexicon is associated with a structural frame. This structural frame consists of a three-tiered unordered tree, specifying the possible structural environment of the particular lexical item (see Fig. 15–3).

The top layer of the frame consists of a single phrasal node (e.g., NP). This so-called root node is connected to one or more functional nodes (e.g., subject, head, direct object) in the second layer of the

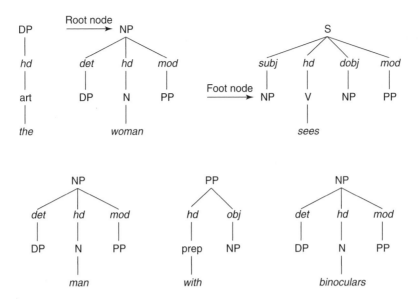

FIGURE 15–3. Syntactic frames in memory. These frames are retrieved on the basis of incoming word form information. DP, determiner phrase; NP, noun phrase; S, sentence; PP, prepositional phrase; art, article; hd, head; det, determiner; mod, modifier; subj, subject; dobj, direct object.

frame. The third layer contains, again, phrasal nodes to which lexical items or other frames can be attached.

This parsing account is "lexicalist" in the sense that all syntactic nodes (e.g., S, NP, VP, N, V, etc.) are retrieved from the mental lexicon. In other words, chunks of syntactic structure are stored in memory. There are no syntactic rules that introduce additional nodes. In the on-line comprehension process, structural frames associated with the individual word forms incrementally enter the unification workspace. In this workspace, constituent structures spanning the whole utterance are formed by a unification operation (see Fig. 15–4). This operation consists of linking up lexical frames with identical root and foot nodes, and checking agreement features (number, gender, person, etc.). It specifies what Jackendoff (2002) refers to as the only remaining "grammatical rule": UNIFY PIECES.

The resulting unification links between lexical frames are formed dynamically, which implies that the strength of the unification links varies over time until a state of equilibrium is reached. Due to the inherent ambiguity in natural language, alternative binding candidates will usually be available at any point in the parsing process. That is, a particular root node (e.g., PP) often finds more than one matching

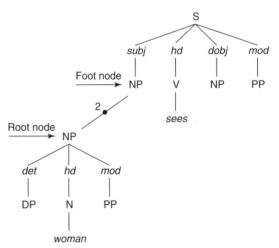

FIGURE 15–4. The unification operation of two lexically specified syntactic frames. The unification takes place by linking the root node NP to an available foot node of the same category. The number 2 indicates that this is the second link that is formed during on-line processing of the sentence "The woman sees the man with the binoculars." (See Fig. 15–3 legend for abbreviations.)

foot node (i.e. PP) with which it can form a unification link (for examples, see Hagoort, 2003).

Ultimately, one phrasal configuration results. This requires that among the alternative binding candidates only one remains active. The required state of equilibrium is reached through a process of lateral inhibition between two or more alternative unification links. In general, due to gradual decay of activation, more recent foot nodes will have a higher level of activation than the ones that entered the unification space earlier. In addition, strength levels of the unification links can vary as a function of plausibility (semantic) effects. For instance, if instrumental modifiers under S-nodes have a slightly higher default activation than instrumental modifiers under an NP-node, lateral inhibition can result in overriding a recency effect.

The unification model accounts for sentence complexity effects known from behavioral measures, such as reading times. In general, sentences are harder to analyze syntactically when more potential unification links of similar strength enter into competition with each other. Sentences are easy when the number of U-links is small and of unequal strength. In addition, the model accounts for a number of other experimental findings in psycholinguistic research on sentence processing, including syntactic ambiguity (attachment preferences; frequency differences between attachment alternatives), and lexical ambiguity effects. Moreover, it accounts for breakdown patterns in agrammatic sentence analysis (see, for details, Vosse and Kempen, 2000).

The advantage of the unification model is that it (1) is computationally explicit, (2) accounts for a large series of empirical findings in the parsing literature and in the neuropsychological literature on aphasia, and (3) belongs to the class of lexicalist parsing models that have found increasing support in recent years (Bresnan, 2001; Jackendoff, 2002; Joshi and Schabes, 1997; MacDonald et al., 1994).

This model also nicely accounts for the two classes of syntax-related ERP effects that have been consistently reported over recent years. One type of ERP effect related to syntactic processing is the P600/SPS (Hagoort et al., 1993; Osterhout and Holcomb, 1992). The P600/SPS is reported in relation to syntactic violations, syntactic ambiguities, and syntactic complexity. Another syntax-related ERP is a left anterior negativity, referred to as LAN or, if earlier in latency than 400 ms, as ELAN (Friederici et al., 1996). In

contrast to the P600/SPS, the (E)LAN has so far only been observed to syntactic violations.

In the unification model, binding (unification) is prevented in two cases. One case is when the root node of a syntactic building block (e.g., NP) does not find another syntactic building block with an identical foot node (i.e. NP) to bind to. The other case is when the agreement check finds a serious mismatch in the grammatical feature specifications of the root and foot nodes. The claim is that the (E)LAN results from a failure to bind, as a result of a negative outcome of the agreement check or a failure to find a matching category node. For instance, the sentence "The woman sees the man because with the binoculars" does not result in a completed parse, because the syntactic frame associated with "because" does not find unoccupied (embedded) S-root nodes that it can bind to. As a result, unification fails.

In the context of the unification model, I propose that the P600/SPS is related to the time it takes to establish unification links of sufficient strength. The time it takes to build up the unification links until the required strength is reached is affected by ongoing competition between alternative unification options (syntactic ambiguity), by syntactic complexity, and by semantic influences. The amplitude of the P600/SPS is modulated by the amount of competition. Competition is reduced when the number of alternative binding options is smaller or when lexical, semantic, or discourse context biases the strengths of the unification links in a particular direction, thereby shortening the duration of the competition. Violations result in a P600/SPS as long as unification attempts are made. For instance, a mismatch in gender or agreement features might still result in weaker binding in the absence of alternative options. However, in such cases the strength and build-up of U-links will be affected by the partial mismatch in syntactic feature specification. Compared with less complex or syntactically unambiguous sentences, in more complex and syntactically ambiguous sentences it takes longer to build up U-links of sufficient strength. The latter sentences, therefore, result in a P600/SPS in comparison to the former ones.

In summary, it seems that the unification model provides an acceptable account for the collective body of ERP data on syntactic processing. It is the computationally most explicit account of the (E)LAN and P600/SPS effects that is currently available (Fig. 15–5).

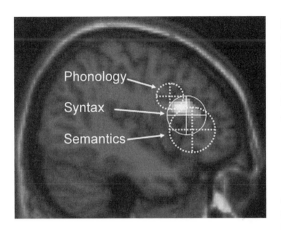

FIGURE 15–5. The gradient in left inferior frontal cortex for activations and their distribution, related to semantic, syntactic, and phonological processing, based on the meta-analysis in Bookheimer (2002). The centers represent the mean coordinates of the local maxima, and the radii represent the standard deviations of the distance between the local maxima and their means (courtesy of Karl Magnus Petersson). The activation shown is from artificial grammar violations in Petersson et al. (2004).

In a recent meta-analysis of 28 neuroimaging studies, Indefrey (2003) found two areas that were critical for syntactic processing, independent of the input modality (visual in reading, auditory in speech). These two supramodal areas for syntactic processing were the left posterior superior temporal gyrus and the left prefrontal cortex. The left posterior temporal cortex is known to be involved in lexical processing (Indefrey and Cutler, 2004). In connection to the unification model, this part of the brain might be important for the retrieval of the syntactic frames that are stored in the lexicon. The unification space, where individual frames are connected into a phrasal configuration for the whole utterance, might be localized in Broca's complex. Presumably, this holds for both language comprehension and language production (Indefrey et al., 2001).

However, unification operations take place not only at the level of syntactic processing. Combinatoriality is a hallmark of language across representational domains. That is, it holds equally for syntactic, semantic, and phonological levels of analyses. In all of these cases, lexical bits and pieces have to be combined and integrated into larger structures. The need for combining independent bits and pieces into a single coherent percept is not unique for syntax. Models for semantic/conceptual unification and phonological unification could be worked out along similar lines as the unification model for syntax, with BA 47 and 45 involved in semantic binding, BA 45 and 44 in syntactic binding, and BA 44 and 6 in phonological binding (see Fig. 15–5).

BROCA'S AREA REVISITED

As I have tried to make clear, despite the large appeal of Broca's area, it is not a very well-defined concept. Instead of "Broca's area," I have therefore proposed to use the term "Broca's complex," to refer to a series of related but distinct areas in the left prefrontal cortex, at least encompassing BAs 47, 45, and 44 and ventral BA 6. This set of areas subserves more than one function in the language domain and almost certainly other nonlanguage functions as well. In the context of language processing, the common denominator of Broca's complex is its role in selection and unification operations by which individual pieces of lexical information are bound together into representational structures spanning multiword utterances. One can thus conclude that Broca's complex has a pivotal role in solving the binding problem for language.

ACKNOWLEDGMENTS   The author is grateful to Katrin Amunts, Michael Coles, Ivan Toni, Harry Uylings, Francisco Aboitiz, Ricardo García, Enzo Brunetti, and Yosef Grodzinsky for their comments on an earlier version of this chapter.

References

Amunts, K., Schleicher, A., Burgel, U., Mohlberg, H., Uylings, H.B., & Zilles, K. (1999). Broca's region revisited: cytoarchitecture and intersubject variability. *Journal of Comparative Neurology, 412*, 319–341.

Amunts, K., Schleicher, A., Ditterich, A., & Zilles, K. (2003). Broca's region: Cytoarchitectonic asymmetry and developmental changes. *Journal of Comparative Neurology, 465*, 72–90.

Amunts, K., & Zilles, K (2001). Advances in cytoarchitectonic mapping of the human cerebral cortex. *Neuroimaging Clinics of North America, 11*, 151–170.

Amunts, K., & Zilles, K. (2005). Broca's region re-visited: A multimodal analysis of its structure and function.

In Y. Grodzinsky & K. Amunts (Eds.), *Broca's region*. Oxford: Oxford University Press.

Basso, A., Lecours, A.R., Moraschini, S., & Vanier, M. (1985). Anatomoclinical correlations of the aphasias as defined through computerized tomography: Exceptions. *Brain and Language, 26,* 201–229.

Bookheimer, S. (2002). Functional MRI of language: New approaches to understanding the cortical organization of semantic processing. *Annual Review of Neuroscience, 25,* 151–188.

Bresnan, J.W. (2001). *Lexical-functional syntax.* Oxford: Blackwell.

Caplan, D. (1987). *Neurolinguistics and linguistic aphasiology.* Cambridge: Cambridge University Press.

Caplan, D. (1992). *Language: Structure, processing, and disorders.* Cambridge, MA: MIT Press.

Caplan, D., Hildebrandt, N., & Makris, N. (1996). Location of lesions in stroke patients with deficits in syntactic processing in sentence comprehension. *Brain, 119,* 933–949.

Caramazza, A., & Zurif, E.B. (1976). Dissociation of algorithmic and heuristic processes in language comprehension: evidence from aphasia. *Brain and Language, 3,* 572–582.

Chomsky, N. (1995). *The minimalist program.* Cambridge, MA: MIT Press.

Decety, J., GrÇzes, J., Costes, N., Perani, D., Jeannerod, M., Procyk, E., et al. (1997). Brain activity during observation of actions. Influence of action content and subject's strategy. *Brain, 120,* 1763–1777.

D'Esposito, M., Aguirre, G.K., Zarahn, E., Ballard, D., Shin, R.K., & Lease, J. (1998). Functional MRI studies of spatial and nonspatial working memory. *Cognitive Brain Research, 7,* 1–13.

Devlin, J.T., Matthews, P.M., & Rushworth, M.F.S. (2003). Semantic processing in the left prefrontal cortex: A combined functional magnetic resonance imaging and transcranial magnetic stimulation study. *Journal of Cognitive Neuroscience, 15,* 71–84.

Fitch, W.T., & Hauser, M.D. (2004). Computational constraints on syntactic processing in a nonhuman primate. *Science, 303,* 377–380.

Friederici, A.D., Hahne, A., & Mecklinger, A. (1996). Temporal structure of syntactic parsing: Early and late event-related brain potential effects. *Journal of Experimental Psychology: Learning, Memory, and Cognition, 22,* 1219–1248.

Fuster, J.M. (1995). Temporal processing. *Annals of New York Academy of Sciences, 769,* 173–181.

Grodzinsky, Y. (2000). The neurology of syntax: Language use without Broca's area. *Behavioral and Brain Sciences, 23,* 1–21; discussion 21–71.

Hagoort, P. (2003). How the brain solves the binding problem for language: A neurocomputational model of syntactic processing. *Neuroimage, 20,* S18–S29.

Hagoort, P., Brown, C.M., & Groothusen, J. (1993). The Syntactic Positive Shift (SPS) as an ERP measure of syntactic processing. *Language and Cognitive Processes, 8,* 439–483.

Hagoort, P., Hald, L., Bastiaansen, M., & Petersson, K.M. (2004). Integration of word meaning and world knowledge in language comprehension. *Science, 304,* 438–441.

Hamzei, F., Rijntjes, M., Dettmers, C., Glauche, V., Weiller, C., & Büchel, C. (2003). The human action recognition system and its relationship to Broca's area: An fMRI study. *Neuroimage, 19,* 637–644.

Haxby, J.V., Gobbini, M.I., Furey, M.L., Ishai, A., Schouten, J.L., & Pietrini, P. (2001). Distributed and overlapping representations of faces and objects in ventral temporal cortex. *Science, 293,* 2425–2430.

Indefrey, P., & Cutler, A. (2004). Prelexical and lexical processing in listening. In M. Gazzaniga (Ed.), *The cognitive neurosciences*, 3rd edition (pp. 759–774). Cambridge, MA: MIT Press.

Indefrey, P., Brown, C.M., Hellwig, F., Amunts, K., Herzog, H., Seitz, R.J., et al. (2001). A neural correlate of syntactic encoding during speech production. *Proceedings of the National Academy of Sciences USA, 98,* 5933–5936.

Jackendoff, R. (1999). The representational structures of the language faculty and their interactions. In C.M. Brown & P. Hagoort (Eds.), *The neurocognition of language* (pp. 37–79). Oxford, UK: Oxford University Press.

Jackendoff, R. (2002). *Foundations of language: Brain, meaning, grammar, evolution.* Oxford, UK: Oxford University Press.

Joshi, A.K., & Schabes, Y. (1997). Tree-adjoining grammars. In G. Rozenberg & A. Salomaa (Eds.), *Handbook of formal languages. Vol. 3: Beyond words* (pp. 69–123). Berlin: Springer Verlag,

Kolk, H.H., & Friederici, A.D. (1985). Strategy and impairment in sentence understanding by Broca's and Wernicke's aphasics. *Cortex, 21,* 47–67.

Kolk, H.H., & Heeschen, C. (1992). Agrammatism, paragrammatism and the management of language. *Language and Cognitive Processes, 7,* 89–129.

Levelt, W.J.M. (1999). Producing spoken language: A blueprint of the speaker. In C.M. Brown & P. Hagoort (Eds.), *The neurocognition of language* (pp. 83–122). Oxford: Oxford University Press.

Linebarger, M.C., Schwartz, M.F., & Saffran, E.M. (1983). Sensitivity to grammatical structure in so-called agrammatic aphasics. *Cognition, 13,* 361–392.

MacDonald, M.C., Pearlmutter, N.J., & Seidenberg, M.S. (1994). Lexical nature of syntactic ambiguity resolution. *Psychological Review, 101*, 676–703.

Mesulam, M.-M. (1990). Large-scale neurocognitive networks and distributed processing for attention, language, and memory. *Annals of Neurology, 28*, 597–613.

Mesulam, M.-M. (1998). From sensation to cognition. *Brain, 121*, 1013–1052.

Mesulam, M.-M. (2002). The human frontal lobes: Transcending the default mode through contingent encoding. In D.T. Stuss & R.T. Knight (Eds.), *Principles of frontal lobe function* (pp. 8–31). Oxford: Oxford University Press.

Miceli, G., Mazzucchi, A., Menn, L., & Goodglass, H. (1983). Contrasting cases of Italian agrammatic aphasia without comprehension disorder. *Brain and Language, 19*, 65–97.

Miller, E.K. (2000). The prefrontal cortex and cognitive control. *Nature Review Neuroscience, 1*, 59–65.

Mohr, J.P., Pessin, M.S., Finkelstein, S., Funkenstein, H.H., Duncan, G.W., & Davis, K.R. (1978). Broca aphasia: Pathologic and clinical. *Neurology, 28*, 311–324.

Nespoulous, J.L., Dordain, M., Perron, C., Ska, B., Bub, D., Caplan, D., et al. (1988). Agrammatism in sentence production without comprehension deficits: Reduced availability of syntactic structures and/or of grammatical morphemes? A case study. *Brain and Language, 33*, 273–295.

Osterhout, L., & Holcomb, P.J. (1992). Event-related brain potentials elicited by syntactic anomaly. *Journal of Memory and Language, 31*, 785–806.

Owen, A.M., Stern, C.E., Look, R.B., Tracey, I., Rosen, B.R., & Petrides, M. (1998). Functional organization of spatial and nonspatial working memory processing within the human lateral frontal cortex. *Proceedings of the National Academy of Sciences USA, 95*, 7721–7726.

Pandya, D.N., & Yeterian, E.H. (1996). Comparison of prefrontal architecture and connections. *Philosophical Transactions of the Royal Society London, 351*, 1433–1444.

Passingham, R.E. (2002). The frontal cortex: Does size matter? *Nature Neuroscience, 5*, 190–192.

Petersson, K.M., Forkstam, C., & Ingvar, M. (2004). Artificial syntactic violations activate Broca's region. *Cognitive Science, 28*, 383–407.

Petrides, M. (2000). Dissociable roles of mid-dorsolateral prefrontal and anterior inferotemporal cortex in visual working memory. *The Journal of Neuroscience, 20*, 7496–7503.

Petrides, M., & Pandya, D.N. (2002). Association pathways of the prefrontal cortex and functional observations. In D.T. Stuss & R.T. Knight (Eds.), *Principles of frontal lobe function* (pp. 31–51). Oxford: Oxford University Press.

Price, C.J., & Friston, K.J. (2002). Degeneracy and cognitive anatomy. *Trends in Cognitive Sciences, 6*, 416–421.

Ryalls, J. (1984). Where does the term "aphasia" come from? *Brain and Language, 21*, 358–363.

Schiller, F. (1992). *Paul Broca: Explorer of the brain.* New York: Oxford University Press.

Shallice, T. (1988). *From neuropsychology to mental structure.* Cambridge: Cambridge University Press.

Thoenissen, D., Zilles, K., & Toni, I. (2002). Differential involvement of parietal and precentral regions in movement preparation and motor intention. *Journal of Neuroscience, 22*, 9024–9034.

Thompson-Schill, S.L., D'Esposito, M., & Kan, I.P. (1999). Effects of repetition and competition on activity in left prefrontal cortex during word generation. *Neuron, 23*, 513–522.

Tomaiuolo, F., MacDonald, J.D., Caramanos, Z., Posner, G., Chiavaras, M., Evans, A.C., et al. (1999). Morphology, morphometry and probability mapping of the pars opercularis of the inferior frontal gyrus: An in vivo MRI analysis. *European Journal of Neuroscience, 11*, 3033–3046.

Uylings, H.B.M., Malofeeva, L.I., Bogolepova, I.N., Amunts, K., & Zilles, K. (1999). Broca's language area from a neuroanatomical and developmentsl perspective. In C.M. Brown & P. Hagoort (Eds.), *Neurocognition of Language* (pp. 319–336). Oxford: Oxford University Press.

Vanier, M., & Caplan, D. (1990). CT-scan correlates of agrammatism. In L. Menn & L.K. Obler (Eds.), *Agrammatic aphasia: A cross-language narrative source book* (pp. 37–114). Amsterdam: John Benjamins.

Vosse, T., & Kempen, G.A.M. (2000). Syntactic structure assembly in human parsing: A computational model based on competitive inhibition and lexicalist grammar. *Cognition, 75*, 105–143.

Whitaker, H.A. (1998). Neurolinguistics from the Middle Ages to the pre-modern era: historical vignettes. In B. Stemmer & H.A. Whitaker (Eds.), *Handbook of Neurolinguistics* (pp. 27–55). San Diego: Academic Press.

Willmes, K., & Poeck, K. (1993). To what extent can aphasic syndromes be localized? *Brain, 116*, 1527–1540.

Zurif, E.B. (1998). The neurological organization of some aspects of sentence comprehension. *Journal of Psycholinguistic Research, 27*, 181–190.

Zurif, E.B., Caramazza, A., & Myerson, R. (1972). Grammatical judgments of agrammatic aphasics. *Neuropsychologia, 10*, 405–417.

16

A Role for Broca's Area Beyond Language Processing: Evidence from Neuropsychology and fMRI

Gereon R. Fink

Zina M. Manjaly

Klaas E. Stephan

Jennifer M. Gurd

Karl Zilles

Katrin Amunts

John C. Marshall

A NEUROPSYCHOLOGICAL AND FUNCTIONAL IMAGING PERSPECTIVE ON THE ROLES OF BROCA'S AREA

Although his paper was only published in 1865 (nearly 30 years after his death), it was Dr. Marc Dax who first associated language functions with the left hemisphere. In 1800, Dax had seen a patient, a captain in the cavalry, who had been wounded in the head by a saber blow and who subsequently suffered from difficulties in remembering words. Dax then read the work of the "organologist" Gall who had made two relevant claims: Gall's first claim was that all mental faculties have their own distinct material substrate in punctate regions of the brain, and his second claim was that each mental faculty is characterized by the content-domain with which it is concerned (Gall, 1822). According to Gall, the cortex is a mosaic of cerebral organs specialized to deal with, for example, language, arithmetic, and music. That is, Gall's organs were defined by the type of material that they analyse and produce rather than by the processes they carry out, irrespective of what was being processed (Marshall, 1984; Marshall and Fink, 2003). For example, "memory of words" and "sense of language and speech," organs 14 and 15 in Gall (1822), were placed side by side in the posterior region of the orbital area of the inferior surface of the frontal lobes. Gall mistakenly thought that the relative sizes (and hence the differential efficiency) of the cortical organs could be inferred from the size of the overlying area of the skull. But more importantly, his craniological (phrenological) localizations could be confirmed (or refuted) by the patterns of impaired and preserved cognitive performance that followed relatively discrete brain lesions: Dax, accordingly, asked where in the head the cavalry officer had been wounded and was told the left parietal region.

Gall, however, had never suggested that language (or any other mental function) could be located in only one side of the brain (frontal or parietal), and hence Dax's observation was puzzling irrespective of its intrahemispheric location: How could a unilateral lesion give rise to such a profound impairment if all mental organs in Gall's scheme were bilaterally represented? Gall's own solution was to conjecture that a sudden insult to one hemisphere could "upset the balance between the two hemispheres, thus affecting the faculties on both sides" (Finger, 2000). Nevertheless, over the following years Dax collected observations on more aphasic patients and eventually concluded that loss of language was indeed preferentially associated with damage to the left half of the brain. Dax presented his paper ["Damage to the left half of the brain associated with forgetting the signs of thought (that is, a loss of words)"] orally at a conference in Montpellier, Le Congrès Méridional in 1836, but died shortly thereafter (McManus, 2002).

Dax's work was only rediscovered some 25 years later, when in 1861 Paul Broca saw two neurological patients with severe language problems. At that time, physicians had already extended the anatomoclinical method (Marshall and Fink, 2003; Marshall and Gurd, 2004) to the study of higher mental functions: brain autopsy at death revealed the pathological changes responsible for the patient's acquired cognitive impairment in life. Paul Broca was an early enthusiast of the method and believed that "if there were ever a phrenological science, it would be the phrenology of convolutions [in the cortex], and not the phrenology of bumps [on the head]" (Broca, 1861). Between Broca (1861) and Liepmann (1900), many cognitive functions were discovered to be impaired after unilateral lesions of the brain. From a physiological point of view these findings were a serious matter: " . . . if it were shown that one particular and perfectly well determined faculty . . . can be affected only by a lesion in the left hemisphere, it would necessarily follow that the two halves of the brain do not have the same attributes—quite a revolution in the physiology of the nervous system. I must say that I could not easily resign myself to accept such a subversive consequence" (Broca, 1861).

Language was the first mental faculty to be studied systematically in terms of its anatomical substrate. From 1825 onward, Jean-Baptiste Bouillaud published many papers on impaired speech after frontal lobe damage in explicit support of Gall's localization of "l'organe du langage articulé" (Bouillaud, 1825) but he never recognized the significance of the laterality of the lesion. Despite his earlier misgivings, Broca himself (1865) eventually became convinced

that unilateral lesions of the *left* third frontal convolution typically gave rise to loss of "the memory of the procedure that is employed to *articulate* language," while equivalent lesions of the right hemisphere did not. Shortly thereafter, Carl Wernicke (1874) observed the association between injury to left temporal cortex and fluent, paraphasic speech combined with impairment of language comprehension. Yet despite these cases many contemporary scientists remained sceptical: "On looking back on brief notes, kept through many years, I find frequent evidences of the conjunction of some form of aphasia with right hemiplegia . . . (nevertheless) . . . I cannot accept—I put no faith in—the theory upheld by M. Broca." As John Hughlings Jackson, the great neurologist, has put it: 'The faculty of language resides nowhere in the brain, because it resides everywhere'" (Watson, 1871).

Nonetheless, many subsequent studies have confirmed the relationship between localized left hemisphere lesions and impairments to core language functions. Over 150 years of research into the neural organization of language based on this anatomoclinical method has stressed the central importance of two regions and their interconnections: Broca's area in inferior frontal cortex and Wernicke's area in the posterior superior temporal region. As a result of this research, the cortical organization of language has long been considered to be largely modular (Bookheimer, 2002). Furthermore, the anatomical substrate of each module was typically large (e.g., Brodmann areas 44/45 or Brodmann's area 22). The story is, however, more complex. For example, small lesions restricted to Broca's area produce few permanent deficits. The wide range of language deficits subsumed under the label of Broca's aphasia usually implicates a larger lesion extending back along the Sylvian fissure. These deficits include problems with articulation, naming, fluent sentence production, morphology, syntax, and the comprehension of some complex syntactic structures. But the range of these impairments makes it difficult to assume that all the underlying functions are indiscriminately computed in one however large area (Bookheimer, 2002). Rather, Alexander et al. (1990) demonstrated with structural magnetic resonance imaging that different lesions around the inferior frontal gyrus correlate with different aphasic symptoms within the overall syndrome of Broca's aphasia.

Finally, there is also neuropsychological evidence that is difficult to reconcile with the claim that left hemisphere language areas are only responsible for language-related functions: Teuber and Weinstein (1956) showed that impairment on the embedded (or hidden) figures task (EFT) could follow injury to any lobe of the brain (frontal, parietal, temporal, and occipital) in either cerebral hemisphere. But, more interestingly, they found that patients with aphasia were significantly more impaired than nonaphasic brain-injured patients, who were in turn more impaired than control subjects. The EFT was originally devised by Gottschaldt (1926; 1929) to study the "influence of past experience upon the perception of visual forms." His findings, however, indicated that the frequency and recency of seeing a target shape had little effect upon the ease of finding that shape when embedded in a more complex figure. Accordingly, subsequent clinical studies have deployed the EFT to investigate the processes of local perception and visual search.

The somewhat unexpected association of a local visual search task with aphasia was replicated by Russo and Vignolo (1967) and Orgass et al. (1972) but no convincing explanation for the association between aphasia and impaired performance on the EFT was put forward. Teuber and Weinstein (1956) suggested that the result may be an artefact of differential severity of brain damage, although ratings of this latter variable in the study of Orgass et al. (1972) were not consistent with this speculation. Furthermore, all the relevant studies took care that the task instructions were understood by the aphasic patients.

Nonetheless, it is not in dispute that Broca's area has language-related functions. Many functional imaging studies support this claim. For example, studies have shown the involvement of inferior frontal cortex in language production (Kim et al., 1997; Petersen et al., 1988), and language comprehension, and in syntactic as well as phonological processing (Chee et al., 1999; Friederici et al., 2003; Zatorre et al., 1996). But recent studies also suggest that Broca's area or parts thereof (Brodmann's area 44) subserve other motor functions in addition to speech and hence may be part of human inferior premotor cortex (Binkofski and Buccino, 2004). Broca's region might thus not only be critical for speech but may also play a more general role in motor control by interfacing external information with the internal motor representations of hand/arm and mouth actions. This claim is based on experiments carried out with brain imaging that showed activation of the inferofrontal gyrus during both the overt and the covert production of actions

(Bonda et al., 1995; Decety et al., 1994; Parsons et al., 1995), mental imagery of grasping movements (Decety et al., 1994; Grafton et al., 1996b), preparation of finger movements to copy a target movement (Toni et al., 1998), and during imagery and execution of visually guided movements (Binkofski et al., 2000; Decety et al., 1994; Stephan et al., 1995).

Common to all these tasks was the preparation of a complex motor act. Furthermore, the involvement of ventral premotor cortex and the pars opercularis of the inferofrontal gyrus in the observation and recognition of actions performed by others (Buccino et al., 2001; Grafton et al., 1996a; Rizzolatti et al., 1996) or in the observation and subsequent imitation of actions (Buccino et al., 2004) has led to the suggestion that the ventral premotor cortex and the pars opercularis of the inferofrontal gyrus in humans might be part of the "mirror neuron system" (Binkofski and Buccino, 2004; Buccino et al., 2004). Thus, functional imaging studies challenge the specificity of the role of Broca's region for language processing. Given the proposal that an observation/execution matching system might provide a necessary bridge from "doing" to "communicating," a role for the mirror neuron system in language evolution has been suggested (Rizzolatti and Arbib, 1998). Such a role would help to reconcile the different results concerning the contribution of Broca's area to language and motor tasks. Yet an involvement of Broca's area in a local visual search task, such as the EFT, would be a mystifying puzzle as no complex motor act is involved and no language-related task component springs to mind.

We accordingly investigated which brain regions are implicated in the EFT. A previous study of the cerebral correlates of the EFT using fMRI (Ring et al., 1999) had contrasted the EFT with a low-level control condition in which subjects fixated on a blank screen. Unsurprisingly, this study design yielded many significant activations that covered all lobes in both hemispheres (Ring et al., 1999). We therefore designed an fMRI experiment (Manjaly et al., 2003) that aimed to isolate the brain regions specifically supporting the EFT compared with both a closely related but easier visual search task and to a high-level baseline (a straightforward shape recognition task). Based on the neuropsychological evidence referred to above, we hypothesized that the EFT would draw specifically upon left hemisphere brain regions that were also involved in language processing. In a second step (Manjaly et al., in press), we analyzed whether any such relationship of the EFT with language-related areas resulted from a yet-to-be-discovered language-related component of the EFT ("hidden language component hypothesis") or rather from a cognitive function unrelated to language but also supported by areas more typically associated with language functions. The latter possibility would strongly suggest that there is no general one-to-one mapping between cognitive functions and the activations of an individual area and thus challenge the notion that language-related areas subserve language-related functions only. It would rather support the importance of "neural context," that is, the hypothesis that the context-dependent binding of a given area into different networks determines the function of that area (McIntosh, 2000). McIntosh (2000) suggests that activation of "a particular region in isolation may not act as a reliable index for a particular cognitive function. Instead, the neural context in which an area is active may define the cognitive function. Neural context emphasizes that the particular spatiotemporal pattern of neural interactions may hold the key to bridge between brain and mind." From this perspective, understanding the potential range of functions of a given area requires us to understand its *context-dependent interactions with other areas*. This view is a challenge to the investigation of functional specialization, as it has been conceived in the large majority of neuropsychological and functional imaging studies to date. It emphasizes the importance of characterizing how *functional integration between different regions* in the brain is achieved (Friston, 1998).

THE ROLE OF BROCA'S AREA IN LOCAL VISUAL SEARCH

Details of our experimental design, data acquisition, and data analysis have been published previously (Manjaly et al., 2003). Here, we briefly summarize the methods, then detail a new analysis of the localization of the activations observed using cytoarchitectonic probability maps, and finally focus on the analysis of effective connectivity, using psychophysiological interactions (PPIs) (see Friston et al., 1997) as reported in Manjaly et al. (in press). Sixteen healthy, right-handed male volunteers (aged 20 to 36 years) with no history of medical illness were studied.

To localize the brain activations that are specific to the local search aspects of the EFT, we compared the EFT with another closely related but easier visual search task (referred to as the "control task") that operated on similar visual stimuli and also engaged visual search, shape analysis, visual matching, decisions about geometrical configurations, and motor responses but that minimized local visual search processes by highlighting the target figure within the complex figure. To investigate whether the spatial arrangement of the stimuli had an influence of how the tasks were performed, we used horizontally and vertically arranged pairs of stimuli equally often. The experimental setup thus constitutes a 2 × 2 factorial design with *task* (EFT versus control) and *stimulus orientation* (horizontal versus vertical) as experimental factors.

In all conditions, each complex figure was accompanied by a simple target figure. These target figures were either embedded into the simultaneously presented complex figures (50% of trials) or were not part of any of the complex figures shown on any trial (50% of trials). To minimize priming effects, each correct target figure was only shown once throughout the entire experiment. Since the incorrect target figures were not embedded in any of the complex figures used in the experiment, they could safely be used twice. Figure 16–1 shows examples of the figures used as stimuli during the EFT and the control task.

For the EFT, subjects were instructed to indicate via right hand button press whether or not the target was embedded in the complex figure. During the control task, subjects were presented with the same stimuli, which were, however, disambiguated: that is, a simple figure within the complex figure was highlighted. For this task, subjects were instructed to indicate via right hand button presses whether or not the target figure matched the simple figure highlighted within the complex figure. The conditions were blocked. Between conditions, a "baseline" was implemented, in which subjects viewed squares or triangles presented centrally and had to indicate via right hand button presses whether or not the figure presented was a square. Before the beginning of each block, instructions for the subsequent task were given, informing the subject of which task to perform and whether the stimuli were arranged horizontally or vertically. The condition sequence was pseudorandomized and counterbalanced across subjects.

Reaction times and error rates were recorded as measures of task difficulty and task performance. Additionally, as the tasks were undertaken in free vision,

Embedded Figures   Control

C1   C3

FIGURE 16–1. Stimuli. Examples of the stimuli used for the embedded figures task (EFT) and the control task. Stimuli were displayed either horizontally or vertically. In the EFT, subjects judged whether the tar- get figure was embedded in the more complex figure. In the control task, subjects judged whether the tar- get figure matched the highlighted figure (indicated in gray) within the complex figure.

we recorded eye movements during the magnetic resonance measurements to assess whether differential eye movements occurred in the EFT and control conditions. Details of the analysis of the behavioral data can be found in our previous article (Manjaly et al., 2003).

Magnetic resonance imaging was performed on a Magnetom Vision 1.5-Tesla scanner (Siemens Medical Systems GmbH, Erlangen, Germany) using a standard head coil. For each subject, a high-resolution, T1-weighted anatomical image was obtained using a MP-RAGE sequence. Functional images were obtained by means of an echo planar imaging (EPI) sequence (for sequence details, see Manjaly et al., 2003)).

Following spatial preprocessing, statistical analysis was performed using a General Linear Model in SPM99 (Friston et al., 1995b). In all statistical analyses, areas of activation were identified as significant only if they passed a threshold of $P_c < 0.05$, corrected for multiple comparisons at the cluster level (Friston, 1997; Friston et al., 1995b). For the fMRI data group analysis, the contrast images from the analyses of the individual subjects were analyzed by one sample t tests. This constituted a random-effects model that allows inference to the population from which the 16 subjects were drawn (Friston et al., 1999). For further details, see Manjaly et al. (2003).

The stereotactic coordinates of the pixels of the local maximum significant activation were determined within areas of significant relative activity change associated with the tasks. The anatomical localization of these local maxima was first assessed with reference to the standard stereotactic atlas (Talairach and Tournoux, 1988). Validation of this method of localization was obtained by superimposition of the SPM maps on the group mean magnetic resonance image calculated after each individual's magnetic resonance image had been stereotactically transformed into the same standard stereotactic space (Friston et al., 1995a).

We then superimposed group activations onto the cytoarchitectonical probabilistic maps of Brodmann's areas 44 and 45, which were brought into stereotactic space (Amunts et al., 2004) and which have been implemented in a toolbox for SPM2, based on in-house software development. The cytoarchitectonic probabilistic maps show for each voxel of the reference brain, the probability with which that voxel can be assigned to Brodmann's areas 44 or 45 (e.g., a probability of 70% for area 44 for a given voxel means that in 7 of 10 postmortem brains this area was found to lie within area 44). We compared the coordinates of the activation maxima found in our functional imaging study with these probabilistic maps.

Finally, for analysis of effective connectivity, we used a variant of psychophysiological interactions (Friston et al., 1997) to determine which brain areas received a context-dependent contribution from the posterior part of the left inferior frontal gyrus (pIFG) cortex and from the intraparietal sulcus (IPS). This procedure is widely used in analyses of effective connectivity (compare, for example, Buchel et al., 1998, and Stephan et al., 2003). The psychophysiological pIFG × task interaction term (referred to as the "PPI regressor") was computed as the element-by-element product of the mean-corrected left pIFG time series (or the mean-corrected left IPS time series, respectively) and a mean-corrected task vector coding for the main effect of task (1 for each scan during the EFT, −1 for each scan during the control task, and

0 elsewhere). In addition to the PPI regressor and the pIFG time series per se, the model of effective connectivity included the main effects of task and stimulus orientation, the highlevel baseline condition, and effects of no interest (instruction periods, movement regressors). Altogether, our analysis of effective connectivity was thus specific for context-dependent pIFG (or IPS) influences that occurred over and above any task effects and context-independent pIFG (or IPS) influences (compare Macaluso et al., 2000, and Stephan et al., 2003). Brain sites receiving contextual pIFG (or IPS) influences that were stronger during EFT than during the control task were determined by testing for positive slopes of the PPI regressor, i.e., by applying a t contrast that was 1 for the PPI regressor and 0 elsewhere. Conversely, areas receiving contextual pIFG (or IPS) influences that were weaker during the EFT than during the control task were found by testing for negative slopes of the PPI regressor, i.e., by applying a t contrast that was -1 for the PPI regressor and 0 elsewhere. The significance of the results was again assessed by correcting for multiple comparisons across the whole brain, using a corrected threshold of $P < 0.05$ at the cluster level (with $P < 0.001$ at the voxel level). For further details, see Manjaly et al. (in press).

Behavioral Results

Analysis of the behavioral data obtained during scanning revealed that subjects performed the EFT significantly more slowly and made significantly more errors than during the control task. Subjects performed the EFT equally well irrespective of display orientation (horizontal/vertical). There was no interaction of the factors *task* and *display orientation*. Eye movement data revealed no significant differences between the EFT and the control task. Any differences in neural activity between the two tasks (see later) thus cannot be ascribed to differential eye movements. Details of all behavioral results can be found in Manjaly et al. (2003).

Neural Activations

As reported in more detail in Manjaly et al. (2003), testing for an overall effect of visual search in geometric figures relative to geometric shape recognition (i.e., the high-level baseline) revealed a mostly sym-

metrical occipitoparietofrontal pattern of activations (Table 16–1A). Bilateral effects ($P_c < 0.05$, corrected) were found in the vermis and lateral cerebellum, lateral occipital cortex, posterior parietal cortex, ventral premotor cortex, and anterior cingulate cortex. Activations specific to the left hemisphere were found in the fusiform and lingual gyri, whereas an activation in the anterior insula was confined to the right hemisphere.

When contrasting the EFT with the control task (i.e., EFT > control task), masked inclusively by control task > baseline (to ensure that activations associated with the EFT were revealed rather than deactivations associated with the control task), the results showed increased neural activity along the left intraparietal sulcus (superior and inferior parietal cortex) and in the left inferior frontal gyrus (Table 16–1B, Fig. 16–2, see color insert).

Comparing the topology of the area of activation in the posterior part of the pIFG (local maximum at x = −42, y = 10, z = 24) with the anatomical probability maps of Brodmann's areas 44 and 45 (Amunts et al., 1999) revealed that 47% of the activated voxels within that area of activation lay in BA 44 (see Fig. 16–3, see color insert). By contrast, only 8% of the activated voxels lay within BA 45.

The reverse comparison, also masked inclusively (i.e., control > EFT masked by EFT > baseline), did not reveal any significant activations associated with the control task relative to the EFT. With regard to factor 2 (*display orientation*), no significant activations were found. Likewise, there was no significant interaction between the factors *task* (EFT, control task) and *display orientation* (horizontal, vertical).

Analysis of Effective Connectivity

The local maximum of the activation in the left pIFG during performance of the EFT served as the starting point for the PPI analysis. For each subject, we determined the local pIFG maximum in the "effects of interest" F contrast that was closest to the group maximum of the EFT > control task contrast and extracted a characteristic regional time series as the basis for the subject-specific PPI analysis. The contrast images resulting from testing for positive and negative regression slopes of the PPI regressor (i.e., the pIFG × task interaction term), respectively, were then entered into standard random-effects group analyses of all six-

TABLE 16–1. Relative Increases in Brain Activity During Performance of the Embedded Figures Task (and the Control Task)

Region	Side	x	y	z	T_{max}	P_c Value
A. Visual search versus baseline: $\frac{1}{4}$ (EFT_h + CT_h + EFT_v + CT_v) > BL						
Vermis + lateral cerebellum	L/R	2	−80	−24	19.34	
Lateral inferior occipital cortex	L	−40	−74	−20	14.40	
	R	46	−70	−18	9.27	
Lateral superior occipital cortex	L	−32	−86	12	13.40	
	R	36	−88	18	11.70	0.0001
Superior posterior parietal cortex	L	−26	−82	36	9.92	
	L	−20	−68	56	9.55	
	R	24	−78	44	11.57	
Fusiform gyrus	L	−28	−54	−20	10.73	
Lingual gyrus	L	−20	−68	−10	8.89	
Ventral premotor cortex (inferior + middle frontal gyrus)	L	−52	12	30	12.50	0.001
	R	56	14	24	8.79	0.0001
Anterior cingulate gyrus	L/R	−2	16	42	8.07	0.012
Right anterior insula	R	40	24	−16	7.42	0.01
B. Embedded Figures Task: EFT_h + EFT_v > CT_h + CT_v						
Ventral premotor cortex (inferofrontal gyrus)	L	−42	10	24	6.77	0.022
Posterior aspect of intraparietal sulcus	L	−24	−58	54	5.15	0.032
Anterior aspect of intraparietal sulcus	L	−36	−38	40	5.01	0.032

Coordinates are in standard stereotactic space and refer to local maxima (distance ≥15 mm) of significant clusters of activated voxels. These maxima were indicated by the locally highest T value (T_{max}) within an area of significant activation (P_c value = corrected P value) associated with the contrasts. k is the number of suprathreshold voxels (each at $P < 0.001$, uncorrected) that together constitute the area of significant activation. x is the distance in millimeters to the right (+) or left (−) of the midsagittal (interhemispheric) line; y is the distance anterior (+) or posterior (−) to the vertical plane through the anterior commissure; and z is the distance above (+) or below (−) the intercommissural line. Anatomical localization is based on the stereotactic atlas and the group mean MR image. R = right, L = left. EFT_h = Embedded Figures Task, horizontal stimulus orientation; EFT_v = Embedded Figures Task, vertical stimulus orientation; CT_h = control task, horizontal stimulus orientation; CT_v = control task, vertical stimulus orientation.

teen subjects (corrected for multiple comparisons across the whole brain, using a corrected cluster-level threshold of $P < 0.05$, with $P < 0.001$ at the voxel level).

In the random-effects group analysis, areas that showed an increased contribution from left pIFG during EFT compared with control task included the left posterior parietal cortex, extrastriate areas bilaterally, and the cerebellar vermis (Fig. 16–4A).

In contrast, areas that received a decreased contribution from the left pIFG during EFT relative to control task included the temporoparietal cortex bilaterally, the posterior cingulate cortex bilaterally, and the left dorsal premotor cortex (Fig. 16–4B).

To complete the characterization of context-dependent functional interactions in our paradigm, we performed analogous PPI analyses for the second area, which, in the conventional SPM analysis, had demonstrated significantly higher activity during the EFT relative to the control task, that is, the left IPS. In this second PPI analysis, the only area that showed an increased contribution from the left IPS during EFT compared with control task was the right posteroparietal cortex (Fig. 16–5a, see color insert). Similar to the PPI results for the left pIFG, the left temporoparietal cortex (Fig. 16–5b, see color insert) was found to receive a decreased contribution from the left IPS during EFT compared with the control task.

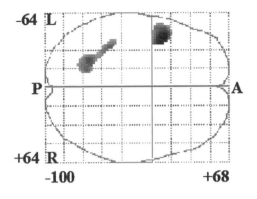
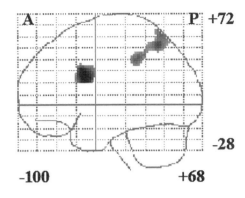

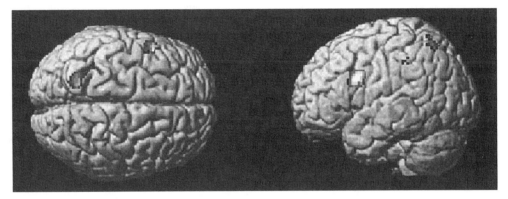

FIGURE 16–2. Main effect of task (EFT versus CT) as reported by Manjaly et al. (2003), random effects analysis (16 subjects). All activations from the EFT versus CT contrast (masked inclusively by the CT versus baseline contrast), significant at a cluster-level corrected threshold of $P < 0.05$, are shown. *Top row:* Maximum intensity projections (glass brains). A, anterior; P, posterior; L, left; R, right. *Bottom row:* Activations overlaid on a rendered template brain.

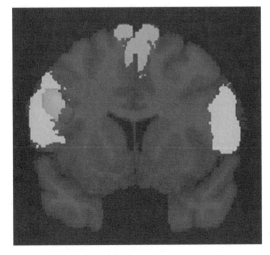

FIGURE 16–3. Overlay of the functional activation of pIFG during EFT (red) with a cytoarchitectonically defined probability map of Brodmann area 44 (light gray).

NETWORKS OF VISUAL SEARCH AND SPATIAL ATTENTION

Previous work has associated visual search (spatial attentional shifts) with activation of superior parietal cortex (Corbetta et al., 1995; Corbetta and Shulman, 2002). Activation of left inferoparietal cortex has been associated with object-based visual attention (Fink et al., 1997a) and with locally directed visual attention in tasks involving hierarchically organized visual stimuli: that is, complex stimuli with both a local and a global organization (Fink et al., 1996, 1997b; Weber et al., 2000). This overall pattern of results is in good accord with our claim that activation of left superior and inferior parietal cortex during performance of the EFT is specifically related to visual search for local targets. More importantly, however, with regard to the association between aphasia and impaired performance on the EFT (Teuber and Weinstein, 1956),

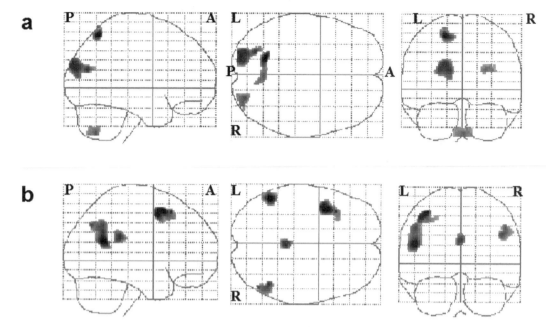

FIGURE 16–4. Results of the PPI analysis, random effects analysis (16 subjects). All areas are shown that receive an increased (*a*) or a decreased (*b*) influence from left pIFG during EFT relative to CT. Cluster-level threshold of $P < 0.05$, corrected for multiple comparisons across the whole brain (voxel-level threshold of $P < 0.001$). Maximum intensity projections (glass brains) of the results: sagittal (*left*), horizontal (*middle*), and coronal (*right*) views. Abbreviations as in Figure 16–2.

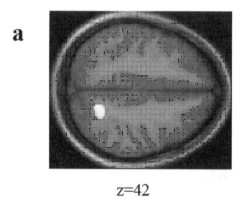

z=42

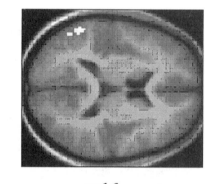

z=16

FIGURE 16–5. Results of the PPI analysis for left IPS, random effects analysis (16 subjects). As in Figures 16–2 through 16–4, results are shown at a cluster-level threshold of $P < 0.05$, corrected for multiple comparisons across the whole brain (voxel-level threshold of $P < 0.001$). (*a*) The only area to receive an increased contribution from left IPS during EFT compared with the control task was the right posterior parietal cortex (18, −62, 42; $t_{max} = 6.69$; $P < 0.001$). (*b*) Similar to the PPI results for the left pIFG (compare with Fig. 16–4), the left temporoparietal cortex (−58, −50, 16; $t_{max} = 4.57$; $P < 0.001$) was found to receive a decreased contribution from the left IPS during EFT relative to the control task.

the region that we found activated in left inferior parietal cortex is relatively close to the posterior language areas of the left hemisphere (Benson, 1979). Furthermore, central disorders of reading and writing may be provoked by lesions of the left supramarginal gyrus (Heilman and Valenstein, 1993).

Likewise, the region of the left inferofrontal gyrus that was activated by performing the EFT is part of the anterior language area as demonstrated by overlying the area of increased neural activity during the EFT with cytoarchitectonically derived probability maps of Brodmann's areas 44 and 45 (Amunts et al., 1999, 2004). Although, in principle, large left hemisphere lesions may result in both aphasia and impairment on the EFT by reason of infarcting two functionally distinct regions (Corkin, 1979), it seems unlikely that the association is simply dependent on the extent of the cerebral pathology, contrary to the claims of Teuber and Weinstein (1956) and Cobrinik (1959). Our results rather imply that two comparatively small regions are associated specifically with local search on the EFT, a finding that is consistent with the observation by Russo and Vignolo (1967) and Orgass et al. (1972) that both large and small lesions can give rise to impairments on the EFT.

The analysis of effective connectivity (i.e., context-dependent functional interactions between different brain regions) of the left pIFG helps to explain the repeatedly observed yet puzzling association between aphasia (due to left hemispheric lesions) and impaired performance on the EFT (Orgass et al., 1972; Russo and Vignolo, 1967; Teuber and Weinstein, 1956). The analysis allows us to distinguish between two possible explanations for why left pIFG, which is usually associated with language processing, might be involved in the execution of the EFT. One hypothesis is that pIFG is activated during the EFT because performing the EFT might involve a "hidden" language-related component that had gone unnoticed by both ourselves and previous researchers. If this "hidden language component hypothesis" was correct and left pIFG function during the EFT was linked to language processes, we would expect to find significant changes in functional interactions with language-related areas, such as the left temporal lobe, during the EFT compared with the control task. The alternative hypothesis is based on the notion of "neural context" (McIntosh, 2000; McIntosh et al., 2003) according to which any given cortical area can contribute to different cognitive processes by participating in multiple networks that are established through context-dependent changes in functional coupling. If this hypothesis is correct and left pIFG can also become involved in local visual search processes, we expected that comparing the functional interactions of left pIFG during the two different visuospatial tasks of our experiment (EFT and the control task) should demonstrate significant changes in coupling with other areas typically involved in visuospatial processing.

In order to assess context-dependent functional interactions and decide between the two hypotheses above, we computed psychophysiological interactions of the left pIFG. Importantly, this method does not determine absolute degrees of coupling, but rather computes the *difference* in the functional contributions of a source area to voxels elsewhere between two different contexts (Friston et al., 1997). Since we had no strong hypotheses on the type of coupling changes induced by the two tasks, we determined the entire set of areas that showed a significant difference in coupling with left IFG between the EFT and the control task, regardless of the direction of this difference.

The results of our PPI analyses suggest that pIFG function is not exclusively linked to language but can cooperate with areas that typically subserve visuospatial functions: during the EFT (relative to the control task), left pIFG increased its contribution to left posterior parietal cortex, bilateral extrastriate cortex, and the cerebellar vermis, and decreased its contribution to left and right temporoparietal cortex, posterior cingulate cortex, and left dorsal premotor cortex (see Figs. 16–4 and 16–5). The involvement of all these areas in various aspects of visuospatial processing has been demonstrated in previous imaging studies (e.g., Corbetta et al., 2000; Corbetta and Shulman, 1998; Fink et al., 1996, 1997a). In contrast, to our knowledge, only two of these areas have also been implicated in language processing: left temporoparietal cortex activation has previously been observed during the processing of spoken language (Binder et al., 1997), and the left dorsal premotor cortex has been linked to verbal working memory (Herwig et al., 2003). These cognitive processes, however, are unlikely to be part of any strategy that could be used to perform either the EFT or the control task: first, spoken words were not part of the stimulus material, and second, the use of verbal working memory was not required to cope with our complex visuospatial displays that remained in full view during task performance (for a more de-tailed discussion, see Manjaly et al., 2003, in press). Moreover, if language-related components had in-deed played a role in our paradigm, one would not have expected the analysis to show higher left pIFG coupling with left temporoparietal and left dorsal pre-motor cortex during the control task than during the EFT. Put the other way around, why should the con-trol task, which was a conventional visual matching task (with minimal visual search), use these putative language-related processes to a greater degree than the more complex EFT?

We thus conclude that the changes in coupling with left pIFG that we have observed in the areas de-scribed earlier reflect functional changes in a more general visuospatial network and are due to the dif-ferent demands that the two tasks place on specific vi-suospatial subprocesses (e.g., direct matching of the target to a "pop-out" element in the control task com-pared to iterative matching during local search in the EFT). This interpretation is supported by additional results from our analysis concerning the context-dependent interactions of the second region that was found to be activated during the EFT relative to the control task, that is, the left IPS (Manjaly et al., 2003, in press). In contrast to left pIFG, there is much pre-vious evidence that left IPS subserves visuospatial functions (e.g., Corbetta et al., 2000; Corbetta and Shulman, 2002; Hopfinger et al., 2000). In our analy-sis, the left IPS showed an increased contribution to the right posterior parietal cortex, another "classic" vi-suospatial area, during EFT compared with the con-trol task (see Fig. 16–5a). Importantly, in analogy to the findings for left pIFG, the reverse comparison demonstrated higher left IPS coupling with the same left temporoparietal region during the control task rel-ative to EFT (Fig. 16–5b).

At a more general level, our findings demonstrate that, depending on the neural context of the task de-mands, left pIFG can contribute to cognitive opera-tions other than language processing. To some extent, this view had previously been suggested by functional imaging experiments of the human "mirror neuron system." These studies have demonstrated that the left pIFG is crucially involved in action understanding and action imitation (Binkofski and Buccino, 2004; Buccino et al., 2001, 2004). Although action under-standing and imitation are not language functions in a strict sense, some proposals have tried to bridge these

two domains by suggesting that the acquisition of lan-guage skills may be linked to the imitation of mouth movements (e.g., Rizzolatti and Arbib, 1998). But our current findings challenge much more radically the traditional view of pIFG as an area exclusively dedi-cated to language than do the results from the above studies of the "mirror neuron system."

CONCLUSIONS

Broca's area (or, more generally, the left inferior frontal region) is undoubtedly implicated in many lan-guage and language-related tasks. The question at is-sue, however, is whether it is legitimate to move from this assertion (supported by very large numbers of le-sion studies and functional neuroimaging experi-ments) to the theoretical claim that the exclusive (or even the core) specialization of Broca's area is the me-diation of language functions. Alternative hypotheses include the possibilities that (1) Broca's area is a mo-saic of many different functional regions, only some of which are directly related to language; (2) Broca's area computes a highly abstract function, such as se-lection from a pool of competing alternative repre-sentations, which subsumes aspects of language pro-cessing and many other cognitive systems, including local visual search (e.g., as in the EFT); and (3) par-ticular neuroanatomical regions, including Broca's area, change their functions consequent upon the si-multaneous activation of other regions that are effec-tively connected to a given region. Our results pro-vide further support for this third conceptual framework in cognitive neuroscience that stresses the importance of context and interactivity for under-standing the functional architecture of the brain (Fris-ton, 1998, 2002; McIntosh, 2000). Although these ap-proaches do not question the existence of specialized computational modules in the brain, they posit that there is no one-to-one mapping between a single anatomical region and a particular cognitive process. Rather, context-dependent interactions within net-works of areas determine the functions of the con-stituent areas. This notion of a distributed architec-ture of brain function implies that a particular area may be part of different networks and hence have dif-ferent functions depending on a given task context. This view is corroborated by neuroanatomical and neurophysiological studies that, collectively, demonstrate that the computational role of any given cortical area cannot be derived from its behavior in a single task or task comparison but is characterized better through its multivariate response profile across a wide range of tasks (Passingham et al., 2002). Such a "functional fingerprint" (Passingham et al., 2002) of a particular area critically depends on its unique pattern of anatomical connections with other areas: That is, the "connectional fingerprint" of an area necessarily constrains its functional interactions. Where an area receives information from and where the processed information can be sent to determine the networks in which the area can participate (Kötter and Stephan, 2003; Passingham et al., 2002).

The notion that a particular area may contribute to more than one cognitive function by participating in more than one functional network represents a one-to-many structure-function relationship. It should be noted that the opposite principle, that is, a many-to-one structure-function relationship, is also realized in the human brain: there are some cognitive functions which can be mediated by means of different (partially overlapping or totally disjoint) networks (Friston and Price, 2003; Price and Friston, 2002). This biological "degeneracy" (Tononi et al., 1999) is found at many different levels, ranging from the genetic code to the systems level of the brain. The degeneracy (in this sense) of the brain, which is believed to be due to sparse structural connectivity patterns ("semiconnectivity") (McIntosh 2000), massively complicates the drawing of reliable causal inferences about structure-function relationships from the study of behavioral deficits consequent upon brain lesions (Price and Friston, 2002; Young et al., 2000). Both types of mapping, that a particular area can participate in different cognitive functions and that a particular cognitive function can be mediated by different networks of areas, demonstrate the highly distributed architecture of the human brain. To disentangle these complex structure-function relationships will be a major challenge for the neurosciences in the twenty-first century (Friston et al., 2003).

ACKNOWLEDGMENTS   J.C.M. and J.M.G. are supported by the Medical Research Council (MRC), United Kingdom. K.Z. and G.R.F. are supported by the Deutsche Forschungsgemeinschaft (DFG-KFO 112), Germany. K.E.S. is funded by the Wellcome Trust, United Kingdom. Additional support from the VolkswagenStiftung to J.C.M., K.Z., and G.R.F. is gratefully acknowledged.

References

Alexander, M.P., Naeser, M.A., & Palumbo, C. (1990). Broca's area aphasias: Aphasia after lesions including the frontal operculum. *Neurology, 40*, 353–362.

Amunts, K., Schleicher, A., Burgel, U., Mohlberg, H., Uylings, H.B., & Zilles, K. (1999). Broca's region revisited: cytoarchitecture and intersubject variability. *Journal of Comparative Neurology, 412*, 319–341.

Amunts, K., Weiss, P.H., Mohlberg, H., Pieperhoff, P., Eickhoff, S., Gurd, J.M., et al. (2004). Analysis of neural mechanisms underlying verbal fluency in cytoarchitectonically defined stereotaxic space—The roles of Brodmann areas 44 and 45. *NeuroImage, 22*, 42–56.

Benson, D.F. (1979). *Aphasia, alexia, and agraphia,*. New York: Churchill Livingstone.

Binder, J.R., Frost, J.A., Hammeke, T.A., Cox, R.W., Rao, S.M., & Prieto, T. (1997). Human brain language areas identified by functional magnetic resonance imaging. *Journal of Neuroscience, 17*, 353–363.

Binkofski, F., Amunts, K., Stephan, K.M., Posse, S., Schormann, T., Freund, H.J., et al. (2000). Broca's region subserves imagery of motion: A combined cytoarchitectonic and fMRI study. *Human Brain Mapping, 11*, 273–285.

Binkofski, F., & Buccino, G. (2004). Motor functions of the Broca's region. *Brain and Language, 89*, 362–369.

Bonda, E., Petrides, M., Frey, S., & Evans, A.C. (1995). Neural correlates of mental transformations of the body-in-space. *Proceedings of the National Academy of Science USA, 92*, 11180–11184.

Bookheimer, S. (2002). Functional MRI of language: New approaches to understanding the cortical organization of semantic processing. *Annual Review Neuroscience, 25*, 151–188.

Bouillaud, J.B. (1825). Recherches cliniques propres à demontrer que la perte de la parole correpond à la lésion des lobuls antérieurs du cerveau et à confirmer l'opinion de M Gall, sur le siège de l'organe du langage articulé. *Archives of General Medicine, 6*, 25–45.

Broca, P. (1861). Nouvelle observation d'aphemic produite per une lesion de la moité postérieur des deuxième et troisième conconvolutions frontales. *Bulletin of the Society of Anatomy of Paris, 36*, 398–407.

Broca, P. (1865). Sur le siège de la faculté du langage articulé. *Bulletin of the Society of Anthropology of Paris, 6*, 377–393.

Buccino, G., Binkofski, F., Fink, G.R., Fadiga, L., Fogassi, L., Gallese, V., et al. (2001). Action observation activates premotor and parietal areas in a somatotopic manner: An fMRI study. *European Journal of Neuroscience, 13*, 400–405.

Buccino, G., Vogt, S., Ritzl, A., Fink, G.R., Zilles, K., Freund, H.-J., et al. (2004). Neural circuits underlying imitation learning of hand actions: An event-related fMRI study. *Neuron, 42*, 323–334.

Buchel, C., Josephs, O., Rees, G., Turner, R., Frith, C.D., & Friston, K.J. (1998). The functional anatomy of attention to visual motion. A functional MRI study. *Brain, 121*, 1281–1294.

Chee, M.W.L., O'Kraven, K.M., Bergida, R., Rosen, B.R., & Savoy, R.L. (1999). Auditory and visual word processing studied with fMRI. *Human Brain Mapping, 7*, 15–28.

Cobrinik, L. (1959). The performance of brain-injured children on hidden-figures tasks. *American Journal of Psychology, 72*, 566–571.

Corbetta, M., Kincade, J.M., Ollinger, J.M., McAvoy, M.P., & Shulman, G.L. (2000). Voluntary orienting is dissociated from target detection in human posterior parietal cortex. *Nature Neuroscience, 3*, 292–297.

Corbetta, M., Shulman, G.L., Miezin, F.M., & Petersen, S.E. (1995). Superior parietal cortex activation during spatial attention shifts and visual feature conjunction. *Science, 270*, 802–805.

Corbetta, M., & Shulman, G.L. (1998). Human cortical mechanisms of visual attention during orienting and search. *Philosophical Transactions of the Royal Society of London B, 353*, 1353–1362.

Corbetta, M., & Shulman, G.L. (2002). Control of goal-directed and stimulus-driven attention in the brain. *Nature Review of Neuroscience, 3*, 201–215.

Corkin, S. (1979). Hidden-figures-test performance: Lasting effects of unilateral penetrating head injury and transient effects of bilateral cingulotomy. *Neuropsychologia, 17*, 585–605.

Decety, J., Perani, D., Jeannerod, M., Bettinard, V., Tadardy, B., Woods, R., et al. (1994). Mapping motor representations with positron emission tomography. *Nature, 371*, 600–602.

Finger, S. (2000). *Minds behind the brain: A history of the pioneers and their discoveries.* Oxford: Oxford University Press.

Fink, G.R., Dolan., R.J., Halligan, P.W., Marshall, J.C., & Frith, C.D. (1997a). Space-based and object-based visual attention: shared and specific neural domains. *Brain, 120*, 2013–2028.

Fink, G.R., Halligan, P.W., Marshall, J.C., Frith, C.D., Frackowiak, R.S.J., & Dolan, R.J. (1996). Where in the brain does visual attention select the forest and the trees? *Nature, 382*: 626–628.

Fink, G.R., Halligan, P.W., Marshall, J.C., Frith, C.D., Frackowiak, R.S.J., & Dolan, R.J. (1997b). Neural mechanisms involved in the processing of global and local aspects of hierarchically organized visual stimuli. *Brain, 120*, 1779–1791.

Friederici, A.D., Ruschemeyer, S.A., Hahne, A., & Fiebach, C.J. (2003). The role of left inferior frontal and superior temporal cortex in sentence comprehension: Localizing syntactic and semantic processes. *Cerebral Cortex, 13*, 170–177.

Friston, K.J. (1997). Testing for anatomically specified regional effects. *Human Brain Mapping, 5*, 133–166.

Friston, K.J. (1998). Imaging neuroscience: Principles or maps? *Proceedings of National Academy of Science USA, 95*, 796–802.

Friston, K.J. (2002). Beyond phrenology: What can neuroimaging tell us about distributed circuitry? *Annual Review of Neuroscience, 25*, 221–250.

Friston, K.J., Ashburner, J., Frith, C.D., Poline, J.-B., Heather, J.D., & Frackowiak, R.S.J. (1995a). Spatial registration and normalization of images. *Human Brain Mapping, 3*, 165–189.

Friston, K.J., Büchel, C., Fink, G.R., Morris, J., Rolls, E.T., & Dolan, R.J. (1997). Psychophysiological and modulatory interactions in neuroimaging. *NeuroImage, 6*, 218–229.

Friston, K.J., Harrison, L., & Penny, W. (2003). Dynamic causal modeling. *NeuroImage, 19*, 1273–1302.

Friston, K.J., Holmes, A., Worsley, K.J., Poline, J.-B., Frith, C.D., & Frackowiak, R.S.J. (1995b). Statistical parametric maps in functional imaging: A general linear approach. *Human Brain Mapping, 2*, 189–210.

Friston, K.J., Holmes, A.P., & Worsley, K.J. (1999). How many subjects constitute a study? *NeuroImage, 10*, 1–5.

Friston, K.J., & Price, C.J. (2003). Degeneracy and redundancy in cognitive anatomy. *Trends in Cognitive Sciences, 7*, 151–152.

Gall, F.J. (1822). *Sur les functions du cerveau et sur cell de chacune de ses parties.*, Paris: Baillière.

Gottschaldt, K. (1926). Über den Einfluss der Erfahrung auf die Wahrnehmung von Figuren, I. *Psychol Forsch, 8*, 261–317.

Gottschaldt, K. (1929). Über den Einfluss der Erfahrung auf die Wahrnehmung von Figuren, II. *Psychol Forsch, 12*, 1–87.

Grafton, S.T., Arbib, M.A., Fadiga, L., & Rizzolatti, G. (1996a). Localization of grasp representation in humans by positron emission tomography: II. Observation compared with imagination. *Exp Brain Res, 112*, 103–111.

Grafton, S.T., Fagg, A.H., Woods, R.P., & Arbib, M.A. (1996b). Functional anatomy of pointing and grasping in humans. *Cerebral Cortex, 6*, 226–237.

Heilman, K.M., & Valenstein, E. (1993). *Clinical neuropsychology.*, Oxford: Oxford University Press.

Herwig, U., Abler, B., Schonfeldt-Lecuona, C., Wunderlich, A., Grothe, J., Spitzer, M., et al. (2003). Verbal storage in a premotor-parietal network: Evidence from fMRI-guided magnetic stimulation. *NeuroImage, 20*, 1032–1041.

Hopfinger, J.B., Buonocore, M.H., & Mangun, G.R. (2000). The neural mechanisms of top-down attentional control. *Nature Neurosciences, 3*, 284–291.

Kim, K.H., Relkin, N.R., Lee, K.M., & Hirsch, J. (1997). Distinct cortical areas associated with native and second languages. *Nature, 388*, 171–174.

Kötter, R., & Stephan, K.E. (2003). Network participation indices: Characterizing component roles for information processing in neural networks. *Neural Networks, 16*, 1261–1275.

Liepmann, H. (1900). Das Krankheitsbild der Apraxie ("motorischen Asymbolie") aufgrund eines Falles von einseitiger Apraxie. *Monatsschrift für Psychiatrie und Neurologie, 8*, 15–44.

Macaluso, E., Frith, C.D., & Driver, J. (2000). Momdulation of human visual cortex by crossmodal spatial attention. *Science, 289*, 1206–1208.

Manjaly, Z.M., Marshall, J.C., Stephan, K.E., Gurd, J.M., Zilles, K., & Fink, G.R. (2003). In search of the hidden: An fMRI study with implications for the study of patients with autism and with acquired brain injury. *NeuroImage, 19*, 674–683.

Manjaly, Z.M., Marshall, J.C., Stephan, K.E., Gurd, J.M., Zilles, K., & Fink, G.R. (2004). Context-dependent interactions of left posterior inferior frontal gyrus in a local visual search task unrelated to language. *Cognitive Neuropsychology*, (in press).

Marshall, J.C. (1984). Multiple perspectives on modularity. *Cognition, 17*, 209–242.

Marshall, J.C., & Fink, G.R. (2003). Cerebral localization, then and now. *NeuroImage, 20*, S2–S7.

Marshall, J.C., & Gurd, J.M. (2004). On the anatomo-clinical method. *Cortex, 40*, 230–231.

McIntosh, A.R. (2000). Towards a network theory of cognition. *Neural Networks, 13*, 861–870.

McIntosh, A.R., Rajah, M.N., & Lobaugh, N.J. (2003). Functional connectivity of the medial temporal lobe relates to learning and awareness. *Journal of Neuroscience, 23*, 6520–6528.

McManus, C. (2002). *Right hand, left hand.*, Cambridge, MA: Harvard University Press.

Orgass, B., Poeck, K., Kirchensteiner, M., & Hartje, W. (1972). Visuo-cognitive performances in patients with unilateral hemispheric lesions. An investigation with three factorial reference tests. *Z Neurol, 202*, 177–195.

Parsons, L.M., Fox, P.T., Hunter Downs, J., Glass, T., Hirsch, T.B., Martin, C.C., et al. (1995). Use of implicit motor imagery for visual shape discrimination as revealed by PET. *Nature, 375*, 54–58.

Passingham, R.E., Stephan, K.E., & Kötter, R. (2002). The anatomical basis of functional localization in the cortex. *Nature Review Neuroscience, 3*, 606–616.

Petersen, S.E., Fox, P.T., Snyder, A.Z., & Raichle, M.E. (1988). Positron emission tomographic studies of the cortical anatomy of single-word processing. *Nature, 331*, 585–589.

Price, C.J., & Friston, K.J. (2002). Degeneracy and cognitive anatomy. *Trends in Cognitive Sciences, 6*, 416–421.

Ring, H.A., Baron-Cohen, S., Wheelwright, S., Williams, S.C.R., Brammer, M., Andrew, C., et al. (1999). Cerebral correlates of perserved cognitive skills in autism. A functional MRI study of embedded figures task performance. *Brain, 122*, 1305–1315.

Rizzolatti, G., & Arbib, M.A. (1998). Language within our grasp. *Trends in Neuroscience, 21*, 188–194.

Rizzolatti, G., Fadiga, L., Matelli, M., Bettinardi, V., Paulesu, E., Perani, D., et al. (1996). Location of grasp representations in humans by PET. 1. Observation versus execution. *Experimental Brain Research, 111*, 246–252.

Russo, M., & Vignolo, L.A. (1967). Visual figure-ground discrimination in patients with unilateral cerebral disease. *Cortex, 3*, 113–127.

Stephan, K.E., Marshall, J.C., Friston, K.J., Rowe, J.B., Ritzl, A., Zilles, K., et al. (2003). Lateralized cognitive processes and lateralized task control in the human brain. *Science, 301*, 384–386.

Stephan, K.M., Fink, G.R., Passingham, R.E., Silbersweig, D.A., Ceballos-Baumann, A.O., Frith, C.D., et al. (1995). Imagining the execution of movements. Functional anatomy of the mental representation of upper extremity movements in healthy subjects. *Journal of Neurophysiology, 73*, 373–386.

Talairach, J., & Tournoux, P. (1988). *Co-planar stereotactic atlas of the human brain,*. Stuttgart: Thieme.

Teuber, H.-L., & Weinstein, S. (1956). Ability to discover hidden figures after cerebral lesions. *Archives of Neurology and Psychiatry, 76*, 369–379.

Toni, I., Krams, M., Turner, R., & Passingham, R.E. (1998). The time course of changes during motor learning: A whole brain fMRI study. *NeuroImage, 8*, 50–61.

Tononi, G., Sporns, O., & Edelman, G.M. (1999). Measures of degeneracy and redundancy in biological networks. *Proceedings of National Academy of Science USA*, 96, 257–326.

Watson, T. (1871). *Lectures on the principles and practice of physic.* London: Jon W Parker.

Weber, B., Schwarz, U., Kneifel, S., Treyer, V., & Buck, A. (2000). Hierarchical visual processing is dependent on the oculomotor system. *Neuroreport*, 11, 241–247.

Wernicke, C. (1874). *Der aphasische Symptomenkomplex.*, Breslau: Cohn & Weigart.

Young, M.P., Hilgetag, C.C., & Scannell, J.W. (2000). On imputing function to structure from the behavioural effects of brain lesions. *Philosophical Transactions of Royal Society of London B*, 355, 147–161.

Zatorre, R.J., Meyer, E., Gjedde, A., & Evans, A.C. (1996). PET studies of phonetic processing of speech: Review, replication, and reanalysis. *Cerebral Cortex*, 6, 21–30.

V

DISCUSSION

The Jülich workshop featured long hours of discussion, inside the conference room as well as outside. The excerpts that follow represent the main issues that arise when one attempts to reconcile the multiple perspectives that currently exist on Broca's region.

17

Jülich Workshop Excerpts

Karl Zilles:

What interested me during this conference is the confusion which comes out when different approaches like the linguistic, the clinical and anatomical are used in the different talks. For example, everybody refers to Broca's region, to Broca's complex, to area 44, to area 45, or to area 47. It is my impression, that this notion is not well defined, more or less chaotic. It is not just a question of nomenclature, but a problem which goes into the interpretation of the data.

For instance, when somebody says that "we found in a clinical study something which is related to a dysfunction of Broca's area 47" and later discusses data from areas 45, this cannot be done, because the "area 47" is not defined. It's rather like "anterior and very ventral" relative to the inferior frontal gyrus, whereas the meaning in the second statement is, let's say cortical area 45, or 44, if it's a bit more posterior. In some cases this notion refers to the mean of a group study, whereas in other cases it is a single brain. The reference system, as well as the way the data came into this system, also differ. Sometimes, it's done by a mathematically controlled elastic warping procedure to a common reference space, whereas in other talks it's just a reference to the Talairach atlas. So we use the definitions of cortical areas in different ways, mixing and matching, and then we end up with theories and statements, which become accepted in the community. But, these statements don't really tell us very much.

So, I would really like to hear your opinion about this because some people tell me "I'm absolutely not interested in these anatomical issues, it's not necessary. I can do my functional studies. I don't need any anatomical atlas, any anatomical basis." This is one viewpoint, but there may be other participants who are interested in knowing whether the blob they see in images is in a structurally homogeneous brain area, or is distributed over different areas. So, what do you think about this situation?

Luciano Fadiga:

I am a neurophysiologist. Usually we believe that anatomical differences correspond to functional differences. For example, if there is an area in which the fourth cortical layer is developed, this differential development is due to a functional reason. It might be, for example, that this particular region of cortex receives a lot of thalamic input, while another region cannot receive this input from the thalamus, hence the differentiation is missing.

So, I think we should really keep in mind that the anatomical subdivision is not simply a classification trick used by neuroanatomists to subdivide the brain. We must remember that there is much confirmation to the claim that for every anatomically classified brain lesion, there is a corresponding function. I think that we can start from this common point of view.

Sergey Avrutin:

I'd like to give an opposite perspective, coming from work with aphasic patients. With my linguistic background, I think that the studies with aphasic patients can actually contribute to the *linguistic* theory independently of the exact knowledge where the damage is. Specifically, suppose that there are two linguistic theories, theory I and theory II. Theory I claims that certain constructions, X and Y, are grouped together. Theory II claims that these are two distinct linguistic constructions. Data from aphasic patients can actually tell us which theory is true. Here is how. Suppose that the patients perform equally well on both constructions. Then it is evidence for theory I, but not II. In this case, we can circumvent the problem of complete localization. We simply don't care. We would care if we were to focus on localization, but then it becomes a question of how one focuses one's research program. If it is on localization, then localization is important; but if your research aims to contribute to a general understanding of language, then it can be ignored.

Francisco Aboitiz:

Sergey's preferred question would be a general understanding of language, and in this way there would be no need to know about localization. But what do you mean by that precisely? I mean, that a general understanding of the organization of language in-

cludes the knowledge of the involved neural processes. If you want to know that you will need to know about localization, anyway.

Sergey Avrutin:

Well, the statement that we don't care is too strong of course. Neurologists tell me that the issue of localization is a mess, and so you can abstract away and approximate. There are Broca's aphasics which are usually classified according to, say, the Boston test, or whatever. Eventually you would like to have of course a very clear connection with localization, to the extent that it exists. What I'm saying is that at the moment, when a typology does not exist, this should not prevent us from working with aphasic patients, and make inferences about function.

Karl Zilles:

I think that there is already a problem. When you look at the classic case of Broca, a lot of people say "Aha, this is Broca's region, where the hole is." But when you have a look to the MR scan of this brain, you will see that—we heard it repeatedly during this meeting—there is much more destroyed tissue in this brain. Then, a question arises whether it is a white matter disease, or a problem of the destroyed connectivity, or a problem of this particular cortical region which includes areas 44, 45, or whether it is a question of subcortical structures. Immediately, you get in trouble with the anatomists, because you have to really define the question. Therefore, I think that the question for structure and functional correlates comes up very early.

Stefano Cappa:

I think that Sergey's point is perfectly legitimate. It depends from what angle you are doing research. Twenty years of cognitive neuropsychology have been basically ignoring the brain completely. I think this is a perfectly legitimate enterprise. It does not detract from the fact that nowadays, especially with functional imaging, many people are asking different kinds of questions, e.g., how language is represented in the brain. At that point, the precision in the anatomy cannot be avoided. To be fair to the field, 15 or 16 years ago it was impossible to be very precise with respect to anatomy, because of positron emission tomography, group studies averaging, a lack of good atlas, etc. Given that, it is appropriate to discuss the data in terms of "slightly more anterior" or "slightly more posterior." I did it, for example, in my talk as well because if you're not very confident about localization, it's only fair to talk in vague terms like anterior, posterior and so on.

Kyle Johnson:

I'd like to talk against Sergey Avrutin. You've got two natural classes, given to you by virtue of the diagnostic criteria for Broca's aphasia, and you know nothing about the physiological basis of these natural classes. But it is still OK, because we've got these two natural classes, by virtue of which we can determine whether the cuts made by linguistic theory or psychological theory are correct. But then there is still a question remaining: What are the diagnostic criteria for distinguishing Broca's aphasics from non-Broca's aphasics?

Sergey Avrutin:

Actually what I meant is that we can just use one group who are diagnosed as Broca's aphasics, and apply the data to two different linguistic theories, without even comparing their performance to a different group. There are tests to classify patients. For some patients, we look at the scans. However, after you work with patients for a while, you just see that a patient is more or less "typical" than another. So there is a bunch of factors to classify patients. There is a difference between patients and I don't even try to say anything about anatomy with these patients.

Stefano Cappa:

There are several points of investigation where you don't need to classify the patients. You don't need classification if you're just testing a psycholinguistic hypothesis on a patient with language disorder.

Gereon Fink:

I think the story is even more complicated. You can't classify many acute stroke patients with lesions of the left hemisphere. They don't fall under Broca's or Wer-

nicke's aphasia or whatever. They are nonclassifiable. After a while, they evolve, e.g., into Broca's aphasics. Thus, when we talk about Broca's aphasia or Wernicke's aphasia, we are talking about something that depends on reconstitution of brain function, on neural plasticity. We often talk about an endpoint, after a lot of changes have happened in the brain, where we have no clue what they are. Such changes occur in the perilesioned areas of the same hemisphere, or in the homologue areas of the other hemisphere. I really think we have to take that into account when we talk about localization of a brain function based on lesions.

Karl Zilles:

With respect to localization and brain maps it seems to me that the probability maps are a fundamental different concept of cytoarchitecture when compared with the maps in the past. The latter suggest that there is a more or less well-defined border. The probability maps tell a different story. You can only choose a probability and then you will see the border here or there. Then you choose a different probability, and you will see the border at another place. We can only make probability statements about the precise location of the border of a cortical area. This is the only—let's say—the only possible way to speak about cytoarchitecture, and how does probability and structure and function fit together. Well, there are experimental studies in animals with extremely high spatial resolution, which show that there is a change in function within 100 micrometers. These studies show that, precisely at the same site, there is a change in the anatomical and cytoarchitectonic structure, in particular. In the somatosensory cortex of rats, for instance, where you have representation of single whiskers, you see abrupt changes at the border of the barrels. For an example in the human brain I refer to the human visual cortex where you have abrupt changes in cytoarchitecture and corresponding changes in function at the border of the striate to the extrastriate cortex. Moreover, you even can identify a small region in between where the meridian is localized. You can see it in the anatomy of the visual cortex. When you look for such areas in different individuals, however, you will see a tremendous variability and therefore when we want to make a general statement about the human cortical brain map, then we can only do it as a probability map.

DIVERSITY OF FUNCTIONAL ANALYSES
OF LANGUAGE

Yosef Grodzinsky:

I would like to shift attention to behavior, if you don't mind. I've been following Karl Zilles' comments very carefully because he tries to keep everybody precise about anatomical statements. I think it's fascinating to see how difficult it is to make a precise anatomical statement as an anatomist, and how it becomes more difficult once you get into lesion data, and on to functional imaging. Anatomical problems keep recurring. The biology is imposing incredibly hard problems on us.

But I want to shift focus because I and many of my colleagues find ourselves in exactly the same situation on the behavioral front. Each and every one of the issues you raise has a parallel in the analysis of behavior. Consider what Zilles said about problems in scoping lesions. Well, look at diagnostic tests of aphasia and you will see practical, conceptual and other problems that similarly arise. While the problem is not limited to language, there are special problems in the case of language. First, what is the framework within which you carve up behavior. And here you discover that if you try to put studies together and interpret them, you quickly discover that people mean very different things when they talk about the lexicon, or phonology, or for that matter the real, the true, the general, diagnostic test. Likewise, when you look at what people do in functional imaging, not only do they use different tasks and different analytic software and different slices and different number of slices, and different blurring filters and so on, but they also use very, very different language tasks. Thus what is fascinating to me about Karl Zilles' presentation is the fact that when you turn to look at the behavioral front, you find an exact parallel to the problems in anatomy you pointed out.

Michael Arbib:

A diversity of linguistic theories came up in the presentations here and in the related papers. I'm firstly struck by the fact that Chomsky for many years was very insistent on the separation between competence and performance and that his theory was a competence theory. I see many people here using straight Chomskian competence grammar as part of a performance theory without any methodological discussion of how it is appropriate to go from what was explicitly declared by the master to be only appropriate for competence.

Yosef Grodzinsky:

Can you give a concrete example of what you mean?

Michael Arbib:

Your trace-deletion hypothesis is an example. There's no processing model there. You simply say, let's consider trees and imagine deleting the traces, which is an absurd notion from a processing point of view because it assumes that the traces are there to be deleted rather than offering a processing account of what an aphasic brain does. I cannot believe that what it does is to construct the traces and delete them. So, it is not a coherent processing account.

Naama Friedmann has a beautiful analysis of production data. What is the thing that connects this beautiful competence account to a processing account for production and perception? What are the ways those trees are constructed? What would it mean to say to "add higher nodes"?

In the same way I'm seeing what maybe coherent linguistic accounts, what may be divergent linguistic accounts, but I see no consistent attempt in the literature to map them to each other. I find each study fascinatingly compelling. Then I go to the next study and there's a completely different linguistic framework and no account of whether those two frameworks really are incompatible, they could be reconciled.

Kyle Johnson:

I wanted to respond to one thing because it's a frustration of anyone coming to the linguistic literature from outside. It's just a living hell for those of us inside, of course. I mean the divergent terminologies and mechanisms offered by different frameworks. But the resolution that you need for the kinds of studies you have here, the sorts of distinctions you need to make, are distinctions that never divide linguistic theory so far as I know or frameworks. So for instance, in each of the papers that I've seen today, different frameworks have been employed. You know in particular the sort of syntax-lexical relationship that Peter Hagoort gave us is quite different from that which would be used by Yosef Grodzinsky's trace-deletion hypothesis. But the distinctions between these two models are for the most part immaterial, as far as I can see. Immaterial to the sorts of questions you're trying to find answers to. I think that for the questions we look at in the neuroscience of language you could really use baby versions of linguistic theory and still get very far.

Look at the principles that grab the phenomena and sort of strip away the terminology that expresses a particular point of view. Take all that extra stuff away, and just look at the phenomena that ground the terminology and that framework, and you'll find that the grounding is exactly the same. So, the same set of phenomena, the same sets of constraints, the models are slightly different, but what's relevant here is the relationship between where you speak this term and some facet of its interpretation. So, I could take the trace-deletion hypothesis, express it in an LFG framework, find the homologue of traces in LFG and I would have the same thesis, empirically, the same thesis that the trace deletion has.

Peter Hagoort:

You have to accept different meanings of cognitive neuroscience. It's very hard to convince people in cognitive neuroscience that, compared to memory and vision, language is a relevant and interesting topic. They say well, we get these linguists, they come and throw their tree structures on the blackboard, make some hand-waving claims about the fact that this all has to be instantiated in some way in the brain, and you neuroscientists go off and tell us exactly that this theory by Mr. Chomsky or whatever version of it is the correct one. That's the perceived attitude in the field of neuroscience.

As a result, people in neuroscience are not willing to go and test a very specific linguistic theory, because they need the vocabulary that allows them to ask the right questions with regard to the brain, and if they're at all interested in whether the address of the account of Mr. Chomsky or Mr. Such and Such, they want an account that would convince not only one particular kind of linguist, but also others.

In addition, you have to specify the nature of the representations being computed. That's part of your processing model, and you need to be explicit about it. Many domains of neuroscience fall in the trap that we don't have an explicit account of what the nature of the representation is being computed.

Yosef Grodzinsky:

I think there are several issues here. First, any theory must accommodate the types of linguistic phenomena we are familiar with. Second, there's an observed aphasic deficit that any theory of language must account for. It doesn't matter whether it's traces or a construct that other theories might use. In this respect, aphasia does not distinguish between linguistic theories.

Moreover, remember that we use this concept (trace) as a descriptive device that carves up behavior. It doesn't mean that we have a neuronal theory of traces and syntactic movement. You use it as a descriptive device and then you go along to see what the next thing that you can discover. Now, there are rare cases which interest Sergey, and interest me, which are those rare cases that do distinguish between linguistic theories. These are extremely interesting cases. But for the most part, these are cases that we don't present to an audience that is interested in brain-language relations. Here we look at core issues which *any* rational linguistic theory must account for. And it doesn't matter what they call it. In other words, the problem of diversity among linguistic theories for the core data here is immaterial and what you have to know is sort of to brush off the terminology and stay with the core conceptions. Furthermore, as long as your claim is used in this theory as a descriptive device, you're not committed to a processing theory because it's not as if you want to derive the behavior from some neuronal theory. You just use it as a descriptive behavior that correlates brain areas with some kind of behavioral distinction. In this respect you simply do the best you can.

Lewis Shapiro:

I absolutely agree that there is a knee jerk reaction to particular kinds of linguistic theories and there are knee jerk reactions from students to neuroscientists. It may simply be because the vocabulary that we use is just outside what you have learned. Same goes for physics: maybe I don't understand the physical vocabulary, but I wouldn't ever say physics isn't important, or physics is the wrong thing to do, or that particular physical theory.

REPRESENTATION AND PROCESSING

Kyle Johnson:

One of the things I found interesting in Naama Friedmann's presentation is that it presented a map of what linguistic theory divides. Linguistic theories, all of them, you know, what they call natural classes. And, her account is based on a syntactic distinction between a high part of a tree and a low part of a tree, given the tree for some sentence. And the characterization of the deficit makes a distinction between the "high part" and "low part" and is tied to a very particular data set. Only a few frameworks model this data set and how she's modeled it would go with any of those frameworks as far as I can see.

But, I do not know of a linguistic theory that makes a divide between high and low. So, the interesting analysis you have uses a method of syntactic representation, but what makes the class—what partitions the data—is something that linguistic theory doesn't make, at least so far as I know.

So, I look at her characterization of the deficit she was studying and I say, that's not a linguistic deficit. It just does not align with what I know to be the general way of carving up nature that linguistic theories give us. But, this is interesting: you have a very specific linguistic theory in which you're describing data, but actually the conclusion should be, I would say, that what's modeled is not only a linguistic deficit. We need some bridge between what's found there and she offered some hypotheses about what that bridge might be, but without the linguistic theories it doesn't matter their particular nature, you wouldn't be able to see that. So, that's what I would claim is the role that linguists can bring here, we have some map of where the natural classes are, how the phenomenon should be divided up, we have some idea about what the phenomena are. And then there is a very big and open question. Is that a correct characterization?

Naama Friedmann:

I think it is, in a way. It is true that I don't see anything in syntactic theory that predicts that high nodes will be more impaired than low nodes, but I can imagine several reasons for that. Based on my data, I have no support for any specific reason for why high nodes are more impaired than low nodes. However, when you look at individual differences and individual patterns,

when you look at recovery patterns, and when you look at treatment results, the data definitely show it.

Why this is so I can only speculate. I can think of several reasons why high nodes would be more impaired. One would be to give it a processing flavor, and to say well, maybe there is a limit to the number of layers we can accumulate and the number of layers are counted from down to up. So, this is one possible way to account for it.

Another way of accounting for it that Sergey Avrutin and I discussed, is to bank on the fact that the higher nodes may be related to discourse. This would, in a way, put Sergey's account and mine together. It would amount to saying that the high nodes are impaired because they are related to discourse, not because they are higher. There are predictions here: To refute this account, we have to find discourse related elements that are lower in the tree, or elements that are not discourse related that are higher in the tree. So that's another way to think about it. One more way might involve syntactic constraints on projection. So, these are three ways to think about it, but what I provided was the data and the generalization, and the next step will be to think why high nodes are more impaired.

Karen Emmorey:

Naama, going back to this "processing issue," what do you think is actually going on when patients are trying to produce these sentences in terms of a processing model of language production?

Naama Friedmann:

I would like to emphasize again that the deficit may not be linguistic—it might be one of the ideas I proposed, or it might be something about processing or about syntactic working memory. But what I think is very important here is that you need a very specific syntactic theory in order to account for the deficit. So if you don't have a well articulated syntactic theory, you are not likely to understand why the patients fail on *wh*-questions but not in Yes-No questions, and so on. In order to know where to look, in order to know what to test, you need a theory. So eventually you might end up with a deficit that is not syntactic, but you definitely need a syntactic theory to know what to do.

The problem with a processing account is that there is no explicit processing theory. What I am then forced to do is take the representational theory of layers within syntactic trees, and try to use it as a processing model. What I get from this is that, you more or less build the syntactic structure from the bottom up, and you get stuck when you have too many nodes to merge.

Karen Emmorey:

Is there any evidence from psycholinguistics, for example, that normal speakers do that – they build from the bottom up? I'm not sure how you'd do this kind of psycholinguistic experiment but that's what you would have to show that in fact that this is the way you produce these kinds of sentences, right?

Naama Friedmann:

I'm not aware of evidence from psycholinguistics.

Peter Hagoort:

This is a very instrumentalist philosophy of science position. You just have a description and as long as this description is adequate, that's fine. I want to know what the psychological reality of this description is.

Lewis Shapiro:

You're missing the point. If the questions you're asking are about the endpoints of behavior—what aphasic patients show – then it's perfectly reasonable to have a linguistic theory that cuts the pie in a particular way. If your question has to do with the processing components that implement this kind of endpoint of behavior, then you would indeed need a full-blown processing theory.

This brings me back to Michael Arbib's comment, about how some of us use linguistic theory terminology in our processing accounts. That's absolutely true. I'm certainly someone who does that. My view is that you take those linguistic objects, and use them as discovery procedures, to suggest what a processing account might look like. In the work that I do, I pick and choose. I pick some vocabulary that seems to be computed in lexical access, I pick some vocabulary that seems to be computed in syntactic parsing. Do

we have a full-blown processing account? No, I don't think so. And would we like to have one? Absolutely. Would it be better to have a really nice processing theory that maps onto linguistic theory? Of course it would.

Yosef Grodzinsky:

I think that what Peter Hagoort is saying is perfectly legitimate: that when you make a descriptive claim, you want to find some kind of coherent construal of it. You have a description which works to some extent—and in Naama Friedmann's tree pruning case it does to an impressive extent, namely it is well-supported across structures and cross-linguistically.

But as a next step, you want to understand what exactly are the neurological underpinnings or the processing underpinnings. Is it possible, given our current understanding? That's where I take issue with the objections that Peter Hagoort, and to an extent Michael Arbib, were voicing. They say that until you come up with a full-fledged processing account, nothing you do is worthwhile (I'm putting it in more extreme terms than you would, of course). But I think that the rational way to go about it is to use the best tools you have at any given moment, and then to try to come up with other, better ones. To my knowledge, parsing theories today perform rather poorly once you try to connect them to the actual empirical reality in neuropsychology. Thus, for the moment, I'd rather stick to an agnostic point of view, and at the same time I am happy to admit that we must make progress and strive to interpret our data in some kind of processing theory.

LANGUAGE DEVELOPMENT

Norbert Herschkovitz:

Last year, Katrin Amunts published a very important paper in the *Journal of Comparative Neurology*, about cytoarchitectonic changes in the asymmetry of area 45 and 44 in the human brain, between ages 3 months to 5 years. It is one of the few developmental studies of anatomical structures. There, an important finding was that area 45 develops asymmetry in a significant way, around 5 years of age, and area 44 later, around 11 years. Now, if you have a theory then you will predict that, there should be some important changes.

Francisco Aboitiz:

And there are changes in child language around this age. One related to more syntactic development, one to more pragmatic development.

Naama Friedmann:

I'm quite excited about it because at the age of 5 we see the relative clauses appear all of a sudden. So at around 5, 5 and a half, you start to see children understanding object relatives. At around 11 they start to understand center embedded object relatives. So it correlates very nicely with the notion of the comprehension of movement at around the age when 45 develops and computation of center embedding around that age.

Peter Hagoort:

I'm still not convinced that this is the ultimate theory we are looking for, because basically it's saying, well, we have something at the level of behavior and yes, we find something at the level of developmental neuroanatomy with which we can correlate the behavior. But it doesn't change anything about our account of linguistic behavior. It also doesn't change anything in our understanding of the neural architecture. It just says: well, these pieces come together, but I'm not sure that essentially we can be thinking that's the ultimate.

Yosef Grodzinsky:

But this is something new. We can learn something from this.

Kyle Johnson:

But it's true, that if you ask for what is the theory, you know, if we had a theory that allowed us, given some range of behaviors, say, to predict where to look anatomically, or visa versa, it doesn't help us develop such a theory. It helps us to develop such a theory in so far as it allows us to see a correspondence. That's important, and we have nothing more than that presently. But maybe Sergey Avrutin's question is, so what else should we have? What other sorts of things should we have?

Yosef Grodzinsky:

I would like to take issue with Kyle Johnson. If you see, if this collusion is true, namely, there are developmental changes that you can tap cytoarchitectonically that correspond to behavioral changes in development, it gives you a new direction for research, that's exactly what it gives you. Because what you have to do now is to start looking for these kinds of correlations and yes, correlations is all we have to go by in science. There's nothing else that I've ever seen or heard about. These things don't exist, there are correlations. If this is true, it gives you a fantastic direction to go by. Well, maybe it's going to happen in 50 years, but it's a new direction.

Sergey Avrutin:

I think it's extremely interesting and extremely important and that it adds something, but I wonder how far you can go. In this example, Naama gave a distinction between types of relative clauses. Well, there is so much in linguistic theory you are not expecting to detect at the neural level at the particular age of 5:2. At the same age, that is around age 4:5, you also find problems with pronouns. It is very interesting, but I don't think we will be able to find neural development that directly correlates with linguistic change.

Michael Petrides:

But you don't know exactly the interaction between brain and language, at some point, you are saying there might be some characteristic of language that are determined by the development and the maturation of certain brain structures.

Sergey Avrutin:

I think everything is determined by brain structures.

Michael Petrides:

That's fine, but you find out, otherwise we wouldn't be in this room, talking about Broca's area.

Katrin Amunts:

You may often find out that the development of language may also influence the brain structure itself. It's a very complex process.

FUNCTIONAL CONNECTIVITY

Karl Zilles:

An important point was mentioned by Michael Petrides with respect to the arcuate fascicle. You can read, in the book by Dejerine from the end of the nineteenth century, a very nice and precise description of the arcuate fascicle connecting the superior temporal region around with the prefrontal and premotor and even the orbital region. I highly recommend these old reports by Dejerine to anyone who looks for connectivity data in the human brain, because these data are so sparse and so rare that we have really to go back to the end of the nineteenth century for the original sources.

The DTI method was mentioned as a hope. I hope you understand that DTI is not the solution to the connectivity in the human brain. DTI shows a preferred direction of water diffusion. "Connectivity" means synaptic connectivity. Fiber tracts do not necessarily mean connectivity. In clinical data, where a fiber tract is disrupted and you have functional deficits, it may be connectivity. Even when an axon has a very intense contact with a cell, it is not necessarily a synapse, because an axon can just pass by and through the area. The strict definition of connectivity requires that you demonstrate the synaptic contact using electron microscopy. This is my personal view point about connectivity, DTI and the hope that we can get more information about connectivity in the human brain in the near future. I think that effective connectivity and other approaches, are more likely to work than the hope that fiber tracking solves all the problems.

Peter Hagoort:

In functional imaging studies, we have the BOLD response which is also no direct measure of the neuronal activity. Nevertheless, we know enough to see whether there is a high correlation between these two components, whatever the mechanism is.

Karl Zilles:

I think this is a comparison of apples and oranges. There is detailed research on the correlation between action potentials and the BOLD effect. This is completely different from the demonstration of some huge fiber, which seems to "connect" areas of the right and the left hemisphere. Whether this leads to a connection in the strict anatomical sense cannot be inferred from DTI, but from animal experiments, where we know that the callosal fibers do synaptic connections between the two hemispheres. In the case of the arcuate fascicle, we don't know how often these fascicles have synaptic connectivity. The arcuate fascicle contains fibers from completely different areas. In DTI you see this fascicle as a continuum, but it's not at all a continuum. This is the problem.

Michael Petrides:

If you read the Dejerine descriptions carefully—and I've read them several times—you realize, for example, that he is not sure as to whether the arcuate fascicle is or isn't the same as the superior longitudinal fascicle. In fact, he is talking about the arcuate fascicle as maybe the superior longitudinal fascicle, with a little branching into the temporal lobe. The point of this story is that we have a general idea about the human pathways, but we don't know where the exact origin is. Are the fibers coming from the posterior part of the supero temporal gyrus, or are they coming from the superotemporal sulcus as well, or are they also coming from the posterior part of the middle temporal gyrus? And Zilles rightly said, if you read Dejerine, you get the impression that they go as far as the orbital frontal cortex. Pandya, trying to make the best picture he could make in the late 1960s based on his reading of the classic human data, and based on what ever was known at the time from monkey work tried to make this diagram including the arcuate fascicle. The arcuate fascicle linking the posterior part of the superotemporal gyrus to the posterior part of the inferofrontal gyrus may not in fact be the way that the language zones of the inferofrontal gyrus and the language zones of the temporal-parietal area are linked.

FUNCTIONAL IMAGING

Michael Petrides:

When you read the work in many areas of cognitive neuroscience, there's lots of functional imaging. You then look at so-called meta-analyses, and you find peaks all over the place. The message that you get out of that is trivial. You read a review of language that basically says that functional neural imaging taught us that besides Broca's area, lots of other areas of the brain are important. This is, at one level, a trivial statement.

We start from the assumption that we have "activated an area." I think that there is something fundamentally wrong with the word "activation." It assumes that the brain was in a baseline state, and somehow when we do a task, we've "activated" that area. In fact, except when we're dead, the brain is never in a baseline state. Even when I'm sitting here and I'm supposed to do nothing, I'm thinking of my girlfriend, my wife, I'm hungry, I want to get out of this place, this place has too much noise. So there are all sorts of activity in the brain, even in the so-called complete base-line state.

Ultimately, what we see is a difference between two states: State A, the experimental state, and State B, the control state. I can take any experimental state, and when I change the baseline I will see completely different sets of activation patterns. I don't think we often think about the implications of that.

For example, I may have seen some parietal activation because in my experimental task, attentional spatial requirements were greater than in my control task. I saw a peak in Broca's area, and in the parietal lobe, and in the cerebellum. To say that this is the network involving this particular task or operation, is at the very least a very naïve way of thinking, because you don't know if those peaks are differences for many different aspects of the task.

If suddenly you saw a cerebellar peak in a working memory task, you may believe that this is not due to some accidental factor. Of course, we always pretend that we can control things, but the truth is that we cannot. I think that we have to be aware of all these kind of problems, the traps, the pitfalls, and I would just like to hear people's views, how we should deal with them.

Yosef Grodzinsky:

When old sages like me who have been around long enough to see the field transform from lesion studies into imaging, I think that it's one of those rare cases where technology has taken science backwards, at least in the beginning. What happened was, and this is completely sociological, that there was this new excitement, new types of researchers came in with a lot of computational muscle and physics muscle, and they thought that behavior was trivial. And what happened was that the same kind of mistakes that were made in aphasiology in the sixties and seventies are now being repeated. That's kind of unfortunate, and I hope it's temporary.

You were saying two kinds of things. First of all you said that you need to do tightly controlled experiments, and secondly you said in order for you to be convinced of the serious involvement of an area, you need generalization across different tasks, and you need replicability. But in this respect, there's nothing special about imaging. The need for generalization and replicability is true of any science.

So why, you might ask yourself, does this issue rise so acutely in the context of imaging? I think that the explanation is purely sociological: There was too much excitement. It's big technology, it's fantastic technology. Not only that, it is another advantage, it is expensive technology, so you get a lot of overhead. And that's exciting. But in the long run, it's very clear to me that things will be straightened out.

Stefano Cappa:

I agree completely with Michael Petrides. But I must say that I was quite impressed by the many functional imaging work presented at this conference, and most of the results which have been important to us have been of the type we call "complex comparison." That is, there was no presentation of data with simple baseline or making some assumption of pure insertion.

At this point, there is no sense in just putting someone in the scanner, give him a task, and wait to see what happens. You must have very specific predictions about the effects you expect from subtle manipulations. In this respect it is important to have constraints such as a specific anatomical partition. I think that a major problem with much of the linguistic work in this area, with some remarkable exceptions, is that you start with a good linguistic theory, but have no prediction about the possible neurological substrate. The trace-deletion hypothesis is one possible exception to this, but there are some other areas of linguistics in which you have a very nice theoretical model but no anatomical prediction. It's totally different from other areas in which you have very strong assumptions from experimental neurophysiology, etc. Language is really special from this point of view.

Luciano Fadiga:

I think that Stefano Cappa's point is a good one—prediction on the activation. This is what we call an experimental hypothesis in science. We cannot run experiments without experimental hypotheses. Otherwise, we make observations; we can also measure phenomena. But in that case, we need very precise methods, and it seems to me that brain imaging is not enough precise for that, at least now.

I would like to make two points: First, we probably have to simplify as much as we can the experimental condition which activates a certain area. So, after a lesion of the pyramidal tract, a violin player is no longer able to play violin. But that doesn't mean that the primary motor cortex serves to play the violin.

Second, we almost never look at the intensity of the response. In the activation, we always look at the statistical maps, which are very useful to give a first look, but after that we extract the region of interest, we measure the intensity, and we lose all information about the intensity of the response in other areas. It seems there is no software that can show the map of the activation in terms of intensity. It's very rare to see papers in which you see the intensity of the response.

Peter Hagoort:

Approaches have been developed, that are a little more informed than before. First, meta-analysis can effectively be used to sum up areas of activation that have been found; it may also be used to distinguish between the accidental and what seems to be the more profound. Second, parametric modulations are crucial, in that they help avoid exactly the problem that Michael Petrides referred to, regarding experimental and control states. I therefore take issue with minimal pair approach that Yosef Grodzinsky was defending, which is based on the pure insertion methodology that compares a kind of type of construction with movement and one without movement, and then claims the difference has to do with movement. In the imaging field, we do have to do parametrical modulations. In this case, you do not only have two conditions, but increase the local parameter in notable steps and see whether the area is sensitive in this behavior to the modulation of that parameter.

Michael Petrides:

There's a problem with minimal pairs if you are going to assume that parametric manipulations is the so-

lution to our problems. For instance, I have two steps to pay attention to I have four steps to pay attention to, or I have ten steps to pay attention to, or whatever. The reaction time increases linearly, perhaps. The problem is, how do you know that the BOLD signal is going to be reflecting your parametric manipulation? For example, suppose that Yosef was able to parametrically these sentences. How do you know that once Broca's area, or whatever region, is activated by that syntactic manipulation, how do you know that the fact that twice as much of that syntactic manipulation should be reflected in twice as much using the BOLD system. Why? When you are increasing these measures in types of complexity, how do you know you are not also increasing the attention of complexity? And also working memory performance? And also x and y which are also going to be reflected as parametric manipulations. My point is that I don't think parametric manipulations solve the problem.

Yosef Grodzinsky:

While I do use parameterization in experiments, it is important to realize that parameterization doesn't solve problems of principle. That is, even if you parameterize conditions in your experiment—which is the right way to go in many instances—you still have to maintain the logical structure of your experiment— the set of basic conditions. So you do need minimal contrasts within which you embed parameters.

Michael Petrides:

Ultimately, I'm not excited about parameterization. It is the catch word in the field now, but I don't think it solves the problems we had before when we only did a comparison between two conditions. Whether you parameterize or you compare two conditions, there will be some activity difference in the brain that were due to your manipulation according to your hypothesis, there are some which are totally irrelevant. There will always be, even when you parameterize, differences in attentional requirements, differences in motor response requirements, differences in conflict resolution, etc. All of these will be reflected in the activity in these other areas. It doesn't necessarily allow you to say that these areas are a network. They could be due to five totally dependent factors that unintentionally were manipulated in your experiment.

Karen Emmorey:

This might make a good transition: One of the things you need in order to try to understand these blobs of activation is a model of the behavior. But the model has to be connected to the neuroscience data that you're looking at. I think that one of the reasons that vision research has been more successful in some sense than language research is because that gap between the cognitive model and neuroscience is smaller for vision than it is for language. If you look at linguistic models, it's not at all obvious in any way how to map that on the brain, as Stefano Cappa commented earlier. There are no predictions about localization. One way is to try to make linguistic theory more compatible with processing models, which in turn can be more compatible with the underlying neural circuitry.

Stefano Cappa:

I noticed that this very interesting development in the field of linguistics. Originally, the typical idea of the linguist who was planning an imaging experiment is, "Let's take this distinction and the view under the imaging experiment. If there is a difference, for me it's enough, wherever it is, who cares, it could be in the toe, wherever it's perfect." This is a logic which is similar to the discussion we were having yesterday about patients. Because, you could take the same computation, just the fact that the patient shows dissociation, it's interesting, and the lesion is developed. There's a whole body of cognitive neuropsychology based on this. Why now I think that there is an interesting development, which is the fact that not only the finding of a difference is relevant, but where you find the difference and whether you have any form of neurological model which connects the two. This is our way of trying to do now. My feeling is that up to now this has not been an extraordinary success, with a few exceptions, this is a meeting on Broca's area and there are some interesting developments here, and there are interesting developments in the area of Wernicke's area. But in the case of Wernicke's area, there are interesting developments because of the interface with the phonology and peripheral processes. In this case you have constraints that is, what you know from audition and recent developments in all the different processing, etc. We seem to have a nice development in two areas which are the interface with, essentially motor and phonological processes. In between, there seems to be much more complicated. And it's not surprising.

Sergey Avrutin:

I want to follow up with what Stefano Cappa said, that the reason why linguists designed the imaging experiment, the reason they first designed the experiment and they said, "Well, let's see what happens," is basically not because people still treat the brain as a black box. Suppose I design a study with central embedded relative clauses, I expect a difference. Should I make such a stupid claim and say that, "Okay, this is the area of the brain that is responsible for all the embedded clauses"? That would be very naïve and primitive. We don't really know how to connect the brain anatomy and behavioral data. Should the theory be formulated in terms of this, we are looking for something that at least encodes a trace or what's left for now? What should the theory look like?

Karen Emmorey:

I was just going to come back to this notion of task, that anatomists and neurophysiologists think about language in terms of tasks. But part of that is because when you try to tap language performance, you have to tap it through some type of task. So, when you look at the early language studies, why did they pick verb generation? It makes no sense from a linguistic point of view, but you can say similar things about grammaticality judgments. The point is in terms of trying to look at the neural systems that underlie language processing, you're looking at processing and you have to tap it with some kind of task. And now the task could be very simple, well, maybe not so simple, some measure of comprehension, type of "did you understand this sentence," etc. In some sense that is really what you want to get at, not whether you decided it was grammatical or not grammatical.

Yosef Grodzinsky:

You're absolutely right, you always have a task. But then, what you have to do is never to forget that the task implements structured behavior. There are principles that govern behavior, and these get implemented in a task. Therefore, you shouldn't think only in terms of task, but remember that the main thing you are after is not the task that you happen to be choosing because you need to be doing an experiment, but rather structured behavior.

In this respect, it is important to go back to David Marr's book on vision. To my knowledge, it is the most explicit statement of the relationship that there should be between structured behavior and cortical tissue. It's very interesting for me to listen to anatomists and physiologists here, because they know a lot about the brain, and their approach to neural tissue is rigorous. But interestingly, for the most part when they talk about behavior, they talk about tasks. That's usually the kind of conception. It seems to me what you have to be talking about is not about tasks, but rather about structured behavior. That's the important thing and what linguistic theory and computation theories of vision give you is exactly a characterization of the kinds of structures that you have to then relate to neural tissue.

So, there's a theory that structures behavior, and everything that there is to know about neural tissue, and the relationship between the two is complex, and you shouldn't expect to try and derive all behavior straight out of neural vocabulary.

Sergey Avrutin:

I agree with you completely. There are these different levels—the algorithm, computational, implementation levels—but the issue with Marr's approach and actually with Chomsky's unification approach is one and the same. When you talk about different levels, there has to be a translation procedure between them. How you translate the description at one level to a description at another level? I do not think David Marr actually answered this question.

Katrin Amunts:

My interest is related to the function of a cortical area. If we want to map complex behavior to the brain, a first prerequisite is to have good brain maps. When we started to map the brain anatomically, we saw a huge variability in the extent of cortical areas. These areas can be defined using different criteria— receptorarchitecture, cytoarchitecture, whatever. You have to be aware, when you map some behavior to some brain area, that there is this variability. Five millimeters or one centimeter difference in the brain can mean a completely different area. And when you have an activation in a different area, perhaps, you also have a different idea or different behavioral concept which you would like to. Here is an example: If you have an activation, which is a little bit above area 44—maybe it's in the region where the inferior frontal sulcus meets the precentral sulcus. Of course, there is a certain overlap with cytoarchitectonic area 44, it is quite variable. Okay, it might be there, but it also might be the case that this is a completely different area. And we have good arguments for this. Our colleagues from the Max Planck Institute in Leipzig, von Cramon and Brass, assume, that there is a little area, in this particular region that is involved in switching of task representations. This is something completely different, not related to language, at least not to overt language. These behavioral differences go in parallel with cytoarchitectonic differences between this little area and the classical Broca's area, or area 44. The question is really, what is a function of an area? I have an anatomy-centered view, of course, but I really would like to prove, or to know, what is the function of a certain cortical area. Such a function cannot be a complex behavior, as language, or movement, or vision. But, maybe these functions are quite more abstract in that sense, like task representation, switching, or whatever. Maybe we should look not only what is language and where it is distributed over the cortex but also from the other angle of view—namely, what means a cortical area? These cortical areas have a very certain cytoarchitecture, receptor architecture, connectivity, transmitters. That is, they have a specific function. I would like to know what's the function of a real, singular anatomical unit in terms of cognitive function or language function.

Luciano Fadiga:

The border is critical. It's not a conceptual problem. If you have area 4, it means that you found the characteristic response of area 4, you will never find the response of an another area.

Peter Hagoort:

So now let's take a more complicated example because we're here for the language system. Is it the case that the movement operations that Yosef is presupposing to be in this particular set of areas, is that something which is essentially different between one individual and the others given certain differences in individual make up of the brain or not? Because that, of course, we abstract away from that and it might not be necessary, but is it also legitimate.

Katrin Amunts:

But there are individual differences in function. Perhaps Yosef's differences in transformations may be very tiny differences. However, we know that they are different capacities of language. Recently, we have analyzed the cytoarchitecture of a language genius, who knew more than 60 languages. Of course, there was not only one single language function which was superior in this human subject than in others, but many. But, at least, this was an extreme point of a distribution of people knowing language. What we found was that the cytoarchitecture is so different from the average population of Broca's regions that we were able to clearly distinguish and to classify this particular brain as compared to all the other brains.

Yosef Grodzinsky:

In what way was it different?

Katrin Amunts:

Remarkable statistically significant cytoarchitecture, not in terms of absolute cell-packing density but rather in terms of connectivity. We at the very beginning to see a correlation between a cognitive ability, e.g., language, and the cytoarchitecture. But, there are such correlations and I could provide additional examples from the developmental perspective. Unfortunately, large intersubject variability both in function and in structure makes these type of analysis difficult. Sometimes, it's not possible to analyze such relationships. But the relationship exists.

Luciano Fadiga:

So you raised the critical point when you told us before the example. You are perfectly right when you say that it was a serendipity discovery. The same was done with single-neuron recordings in the monkey. So the technique allowed the serendipity in other terms, with brain imaging it would never been possible to discover the same effect. But, if you can find the same cell that responds during observation and execution, you can try to formulate a hypothesis; otherwise, it's very difficult to.

LESION STUDIES

Kyle Johnson:

Let's come to the next part of the discussion. The target here is the units of analysis at the anatomical level, the physical level. What are those units? Does it make sense to talk about them, how do we demarcate them, and so on.

Luciano Fadiga:

I've learned something from patients studies concerning these issues. The study of patients was really very important in the last century, considering, for instance, technical limitations. There were no other possible approaches to the problem. As neurophysiology developed, lesion studies were gradually abandoned, because we know that they are quite unspecific. I would like to ask those who study patients, what in their view they can say to neuroscience, neurophysiology, and neuroanatomy. What they can tell us about Broca's area?

Stefano Cappa:

I think it's still extremely important. For example, going to Yosef Grodzinsky's sentence data, about different kinds of movement, and finding right hemisphere activation. Of course, it would the best thing at this point to go back to patient with right hemispheric lesion and see what happens with this kind of structure. I don't think so far anybody has been doing this. Of course, there are other complications that have been mentioned several times. You have a distance effect, the stage of the deficit, etc. However, I think this remains a very important tool to test the necessity of a given structure for a function. Another interesting technology is TMS, but, as you know TMS has also problems. The effects might complicate the data, for example for repetition and match on the rate of stimulation. And there, too, you have distance effect. The only difference is that you don't expect to see much organization because it's such a time-locked procedure.

Michael Petrides:

I'll defend the lesion studies. A problem with language, of course, is that unfortunately you cannot get beautiful lesions and precise lesions. But, for example in monkeys, in the prefrontal cortex where I started in neurophysiology, I could stick a microelectrode in there, do a complex task, and see all sorts of crazy activity, which I could never be able to interpret because I had no constraints. So, by going there and making a tiny lesion in the monkey brain bilaterally, and I emphasize the precision, the bilateral character, and the smallness, that are targeting architectonic areas. For all intensive purposes, the monkey's behavior in 99.9% of the cognitive tasks was normal. And then, there comes a task, BOOM, and it cannot do it. Then you can manipulate the requirements and get some fundamental ideas about what kind of area might be doing. I don't think you would ever get such data from neurophysiology, particularly recording studies. You can only get from the lesion data. Now, we get into recording areas, medial lateral-prefrontal cortex. Lesion studies have enabled me to constrain the hypothesis, and now we have very precise hypothesis to test. I think lesion studies are wonderful, in the language area they are problematic not because the methodology is the problem, it's just often difficult to have precise lesions. If you could have precise lesions of, let's say area 44 in humans, bilaterally, you would have done wonderful studies.

Lewis Shapiro:

When I do lesion studies, I look for particular kinds of behavioral profiles of patients. Let's say, they are Broca's aphasia patients. Now what I want to do is find out the online processing antecedents to off-line comprehension behavior. I want to know how the operations work in real time, rather than just finding the endpoint. So, I select these patients by a priori selection criteria, and then I test them in reaction time experiments, and find differences between them and healthy subjects. Now the critical question regards the claim am I going to make. One possibility is that Broca's area is responsible for the normal functioning of the process I isolated. It's a grain-size thing, that is, it is located in the left anterior frontal lobe somewhere around Broca's area. Then you find that other patients that you have selected don't exhibit the same effect — they show some other pattern, and they have damage elsewhere.

The next step might be, "Okay, now we image these patients." The problem is that there are tasks that you can't use in the magnet. Simple online tasks, reaction time tasks, are sometimes very difficult to translate into imaging tasks or in evoked potential experiments, due to all sorts of constraints on the method. So, that's what you get.

Sergey Avrutin:

One thing to do, with for example, Broca's aphasics, is to see not only what they cannot do, but what they can do. When we design an experiment with aphasic patients, we always have a minimal pair, a linguistic minimal pair, that will tell you, that the two constructions are different in this specific way. Then you look and these patients with sometimes very severe damage perform very well, above chance, at least, compared to other conditions. So, one interesting conclusion for neurophysiology, maybe, is that for this particular linguistic operation, your Broca's area or whatever is not really that important. Because, even with this part of the brain completely gone, they can still do it at an above chance level, almost like normal. This seems to be important, too.

Peter Hagoort:

I represent the villains. Take a precise lesion in area MT in the monkey, for which we know it's involved in motion processing. You create a precise lesion in the monkey, and find that there is no behavioral impairment visible in the monkey in terms of perceived motion. And that is what Edelman and others call the issue of degeneracy, the brain might have multiple ways to solve a particular problem. Thus, information all based on lesions does not allow us to say that this area, therefore, is not involved in motion processing.

Michael Petrides:

I agree with all you say. If I was to do this experiment, and I tested the monkey in motion perception, and the monkey was not impaired, then I would go back and ask myself the question that there is some fundamental contribution that that MT area is doing to motion, that none of my simple motion detection experiments are capturing. So, what essentially you are showing, is that subcortical and other cortical areas are capable of resolving and allowing the animal to say yes, I see these things moving, no, I don't see those moving. And, in fact, the motion properties at the cell level in the MT, are not just to detect motion, as we perhaps simple mindedly, originally thought. In 10 years' time, when more sophisticated experiments are done in that area, perhaps the detection of form from motion, or some higher level use of motion in perception, either of space or whatever, then people will suddenly, BOOM, detect different a fantastic and clear deficit in there. These deficits then it will be very useful to go back to the argument just previously made, when you contrast it with all the motion tasks that the monkey is capable of doing. And actually all cognition is done is multiple areas, but there must be some fundamental computations that are going there, otherwise God or nature would not have created a structure there. But, when you start searching suddenly you realized that a certain aspects of working memory that have been impaired, which now enables you to go back and record and ask new questions of those neurons and instead of interpreting them as simply neurons that hold information online, which incidentally is happening in many other parts of the cortex, you are able to say there are certain decision making requirements down there. So, that's my way of thinking. I would make a strong claim that if you, at some point, if you do the right experiments that really tap the specific contribution of that area to motion, you'll find it.

Peter Hagoort:

So there's no redundancy in the brain?

Michael Petrides:

There is redundancy in the sense, that all cognitive tasks can be solved in alternative ways, to a lesser or greater degree. In that case, we do rely on other structures. But I think if you really shape the right kind of manipulation, you are going to see a massive impairment from a given lesion in a certain area.

Stefano Cappa:

I think that it's clear there are limitations in lesion methods, but why does one wish to continue to rely on very lousy anatomy. There are a lot of very interesting developments in the field, and if you think that studying patients will still bring some contribution, which I think is the case, it's quite important at this point to have precise lesion localization taking into account the developments in the mapping methods, etc. I think it's very important to go back from the results of imaging to lesion studies. But in order to do

that in any reasonable way, we should be able, at the minimal, to map activation and lesion in the same space. Otherwise, this is a topic open to wide array of different possible interpretations. I think it's quite important to try to take advantage now of what is available and to have, for example, something we don't have except in a few places in which they've been working very systematically and use a large database of lesion cases with very precise localization, this is very helpful.

Luciano Fadiga:

I would like to ask Michael Petrides a question. You raised the point of the bilateral of the lesion, and this is very rare in a physician office. But we know that almost all of the frontal lobe is connected with homologous contralateral part, apart from the hand area of the primary motor cortex, so I couldn't comment on your view why so it's so necessary, this bilateral lesion. Do you think that there is a compensatory effect of the contralateral area every time you remove only one?

Michael Petrides:

The striking example is the mediotemporal lobe. You remove the amygdala-hippocampal area, and let's not get into the argument whether or not it's the hippocampus, entorhinal, or perirhinal, cortex bilaterally, you have massive amnesia that lasts a lifetime, H.M. is a classic example. You then remove the left mediotemporal lobe areas, the amygdala, hippocampus, entorhinal, perirhinal cortex etc., you get a significant verbal memory, but not as severe as that of H.M. This implies that to some extent, both the left hippocampus of capable of processing non verbal stimuli and the right one is capable of, to some extent, of verbal stimuli. The maximal effect is when you have bilateral lesions.

Karl Zilles:

We should stop here. For me, the major points of the discussion are that we cannot draw any conclusions from patient studies without a careful and critical approach. This is so because in our study we knock-out neither a specific anatomical area nor a well-defined functional unit. It's a mixture: lesions are rather large and don't care about borders of anatomical areas, or definitions of functional units.

VI

HISTORICAL ARTICLES

Choices We Made: An Introduction to the Historical Section

Katrin Amunts

Yosef Grodzinsky

Broca's region was among the first pieces of brain tissue to which a circumscribed function—articulated language—was specifically related. Modern neuropsychology is believed to have begun when Paul Broca delivered a short presentation at the Anthropological Society of Paris in 1861. This famous paper, and the more detailed ones that followed, are often seen as the beginning of modern research on the localization of language in the brain and of investigations into cognitive functioning in general.

This section seeks to give the reader a flavor of the history of the investigation into the neurological underpinnings of language, so that current-day research achievements can be situated in a broader context. To this end, we collected papers we deem to be of major historical importance, which we present in chronological order (some as a whole, others just in excerpts). These papers—whose detailed descriptions of neurological symptoms and anatomical features are stunningly accurate even by current standards—cover mainly two topics: language (studied through apha-

sia) and anatomy. Some papers are famous and frequently cited; others are less well known. Many are kept in only a few libraries, and some are originally written in languages other than English. Our goal here was to make all these accessible. Below we tell the reader what we chose and why.

Broca's first paper was published one day after the death of his famous patient "Tan" and the removal of Tan's brain at an autopsy. The paper contains Broca's ideas about localization of language, which he then continued to develop. While his first paper is famous, less well known is the fact that Broca actually published analyses of patients other than Leborgne (some with smaller and more circumscribed lesions than Tan's) and that during the 1860s, he wrote a series of papers about the localization of function, on the clinical description of the effects of brain damage, and on the neuroanatomy of lesion sites. Equally important is the fact that Broca did not start a field from scratch. Interest in the relation between brain and cognitive capacity began earlier. Broca was preceded by Franz

Josef Gall and his pupil Johann Casper Spurzheim and by Gustav Dax, Louis P. Gratiolet, Jean Baptiste Bouillaud, Ernest Aubertin, and several others who had published earlier observations of patients with aphasia after brain injury. Later studies supplemented these early findings but also provided contradictory evidence.

Indeed, Broca's modular view of language and its cerebral representation (more clearly articulated by Carl Wernicke and his disciples) did not pass without reaction. The localizationist approach was criticized almost at once. First and foremost among the opponents of the localizationist group was John Hughlings-Jackson, the great British neurologist who is probably best known for his description of epileptic convulsions. Hughlings-Jackson wrote a series of papers in which he argued that language is not localizable in any specific area of the cerebral cortex. His writings on aphasia, published from the mid-1870s on, represent the first attack on the localizationist school from an antimodular point of view—one that views cognitive deficits as a domain-general "asymbolia." What is special about Hughlings-Jackson is not just his approach but also his attempt—the first ever to our knowledge—to make contact with some principled way to think about language as an entity by itself. As can be seen from the excerpts we selected, he was very much influenced by the ideas of philosopher Herbert Spencer about language. And while modern linguistics was not born yet, Hughlings-Jackson's attempt is the first to connect language structure to brain disease.

We did not select a paper by Broca's successor, Carl Wernicke, simply because his views are well represented by a famous article on brain/language relations by Ludwig Lichtheim, which we excerpted. Yet, it was Wernicke who in 1874 described temporal lobe aphasia, which he related to a posterior language center and juxtaposed it to the anterior aphasia—and language center—that Broca had discovered. Wernicke proposed the first detailed model for how language is organized in the left hemisphere, consisting of the anterior (Broca) and the posterior (Wernicke) connected via the arcuate fascicle. This model is the basis of a schema drawn by Ludwig Lichtheim, who in 1885 published a comprehensive review paper on aphasia that contained diagrams of the cerebral representation of language processing. All of these schema and diagrams—gathered by Wernicke's disciples, who became known as Connectionists or diagram makers— were inspired by Wernicke's ideas and hypotheses about how the brain has nodes and connections and about how these can be injured to produce the various types of aphasia. These diagrams are still widely used in behavioral neurology and aphasia research.

The historical section then shifts focus to studies of the brain's cytoarchitecture, which intensified around the turn of the twentieth century, subsequent to Golgi's discovery of methods that stain selectively neural tissue. We present Korbinian Brodmann's 1908 cytoarchitectonic paper, which contains the first complete description of a parcellation of the whole cortical surface, one that is still widely used today. The paper is a shorter version of Brodmann's famous 1909 book. We chose another important cytoarchitectonic study with respect to Broca's region, by Brodmann's contemporary, L. Riegele, who was, like some years earlier Brodmann, a co-worker of the Vogts at the Kaiser Wilhelm Institute for Brain Research in Berlin. At the time, this institute was one of the most advanced centers for neuroscience, featuring a modern multidisciplinary approach to the brain that consisted of neuropathology, psychiatry, electrophysiology, comparative anatomy, and genetics. Many of Riegele's criteria for cytoarchitectonic borders can still be used in mapping efforts today.

The next paper is by Carl Wernicke's contemporary, Arnold Pick, who studied medicine in Vienna and also worked in Berlin for some time. Pick, who studied agrammatism (although it was Kußmaul who coined the term), was the first to put the study of language disturbances in the context of modern psycholinguistic research. Agrammatism is now recognized as a central feature of Broca's aphasia. Pick's recognition of the centrality of the grammatical aspect in the deficit in Broca's aphasia paved the way to later linguistic analyses of aphasic syndromes, and thus made linguistic investigations of brain–language relations possible.

For linguistic concepts to enter the arena, it would still take time. Indeed, linguists first entered the field late, perhaps too late. A first step was made almost 30 years after Pick's observations. At this point, clinically based notions as to how one should analyze language were already deeply entrenched, and exceedingly difficult to change. The first to try was structural linguist Roman Jakobson. His 1941 seminal monograph *Kindersprache, Aphasie und allgemeine Lautgesetze* [*Child Language, Aphasia, and Phonological Universals*] was an attempt to identify universal dimensions to phonological analysis and to show that these unfold at a fixed order in language development and break down at a reverse order in aphasia (the regression hypothesis). We present some of Jakobson's later ideas in an excerpt from *Fundamentals of Language* (co-authored with Morris Halle).

The notion of a controlled experiment also entered the scene at a delay. Harold Goodglass was among the first psychologists to investigate aphasia, and he should most likely be credited with the introduction of controlled experimental methods into the field. In one of his first studies, he operationalized an idea conveyed to him by Massachusetts Institute of Technology linguist Morris Halle and, with the help of J. Hunt, incorporated the notion of grammatical transformation into an experiment of language production in aphasia. Readers can thus observe the results of the first study of transformational grammar (perhaps a precursor of much work that followed and is represented in this book).

Finally, we present two more recent papers written by neurologists. While interest in brain–language relations was low in the 1940s–1950s, the charisma of Norman Geschwind helped revive it. His work on the cerebral representation of language resulted in an enriched Connectionist model, which he explored in the context of other disorders such as apraxia and agnosia. Later, in 1978, Jay P. Mohr published a paper, which quickly became a classic, in which he correlated Broca's aphasia with infarction in Broca's region. He showed that speech disturbances resulting from infarction limited to the Broca region differ from the clinical characteristics in Broca aphasia and concluded that the latter is observed subsequent to damage that extends beyond Broca's region.

The papers of this chapter cover single aspects of the history of language and do not mention many others. We hope, however, that they illustrate the spectrum of studies from different disciplines, articulate different points of views with respect to the localization of a complex function, and reflect the changes in the understanding of language and in neuronal correlates during more than 140 years. And perhaps they raise the wish to go back to the original, complete sources and to read more about the beginnings of the science of language.

Space limitations precluded a comprehensive historical survey, so we should just mention a few twentieth-century scientists and clinicians who influenced our thinking about brain and language, and who were unfortunately left out: Joseph Jules Dejerine, Henry Head, Theodore Weisenburg and Katharine McBride, Kurt Goldstein, Alexander R. Luria, and Hildred Schuell on the neuropsychological side, as well as Friedrich Sanides, Constantin von Economo, Oskar and Cecile Vogt, Ottfried Foerster, and E. Kononova on the anatomical side.

It should be clear from this short selection that the study of brain and language initially revolved around several geographical locations: in the early phase, the second half of the nineteenth century, Europe was at center stage for both clinical neurology and neuroanatomy. The influence of the early heroes persists, as can be seen from the current papers published earlier in this book. Later, the study of aphasia gravitated to the United States, where, starting in the early 1960s, it was primarily conducted in the Aphasia Unit, later the Aphasia Research Center, at the Boston VA Hospital, co-directed by Norman Geschwind and Harold Goodglass. Many current leaders in cognitive neuroscience passed through the VA Hospital and its various wards and programs, where they encountered scientists such as Sheila Blumstein and Edgar Zurif, who pioneered the use of psycholinguistic methods in the study of aphasia. We thus see ourselves as part of a long line that we hope will stretch far into the future.

18

Comments Regarding the Seat of the Faculty of Spoken Language, Followed by an Observation of Aphemia (Loss of Speech)

Paul Broca

The case and observation that I present to the Anatomical Society come in support of the ideas propagated by Mr. Bouillaud on the seat of the faculty of language. The question at hand, partly a physiological and partly a pathological one, deserves more attention than most doctors have accorded it to date, and the matter is delicate enough, the subject obscure and complicated enough, that it seems useful to me to start with a few comments on that which I have observed.

I.

We know that the school of phrenology placed the seat of the faculty of language in the anterior part of the brain, on one of the convolutionsthat rests in the

Translated by Simran Karir. From "Remarques sur le Siége de la Faculté du Langage Articulé, Suivies d'une Observation d'aphémie (Perte de la Parole)," in *Bulletin de la Société Anatomique de Paris* 6:330–357, 1861. The author was Surgeon at the Bicêtre Hospital.

orbital arch. This opinion, which was offered, like so many others, without sufficient proof and which, by the way, was based only on a very imperfect analysis of phenomena occurring in language, would no doubt have disappeared with the rest of the system, had Mr. Bouillaud not modified and surrounded it by a cortege of proof, borrowed especially from pathology, thereby saving it. Without considering language to be a simple faculty, dependent on only one cerebral organ, and without looking to circumscribe the location of this organ in a space of a few millimeters, as the school of Gall did, this professor was led by an analysis of a great number of clinical facts, followed by autopsies, to acknowledge that certain lesions on the hemispheres abolish the ability of speech, without destroying intelligence, and that these lesions are always located in the anterior lobes of the brain. He concluded that there are somewhere on these lobes one or several convolutionsthat hold one of the essential elements of the complex phenomenon of speech, and this is why he therefore, less exclusively than the school of Gall, placed in the anterior lobes, without further specifying, the seat of the *faculty of spoken language*, which must not be confounded with the *general faculty of language*.

There are, in effect, several types of languages. All systems of signsthat permit one to express ideas in a more or less intelligible, more or less complete, more or less rapid manner are a language in the most general sense of the word: speech, mimicry, dactylology, pictorial writing, phonetic writing, etc., are all types of languages.

There is a general faculty of language that presides over all these ways of expressing thought, and which can be defined as: the faculty for establishing a constant relationship between an idea and a sign, be it sound, a movement, a picture, or whatever sort of sketch. In addition, every type of language necessitates the play between certain organsthat are responsible for *emitting* and *receiving* information. Organs [sic] receiving information are sometimes the ear, sometimes sight and sometimes even touch. As to the organs emitting information, these are set in play by muscles, which can be controlled by will, like the ones in the larynx, the tongue, the soft palate, the face, upper extremities, etc. All regular language therefore requires the soundness of: (1) a certain number of muscles, motor nerves leading up to these, and part of the central nervous system, where these nerves stem from; (2) a certain number of external sensorial devices, the sensory nerve leading from this device, and the part of the central nervous system, where this nerve will be directed to; (3) and finally the part of the brain, which holds the general faculty of language, as was defined above.

The absence or abolition of this faculty renders any type of language an impossibility. Hereditary or accidental lesions on organs of reception and emission can prevent a certain type of language for which the contribution of these organs is necessary; but if the general faculty of language still functions with a sufficient degree of intelligence, then we can supplement this lost one with another type of language.

The pathological causes, which deprive us of our means of communication, usually only have us lose half of these, because it is very rare that both organs of emission and reception are afflicted at the same time. For example, the adult who becomes deaf continues to express himself by speaking, but to transmit an idea to him, we use a different kind of language, like a gesture or writing. The opposite takes place, when the muscles involved in speech are paralyzed; the patient we address by spoken language will answer us using a different kind of language. This is how the different types of languages can mutually supplement each other.

This is but elementary physiology, pathology permits pushing even further the analysis of spoken language, which is the most important and probably the most complex of all languages.

There are cases where the general faculty of language continues to exist in an unaltered state, where the auditory apparatus, where the muscles, even those having to do with the voice and with articulation, can be moved at will, and yet where a cerebral lesion abolishes spoken language. This abolition of speech in individuals who are neither paralyzed nor idiots constitutes such a unique symptom that I deem it useful to designate it by a special term. I will therefore give it the name *aphemia* (α deprive; $\varphi\eta\mu\iota$, I speak, I pronounce), as all these patients are missing is the faculty to articulate words. They hear and understand everything one tells them; they are fully intelligent; they easily emit vocal sounds; they move their tongues and lips, producing movementsthat are much more expansive and energetic than it would take to articulate sounds, and yet the intended answer they would like to give is reduced to a very small number of articulated sounds that are always the same and always produced in the same manner; their vocabulary, if one can call it that, is made up of a short series of syllables, sometimes of monosyllables, that express everything or rather express nothing, as this distinct word is most often not to be found in any vocabulary. Some patients do not even have this trace of spoken language; they make efforts, which are in vain, without pronouncing one single syllable. Others have, in some ways, two degrees of articulation. Under ordinary circumstances, they invariably pronounce their word of choice; but when they experience a fit of anger, they become able to articulate a second word, more often a vulgar swear word, which they were probably familiar with before their sickness; they then stop after this last effort. Mr. Auburtin observed a patient who is still alive and who needs no other stimulus in order to pronounce this common swear word. All his answers started with a strange word comprised of six syllables and invariably ended with this supreme invocation: *Sacred name of G . . .*

Those who have studied these strange occurrence for the first time, might have thought, due to insufficient analysis, that the faculty of language, in similar cases, had been abolished; but it evidently exists, since the patients perfectly understand spoken and written language; since those, who do not know or cannot write are intelligent enough (and one needs a lot in both cases) to find a way to communicate their thoughts, and finally since those people, who are literate and who are able to use their hands, clearly put their ideas to paper. They therefore know the sense and meaning of words, in an oral as well as in a graphic form. The language they spoke not long ago is still familiar to them, but they cannot execute the series of methodical and coordinated movements, which correspond to the syllables they search for. That, which has perished in them, is therefore not the faculty of language, it is not the memory of words, it is not the actions of the nerves, the muscles responsible for phonation and articulation either, it is something else, it is a particular faculty considered by Mr. Bouillaud as the faculty of coordinated movements, responsible for spoken language [*faculté de coordonner les mouvements propres au langage articulé*] or simply the faculty of spoken language [*faculté du langage articulé*], since there is no articulation possible without it.

The nature of this faculty and the place it must be assigned in the cerebral hierarchy may be cause for some hesitation. Is it but a kind of memory, and those individuals, who have lost it, have they simply lost, not the memory of words, but the memory of the process, which has to take place to be able to articulate words? Have they regressed to a condition comparable to that of a young child, who already understands the language spoken by those close to him, who is sensitive to blame and praise, who can point out all objects that are named, who has gathered a bunch of simple ideas, and who, to express them, only knows to babble but one syllable? Little by little, after countless efforts, he is able to articulate a few new syllables. But it still happens, that he often makes mistakes and says *papa*, for example, while he meant to say *mama*, because at the moment of pronouncing this last word, he could not remember the position his tongue and lips had to be in. Soon he knows the mechanism of some simple and easy syllables quite well, so much so, that he can instantly pronounce them without making a mistake and without hesitation; but he still hesitates and makes mistakes with syllables, that are more complicated and difficult, and when he has finally mastered several monosyllables, he needs to ac-

quire a new experience in order to all of a sudden move from one syllable to another and to pronounce, instead of repeating monosyllables, which constituted his vocabulary, words composed of two or three different syllables. This gradual perfecting of spoken language in children is due to developments of a type of memory, which is not the memory of words, but one concerning the necessary movements in order to articulate words. And this particular memory has no rapport with other memories, nor with the remaining intelligence. I knew a child of three, who was intelligent and willful beyond his age, who had a well-developed language, and who did not yet know how to speak. I know another very intelligent child who, at twenty-one months, understands two languages perfectly, who consequently possesses a very good memory of words, and who, to date, has not been able to progress past the stage of pronouncing monosyllables.

If those adults, who lose their ability of speech, have simply forgotten the art of articulation, if they simply reverted back to a state they were at, before having learned to pronounce words, then one has to classify the faculty, which they have been deprived of due to sickness, as an intellectual faculty. This hypothesis seems quite plausible to me. It could be possible however, that something else occurred and that the aphasia was the result of a *locomotor ataxia*, which is limited to that part in the central nervous system, which presides over the movements with which sounds are articulated One objects, it is true, that these patients can freely carry out with their tongue and lips all movements except those of articulation; that they immediately, when asked, can point their tongue up, down, to the right and the left, etc.; but these movements, no matter how precise they might seem, are far less so than the very delicate movements necessary for speech. When extremities are inflicted with a locomotor ataxia, we observe the patient executing at will all the big movements: when we ask them to lift their hand, to open it, to close it, they will almost always do so without hesitation; but when they want to carry out a more precise movement, for example, grabbing something very small in a certain manner, they reach over or below it; they do not know how to coordinate their muscle contractions in a manner as to obtain the desired results, and they err a lot less on the direction their movement should take than on the amount of force it would take and the successive order of partial movements that constitute the action of grabbing an object. We can thus ask ourselves if aphemia is not a kind of locomotor ataxia limited to the muscles responsible for sound articulation, and if this is the case, the faculty the patients lost is not an intellectual one, that is a faculty belonging to the 'thinking' part of the brain, rather it would simply be a case, particular to the general faculty governing the coordination of muscle actions, a faculty, which depends on the motor part of nervous centers.

We can thus set up at least two hypotheses on the nature of the special faculty of spoken language. In the first hypothesis, it would be a higher faculty, and aphemia would be an intellectual disorder; in the second hypothesis, it would be a lesser faculty, and aphemia would be no more than a disorder of locomotion. Although the latter interpretation seems to me a lot less likely than the other, I would nonetheless not dare categorically appoint one over the other, if all was based only on clinical observations.

Whatever the case may be, based on the functional analysis, the existence of the special faculty of spoken language, as I defined it, cannot be denied, since a faculty, which can perish in isolation, without affecting neighboring ones, is evidently a faculty, independent of all others, that is, a special faculty.

If all cerebral faculties were this distinct, as neatly circumscribable as this one, we would finally have a positive starting point for answering the controversial question concerning cerebral localization. This is unfortunately not the case, and the biggest obstacle hindering progress in this part of physiology results from the insufficiency and uncertainty of the functional analysis, which must precede the search for identifying organs in relation to each function.

Science is so behind in this respect, that it has not even found its foundation yet, and that, which is being contested today, is not this or that phrenological system, but the principle of localization itself, i.e. the preliminary question of knowing if all the parts of the brain, which are affected during thought have identical attributes or different attributes.

A report by Mr. Gratiolet concerning cerebral and intellectual similarities among the human races has, some time ago, spurred the Anthropological Society of Paris to examine this important question, and Mr. Auburtin, partisan of the localization principle, thought, and rightly so, that the localization of *one* faculty would suffice to prove this principle to be true; he therefore sought to demonstrate, conforming to the doctrine of his teacher Mr. Bouillaud, that the faculty of spoken language is located in the anterior lobes of the brain.

For this, he first examined a series of cases, where a spontaneous cerebral affliction had destroyed the faculty of spoken language without destroying the other cerebral faculties, and where, during the autopsy, one found a deep lesion on anterior convolutions in the brain. The special nature of the symptom of aphemia did not depend on the nature of the ailment, but rather on its location, since the lesion was in one case a softening, in another an apoplexy, in another an abscess or a tumor. In conclusion, Mr. Auburtin referred to another series of cases, where aphemia was the result of a lesion on the anterior lobes in the brain caused by trauma; these facts, according to him, were equivalent to a vivisection, and he concluded by saying that to his knowledge one has never found anterior lobes of the brain in a state of complete intactness, not even in a state of being somewhat intact, in autopsies of those individuals, who had lost the faculty of spoken language without losing the rest of their intelligence.

He was confronted by several remarkable facts concerning individuals who had spoken up to their dying day, but whose anterior lobes were the seat for deep spontaneous or traumatic lesions; but he responded, that this did not prove anything, that a lesion on the anterior lobes, even if widespread, did not necessarily have to reach the part of these lobes where the seat of the faculty of spoken language is situated; that the objection would only be valid if all the frontal convolutions had been destroyed on both sides and all along their expansion, i.e. all the way to the fissure of Rolando, and that in the cases he was being confronted with, the destruction of these convolutions was only partial. He thus recognized that a lesion on the anterior lobes does not necessarily lead to a loss of speech, but he maintained that this was a sure clue for allowing it to be diagnosed; that this diagnosis had been made many times during life, and has never been denied at the autopsy; at last, after having presented the case of a still living individual, who for several years showed very distinct symptoms of aphemia and who is actually at the *Hospice des Incurables*, he declared that he would completely renounce Mr. Bouillaud's doctrines if the autopsy of this patient did not confirm the diagnosis of a cerebral lesion that was exclusively or mainly located on the anterior lobes. (Cf. *Bulletin de la Société d'anthropologie*, 1, II, session of April 4th, 1861.)

I thought it necessary to briefly repeat this discussion in order to underline the interest and relevance of the observation I am presenting to the Anatomical Society today. No doubt the value of the facts is not bound by the circumstances in which we observe them, but the impression they make on us depends greatly on them, and when, a few days after having heard Mr. Auburtin's arguments, I found one morning in my care a deadly sick man, who twenty-one years ago had lost the faculty of spoken language, I treated with the greatest care this case that seemed to come especially to serve as a touchstone for the theory upheld by my colleague.

Up until now, without refuting this theory and without underestimating in any way the importance of the facts that favor it, I was quite hesitant in light of the many contradictions that exist in science. Although a partisan of localization, I asked myself, and still ask myself, to what extent is this principle applicable? There is a point, which seems to me, to be almost established by comparative anatomy, by anatomical and physiological similarities in human races, and lastly by the comparison of individual groups of normal, abnormal of pathological humans belonging to the same race, that is we know, that the highest cerebral faculties, those which, very plainly put, constitute reasoning, like judgement, thought, and the faculties responsible for comparing and abstraction have their seat on the frontal convolutions, whereas the convolutions located on the temporal, parietal and occipital lobes are responsible for emotions, for likes and for passion. In other words, there are groups of faculties in the mind [esprit] and in the brain there are groups of convolutions; and the facts gathered in science up until now permit one to admit, that, as I have stated elsewhere, the largest regions of the mind [esprit] correspond to the largest regions of the brain. It is in this sense, that I see the principle of localization, even if it has not been rigorously proven, to be at least extremely probable. But to know if every particular faculty is located on a particular convolution, is a question, which seems quite unanswerable to me in the current state science is in.

The study of the facts concerning the loss of spoken language is one of those, which have the best possibility of guiding us to a positive or negative solution. The independence of this faculty is proven by pathological observations, and although we may have some doubts as to its nature, although we may ask ourselves, as we saw further up, if it is part of the intellectual functions or part of the cerebral functions, which are connected to the muscles, it is permitted to side with the first hypothesis, at least temporarily, which already at first glance seems to be the most probable and in favor of which the pathological anatomy of aphemia places its strongest suppositions. In fact in all cases to date, where an autopsy could be performed, the substance of the entire convolutions were found to be strongly altered; in some patients the lesions were located *exclusively* on the convolutions: which leads us to believe, that the faculty of spoken language is one of the functions located on the convolutions. We generally admit, that all faculties we consider being intellectual, have their seat in this region of the brain, it therefore seems very probable, that all faculties, located on cerebral convolutions, are faculties of the intellectual order.

In choosing this point of view, we will easily recognize, that the pathological anatomy of aphemia renders more, than simply the answer to a particular question and that it can shed a lot of light on the general question of cerebral localization, by offering the physiology of the brain a starting point or rather a very precious point of comparison. If it is proven, for example, that aphemia might result from lesions, which randomly affect any convolution in any lobe, we would have the right to conclude, that not only is the faculty of language not localized, but that it is very likely, that the other faculties *of the same order* are not localized either. If it were proven, on the other hand though, that the lesions, which abolish speech constantly occupy a determined convolution, we could not do otherwise but to admit, that that convolution is the seat of the faculty of spoken language and having once admitted the existence of a first localization, the principle of localization by convolutions will have been established. Lastly, between these two extreme alternatives, there is a third one, which could lead to a mixed doctrine. Let's suppose, in effect, that the aphemic lesions constantly occupy the same cerebral lobe, but that in this lobe, they did not constantly occupy the same convolution; the result would be, that the faculty of spoken language would have its seat in a certain region, on a certain group of convolutions but not on a particular convolution, and it would thus become very probable, that the cerebral faculties are localized by region and not by convolution.

Consequently, it is important to examine, with the greatest care, one particular question, which may have very general as well as very important doctrinal consequences. It is not only about searching for that region of the brain, where the aphemic lesion is located; in addition, the affected convolutions must be designated by their name and row and to what degree each one was affected. This is not how we have proceeded up until now. We have limited ourselves, even in the most complete observations, to saying that the lesion started and ended at so many centimeters from the anterior extremity of the hemisphere, at so many centimeters from the big median fissure or from the fissure of Sylvius. But this is quite insufficient, because with these indications, no matter how detailed they are, the reader cannot guess what affected convolution this is. Thus, there are cases, where the affliction is situated in the anterior most region of the hemisphere; others, where it is situated 5 or even 8 centimeters behind this point and it seems, according to this, that the seat of the lesion is very different; but if we imagine, that the three anterio-posterior convolutions of the arch of the frontal lobe start at the level of the superciliary arch and progress side by side, from the front to the back, and all three merge into the frontal transversal convolution, which forms the anterior border of the fissure of Rolando; if one imagines, that this fissure is situated 4 centimeters behind the coronal suture[1] and that the three antero-posterior frontal convolutions occupy more than two-fifths of the length of the total brain, — we will understand, that the same convolution may be affected by lesions in places, situated at very different points and very distant from one another. It is thus much less important to indicate the level of the affliction, than to state what convolution is affected.

This type of description is no doubt much less convenient than the other, since the classical works in anatomy have, up till now, not popularized the study of the cerebral convolutions, which the phrenologists themselves have unfortunately neglected as well. We have let ourselves be dominated by this old prejudice, that cerebral convolutions have nothing fixed about them, that they are simple folds, randomly produced, comparable to the disordered twists and turns in the loops of the intestine, and what has sustained this idea is, that the *secondary* folds, which depend on the degree of development of the *fundamental* convolutions,

vary not only from individual to individual but often also, in the same individual, from one hemisphere to the other. It is no less true, that the primary [*fondamentales*] convolutions are fixed and constant in animals of the same species, and that in the animal hierarchy, they are considered to behave like any other perfectly distinct organ. The description and inventory of all these primary convolutions, of their connections and of their combinations will not take place here. They can be found in the special works of MM. Gratiolet and Rodolphe Wagner.[2]

And since I expressed regret about how imprecise the descriptions of lesions on the cerebral hemispheres were, I will bring to your attention a vexing mistake, which has led many observers astray. Many people, who are used to specifically examining the brain from its inferior side, imagine that the anterior lobes comprise only that part of the hemispheres, which is situated in front of the chiasma of the optic nerves and of the anterior extremity of the temporosphenoidal lobe. This, in fact, is where the *inferior* side of the anterior lobes end; but, on the side of the hemispherical convexity, these lobes have a length at least double that of the preceding one and extend beyond the fissure of Sylvius, of which they form the upper border up to the fissure of Rolando, which separates them from the parietal lobes. When one reads in certain observations, that patients, whose two anterior lobes were *completely destroyed*, continued to speak up until their death, it is permitted to think, in the absence of other indications, that the author had specifically wanted to talk about that part of the lobes, which covers the orbital arch. It is stated, for example, in the most famous of these observations, that a man, hit on the forehead by a mine explosion, had both anterior lobes *completely crushed* and *reduced to a pulp*. But is clear, that no trauma can immediately, completely and in one single shot reduce both entire anterior lobes to a pulp, without at the same time crushing all the anterior half of the brain, including the insula, the striate body, the corpus callosum, the fornix cerebri, etc and such a lesion is not admissible in a man, who was able to walk to his bed, who had retained all his intelligence, and who had survived for twenty-four hours without showing signs of contracture or of paralysis. Likewise, when I, in a meeting of doctors, for the first time showed the brain of the man, who is the subject of the case I am presenting today, several people protested, that this specimen contradicted Mr. Bouillaud's ideas, that the anterior lobes were quite healthy, that the lesion was almost completely situated behind these lobes. We will see though, that frontal (or anterior) convolutions were destroyed on a considerable part of their extension.

But I am to apologize for having gotten ahead of myself in these preliminary comments. It is time to turn to the description of my observation of aphemia.

II.

Aphemia Dating Back Twenty-one Years Produced by a Chronic and Progressive Softening of the Second and Third Convolution of the Upper Part of the Left Frontal Lobe

On 11 April 1861, a man of fifty-one years of age and named Leborgne was transported to the general infirmary at Bicêtre, into the care of surgery, afflicted with a gangrenous diffuse phlegmon of all his lower right extremity from the instep up to the buttocks. In response to the questions I asked him the following day, concerning the origin of his pain, he replied only using the monosyllable *tan*, which he repeated two times in a row, and accompanied by a movement of his left hand. I gathered all the information in the history of this man, who had been at Bicêtre for twenty-one years. We questioned those people looking after him, his friends in the ward and those of his parents, who came to see him, and this is the result of this investigation.

Since his youth he had been subjected to attacks of epilepsy; but he was able to take up the trade of milner, which he carried out until the age of thirty. At that time he lost the ability to speak, and it is for this reason, that he was admitted as an invalid to the Bicêtre hospital. We could not find out if the loss of speech came about slowly or gradually, nor if any other symptoms had accompanied the beginning of this affliction.

When he came to Bicêtre, he had not been able to speak for two or three months already. He was at this time perfectly healthy and intelligent and differed from a healthy person only by the loss of spoken language. He went about the hospital, where he was known as *Tan*. He understood everything one told him; he even had a very sensitive sense of hearing; but no matter what question we asked him, he always answered: *tan, tan*, and accompanied this with vary-

ing movements with which he was able to express most of his ideas. When his partners in conversation did not understand hispantomime, he would quickly become angry and then added to his vocabulary a very vulgar swear word, only one, and precisely the same one, which I have indicated above, when discussing a patient observed by Mr. Auburtin. *Tan* was thought to be egotistical, vengeful, mean, and his fellow patients, who hated him, even accused him of being a thief. These faults could, for the most part, be due to the cerebral lesion; nevertheless they were not pronounced enough, to appear to be pathological, and although the patient was at Bicêtre, the thought never occurred to us to place him in the ward for patients with mental deficiencies. On the contrary, we considered him to be a man, who took absolute responsibility for his actions.

It had been ten years since he had lost his speech, when a new symptom manifested itself: the muscles in his right arm gradually weakened, and ended up being completely paralyzed. *Tan* continued to walk without difficulty but his paralysis spread little by little to the inferior right extremity, and after having dragged his leg around for some time, the patient had to resign himself to remain constantly in bed. About four years had passed since the start of the paralysis of the arm up to that of the abdominal extremity had advanced to the point, where the situation was intolerable. It was thus about seven years, that *Tan* had been bed-ridden, when he was brought to the infirmary. This last period of his life is the one, we have the least information about. As he became incapable of being a nuisance, his fellow patients did not bother with him any more, and if so, then only to sometimes amuse themselves at his expense (which pushed him into fits of rage), and he lost the little notoriety that the singularity of his sickness accorded him in the hospital before. We noticed that his sight had weakened considerably since about two years. That was the only aggravation we noticed, since he had been confined to his bed. As to the rest, he was never picky; his sheets were only changed once a week, so that the diffuse phlegmon for which he was brought to the infirmary on April 11, 1861, was only discovered by the nurse when it had spread considerably and had completely taken over the right abdominal extremity, from the foot up to the buttocks.

The examination of this poor fellow, who could not speak and who, being paralyzed in the right hand, could not write, proved to be difficult. He was further more in such a perilous general state, that it would have been cruel to have tortured him with long examinations.

I did, however, ascertain that his general sensation was still intact everywhere, even if not equally everywhere. The right side of the body was less sensitive than the other, and this had undoubtedly contributed to attenuating the pain of the diffuse phlegmon. The patient did not suffer much from it as long as we did not touch it, but the palpation was painful and some incisions, which I had to undertake, provoked agitation and screams.

The two right extremities were completely paralyzed; the two other extremities could be moved at will and although weak, could without any hesitation, execute all the movements. The emission of urine and fecal matter was natural, but swallowing posed some difficulty; mastication, on the contrary, went well. The face was not disfigured; nonetheless, while blowing, the left cheek seemed to bulge out more than the right one, which indicated that the muscles on this side of the face were a little weaker. There was no tendency towards being cross-eyed. The tongue was absolutely free; it was not deformed in any way; the patient could move it in every direction and stick it out of his mouth. The two halves of this organ were of the same thickness. The difficulty in swallowing I mentioned, was due to a paralysis, which was beginning at the pharynx, and not due to a paralysis of the tongue, as it was hard to swallow the third time. The muscles of the larynx did not seen to be altered, the timbre of the voice was natural, and the sound the patient produced, to pronounce his monosyllables, was completely pure.

The sense of hearing remained very good: *Tan* heard the noise of the watch very well, but his sight was very weak; when he wanted to see the time, he had to take the watch himself into his left hand and hold it about 20 centimeters from his right eye, which seemed to be better than the left.

The state of his intelligence could not exactly be determined. It is certain that *Tan* understood almost everything that was said to him; but as he could only express himself by moving his left hand, our dying man could not make himself understood as well as he could understand others. The numerical answers were the ones he did the best with, by opening or closing his fingers. I asked him many times, for how long had he been sick? He would answer sometimes five days, sometimes six days. How many years had he been at Bicêtre? He opened his hands four times in a row and added the rest with a single finger; this came out to twenty-one years, and as we have seen above, this information is absolutely exact. The next day, I repeated the same question, and got the same answer; but when I had wanted to do it a third time, *Tan* understood that I was making him do an exercise; he became angry and uttered the swear word already mentioned, which I heard come out of his mouth only once. I showed him my watch two days in a row. The second hand did not work; consequently, he could distinguish the three hands only by their form or their length; nonetheless, after having examined the watch for a while, he could indicate the exact time every time. It is indisputable that this man was intelligent, that he could think, and that he had maintained, to a certain extent, the memory of old things. He could even understand quite complicated ideas: thus I asked him in what order his paralyses succeeded each other; he first made a little horizontal movement with the index of his left hand, which meant: understood! Then he successively showed me his tongue, his right arm and his right leg. This was absolutely correct; that he attributed the loss of speech to a paralysis of the tongue, was very natural.

Nonetheless, diverse questions that a man of ordinary intelligence would have found a way to answer using a gesture, even with one hand, were left unanswered. Other times, we were unable to grasp the meaning of some answers, which seemed to make the patient very impatient; and other times, the answer was clear but wrong: for example, although he never had children, he pretended to have children. Thus, without a doubt the intelligence of this man had been affected quite deeply, be it due to his cerebral affliction, be it due to the fever, which devoured him; but he was evidently more intelligent than it is necessary to be in order to speak.

From the information gathered and the present state of the patient it was clear, that there existed a progressive cerebral lesion, which at the beginning and during the last six years of the sickness had stayed limited to a region, which was quite bounded and which in this first period had not attained the organs of motility, nor the sensory organs; that after ten years, the lesion had spread to one or several organs of motility, still without touching the sensory organs; and that finally more recently, the general sensation had numbed at the same time as the vision, especially the vision in the left eye. Seeing as the complete paralysis of movement was located in the two extremities on the *right* side, and the sensation of both these extremities being somewhat weakened, the main cerebral lesion had to occupy the *left* hemisphere, and that which confirmed this opinion, was the complete paralysis of the muscles of the *left* cheek and of the retina of the same side, since it is superfluous to reiterate, that paralyses caused by the brain manifest themselves cross wise in the torso and the extremities and directly in the face.

The cause at hand now was to determine more exactly, if possible, the seat of the first lesion and although the last discussion of the Anthropological Society left some doubt as to Mr. Bouillaud's doctrines, I wanted to, while waiting for the next autopsy, reason as if the doctrine were true; this was the best way to put it to the test. I invited Mr. Auburtin, who having declared some days before, that he would renounce it if someone showed him a single case of well discernable aphemia, without lesions on the anterior lobes, to come see my patient in order to see, what his diagnosis would be, and if this case would be one to offer a concluding result. Despite the complications, which had ensued for the past eleven years, my colleague found the actual state and the preceding ones clear enough to affirm, without hesitation, that the lesion had to have started on one of the anterior lobes.

Reasoning from this fact in order to complete the diagnosis, I considered the striate body to be the motor organ closest to the anterior lobes; it was no doubt by gradually spreading to this organ, that the first lesion had caused the hemiphlegia. The probable diagnosis was thus: original legion on the left anterior lobe, then spreading to the striate body on the same side. As to the nature of this lesion, everything indicated a chronic softening, which was progressing, but very slowly, since the absence of all phenomenon of pressure excluded the possibility of an intracranial tumor.

The patient died on April 17, at eleven o'clock in the morning. The autopsy was performed as soon as possible, i.e. after twenty-four hours. The temperature was cool. The cadaver showed no signs of putrefaction. The brain was shown a few hours later to the Anthropological Society, then immediately put into alcohol. This organ was so altered that it took very great precautions to conserve it. It was only after two months, and after having changed the liquid many times, that the specimen started to become firm. To-

day it is in perfect condition and is deposited in the Dupuytren museum under the number 55*a*, *of the nervous system.*

I will not go into the details concerning the diffuse phlegmon. The muscles of both extremities on the right hand side were completely fatty and reduced in size. All the internal organs were healthy except the brain.

The skull was sawed open with great care. All the sutures were joined; the bone was a little thicker; the diploë was replaced by compact tissue. The inside surface of the cranial arch had indications of small wormholes all along its surface, a sure indication of a chronic osteitis (no. 55*b*).

The outside surface of the dura mater was red and very vascularized; this membrane was very thick, very vascular, almost fleshy and on the inside covered by a pseudo-membranous layer, permeated by serous fluid and greasy looking. The dura mater and the false membrane together had a thickness of about 5 millimeters (min. 3 millimeters; max. 8), which indicates that the brain must have lost a considerable amount of its original size.

The dura mater removed, the pia mater seemed to be very pierced in certain spots, thick everywhere, and opaque in certain places, infiltrated by an unnaturally yellow material, the color of pus, but which is solid and which, when examined under the microscope, did not hold any purulent globules.

On the lateral side of the left hemisphere, at the level of the fissure of Sylvius, the pia mater is raised by a pool of transparent serous fluid, which is lodged in a large and deep depression in the cerebral substance. Having removed this liquid by puncturing it, the pia mater sinks very deeply, resulting in a cavity with a capacity for holding a chicken's egg, located at the level of the fissure of Sylvius and consequently separating the frontal lobe from the temporal lobe. The cavity extends in the back up to the fissure of Rolando, which separates, as we know, the anterior or frontal convolutions from the parietal convolutions. The lesion is thus completely situated in front of this fissure, and the parietal lobe is healthy, relatively at least, since no part of the hemisphere is in a state of complete health.

By cutting into and pushing aside the pia mater at the level of the cavity, I just mentioned, one recognizes at first glance, that this is not a depression, but a loss of substance of the cerebral mater; the liquid, which filled it, was consecutively drawn into it, to fill the void as it was being formed during the chronic softening of the upper layers of the brain or of the cerebellum. The examination of the convolutions, which bound the cavity, show, that they are the seat of one of this chronic softening, whose progress is slow enough for the cerebral molecules, in some ways dissociated from each other, to be reabsorbed and replaced by an emission of serous fluid.[3] A large part of the left hemisphere had gradually been destroyed like this; but the softening extends much further than the cavity; the softening is bound nowhere and can in no way be compared to a cyst. Its inner surfaces, irregular almost everywhere, full of holes, are made up of the cerebral substance itself, extremely soft at this level and whose inner-most layer in contact with the emitted serous fluid, was on the path of a slow and gradual dissolution, at the time the patient succumbed to his sickness. Only the inferior inner surface is smooth and is of a quite firm consistence.

It is consequently clear that the original location of the softening was located there, where today substance is lost; that the waste then spread from tissue to neighboring tissue; and that the starting point of this waste must be searched for not among the organs, which are actually soft or in the process of softening, but among those that are more or less completely destroyed. We will thus, according to the examination of the parts that neighbor the lost substance, set up the list of those that have disappeared.

The cavity, which we will describe, is situated, as we have already seen, at the level of the fissure of Sylvius; it is consequently situated between the frontal lobe and the temporo-sphenoidal lobe and if the organs, which surround it, were only pushed back, without being destroyed, we should find on its upper or temporal border the *marginal inferior convolution*, on its upper or frontal border the *third frontal convolution*,[4] and lastly, on its deep inner surface, the *lobe of the insula*. The following is not unimportant either. (1) The inferior border of the cavity is bound by the second temporo-sphenoide convolution, which, by the way, is complete and which has a quite firm consistence. The inferior marginal convolution has thus been destroyed in all its thickness, that is up to the *parallel fissure*. (2) The deep inner surface of the cavity does not show any trace of the lobe of the insula anymore; this lobe is entirely destroyed, as well as the inner half of the extra-ventricle core of the striate body; lastly, the loss of substance reaches into the an-

terior part of the ventricle core of the striate body on this side, in such a manner, that our cavity connects, by way of a long opening, half a centimeter long and with irregular borders, with the lateral ventricle of the brain. (3) Lastly, the upper border or rather the upper inner surface of the cavity considerably infringes into the frontal lobe, which, at this level, is a large and deep depression. The posterior half of the third frontal convolution is completely destroyed in all its thickness; the second frontal convolution is affected a little less. At least two thirds of its external part has disappeared, and the remaining external third is extremely soft. In back, the inferior third of the frontal transversal convolution is destroyed in all its thickness up to the fissure of Rolando.

To sum up, the destroyed organs are the following: The small inferior marginal convolution (temporo-sphenoidal); the small convolutions on the lobe of the insula and the subjacent part of the striate body; lastly, on the frontal lobe, the inferior part of the transversal convolution, and the posterior half of the two big convolutions known as the second and third frontal convolutions. Of the four convolutions that form the upper level of the frontal lobe, only one, the first and inner most one, is not intact, since it is soft and small, but has kept on existing; and if we recall all the parts, which have disappeared, we find that at least three thirds of the cavity has been dug up at the expense of the frontal lobe.

We must now determine the place where, the lesion must have started. We know, that by examining the cavity left behind by the loss of substance first of all shows, that the center of the place of origin corresponds to the frontal lobe. Consequently, if the softening had spread uniformly in all directions, this lobe would have been the starting point for the destruction. We should not only be guided by studying the cavity, but also must take into account the state of the surrounding parts. These parts are very unevenly softened, and to very different extents. As such, the second temporal convolution, which borders below the place of origin, has a soft surface and a quite firm consistency; it is no doubt softened, but not very much and only on its upper layers. On the other side, on the frontal lobe, the softening has, on the other hand, almost taken on a liquid form near the place of origin; moving away, the cerebral substance gradually becomes firmer, but, in reality, the softening extends a considerable distance, and almost reaches the frontal lobe. So it is especially into this lobe, that the softening has spread and it is quite certain, that the other parts have only been invaded consecutively.

If we wanted to go into it in greater detail, we would see that the third frontal convolution has lost the most substance, that it is not only cut in half at the level of the anterior extremity of the fissure of Sylvius, but also that its posterior half is entirely destroyed, such that it alone witnessed a loss of substance equaling half of the entire loss of substance; that the second convolution or middle convolution, although deeply damaged, still upholds its continuity in its most internal part, and that by consequence, according to all probability, it is in the third frontal convolution, that the destruction started.

The other parts of the hemisphere are relatively intact; they are, it is true, a little less firm than usual, and we can say, that the exterior parts of the brain have undergone a notable shrinkage, but they have conserved their shape, their continuity and their normal characteristics. As to the parts located deeper inwards, I have given up examining these, in order not to destroy the specimen, which I consider to be very important to donate to the museum. Nevertheless, the opening, which connected the anterior part of the left lateral ventricle with the exterior, having widened, despite my efforts?, during the dissection of the pia mater, allowed me to half examine the internal surface of the this ventricle, and I saw that the striate body was more or less softened, but that the thalamus had retained its color, its normal size and its normal consistence.

The entire brain *weighed with the pia mater,* after the liquid, which filled the cavity, was removed, no more than 987 grams. It thus weighed about 400 grams less than the average weight of a brain of a *male* of fifty years. This considerable loss is almost entirely carried by the cerebral hemispheres. We know, in fact, that the rest of the brain in a normal state never weighs 200 grams, and remains almost constantly under 180. We know, that the cerebellum, the protuberance and the bulb, although not very big in our subject, are certainly not very much below the average, and supposing the impossible, that they had lost a quarter of their weight, that would only account for a very small part of the total loss.

The destruction of the organs surrounding the fissure of Sylvius in the left hemisphere no doubt contributes a lot to diminishing the weight of the brain;

but I extracted the same mass of substance from a healthy brain and the amount I took did not quite weigh 50 grams. It is thus very probable, that the cerebral hemispheres shrunk a great deal and this probability changes to certainty, if one thinks about how thick the meninges and false arachnoid membrane are, in certain points reaching up to 5 or 6 millimeters.

After having described the lesion and searched to determine the nature, seat and anatomical path it took, it is important to compare these results with the clinical observation, in order to establish, if possible, a rapport between the symptoms and the material disturbance.

The anatomical examination shows that the lesion was still spreading when the patient died. This lesion has thus been progressive, but very slow, since it took twenty-one years to destroy a rather limited part of the cerebral mass. Consequently, it is permissible to think that there was a long period in which the lesion had not reached beyond the limits of the organ it originated in. We know that the destruction started in the frontal lobe, and very probably in the third frontal convolution. This leads us to admit that in point of view of anatomical pathology, there were two periods: one in which only one frontal convolution (probably the third) was altered; the other in which the destruction propagated itself more and more onto other convolutions of the lobe of insula or of the core of the extra-ventricle of the striate body.

Now if we examine the succession of symptoms, we equally find two periods: a first one, which lasted ten years, in which the faculty of spoken language was abolished and where all other functions of the brain were intact; and a second period of eleven years, in which a paralysis at first partially, then completely set in, invading the upper extremity and then the lower extremity on the right side.

This stated, it is impossible to overlook that there was a connection between the anatomical periods and the two symptomatological periods. No one is ignorant of the fact, that the cerebral convolutions are not motor organs. The striate body in the left hemisphere is thus, from all organs touched by the lesion, where we can look for the cause of the paralysis of both right extremities and the second clinical period, the one in which the motility was altered, therefore correspond to the second anatomical period, i.e. the one, in which the softening, reaching beyond the limits of the frontal lobe, spread into the insula and the striate body.

Therefore, the first period of ten years, clinically characterized by the unique symptom of aphemia, must correspond to the period when the lesion was still limited to the frontal lobe.

Until now, in this parallel of lesions and symptoms, I have not spoken of the problems concerning intelligence, nor of their anatomical causes. We saw, that our patient's intelligence was perfectly maintained for a long time, and that it had strongly deteriorated, when we saw him for the first time. We have in the autopsy alterations, which more than suffice to explain this state. Three out of four frontal convolutions were deeply lesioned to a considerable extent, almost all of the frontal lobe was more or less softened; finally, all the mass of the convolutions of both hemispheres was atrophied, collapsed and softer than in the normal state. It is difficult to believe that the patient was able to still maintain some intelligence, and it does not seem probable that one can live for very long with such a brain. For my part, I think, that the general softening of the left frontal lobe, the general atrophy of both hemispheres and the general chronic meningitis do not go too far back; I am disposed to believe, that these lesions came about a long time after the softening of the striate body, so that one could subdivide the second period into two secondary periods, and resume the patient's history thus.

Facts, which, like this one, are attached to grand doctrinal questions, cannot be described with much detail, nor discussed with much care. I need this excuse in order to pardon the dryness of the descriptions and the length of the discussion. I now only have a few words to add, with which the conclusions, I have drawn from this case, may be stated.

1. Aphemia, i.e. the loss of speech, before all other intellectual disturbances and before any paralysis, was the result of a lesion in the anterior lobes of the brain.
2. Thus, our case just confirmed Mr. Bouillaud's opinion, which places the seat of the faculty of spoken language in these lobes.
3. The observations gathered up until now, those which at least are accompanied by a clear and precise anatomical description, are too few in order that we may consider this localization of a particular faculty in a determined lobe as definitely proven, but we can at least consider it as highly likely.
4. It is a much harder question to ask whether the faculty of spoken language depends on the whole anterior lobe or only specifically on one of the convolutions in this lobe; to know, in other words, if the localization of cerebral faculties takes place by faculty and by convolution, or only by group of faculties and group of convolutions. The future observations should be gathered in light of answering this question. For this, one needs to indicate the exact name and the row of afflicted convolutions, and if the lesion is very extensive, try to determine as much as possible, by way of anatomical examination, the point or rather the convolution, where the affliction seems to have started.
5. In our patient, the original seat of the lesion was in the second or third frontal convolution, most probably in the latter. It is thus probable, that the faculty of spoken language is located in one or the other of these two convolutions; but we cannot know it yet, as previous observations are silent about the particular state of each convolution, and we cannot even theorize on it, since the principle of localization by convolution does not rest on a certain foundation yet.
6. In any case, it suffices to compare our case with others, which have preceded it, to push aside the idea today, that the faculty of spoken language lies in a point that is fixed, circumscribed and situated under any bump on the skull; the lesions of aphemia were most often found in the most anterior part of the frontal lobe, not far from the eyebrows and above the orbital arch; whereas with my patient, they existed much further back and a lot closer to the coronal suture of the superciliary arch. This difference in seat is incompatible with the system of bumps: on the other hand, it would be perfectly reconcilable with the system of localization by convolutions, since every one of the three big convolutions on the upper level of the frontal lobe successively run through, in its anterio-posterior path, all regions, where one, up until here, found the lesions causing aphemia.

Notes

1. It is generally thought that the fissure of Rolando is situated directly under the coronal suture, and Mr. Gratiolet therefore grants the study of this suture much importance, which would permit to establish a very precise relationship between the frontal region of the skull and the anterior lobes of the brain. This would be very important data in the comparison of human races. Unfortunately, the data is arrived at in a very inexact way: the

brain, removed from the skull and placed onto a table, spreads and stretches out, and if one then measures the length of the anterior lobe of the hemisphere, one finds that it is about the same as the frontal bone. But in examining the organ in place, I came to a completely different result. This is how I proceeded. After having removed the integument and the pericranium, I drill bits into different points along the coronal suture and push little wooden pins into these holes and into the cerebral substance. The skull is then sawed open; the brain is removed and cleaned of its membranes, and I examine the location of the wooden pins in relation to the fissure of Rolando. I have done this with eleven subjects of the male gender who had attained or passed the age of adulthood, and I constantly found that the fissure of Rolando starts, on the median line, at least 4 centimeters behind the coronal suture (minimum 40 millimeters; maximum 63 millimeters). On its external surface, this fissure, *which is oblique and not transverse*, nears the coronal suture; at 4 centimeters of the median line, it is situated only about 2 centimeters, max. 3, behind this suture. The same procedure allowed me to find that, on the other hand, there is a constant enough relationship between the lambdoid suture and the transverse occipital fissure that separates the parietal lobe from the occipital lobe of the hemisphere. The pins thrust into the lambdoid suture ordinarily penetrate the occipital fissure or very close to there. I never found it more than 15 millimeters from this fissure, and the difference is rarely more than 5 millimeters.

2. Gratiolet and Leuret, *Anatomie comparée du système nerveux*, 1. II, p. 110. Paris, 1857, in –8. This second volume is the exclusive work of Mr. Gratiolet.—Gratiolet, *Mémoire sur les plis* cérébraux *de l'homme et des primates*, Paris, 1854, in-4, with atlas in-folio.—Rodolphe Wagner, *Abhandlung über die typischen Verschiedenheiten der Windungen der Hemisphaeren*, etc. Göttingen, 1860, in-4, with atlas, pp. 13 to 25. We will find further on, in another note, an abridged description of the anterior or frontal convolutions.

3. This is not how it happens with the softening, which starts in the medullary layer of the convolutions: its only when the lesion starts under the pia mater, i.e. the cortical layer of convolutions, that the substance, softened and slowly reabsorbed, is replaced by serous fluid. I observed the diverse phases of this procedure on the cerebellum as well as on the brain. The first specimen I took (and which I presented in January 1861 to the Anatomical Society) had first baffled me; but many others have since laid my doubts to rest.

4. It had seemed necessary to me, for the sake of understanding that which will follow, to briefly remind here the nature of and rapport amongst the cerebral organs, which I will mention.

The anterior lobe of the brain makes up all that part of the hemisphere, situated above the fissure of Sylvius, that separates it from the temporo-sphenoidal lobe, and in front of the fissure of Rolando, that separates it from the parietal lobe. The location of this latter fissure has been specified in a previous note (p. 340). Its path is almost transversal; starting from the median line, it follows an almost straight line, hardly deviating in slight turns, ending at the bottom and beyond the fissure of Sylvius, which it meets almost at a right angle behind the posterior border of the lobe *of the insula*.

The anterior lobe of the brain is comprised of two *levels*, one inferior or orbital, formed by many said *orbital* convolutions, which lie on the orbital arch and which I will not discuss; the other, superior one, is situated under the shell of the frontal bone and under the most anterior part of the parietal.

This superior level is comprised of four main convolutions simply called *frontal convolutions*: one is located in the posterior, the others in the anterior. The posterior one, not very winding, forms the anterior border of the fissure of Rolando; it thus almost lies transversely and comes up from outside going inwards from the fissure of Sylvius to the great median fissure, which receives the falx of the brain: that is why it is indifferently known under different terms as the *frontal posterior, transversal or ascending convolution*. The other convolutions on the superior level are very winding, very complicated and it takes getting used to, in order to distinguish them in all their length, without confusing the main fissures that separate them with the secondary fissures that separate the folds of the second order and which changes, following the individual, according to the degree of complication, i.e. according to how developed the frontal convolutions are. These three anterior convolutions are anterio-posterior, and running side by side, follow a path going from the front to the back all along the length of the frontal lobe. They start at the level of the sourciliary arcade, where they bend back, in order to continue with the convolutions on the inferior layer, and they end, in back, at the frontal transversal convolution, in which all three merge into. They are termed the *first, second, and third frontal convolution*. They can also be called *inner, middle, and external*; but the ordinal names have prevailed.

The *first* follows the grand fissure of the brain; in humans, it constantly presents an antero-posterior fissure that is more or less complete and divides into two folds of the second order. It has thus been subdivided into two convolutions; but comparing the anatomy shows that these two folds only form one main convolution.

The *second frontal convolution* is not very distinguishable; it is different from the *third* one, which lies the most externally. This one forms an upper or inner contiguous border with the winding border of the middle convolution, and an inferior or external border, of which the relationships differentiate according to where they are examined in front or in back. In its anterior half, the border is in contact with the external border of the most external orbital convolution. In its posterior half, on the other hand, it is free and separated from the temporosphenoidal lobe by the fissure of Sylvius, for which it forms the superior border. It is due to this last relationship that the third frontal convolution is sometimes referred to as the *superior marginal convolution*.

Let's add that the inferior border of the fissure of Sylvius is formed by the superior convolution of the temporo-sphenoidal lobe, which is therefore called the *inferior marginal convolution*. It is a thin and almost straight antero-posterior fold that is separated by the second temporo-sphenoidal convolution by a fissure parallel to the fissure of Sylvius. This fissure is designated under the term *parallel fissure* (as implied in relation to the *fissure of Sylvius*).

Finally, when we push aside the two marginal convolutions, the superior and inferior one, from the fissure of Sylvius, we recognize a large but not very protruding bump whose summit gives birth to five simple little convolutions, or rather to five straight lined folds, spread out in the shape of a fan: this is the *lobe of the insula*, which covers the extraventricle core of the striate body, and which, emerging from the bottom of the fissure of Sylvius, is connected to the most sunken part of both marginal convolutions by its cortical layer and to the extra-ventricle core of the striate body by its medullary layer. The result of this connection is that a propagating lesion has to pass by the *insula* lobe, and that from there, it has a big opportunity to spread to the extra-ventricle core of the striate body, that is if the substance of the *insula*, which separates this core from the surface of the brain, is but a very thin layer.

19

On Affections of Speech from Disease of the Brain

John Hughlings-Jackson

It is very difficult for many reasons to write on Affections of Speech. So much, since the memorable researches of Sax and Broca, has been done in the investigation of these cases of disease of the brain, that there is an *embarras des richesses* in material. To refer only to what has been done in this country, we have the names of Gairdner, Moxon, Broadbent, William Ogle, Bastian, John W. Ogle, Thomas Watson, Alexander Robertson, Ireland, Wilks, Bristowe, Ferrier, Bateman, and others. To Wilks, Gairdner, Moxon, Broadbent and Ferrier, I feel under great obligations. Besides recognising the value of Broadbent's work on this subject, I have to acknowledge a particular indebtedness to him. Broadbent's hypothesis—a verified hypothesis—is, I think, essential to the methodical investigation of affections of speech. Let me give at once an illustration of its value. It disposes of the difficulty there otherwise would be in holding

From *Brain*, vol. i, 1878–79, pp. 304–330. (Reprinted in *Brain*, 1915, vol. xxxviii.)

(1) that loss of speech is, on the physical side, loss of nervous arrangements for highly special and complex articulatory *movements*, and (2) that in cases of loss of speech the articulatory *muscles* are not paralysed, or but slightly paralysed. I shall assume that the reader is well acquainted with Broadbent's researches on the representation of certain movements of the two sides of the body in each side of the brain; the reader must not assume that Broadbent endorses the applications I make of his hypothesis. The recent encyclopaedic article on Affections of Speech, by Kussmaul, in Ziemssen's *Practice of Medicine*, is very complete and highly original. It is worthy of most careful study.

The subject has so many sides—psychological, anatomical, physiological and pathological—that it is very difficult to fix on an order of exposition. It will not do to consider affections of speech on but one of these sides. To show how they mutually bear, we must see each distinctly. For example: we must not confound the physiology of a case with its pathology, by using for either the vague term "disease." Again, we must not ignore anatomy when speaking of the physical basis of words, being content with morphology, as in saying that words "reside" in this or that part of the brain. Supposing we could be certain that this or that grouping of cells and nerve-fibres was concerned in speech, from its being always destroyed when speech is lost, we should still have to find out the anatomy of the centre. Even supposing we were sure that the physical states called words, and the nervous states in the "centre for words," were the same things, we should still have the anatomy of that centre to consider. The morphology of a centre deals with its shape, with its "geographical" position, with the sizes and shapes of its constituent elements. A knowledge of the anatomy of a centre is a knowledge of the parts of the body represented in it, and of the ways in which these parts are therein represented. Whilst so much has been learned as to the morphology of the cerebrum—cerebral topography—it is chiefly to the recent researches of Hitzig and Ferrier that we are indebted for our knowledge of the anatomy of many of the convolutions, that is, a knowledge of the parts of the body these convolutions represent. It is supposed that the anatomy of the parts of the brain concerned with words is that they are cerebral nervous arrangements representing the articulatory muscles in very special and complex movements. Similarly, a knowledge of the anatomy of the centres concerned during visual ideation is a knowledge of those regions of the brain where certain parts of the organism (retina and ocular muscles) are represented in particular and complex combinations. A merely materialistic or morphological explanation of speech or mind, supposing one could be given, is not an anatomical explanation. Morphologically, the substratum of a word or of a syllable is made up of nerve-cells and fibres: anatomically speaking, we say it is made up of nerve-cells and fibres representing some particular articulatory movement.

Unless we most carefully distinguish betwixt psychology and the anatomy and physiology of the nervous system in this inquiry, we shall not see the fundamental similarity there is betwixt the defect often described in psychological phraseology as "loss of memory for words," and the defect called ataxy of articulation. A method which is founded on classifications which are partly anatomical and physiological, and partly psychological, confuses the real issues. These mixed classifications lead to the use of such expressions as that an *idea* of a word produces an articulatory *movement*; whereas a psychical state, an "idea of a word" (or simply "a word") cannot produce an articulatory movement, a physical state. On any view whatever as to the relation of mental states and nervous states such expressions are not warrantable in a *medical* inquiry. We could only say that discharge of the cells and fibres of the anatomical substratum of a word produces the articulatory movement. In all our studies of diseases of the nervous system we must be on our guard against the fallacy that what are physical states in lower centres fine away *into* psychical states in higher centres; that, for example, vibrations of sensory nerves *become* sensations, or that somehow or another an idea produces a movement.

Keeping them distinct, we must consider now one and now another of the several sides of our subject: sometimes, for example, we consider the psychical side—speech—and at other times the anatomical basis of speech. We cannot go right on with the psychology, nor with the anatomy, nor with the pathology of our subject. We must consider now one and now the other, endeavouring to trace a correspondence betwixt them.

I do not believe it to be possible for anyone to write methodically on these cases of disease of the nervous system without considering them in relation to other kinds of nervous disease; nor to be desirable in a medical writer if it were possible. Broadbent's hypothesis is exemplified in cases of epilepsy and hemiplegia, as well as in cases of affections of speech, and can only be vividly realised when these several diseases have been carefully studied. Speech and perception ("words" and "images") co-operate so intimately in mentation (to use Metcalfe-Johnson's term) that the latter process must be considered. We must speak briefly of imperception—loss of images—as well as of loss of speech—loss of symbols. The same general principle is, I think, displayed in each. Both in delirium (partial imperception) and in affections of speech the patient is reduced to a more automatic condition; respectively reduced to the more organised relations of images and words. Again, we have temporary loss or defect of speech after certain epileptiform seizures: temporary affections of speech after these seizures are of great value in elucidating some difficult parts of our subject, and cannot be understood without a good knowledge of various other kinds of epileptic and epileptiform paroxysms, and post-paroxysmal states. After a convulsion beginning in the (right) side of the face or tongue, or in both these parts, there often remains temporary speechlessness, although the articulatory muscles move well. Surely we ought to consider cases of discharge of the centres for words as well as cases in which these centres are destroyed, just as we consider not only hemiplegia but hemispasm. Before trying to analyse that very difficult symptom called ataxy of articulation, we should try to understand the more easily studied disorder of co-ordination, locomotor ataxy; and before that, the least difficult disorder of co-ordination of movements resulting from ocular paralysis. Unless we do, we shall not successfully combat the notion that there are centres for co-ordination of words which are something over and above centres for special and complex movements of the articularly muscles, and that a patient can, from lesion of such a centre, have a loss of co-ordination, without veritable loss of some of the movements represented in it.

It might seem that we could consider cases of aphasia, as a set of symptoms at least, without regard to the pathology of different cases of nervous disease. We really could not. It so happens that different morbid processes have what, for brevity, we may metaphorically call different seats of election; thus, that defect of speech with which there are frequent mistakes in words is nearly always produced by local cerebral softening; that defect which is called ataxy of articulation, is, I think, most often produced by haemorrhage. Hence we must consider hemiplegia in relation to affections of speech; for it so happens that the first kind of defect mostly occurs, as Hammond has pointed out, without hemiplegia, or without persistent hemiplegia, a state of things producible by embolism and thrombosis, and the latter mostly with hemiplegia and persistent hemiplegia, a state of things usually produced by haemorrhage. From ignoring such considerations, the two kinds of defects are by some considered to be absolutely different, whereas on the anatomicophysiological side they are but very different degrees of one kind of defect.

There are certain most general principles which apply, not only to affections of speech, but also to the commonest variety of paralysis, to the simplest of convulsive seizures, and to cases of insanity.

The facts that the speechless patient is frequently reduced to the use only of the most general propositions "yes" or "no," or both; that he may be unable to say "no" when told, although he says it readily in reply to questions requiring dissent; that he may be able ordinarily to put out his tongue well, as for example to catch a stray crumb, and yet unable to put it out

when he tries, after being asked to do so; that he loses intellectual language and not emotional language; that although he does not speak, he understands what we say to him; and many other facts of the same order, illustrate exactly the same principle as do such facts from other cases of disease of the nervous system as—that in hemiplegia the arm suffers more than the leg; that most convulsions beginning unilaterally begin in the index finger and thumb; that in cases of post-epileptic insanity there are degrees of temporary reduction from the least towards the most "organised" actions," degrees proportional to the severity of the discharge in the paroxysm, or rather to the amount of exhaustion of the highest centres produced by the discharge causing the paroxysm. In all these cases—except in the instance of convulsion, which, however, illustrates the principle in another way—there are, negatively, degrees of loss of the most voluntary processes with, positively, conservation of the next most voluntary or next more automatic; otherwise put, there are degrees of lost of the latest acquirements with conservation of the earlier, especially of the inherited, acquirements; speaking of the physical side, there are degrees of loss of function of the least organised nervous arrangements with conservation of function of the more organised. There is in each reduction to a more automatic condition: in each there is Dissolution, using this term as Spencer does, as the opposite of Evolution.[1]

In *defects* of speech we may find that the patient utters instead of the word intended a word of the same class in meaning as "worm-powder" for "cough-medicine"; or, in sound, as "parasol" for "castor oil." The presumption is that the patient uses what is to him a more "organised" or "earlier" word, and if so, Dissolution is again seen. But often there is no obvious relation of any sort betwixt the word said and the one appropriate, and thus the mistake does not appear to come under Dissolution. If, however, we apply the broad principles which we can, I think, establish from other cases of Dissolution, *viz.* from degrees of insanity—especially the slight degrees of the post-epileptic insanity just spoken of—we shall be able to show that many of the apparently random mistakes in words are not real exceptions to the principle of Dissolution.

For the above reasons I shall make frequent references to other classes of nervous disease. The subject is already complex without these excursions, but we must face the complexity. Dr. Curnow has well said

(*Medical Times and Gazette*, November 29, p. 616), "The tendency to appear exact by disregarding the complexity of the factors is the old failing in our medical history."

Certain provisional divisions of our subject must be made. The reader is asked to bear in mind that these are admittedly arbitrary; they are not put forward as scientific distinctions. Divisions[2] and arrangements are easy, distinctions and classifications are difficult. But in the study of a very complex matter, we must first divide, and then distinguish. This is not contradictory to what was said before on the necessity of encountering the full complexity of our subject. Harm comes, not from dividing and arranging, but from stopping in this stage, from taking provisional divisions to be real distinctions, and putting forward elaborate arrangements, with divisions and subdivisions, as being classifications. In other words, we shall, to start with, consider our subject empirically, and afterwards scientifically; we first arbitrarily divide and arrange for convenience of obtaining the main facts which particular cases supply, and then try to classify the facts, in order to show their true relations one to another, and consider them on the psychical side as defects of mind, and on the physical side as defects of the nervous system. Empirically we consider the cases of affection of speech we meet with, as they *approach* certain nosological types (most frequently occurring cases), scientifically we classify the facts thus obtained, to show how affections of speech are *departures from* what we know of healthy states of mind and body. The latter study is of the cases as they show different degrees of nervous dissolution.

Let us first of all make a very rough popular division. When a person "Talks" there are three things going on—speech, articulation and voice. Disease can separate them. Thus from disease of the larynx, or from paralysis of its nerves, we have loss of voice, but articulation and speech remain good. Again, in complete paralysis of the tongue, lips and palate, articulation is lost, but speech is not even impaired; the patient remains able to express himself in writing, which shows that he retains speech—internal speech—that he propositionises well. Lastly, in extensive disease in a certain region in one half of the brain (left half usually) there is loss of speech, internal and external, but the articulatory muscles move well.

Let us make a wider division. Using the term language, we make two divisions of it, intellectual and emotional. The patient, whom we call speechless (he is also defective in pantomime), has lost intellectual language and has not lost emotional language.

The kind of case we shall consider first is that of a man who has lost speech, and whose pantomime is impaired, but whose articulatory muscles move well, whose vocal organs are sound, and whose emotional manifestations are unaffected. This is the kind of case to be spoken of as No. 2 (p. 161).

The term Aphasia has been given to affections of speech by Trousseau; it is used for defects as well as for loss of speech. I think the expression Affections of Speech (including defects and loss) is preferable. Neither term is very good, for there is, at least in many cases, more than loss of *speech*; pantomime is impaired; there is often a loss or defect in symbolising relations of things in any way. Dr. Hamilton proposes the term Asemasia, which seems a good one. He derives it "from ἀ and σημαίνω, an inability to indicate by signs or language." It is too late, I fear, to displace the word aphasia. Aphasia will be sometimes used as synonymous with affections of speech in this article.

We must at once say briefly what we mean by speech, in addition to what has been said by implication when excluding articulation, as this is popularly understood, and voice. To speak is not simply to utter words, it is to propositionise. A proposition is such a relation of words that it makes one new meaning; not by a mere addition of what we call the separate meanings of the several words; the terms in a proposition are modified[3] by each other. Single words are meaningless, and so is any unrelated succession of words. The unit of speech is a proposition. A single word is, or is in effect, a proposition, if other words in relation are implied. The English tourist at a French *table d'hôte* was understood by the waiter to be asking for water when his neighbours thought he was crying "oh!" from distress. It is from the use of a word that we judge of its propositional value. The words "yes" and "no" are propositions, but only when used for assent and dissent; they are used by healthy people interjectionally as well as propositionally. A speechless patient may retain the word "no," and yet have only the interjectional or emotional, not the propositional, use of it; he utters it in various tones as signs of feeling only. He may have a propositional use of it, but yet a use of it short of that healthy people have, being able to reply "no," but not to say "no" when told; a speechless patient may have the full use of it. On the other hand, elaborate oaths, in spite of their propositional structure, are not propositions, for they have not, either in the mind of the utterer or in that of the person to whom they are uttered, any meaning at all; they may be called "dead propositions." The speechless patient may occasionally swear. Indeed he may have a recurring utterance, *e.g.* "Come on to me," which is propositional in structure but not, to him, propositional in use; he utters it on any occasion, or rather on no *occasion*, but every time he tries to speak.

Loss of speech is therefore the loss of power to propositionise. It is not only loss of power to propositionise aloud (to talk), but to propositionise either internally or externally, and it may exist when the patient remains able to utter some few words. We do not mean, by using the popular term power, that the speechless man has lost any "faculty" of speech or propositionising; he has lost those words which serve in speech, the nervous arrangements for them being destroyed. There is no "faculty" or "power" of speech apart from words revived or revivable in propositions, any more than there is a "faculty" of co-ordination of movements apart from movements represented in particular ways. We must here say too that besides the use of words in speech there is a service of words which is not speech; hence we do not use the expression that the speechless man has lost words, but that he has lost those words which serve in speech. In brief, Speechlessness does not mean entire Wordlessness.

It is well to insist again that speech and words are psychical terms; words have of course anatomical substrata or bases as all other psychical states have. We must as carefully distinguish betwixt words and their physical bases, as we do betwixt colour and its physical basis; a psychical state is always accompanied by a physical state, but nevertheless the two things have distinct natures. Hence we must not say that the "memory of words" is a *function* of any part of the nervous system, for function is a physiological term (*vide infra*). Memory or any other psychical state arises *during* not *from*—if "from" implies continuity of a psychical state with a physical state—functioning of nervous arrangements, which functioning is a purely physical thing—a discharge of nervous elements representing some impressions and movements. Hence it is not to be inferred from the rough division we just made of the elements of "talking," and from what was said of their "separation" by disease, that there is anything in common even for reasonable contrast, much less for comparison, betwixt loss of speech (a psychi-

cal loss) and immobility of the articulatory muscles from, say disease of the medulla oblongata, as in "bulbar paralysis" (a physical loss). As before said, we must not classify on a mixed method of anatomy, physiology and psychology, any more than we should classify plants on a mixed natural and empirical method, as exogens, kitchen-herbs, graminaceae and shrubs. The things comparable and contrastable in the rough division are (1) the two physical losses: (*a*) loss of function of certain nervous arrangements in the cerebrum, which are not speech (words used in speech), but the anatomical substrata of speech; and (*b*) loss of function of nervous arrangements in the medulla oblongata. (2) The comparison, on the psychical side, fails. There is no psychical loss in disease of the medulla oblongata to compare with loss of words, as this part of the nervous system, at least as most suppose,[4] has no psychical side; there is nothing psychical to be lost when nervous arrangements in the medulla oblongata are destroyed.

The affections of speech met with are very different in degree and kind, for the simple reason that the exact position of disease in the brain and its gravity differ in different cases; different amounts of nervous arrangements in different positions are destroyed with different rapidity in different persons. There is, then, no single well-defined "entity"—loss of speech or aphasia and thus, to state the matter for a particular practical purpose, such a question as, "Can an aphasic make a will?" cannot be answered any more than the question, "Will a piece of string reach across this room?" can be answered. The question should be, "Can this or that aphasic person make a will?" Indeed, we have to consider degrees of affection of Language, of which speech is but a part. Admitting the occurrence of numerous degrees of affection of Language, we must make arbitrary divisions for the first part of our inquiry, which is an empirical one.

Let us divide roughly into three degrees: (1) *Defect of Speech*.—The patient has a full vocabulary, but makes mistakes in words, as saying "orange" for "onion," "chair" for "table"; or he uses approximative or quasi-metaphorical expressions, as "Light the fire up there," for "Light the gas." "When the warm water comes the weather will go away," for "When the sun comes out the fog will go away." (2) *Loss of Speech*.— The patient is practically speechless and his pantomime is impaired. (3) *Loss of Language*.—Besides being speechless, he has altogether lost pantomime, and emotional language is deeply involved.

To start with, we take the simplest case, one of *loss of speech*, No. 2 ("complete aphasia"). Cases of defect of speech (1) are far too difficult to begin with, and so, too, are those cases (3) in which there is not only loss of speech, but also deep involvement of that least special part of language which we call emotional language. Moreover, we shall deal with a case of permanent speechlessness. I admit that making but three degrees of affection of language, and taking for consideration one kind of frequently occurring case, is an entirely arbitrary proceeding, since there actually occur very numerous degrees of affection of language, many slighter than, and some severer than, that degree (No. 2) we here call one of loss of speech. But, as aforesaid, we must study subjects so complex as this empirically before we study them scientifically; and for the former kind of study we must have what are called "definitions" by type, and state exceptions. This is the plan adopted in every work on the practice of medicine with regard to all diseases. Let us give an example of the two-fold study. Empirically or clinically, that is for the art of medicine, we should consider particular cases of epilepsy as each *approaches this or that nosological type* (*le petit-mal, le grand-mal,* etc.). For the science of medicine we should, so far as is possible, consider cases of epilepsy as each is dependent on a "discharging lesion" of this or that part of the cortex cerebri, and thus as it is a *departure from healthy states* of this or that part of the organism. We cannot do the latter fully yet, but the anatomico-physiological researches of Hitzig and Ferrier have marvellously helped us in this way of studying epilepsies, as also have the clinical researches of Broadbent, Charcot, Duret, Carville, and others.[5]

The following are brief and dogmatic statements about a condition which is a common one—the kind of one we call loss of speech, our second degree (No. 2) of Affection of Language. The statements are about two equally important things: (1) of what the patient has lost in Language—his negative condition, and (2) of what he retains of Language—his positive condition. Here, again, is an illustration of a general principle which is exemplified in many if not in all cases of nervous disease, and one of extreme importance when they are scientifically considered as instances of nervous Dissolution. We have already stated the duality of many symptomatic conditions in the remarks on p. 157. Without recognising the two elements in all cases of affections of speech, we shall not be able to classify affections of speech methodically. If we do

not recognise the duplex (negative and positive) condition, we cannot possibly trace a relation betwixt Nos. 1, 2 and 3 (p. 161). There can be no basis for comparison betwixt the wrong utterances in No. 1 and the non-utterances in Nos. 2 and 3—betwixt a positive and a negative condition—betwixt speech, however bad, and no speech. There is a negative and a positive condition in each degree; the comparison is of the three degrees of the negative element and the three degrees of the positive element; the negative and positive elements vary inversely. The condition of the patient No. 1, who made such mistakes as saying "chair" for "table" was duplex; (*a*) negatively in not saying "table," and (*b*) positively, in saying, "chair" instead; there is in such a case *loss* of some speech, with *retention* of the rest of speech. Hence the term defect of speech applied to such a case is equivocal; it is often used as if the actual utterance was the *direct* result of the disease. The utterance is wrong in that the words of it do not fit the things intended to be indicated; but it is the best speech under the circumstances, and is owing to activity of healthy (except perhaps slightly unstable) nervous elements. The real, the primary, fault is in the nervous elements which do not act, which are destroyed, or are for the time *hors de combat.* If then we compare No. 1 with No. 2, we compare the two negative conditions, the inability to say "table," etc. (the loss of some speech) in No. 1, with the loss of nearly all speech in No. 2, saying the latter is a greater degree of the former, and we compare the two positive conditions, the retention of inferior speech (the wrong utterances) in No. 1, with in No. 2 the retention of certain recurring utterances and with the retention of emotional language, saying the latter is a minor or lower degree of language than the former. Unless we take note of the duplex condition in imperception (delirium and ordinary insanity), we shall not be able to trace a correspondence betwixt it and other nervous diseases. There are necessarily the two opposite conditions in all degrees of mental affections, from the slightest "confusion of thought" to dementia, unless the dementia be total.

THE PATIENT'S NEGATIVE CONDITION

1. *He does not speak.*—He can, the rule is, utter some jargon, or some word, or some phrase. With rare exceptions, the utterance continues the same in the same patient: we call these Re-

curring Utterances. The exceptions to the statement that he is speechless are two. (*a*) The recurring utterance may be "yes," or "no," or both. These words are propositions when used for assent or dissent, and they are so used by some patients who are for the rest entirely speechless. (*b*) There are Occasional Utterances. Under excitement the patient may swear: this is not speech, and is not exceptional; the oath means nothing; the patient cannot repeat it, he cannot "say" what he has just "uttered." Sometimes, however, a patient, ordinarily speechless, may get out a phrase appropriate to some simple circumstance, such as "good-bye" when a friend is leaving. This is an exception, but yet only a partial exception; the utterance is not of high speech value;[6] he cannot "say" it again, cannot repeat it when entreated; it is inferior speech, little higher in value than swearing. However, sometimes a patient, ordinarily speechless, may get out an utterance of high speech value; this is very rare indeed.

2. *He cannot write*; that is to say, he cannot express himself in writing. This is called Agraphia (William Ogle). It is, I think, only evidence of the loss of speech, and might have been mentioned in the last paragraph. Written words are symbols of symbols. Since he cannot write, we see that the patient is speechless, not only in the popular sense of being unable to talk, but altogether so; he cannot speak internally. There is no fundamental difference betwixt external and internal speech; each is propositionising. If I say "gold is yellow" to myself, or think it, the proposition is the same; the same symbols referring to the same images in the same relation as when I say it aloud. There is a difference, but it is one of degree; psychically "faint" and "vivid," physically "slight" and "strong" nervous discharges. The speechless patient does not write because he has no propositions to write. The speechless man may write in the sense of penmanship; in most cases he can copy writing, and can usually copy print into writing, and very frequently he can sign his name without copy. Moreover he may write in a fashion without copy, making, or we may say drawing, a meaningless succession of letters, very often significantly the simplest letters, pothooks. His handwriting may be a very bad scrawl, for he may have to write with his left hand. His inability to write, in the sense of expressing himself, *is* loss of speech; his ability to make ("to draw") letters, as in copying, etc., shows that his

"image series" (the materials of his perception) is not damaged.

Theoretically there is no reason why he should not write music without copy, supposing of course that he could have done that when well; the marks (artificial images) used in noting music have no relation to words any way used. On this matter I have no observations. Trousseau writes in his "Lecture on Aphasia" (*Sydenham Society's Transactions*, vol. i, p. 270), "Dr. Lasegue knew a musician who was completely aphasia, and who could neither read nor write, and yet could note down a musical phrase sung in his presence."

3. In most cases the speechless patient *cannot read at all*, obviously not aloud, but not to himself either, including what he has himself copied. We suppose our patient cannot read. This is not from lack of sight, nor is it from want of perception; his perception is not itself in fault, as we shall see shortly.

4. His power of making signs is impaired (pantomimic propositionising). We must most carefully distinguish pantomime from gesticulation. Throwing up the arms to signify "higher up," pantomime, differs from throwing up he arms when surprised, gesticulation, as a proposition does from an oath.

So far we have, I think only got two things, loss of speech (by simple direct evidence, and by the indirect evidence of non-writing and non-reading) and defect of pantomime. There are in some cases of loss of speech other inabilities; the most significant are that a patient cannot put out his tongue when he tries, or execute other movements he is told, when he can move the parts concerned in other ways quite well.

THE PATIENT'S POSITIVE CONDITION

1. He can understand what we say or read to him; he remembers tales read to him. This is important, for it proves that, although Speechless, the patient is not Wordless. The hypothesis is that words are in duplicate; and that the nervous arrangements for words used in speech lie chiefly in the left half of the brain; that the nervous arrangements for words used in understanding speech (and in other ways) lie in the right also. Hence our reason for having used such expressions as "words serving in speech"; for there is, we now see, another way in which

they serve. When from disease in the left half of the brain speech is lost altogether, the patient understands all we say to him, at least on matters simple to him. Further it is supposed that another use of the words which remain is the chief part of that service of words which in health precedes speech; there being an unconscious or subconscious revival of words in relation before that second revival which is speech. Coining a word, we may say that the process of Verbalising is duel; the second "half" of it being speech. It is supposed also that there is an unconscious or subconscious revival of relations of images, before that revival of images in relation which is Perception.

2. His articulatory organs move apparently well in eating, drinking, swallowing, and also in such utterances as remain always possible to him (recurring utterances), or in those which come out occasionally. Hence his speechlessness is not owing to disease of those centres in the medulla oblongata for immediately moving the articulatory muscles; for in other cases of nervous disease, when these centres are so damaged that the articulatory muscles are so much paralysed that *talking* is impossible, the patient remains able to *speak* (to propositionise) as well as ever; he has internal speech, and can write what he speaks.

   The following dicta may be of use to beginners. Using the popular expression 'talk," we may say that if a patient does not talk because his brain is diseased, he cannot write (express himself in writing), and can swallow well; if he cannot talk because his tongue, lips and palate are immovable, he can write well and cannot swallow well.

3. His vocal organs act apparently well; he may be able to sing.

4. His emotional language is apparently unaffected. He smiles, laughs, frowns and varies his voice properly. His recurring utterance comes out now in one tone and now in another, according as he is vexed, glad, etc.; strictly we should say he sings his recurring utterance; variations of voice being rudimentary song (Spencer); he may be unable to sing in the ordinary meaning of that term. As stated already, he may swear when excited, or get out more innocent interjections, simple or compound (acquired parts of emotional language). Although he may be unable to make any but the simplest signs, he gesticulates apparently as well as ever, and probably he does so more frequently and more copiously than he used to do. His gesticulation draws attention to his needing something, and his friends guess what it is. His friends often erroneously report their guessing what he wants when his emotional manifestations show that he is needing something, as his expressing what thing it is that he wants.

So far for the negative and positive conditions of language in our type case of Loss of Speech—No. 2 in Defect of Language.

Words are in themselves meaningless, they are only symbols of things or of "images" of things; they may be said to have meaning "behind them." A proposition symbolises a particular relation of some images.[7]

We must then briefly consider the patient's condition in regard to the images symbolised by words. For although we artificially separate speech and perception, words and images co-operate intimately in most mentation. Moreover, there is a morbid condition in the image series (Imperception), which corresponds to aphasia in the word series. The two should be studied in relation.

The speechless patient's perception (or "recognition," or "thinking" of things) (propositions of images) is unaffected, at any rate as regards simple matters. To give examples: he will point to any object he knew before his illness which we name; he recognises drawings of all objects which he knew before his illness. He continues able to play at cards or dominoes; he recognises handwriting, although he cannot read the words written; he knows poetry from prose, by the different endings of the lines on the right side of the page. One of my patients found out the continuation of a series of papers in a magazine volume, and had the right page ready for her husband when he returned from his work; yet she, since her illness, could not read a word herself, nor point to a letter, nor could she point to a figure on the clock. There is better and simpler evidence than that just adduced that the image series is unaffected; the foregoing is intended to show that the inability to read is not due to loss of perception nor to non-recognition of letters, etc., as particular marks or drawings, but to loss of speech. Written or printed words cease to be symbols of words used in speech for the simple reason that those words no longer exist to be symbolised; the written or printed words are left as symbols of nothing, as mere odd drawings. The simplest example showing the image series to be undamaged is that the patient finds his way about; this requires preconception, that is, "propositions of images" of streets, etc. Moreover, the patient can, if he retains the propositional use of "yes" and "no," or if he has the equivalent pantomimic symbols, intelligently assent or dissent to simple statements, as that "Racehorses are the swiftest horses," showing that he retains organised nervous arrangements for the images of the things "swiftness" and "horse"; this has already been implied when it was asserted that he understands what we say to him, a process requiring not some of his words only, but also some of his "images" of things, of which the words are but symbols.

Such facts as the above are sometimes adduced as showing that the patient's "memory" is unaffected. That expression is misleading, if it implies that there is a general faculty of memory. There is no faculty of memory apart from things being remembered; apart from having, that is, now and again, these or those words, or images, or actions (faintly or vividly). We may say he has not lost the memory of images, or, better, that he has the images actually or potentially; the nervous arrangements being intact and capable of excitation did stimuli come to them; we may say that he has lost the memory of those words which serve in speech. It is better, however, to use the simple expression that he has not lost images, and that he has lost the words used in speech.

These facts as to retention of images are important as regards the writing of speechless patients. The printed or written letters and words are images, but they differ from the images of objects, in being artificial and arbitrary, in being acquired later; they are acquired after speech and have their meaning only through speech; written words are symbols of symbols of images. The aphasic patient cannot express himself in writing because he cannot speak; but the nervous arrangements for those arbitrary images which are named letters are intact, and thus he can reproduce them as mere drawings, as he can other images, although with more difficulty, they, besides lacking their accustomed stimulus, being less organised. He can copy writing, and he can copy print into writing. When he copies print into writing, obviously he derives the images of letters from his own mind (physically his own organisation). He does not write in the sense of expressing himself, because there are no words reproduced in speech to express. That series of artificial images which makes up the signature of one's name has become almost as fully organised as many ordinary images; hence in many cases the speechless

man who can write nothing else without copy can sign his name.

For the perception (or recognition or thinking) of things, at least in simple relations, speech is not necessary, for such thought remains to the speechless man. Words are required for thinking, for most of our thinking at least, but the speechless man is not wordless; there is an automatic and unconscious[8] or subconscious service of words.

It is not of course said that speech is not required for thinking on novel and complex subjects, for ordering images in new and complex relations (*i.e.* to the person concerned), and thus the process of perception in the speechless but not wordless man may be defective in the sense of being inferior from lack of co-operation of speech: it is not itself in fault, it is left unaided.

To understand anything novel and complex said to him, the healthy man speaks it to himself, *e.g.* repeats, often aloud, complex directions of route given to him.

The word "thing" has not been used as merely synonymous with "substance"; nor is it meant that anybody has nervous arrangements for the images of "swiftness" and "horse," but only for images of some swiftly-moving thing or things, and for images of some particular horse or horses.

It may be well here to give a brief recapitulation of some parts of our subject and, also very briefly, an anticipation of what is to come; the latter is given partly as an excuse for having dwelt in the foregoing on some points not commonly considered in such an inquiry as this, and partly to render clearer some matters which were only incidentally referred to.

The division into internal and external speech (see p. 163) is not that just made into the dual service of words. Internal and external speech differ in degree only: such a difference is insignificant in comparison with that betwixt the prior unconscious, or subconscious, and automatic reproduction of words and the sequent conscious and voluntary reproduction of words; the latter alone is speech, either internal or external. Whether I can show that there is this kind of duality or not, it remains certain that our patient retains a service of words, and yet ordinarily uses none in speech. The retention of that service of words which is not a speech use of words, is sometimes spoken of as a retention of "memory of" words, or of "ideas of" words. But as there is no memory or idea of words apart from having words, actually or potentially, it is better to say that the patient retains words serving in other ways than in speech; we should say of his speechlessness not that he has lost the memory of words, but simply that he has lost those words which serve in speech.

When we consider more fully the duality of the Verbalising process, of which the second "half" is speech, we shall try to show that there is a duality also in the revival of the images symbolised; that perception is the termination of a stage beginning by the unconscious or subconscious revival of images which are in effect "image symbols"; that we think not only by aid of those symbols, ordinarily so-called (words), but by aid of symbol-images. It is, I think, because speech and perception are preceded by an unconscious or subconscious reproduction of words and images, that we seem to have "faculties" of speech and of perception, as it were, above and independent of the rest of ourselves. We seem to have a memory or ideas[9] of words *and* words; having really the two kinds of service of words. The evidence of disease shows, it is supposed, that the highest mentation arises out of our whole organised states, out of ourselves—that will, memory, etc., "come from below," and do not stand autocratically "above," governing the mind; they are simply the now highest, or latest, state of our whole selves. In simple cases of delirium (partial imperception with inferior perception) as when a patient takes his nurse to be his wife, we find, I think, a going down to and a revelation of what would have been when he was sane, the lower and earlier step towards his true recognition or perception of the nurse.

The first step towards his recognition of her when he was sane would be the unconscious, or subconscious, and automatic reproduction of his, or of one of his, well-organised symbol-images of woman; the one most or much organised in him would be his wife. To say what a thing is to say what it is like; he would not have known the nurse even as a woman, unless he had already an organised image of at least one woman. The popular notion is, that by a sort of faculty of perception, he would recognise her without a prior stage in which, he being passive, an organised image was roused in him by the mere presence of the nurse; the popular notion almost seems to imply the contradiction that he first sees her, in the sense of recognising her, and then sees her as like his already acquired or organised image of some woman. We seem to ourselves to Perceive, as also to Will and to

Remember, without prior stages, because these prior stages are unconscious or subconscious. It seems to me that in delirium the patient is reduced to conditions which are revelations of, or of parts of, the lower earlier and prior stages; the lower or earlier stages are then conscious. They are the *then* highest or latest conscious states. When the patient becomes delirious, he takes the nurse to be his wife. More or fewer of the highest nervous arrangements being then exhausted, the final stage is not possible; there is only the first stage; the reproduction of his well-organised symbol-image is all there is, and that is all the nurse can be to him; she is, to him, his wife. The symbol-image is then vividly reproduced because the centres next lower than those exhausted are in abnormally great activity (note, that there are two conditions, one negative and the other positive). There is a deepening of consciousness in the sense of going down to lower earlier and more organised states, which in health are mostly unconscious or subconscious, and precede higher conscious states; in other words with loss or defect of object-consciousness, even in sleep with dreaming, there is increasing subject consciousness; on the physical side, increasing energising of those lower centres which are in the day time more slightly energising during that unbroken subconscious "dreaming" from which the serial states, constituting our latest or highest object-consciousness, are the continual "awakenings."

It is supposed that the well-organised images spoken of—in effect arbitrary images, symbol-images, those which *become* vivid and are "uppermost" in delirium, and then cease to be mere symbols—constitute what seems to be a "general notion" or "abstract idea" of such things as "horse," "swiftness," etc.; their particularity (that they are only images of some horse or horses, of some swift moving thing or things) not appearing, because they are unconscious or subconscious; they served once as images of particular things, and at length as symbol-images of a class of images of things, as well as images of the particular things.

At page 164 we spoke of the right half of the brain as being the part during the activity of which the most nearly unconscious and most automatic service of words begins, and of the left as the half during activity of which there is that sequent verbal action which is speech. The division is too abrupt; some speech—voluntary use of words—is, as we have seen, when alluding to occasional utterances, possible to the man who is rendered practically speechless by disease in the left half. Again, from disease of the right half, there is not loss of that most automatic service of words which enables us to understand speech. The thing which it is important to show is, that mentation is dual, and that physically the unit of function of the nervous system is double the unit of composition; not that one half of the brain is "automatic" and the other "voluntary."

Having now spoken of the kind of case we shall consider, and having added remarks, with the endeavour to show how the several symptoms—negative and positive—are related one to another, we shall be able to give reasons for excluding other kinds of cases of speechlessness.

We are not concerned with cases of all persons who do not speak. We shall not, for example, deal with those untrained deaf-mutes who never had speech, but with the cases of those persons only who have had it, and lost it by disease. The condition of an untrained deaf-mute is in very little comparable with that of our arbitrarily-taken case of loss of speech. The deaf-mute's brain is not diseased, but, because he is deaf, it is uneducated (or in anatomical and physiological phraseology undeveloped) so as to serve in speech. Our speechless patient is not deaf. Part of our speechless patient's brain is destroyed, he has *lost* nervous arrangements which had been trained in speech. Moreover, our speechless man retains a service of words which is not speech; untrained deaf-mutes have no words at all. Further, the untrained deaf-mute has his natural system of signs, which to him is of speech value so far as it goes. He will think by aid of these symbols as we do by aid of words.[10] Our speechless patient is defective even in such slight pantomime as we may reasonably suppose to have been easy to him before his illness. The deaf-mute may have acquired for talking and thinking the common arbitrary system of deaf-mute signs (finger-talk), or he may have been taught by the new method to speak as we do, and thus have ceased to be mute. But when not taught to speak, he is not in a condition even roughly comparable with that of a man who has *lost* speech. No doubt by disease of some part of his brain the deaf-mute might lose his natural system of signs, which are of some speech value to him, but he could not lose speech, having never had it. Much more like our speechless patient's condition is that of the little child which has

been taught to understand speech, and has not yet spoken.

There is another set of cases of so-called loss of speech, which we shall not consider as real loss of speech. I prefer to say that these patients *do* not speak: cases of some persons are meant, who do not talk and yet write perfectly. This may seem to be an arbitrary exclusion. There is in most of these cases an association of symptoms, which never arises from any local disease of any part of the nervous system; the so-called association is a mere jumble of symptoms. Let us state the facts. The patients are nearly always boys or unmarried women. The bearing of this is obvious. The so-called loss of speech is a total non-utterance, whereas it is an excessively rare thing for a patient who does not speak, because his brain is locally diseased, to have no utterance whatever; I do not remember seeing one such case in which there was not some utterance (recurring utterance) a few days or a few weeks after the onset of the illness; the absolute pseudo-speechlessness may remain for months. They cannot be mute from paralysis of the articulatory muscle, because they swallow well. Frequently there is loss of voice also—they get out no sounds except, perhaps, grunts, etc.—and yet they cough ringingly and breathe without hoarseness or stridor; there is no evidence of laryngeal disease. Now loss of voice never occurs with loss of speech from local disease of one side of the brain. No disease of the larynx would cause loss of speech or loss of articulation. The patients often "lose" their speech after calamity or worry. In these cases there is no hemiplegia and no other one-sided condition from first to last. They often, after months of not-speaking, recover absolutely and immediately after some treatment which can have no therapeutical effect, *e.g.* a liniment rubbed on the back, a single faradaic stimulation of the vocal cords or of the neck. Dr. Wilks has reported a case of "cure" of a girl who had not spoken for months; she had also "lost" the use of her legs. Knowing well what was the general nature of the case, Dr. Wilks, by speaking kindly to her, and giving her an excuse for recovery in the application of faradisation, got her well in a fortnight. Sometimes the so-called speechless patient speaks inadvertently when suddenly asked a question, and then goes on talking; is well again. Sometimes speech is surprised out of her. Thus a woman, whose case is recorded by Durham, when told to cry "ah!" when the spatula was holding down her tongue, pushed his hand away, saying, "How can I, with that thing in my mouth?" She then said, "Oh! I have spoken." She was "cured." I believe that patients, "speechless" as described, might be "cured" by faradisation of the vocal cords, or by a thunderstorm, or by quack medicines, or appliances, or by mesmerism, or by wearing a charm, or—not speaking flippantly—by being "prayed over."

Sometimes these cases are spoken of as cases of "emotional aphasia"—the speechlessness is said to be "caused by" emotional excitement, because it often comes on *after* emotional disturbance.

I submit that the facts that the patients do not talk, and *do* write and *do* swallow are enough to show that there is no disease at all, in any sense except that the patients are hysterical (which is saying nothing explanatory), or that they are pretending. There can be no *local* disease, at any rate.

These cases are spoken of at length, although they are excluded, because they are sometimes adduced as instances of aphasia, or loss of speech proper, with ability to write remaining. I confess that were I brought face to face with a man whom I believed to *have* local disease of his brain, who did not *talk*, and yet wrote well, I should conclude that he did *speak* internally although he could not talk. To say that *he* cannot speak and yet can express himself in writing is equivalent, I think, to saying *he* cannot speak and yet *he* can speak.

Notes

1. Here I must acknowledge my great indebtedness to Spencer. The facts stated in the text seem to me to be illustrations from actual cases of disease, of conclusions he has arrived at deductively in his *Psychology*. It is not affirmed that we have the exact opposite of Evolution from the apparently brutal doings of disease; the proper opposite is seen in healthy senescence, as Spencer has shown. But from disease there is, in general, the corresponding opposite of Evolution.

2. "How often would controversies be sweetened were people to remember that 'Distinctions and Divisions are very different things,' and that 'one of them is the most necessary and conducive to true knowledge that can be; the other, *when made too much of*, serves only to puzzle and confuse the understanding.' Locke's words are the germ of that wise aphorism of Coleridge: 'It is a dull or obtuse mind that must divide in order to distinguish; but it is a still worse that distinguishes in order to divide.' And if we cast our eyes back over time, it is the same spirit as that which led Anaxagoras to say, 'Things in this one connected world are not cut off from one another as if with a hatchet.'"—*Westminster Review* (art. Locke), January 1877 (no italics in original).

3. On this matter see an able article in the *Cornhill Magazine*, May 1866. See also Waitz, *Anthropology* (Collingwood's Translation), pp. 241 *et seq.*

4. I, however, believe, as Lewes does, that in so far as we are physically alive, we are psychically alive; that some psychical state attends every condition of activity of every part of the organism. This is, at any rate, a convenient hypothesis in the study of diseases of the nervous system.

5. See Moxon, "On the Necessity for a Clinical Nomenclature of Disease," *Guy's Hospital Reports*, vol. xv. In this paper Moxon shows conclusively the necessity of keeping the clinical or what is above called empirical—not using that term in its popular bad signification—and scientific studies of disease distinct. After reading this paper, my eyes were opened to the confusion which results from mixing the two kinds of study. It is particularly important to have both an empirical arrangement and a scientific classification of cases of insanity.—An example of the former is the much-criticised arrangement of Skae; the scientific classification of cases of insanity, like that of affections of speech, would be regarding them as instances of Dissolution; the Dissolution in insanity begins in the highest and most complex of all cerebral nervous arrangements, the Dissolution causing affections of speech in a lower series. The one kind of classification is for diagnosis (for direct "practical purposes"), the other is for increase of knowledge, and is worthless for immediate practical purposes. The fault of some classifications of insanity is that they are mixed, partly empirical and partly scientific.

6. What is meant by an utterance of high speech value and by inferior speech will later on be stated more fully than has been just now stated by implication. When we cease dealing with our subject empirically and treat it scientifically, we hope to show that these so-called exceptions come in place under the principle of dissolution. We may now say that speech of high value, or superior speech, is new speech, not necessarily new words and possibly not new combinations of words; propositions symbolising relations of images new to the speaker, as in carefully describing something novel; by inferior speech is meant utterances like, "Very well," "I don't think so," ready fitted to very simple and common circumstances, the nervous arrangements for them being well organised.

7. The term "image" is used in a psychical sense, as the term "word" is. It does not mean "visual" images only, but covers all mental states which represent things. Thus we speak of auditory images. I believe this is the way in which Taine uses the term image. What is here

called "an image" is sometimes spoken of as "a perception." In this article the term perception is used for a *process*, for a "proposition of images," as speech is used for propositions, *i.e.* particular inter-relations of words. The expression "organised image" is used briefly for "image, the *nervous arrangements for which* are organised," correspondingly for "organised word," etc.

8. The expression "*un*conscious reproduction of words" involves the same contradiction as does the expression "unconscious sensation." Such expressions may be taken to mean that energising of lower, more organised, nervous arrangements, although unattended by any sort of conscious state, is essential for, and leads to, particular energisings of the highest and least organised—the now-organising—nervous arrangements, which last-mentioned energising is attended by consciousness. I, however, think (as Lewes does) that some consciousness or "sensibility" attends energising of all nervous arrangements (I use the term subconscious for slight conscious-

ness). In cases where from disease the highest nervous arrangements are suddenly placed *hors de combat*, as in sudden delirium, the next lower spring into greater activity; and then, what in health was a subordinate sub-consciousness, becomes a vivid consciousness, and is also the highest consciousness there then can be.

9. The so-called *idea* of a word, in contradistinction to *the* word, is itself a word subconsciously revived, or revivable, before the conscious revival, or revivability of the same word, which latter, in contradistinction to the so-called *idea* of a word, is the so-called *word itself*—*the* word.

10. We must not confound the finger-talk with the "natural" system of signs. They are essentially different. No one supposes that words are essential for thought, but only that some symbols are essential for conceptual thought, although it may be that people with "natural" symbols do not reach that higher degree of abstract thinking which people do who have words.

20

On Aphasia

Ludwig Lichtheim

When we read the recent controversies concerning the symptoms of Aphasia and their explanation, we might readily come to the conclusion, that there exist differences between the methods of investigation adopted by the chief authorities, and that it would be, therefore, desirable first to reach unanimity upon this fundamental question of method.

Happily such an opinion would be erroneous, and we can have no doubt as to the way to follow in our investigations, as there is no such divergence. The method which has hitherto yielded the results does not differ from those used in the natural sciences. Starting from the observation of facts, it culminates in the explanation of these facts. The correctness of our explanations must be subjected to the control of further observations. Precisely the same course is followed in experimental research, with the exception that, in our present subject, the experiments are not instituted at the will of the investigator, but are supplied to him by nature, and that he thus depends for them upon a happy chance. The erection of the building can therefore proceed at a slow pace only, and must rise by degrees as the result of many toilers' work.

Nor do we meet with any divergence of opinion as to the end to be attained. Our task is to determine the connections and localisation of the paths of innervation subservient to language and its correlated functions. On the supposition of our having reached this end, we should then be able to determine the exact place of any solution of continuity in these paths, and account for its symptomatic manifestations with the same precision as we do for those of a motor or

Excerpts from *Brain: A Journal of Neurology* (January 1985). The author was Professor of Medicine at the University of Berne.

This paper has been translated by me from the German manuscript; but our limits required that the original should be condensed. The whole task was by no means an easy one; the careful revision bestowed by Professor Lichtheim on the proofs, and for which I beg to return him my best thanks, has, however, materially relieved me from the responsibility I had assumed.—A. DE W.

sensory paralysis depending on a lesion of the peripheral nerves.

Now, although all are agreed that we have by no means as yet reached this point, opinions differ as to how near we have arrived. We may, however, congratulate ourselves upon the simple fact of there being some agreement as to the fundamental meaning of disturbances of speech from cerebral causes. The amount of superstructure which will be raised on such a foundation must depend, in individual instances, upon the personal temperament of the architect. There is room both for the enthusiast and the sceptic, who both have their function to fulfil in the race for truth. The only necessary condition for the successful building up of the edifice, is that the one should not deny, the other not distort, acquired facts.

It follows from what I have already said, that every step which brings us nearer the fulfilment of the task before us must enable us to differentiate more accurately the clinical forms of aphasic disturbance. What to-day appears to us as a curiosity, as a case aberrant from the ordinary type, will tomorrow be classified as an instance of conformity to the law. This we shall find illustrated in the history of the previous researches into the nature of Aphasia. Broca was led, after many mistakes had been made, to bring into sharp relief aphasia in its narrower sense. Wernicke[1] was the first, to my knowledge, who distinguished between the latter symptom and those due to an interruption in the centripetal afferent paths. Besides these two chief forms, which he calls motor and sensorial aphasia respectively, Wernicke describes a third, and designates it as commissural aphasia (*Leitungsaphasie*). The following discussion, the object of which is to establish a further differentiation, will bear upon this triple division of Wernicke's, and give me the opportunity of mentioning the other categories of aphasia. I abstain from any further reference to the historical aspect of the question, which has been treated by Kussmaul[2] in a way which leaves nothing to be desired.

The morbid types which I intend to discuss in the following remarks have been determined, in as far as they are new, deductively: it was the task of subsequent clinical observations to test the validity of the inferences. The necessity of differentiating still further the types of aphasia struck me on attempting to schematize the forms hitherto known, for the purposes of instruction. But I did not consider that my schema should be published until cases had been observed which coincided with the new types postulated

therein. The important element of my task lies in the observations themselves and in their interpretation. Still I thought it advisable, in presenting my results, to follow the same path which I had myself trodden, giving in the first place the schematic representation from which I started in elaborating my views of aphasia. It will be seen that my conception is intimately connected with previous ones, especially with that of Wernicke: the points of difference will appear in the course of the argument.

The schema is founded upon the phenomena of the acquisition of language by imitation, as observed in the child, and upon the reflex arc which this process presupposes. The child becomes possessed, by this means, of auditory memories of words (auditory word-representations[3]) as well as of motor memories of co-ordinated movements (motor word-representations).[4] We may call "centre of auditory images" and "centre of motor images," respectively,[5] the parts of the brain where these memories are fixed. They are designated in the schema by the letters A and M. The reflex arc consists in an afferent branch *a* A, which transmits the acoustic impressions to A; and an efferent branch M *m*, which conducts the impulses from M to the organs of speech; and is completed by the commissure binding together A and M.

When intelligence of the imitated sounds is superimposed, a connection is established between the

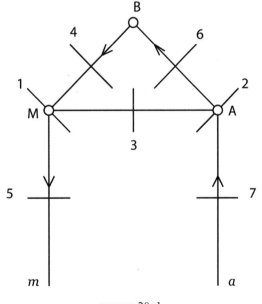

FIGURE 20–1.

auditory centre A, and the part where concepts[6] are elaborated, B. All the diagrammatic representations of these phenomena agree so far, at least those given by German authors; beyond this, controverted points are found. The next step in the formation of volitional, or intelligent, speech involves a centrifugal connection between B and M. Our schema introduces, in consonance with most others, a direct commissure, whilst Kussmaul makes it pass from B through A to M. We shall soon return to this point. Leaving aside the point B for the present, we see from the diagram that seven different interruptions may occur in the paths therein assumed. It is manifest at first sight how variously the function of language may be disturbed by some of them; yet it is necessary, in order to gain a clear conception of the various types so produced, that we should include in our survey the disturbances of the functions of language involved in the acts of reading and writing. These are acquired in connection with the exercise of speech, and are hence intimately connected with it; the same nervous paths are, to some extent, brought into play. Reading postulates the existence of visual memories of letters and of groups of letters. We may learn to understand writing through the connection between such visual representations (centre O) and auditory representations: by spelling aloud we bring the auditory centre into action, and thus establish a connection, through the path O A, between O and B; in reading aloud, the tract *o* A M *m* is thrown into activity.

The problem with reference to writing is more complicated. The necessary movements have to be learnt, and associated with the visual representations; this is done through the commissure O E, designating by E the centre from which the organs of writing are innervated.

It is more difficult to determine the path through which volitional, or intelligent writing is executed. This tract must united B with E, and clinical facts leave no doubt that it passes through M. There may be some doubt as to whether it leads directly hence to E, or passes round through A on its way thither. I shall return to this question presently; and adopt provisionally the former view, according to which Diagram 2 is constructed.

This figure makes it easy to derive the symptomatic type characteristic of each of the several possible interruptions in the reflex arc. I have been in the habit of using it for several years past in my lectures, and have found that it greatly facilitates to beginners the

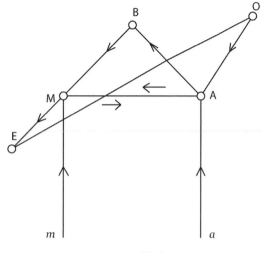

FIGURE 20–2.

mastering of an otherwise very complicated subject. But if the schema is to have any value beyond that of an aid to teaching, it must be shown that the seven derivable types do really correspond to existing forms of aphasia, and that clinical observations are fairly reducible to them. I shall begin my discussion with an *exposé* of the several types.

1. Interruptions in M—the centre of motor representations of words, or motor centre of speech—give rise to the following association of symptoms:
   Loss of (*a*) volitional speech;
   (*b*) repetition of words;
   (*c*) reading aloud;
   (*d*) volitional writing;
   (*e*) writing to dictation.
   There still exist:—
   (*f*) understanding of spoken words;
   (*g*) understanding of written words;
   (*h*) faculty of copying.

This constitutes the true "aphasia" of Broca, as well as the "motor aphasia" of Wernicke, and the "ataxic aphasia" of Kussmaul. The interpretation usually given of this trouble of speech is the same as that involved in my plan. It is this aphasia which rests upon the firmest basis, and I need not adduce examples from the large number of those on record, such as, for instance, the two celebrated cases of Broca's. I believe I have seen some pure cases of this description, but I have no notes of them, and their investigation was not conducted with the fulness of detail necessary to clear up the only point among the symptoms which still remains to be elucidated. I am referring to the question, whether there is understanding of written language in such cases. According to the diagram, the power of reading aloud should be lost, but that of silent reading preserved intact. I am sure that in uncomplicated instances this must be so, but I much regret that I have not had such a case to observe during the last few years; for the study of the literature of the subject has not afforded me any positive proof. In the majority of published cases no sufficient attention has been bestowed upon this question. It has indeed often been specified that the faculty of reading was intact: on the other hand, Trousseau[7] has shown that many 'aphasics' appear eager in their reading and yet do not understand what they read. He makes this observation precisely with reference to patients in whom the symptom of deficient understanding of writing was associated with the typical signs of Broca's aphasia. I shall return to this point, and show by personal observations how I think this contradiction may be explained.

2. If the continuity be broken at the point A, in the acoustic word-centre we find loss of:—
(a) understanding of spoken language;
(b) understanding of written language;
(c) faculty of repeating words;
(d) faculty of writing to dictation;
(e) faculty of reading aloud.
There is preservation of:
(f) faculty of writing;
(g) faculty of copying words;
(h) faculty of volitional speech.

This type corresponds with the "sensorial aphasia" of Wernicke, who has himself shown that though the faculty of volitional language is not lost, yet there are considerable disturbances in it. The latter is incorrect, inasmuch as wrong words are used, the words themselves are altered by the introduction of wrong syllables, occasionally to such an extent that the language becomes wholly unintelligible. This form has been called also "paraphasia." The explanation given by Wernicke of the fact, that in sensorial aphasia such disturbances occur in spite of the preservation of the tract for voluntary speech, appears at first sight rather forced. He assumes that the nervous influx descending along the path B M m sends a branch current to A, and that this *subconscious* innervation of the audi-

tory memories of words secures the correct choice and expression of them; and that irregularities occur as soon as the co-operation of these elements ceases to take place.

I accept this interpretation, but with a modification, namely, that the mere excitation of the auditory representation is not sufficient to secure correct speech, but that this representation must enter into relationship with the concept; that therefore the commissure A B must necessarily be intact for the same purpose. Paraphasia will be observed when in the arc B M A B, an interruption has occurred in such a way that language is not altogether arrested. The causes of such a modification will be pointed out presently.

It is by no means difficult to ascertain through self-observation, that such an innervation of the auditory word-centre does really take place. When speaking aloud, we cannot control the fact, because the words are actually heard, and the innervation of A from *a* being much more powerful, conceals that of A from M. But if we perform only the movement of the mouth necessary to the emission of a monosyllable, without issuing it, we shall be most distinctly conscious of the corresponding auditory representation. This observation has perhaps given rise to the assumption of Kussmaul, that the path from the concept- to the movement-centre passes through the auditory centre. This is one of the points on which his schematic representation differs from the one given above. His diagram corresponds to the one given here (Fig. 20–3), and his path for voluntary language would be B A M *m*.

But it seems to me that this view does not correspond to the facts; the disagreement begins already in the case of Broca's aphasia, of which Kussmaul refers the seat, as we do, to the motor centre M. He assumes that the auditory representations are intact, and may be innervated from the concept-sphere; but this is, I believe, not the case. Trousseau, intending to prove that in aphasia words were forgotten, showed that in numerous cases the "inner speech" had disappeared. I have obtained evidence of this in a patient suffering from a form of the disease allied to Broca's type, and which will be adduced further on. It will generally be found a difficult task to elucidate this point satisfactorily; this is the method I use: I ask the patient to press my hand as often as there are syllables in the word to which an object corresponds. Those who have not lost the auditory representations can do this, even if their intelligence be limited, as I have been able to satisfy myself even under the least favourable cir-

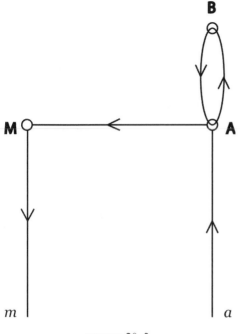

FIGURE 20–3.

rial aphasia. I cannot refer to any typical instance of sensorial aphasia from my own experience; but Wernicke has given one,[9] carefully and minutely described, and in which the symptoms coincided[10] with the deductions from our schema.

3. The third form of aphasia, caused by the interruption of the commissure M A, has also been described by Wernicke, and corresponds with what we find in the diagram.

There are preserved:
(*a*) Understanding of spoken language;
(*b*) understanding of written language;
(*c*) copying words.

Paraphasia and paragraphia are present; showing, in accordance with what has been said previously, the existence of:
(*d*) volitional language; and
(*e*) volitional writing.

Similar disturbances are observed in the
(*f*) repetition of words;
(*g*) reading aloud;
(*h*) writing to dictation.

The path generally used in these acts (from A to M) is interrupted; still they are not completely in abeyance, because the tract A B M may be substituted for it. These actions, therefore, are not those of repeating, reading, and writing to dictation, properly so called, but are the result of impulses from the concept-centre; hence they manifest the same disturbances as volitional speech.

Cases of this sort do not appear to be very rare, though I am not acquainted with any observation of the kind as complete as could be wished. This is the more to be regretted, that it is precisely here that I have some doubts as to whether the construction of the path of volitional writing is correct. I have mentioned previously that I hold it as doubtful whether the path B M E be really used in volitional writing, or whether the channel of innervation be not from B through M and A to E (Fig. 20–4). The circumstance, that in volitional writing we are conscious of the excitation of auditory representations, does not prove that the *direct* innervation current really passes through the centre for the latter. The conditions are the same here as for the relation existing between these word-representations and volitional speech; whilst the chief current flows along B M directly to E, a secondary current may diverge from M through A to B, in order to secure the correctness of writing, as it

cumstances. For instance, a patient who, besides a focal lesion of the right hemisphere, had had a hemorrhage in the left half of the pons, and suffered, among other pseudo-bulbar symptoms, from complete speechlessness, preserved the faculty of fulfilling the test to the very last.

I have unfortunately, as was just said, not observed recently any pure cases of Broca's aphasia, but I have had a series of mixed cases in which this type predominated at least, and of pure cases of allied forms. I always found that the patients had lost the innervation of the auditory word-representations. These observations correspond so accurately to those of Trousseau, that I feel convinced that in ordinary cases of ataxic aphasia, the path from concept- to sound-centre must be interrupted.[8] Hence the diagram of Kussmaul cannot be correct, nor can a lesion in the path B A (Fig. 20–3) explain what occurs, for then the arc *a* A M *m*, and the power of repeating words would remain intact; whereas the latter, in Broca's aphasia, suffers as much as that of volitional language.

These considerations show that our schematic diagram may be considered as accurate, and that the co-operation of the auditory representations in speech is calculated to support the interpretation given by Wernicke of the paraphasic phenomena in his senso-

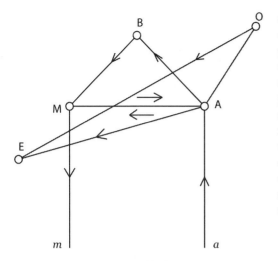

FIGURE 20–4.

does in the ease of speaking. Clinical observations are necessary to decide on this point also; and the solution will be found in cases (described under 2) of Wernicke's sensorial aphasia, and of aphasia due to an interruption in the path M A. If localising the lesion of sensorial aphasia in A, we consider Diagram 4, the faculty of writing must have been lost too; whereas paragraphia only will be present, on the assumption that the relation of parts is as in Figure 2.

Though the question, when framed in these terms, appears a simple one, yet it is far from being easy to find an answer to it, because the published material at our disposal scarcely contains any sufficiently precise data to give us certainty on this point. The only case which we may adduce is the one already quoted of Wernicke's;[11] the patient could not write: "When sitting at the table to write, she takes the pencil presented to her point upwards, looks at it, turns it round, holds it properly, but makes only up and downwards strokes. When the pen is given to her in the same way, she turns it round, dips it properly into the inkstand, holds it properly, but with no better result." The agraphia persisted throughout, whilst the disturbance in the expression and intelligence of speech had disappeared. This case points to the correctness of Diagram 4 (Fig. 20–4); but it is not safe to draw a definite conclusion from a single instance, and unfortunately all other published cases of word-deafness fail us here, as will be seen on reading the thesis of Skwortzoff.[12]

Precisely in the same way the form of aphasia arising from an interruption in the path M A, ought, ac-

cording to Diagram 4, to be accompanied with a loss of volitional writing; whilst, according to Diagram 2, paragraphia ought to be present: but we cannot decide with absolute certainty from the observations at our disposal. In both of Wernicke's cases agraphia was present; whilst others, scarcely reported with sufficient accuracy however, leave room for doubts. In a case of my own the clinical aspects clearly corresponded to this type, whilst the post-mortem appearances coincided with Wernicke's description. I relate it here, because such autopsies are rare; but, owing to the insufficiency of the notes, it cannot serve in deciding on the point we are discussing.

Case I.—Right Hemiplegia; Aphasic Disturbances.—Obliteration of the Sylvian Artery; Brown Softening of the Left Insula and Neighbouring Portions of Frontal and Temporal Convolutions.—Pachymeningitis Interna.—Valvular Heart-Disease, &c.

J. S. B., aged 46, a labourer in Thun, was brought into hospital at Berne on the 3rd of April, 1883. We failed to obtain any clue to the beginning and course of the disease.

Sensorium normal. *Speech* much altered. When asked to relate his history, he strings together in a fluent manner numerous words, of which scarcely one now and then can be made out. The following were noted: "Evening, five and twenty, and." Patient is aware of the incorrectness of his diction, and tries to assist himself by gestures. He succeeds better with single short words and answers; thus, in answer to the question, "What was there for supper?" he answered, "Bread, meat, potatoes," with only two mistakes. His own name he mutilates.

Repeating.—When he repeats connected sentences he manifests the same defects as in volitional speech; single short words are pretty correctly rendered. No note taken of the way the patient names objects.

Understanding of Speech entire.—*Understanding of Writing*, whether printed or hand-written, is preserved. On reading aloud he makes the same mistakes as in talking.

Writing very imperfect. He mixes up the order of the letters in a word; and usually stops after an attempt of short duration. He can copy what is set before him with absolute correctness.

Motility.—Slight paralysis of the right arm and leg; apparent on simultaneous action of both sides of the body. Paresis in buccal region of right facial.

Sensation normal. The tongue deviates to the right, and is the seat of tremors. We pass over the symptoms in the chest and other organs. Symptoms remained unaltered until the beginning of May. Then consciousness became obscured during the next few days, and he died in the night of the 8th to 9th of May.

The autopsy was made, and a full report drawn up, by Professor Langhans. The brain presented the following appearances:

Inflammatory membranous deposits on the inner surface of the dura-mater on the left side. Pia-mater somewhat opaque and whitish, especially over ascending, and apex of temporal convolutions, where it is adherent.

A good deal of serum at the base of the brain. There is a considerable depression of the convolutions bordering the upper and posterior part of the left Sylvian fissure, as well as of the ascending frontal and parietal convolutions. The Island of Reil is sunken, forming a depression into which the second frontal convolution falls suddenly to a depth of 1½ ctm.; the third (lowest) frontal convolution terminates into it likewise. Here the pia is inflamed with yellow discoloration. The depression is bounded posteriorly by the fissure of Sylvius. The middle portion of the first temporal convolution is somewhat sunken opposite the depression of the Insula, in which the consistence of the cerebral matter is soft, with harder patches around.

It is difficult to follow the Sylvian artery beyond the point where it reaches the Insula, and presents on the length of 1½ ctm. a tough whitish appearance; it is occluded just before the division and a short way up the posterior branch.

The softened patch occupies the bottom of the Sylvian fissure and extends to about 1½ ctm. of the posterior part of the inferior frontal convolution, and to the neighbouring portions of the ascending frontal convolution. A fragment of the cortex of the ascending temporal is also wanting, but there is no yellow discoloration here.

The case just described is undoubtedly one of the third kind of aphasia; the symptoms tally with the theoretical postulates established previously. But the point which to us is most interesting, the capacity of the patient for volitional writing, is not established in the notes, because it is not sufficiently distinguished from writing to dictation.

In the absence of more definite data than those already adduced, whereby to decide which course the impulses follow in volitional writing, it appears to me more probable that Diagram 4 gives the more correct construction. There is one difficulty, however, and it is that in Broca's aphasia, writing to dictation is disturbed, a fact not deducible from Diagram 4, but with which Diagram 2 appears more consonant. On the other hand, as we shall see, in some cases where volitional speech is lost, but not the faculty of repeating words, the first syllables only are repeated correctly; when the patient is to repeat a sentence it is necessary to say it word by word. The explanation of this phenomenon is easy. If four or five words are given together, the patient must retain them in his memory, and thus what he says ceases to be a repetition, properly so called, but is an effect of volition. This is still more the case with reference to writing, an act which takes a much longer time; but few letters are written really to dictation, and indeed one finds in many cases of Broca's aphasia that the first letter of a word can be written down, the rest of the word being unreadable.

Further observations cannot fail to throw light on the question. This controverted point does not apply to the remaining forms of aphasia.

4. A variety of motor aphasia is created by interruption of the path B M, of which we have many examples. From the diagram we should expect the loss of

(*a*) volitional speech;

(*b*) volitional writing;

whilst there are preserved—

(*c*) understanding of spoken language;

(*d*) understanding of written language;

(*e*) the faculty of copying.

So far the symptoms coincide with those of Broca's aphasia. They differ inasmuch as there is preservation of

(*f*) faculty of repeating words:

(*g*) writing to dictation;

(*h*) reading aloud.

As an example of this kind of aphasia, characterised by loss of volitional speech and preservation of power of repeating words, I may mention a case of Hammond.[13]

Still more striking is the faculty of reading aloud. Most recorded cases are incomplete in this respect. I therefore give a case of my own which beautifully illustrates this point.

Case II.—Traumatic Aphasia.

Dr. C. K., a busy medical practitioner, had a carriage accident, and was carried home unconscious. Three hours afterwards he was bled, when consciousness returned. There were severe bruises on the right side of the body, and of the head, which was ecchymosed. The movements of the right arm and leg were never absent, but weakened, whether through paralysis or injury is not certain. Immediately after venesection the right hand could be stretched firmly, only lifting it was difficult. Sensation normal. Difficulty of swallowing during the first two days; fluids readily got into the air-passages; mouth not easily opened; tongue difficult to pull out. Patient got up after about a week, when it was noticed that he dragged the right leg and swayed a little.

Speech was much affected: the first day he only said "yes" or "no," but quite appositely. Gradually, more and more words returned, at first imperfect. Whilst his vocabulary was still very meagre, it was observed that he could repeat everything perfectly. Soon after the accident he began to read with perfect understanding. It was established beyond doubt that he could *read aloud* perfectly at a time when he could scarcely speak at all. The statements of his wife are most positive and trustworthy on this point, though he himself does not remember what took place just after the accident. She states that after much difficulty in making himself understood by gestures, he obtained a newspaper, and to the great astonishment of all present he began to read fluently. She herself thought it most strange and inexplicable.

He could not write voluntarily at all; but this faculty returned slowly and imperfectly, as did speech. On the other hand, he could, soon after he had left his bed, *copy and write to dictation*. He spoke German and French fluently before the injury; but German rather the better of the two. As the aphasia diminished, German words returned before French.

Immediately after the accident the right pupil was dilated and immovable; no troubles of vision. I saw the patient six weeks afterwards, at a time when the loss of speech had to a great extent disappeared. One could observe a slight paresis in the right lower facial region; some weakness of the right leg, but nothing noticeable in the right arm. Sensation was normal, except that he did not so readily recognise objects with his right as with his left hand. The right pupil sluggish; no disturbance of vision nor hemiopia.

In every other respect he is in a normal condition, with the exception of speech. His vocabulary is copious, but he does not talk much, and speaks in a drawling manner. From time to time he misses a word or construction; he then tries to express himself with gestures. Speech much more defective when he must name objects shown to him; then many names escape him, and he also makes mistakes (*e.g.* for "Bild," he says "Milbe," then corrects himself and says "Portrait"; for "Stahlfeder" he says first "Bleifeder," then "Tintenfeder"). Many words are missed in French also; he finds the French equivalents of the words he can say in German. Patient says himself that the auditory representations of the words he cannot find are missing; he cannot tell the number of syllables in them. If these words are spoken to him or written before him he says them at once, but forgets them immediately. He repeats correctly whole sentences, if not too long.

He understands spoken and written language perfectly. He can read aloud with the greatest fluency, and with scarcely any stoppage. Writing very imperfect. Asked to write the history of his illness, he puts down mutilated, meaningless words, in which it is impossible to discover any sense. Writing single words, names of objects shown, gives a somewhat better result. There is a parallelism here between writing and speech; such names as he cannot say, neither can he write.

On dictation, he writes fluently and without faults. The strokes are somewhat clumsy. He copies equally well. Intelligence normal. His wife assures me that he manages business perfectly, thinks of things in time, &c.

I saw the patient again a month later. Great improvement in his speech, which is fluent, and with almost no hesitation; he names objects with much less difficulty; words are rarely mutilated. Writing is still deficient, though much improved. What he writes is perfectly legible.

5. Still better known than the preceding is the type of aphasia arising in an interruption of the path M *m*. The diagram indicates loss of:—
   (*a*) Volitional speech;
   (*b*) repetition of words;
   (*c*) reading aloud.
      Preservation of:—
   (*d*) Understanding of speech;
   (*e*) understanding of writing;
   (*f*) faculty of copying.
      Again, and as a distinguishing feature between this and Broca's type, there remain:—

(*g*) Faculty of volitional writing;
(*h*) of writing to dictation.

There are numerous examples of patients who had lost the faculty of speaking, and could yet make themselves understood by writing. I have seen several cases of this description, and possess the notes of one in which the patient was under my care several years ago, and wrote his history himself. But it would be useless to relate it here, in presence of the material already at hand.

According to Kussmaul, such cases present the true uncomplicated type of ataxic aphasia, that is, of that form of speechlessness, "in which patients, with freedom of intellect and of movement of the tongue, have the memory of words as acoustic signs, but are unable to emit them. The proof that they really possess these signs is found in the fact, that they can embody them in writing. When asked to articulate them as sounds or words, they cannot, even if they are shown how to shape their tongue and lips."

It is obvious that this description includes the type now before us, and Kussmaul gives a series of most pregnant instances in this chapter on ataxic aphasia. But the aphasia he so designates extends over a wide range of cases, such as those of Broca's aphasia, which we have discussed under our first heading. In these cases there is ataxic agraphia also, owing to the implication of the centre of co-ordination for written signs, which is distinct from, though connected with, that for spoken signs. The close relationship between these centres explains the fact, that the two symptoms so often co-exist.

Kussmaul's views rest on the assumption that, as the motor tract of spoken language is innervated by the left hemisphere only, so is the tract of written language; for it is only under such circumstances that a lesion of the left hemisphere could cause agraphia by an injury to the writing centre. I cannot accept this interpretation, but hold it more probable that the innervation of the movements of writing originates in both cerebral hemispheres.

When we learn how to write, we apparently employ the left hemisphere only; but we must assume that the right hemisphere is the seat of slight nervous action as well, for it can be shown that a certain amount of facility is also imparted for the same movements with the left hand. When the left hand executes "mirror-writing," it performs the same movements as the right hand in ordinary writing, and it is easy to show that the left hand writes mirror-wise bet-

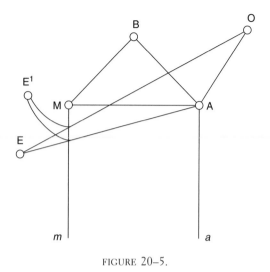

FIGURE 20–5.

ter than it does the usual type. In my own case, even, the strokes are more correct if I write in English characters. Now it could be objected that this innervation of the left hand flows from the left hemisphere; but this is improbable, for in some lesions of the left hemisphere it happens that this tendency of the left hand to execute mirror-writing becomes manifest. Moreover, the fact, that in complete right hemiplegia the power to write with the left hand is not diminished, is opposed to the unilateral innervation of the movements of writing. Therefore the point E, which in our diagram represents the centre of writing movements, must not be looked upon as single; in addition to the point E in the left hemisphere, there is a corresponding spot, E in the right, to which commissures go, and which can come into action when there is some lesion of E. There are other proofs that in agraphia the motor innervation of the movements of writing is not involved. In pure cases of Broca's aphasia the faculty of copying is preserved,[14] whilst that of reading aloud, and of every kind of repetition, is lost. On the other hand, these patients are not only unable to write, but cannot even compose words with letters placed before them. The real cause of the agraphia does not depend on any lesion of the motor apparatus, but on the impossibility of reproducing voluntarily the auditory representations.[15] I have already shown how one can convince oneself that such patients are wanting in the faculty of volitional recall of the auditory representations, and have stated how far I had reached certainty on this point.

Since the above has been written, a case of Pitres[16] has been published, which gives direct evidence of the correctness of my views on agraphia. The patient was suffering from agraphia, the residual sequel of an apoplectic seizure; speech, understanding of language and writing were intact, whilst volitional writing and writing to dictation were impossible, the faculty of copying being preserved. The lesion would be referred by me in the path A E (Fig. 4). The interesting point about the case is, however, that this agraphia affected solely the right hand; the patient could write correctly with the left hand, and copy with his right what he had written with his left hand. This shows the correctness of the diagram in which the centre E is represented as existing in both hemispheres, and the path A E as being double.

It is obvious that this agraphia has nothing in common with that occurring in Broca's aphasia. As could be expected, the patient could make up words from their component letters, a feat impossible to those suffering from Broca's aphasia.

Pitres adduces two more cases of isolated agraphia. The first, quotes from Ogle, is apparently much more complex. The patient could not even copy, nor make up his name with the letters, and had serious embarrassment of speech. The lesion was probably a more extensive one, and took its origin in an injury received eight years previously. In the second case (from Charcot) the conditions were likewise less simple. We are not told whether the agraphia was bilateral. I may add, that the paths A E and A C may be interrupted at the same time, as they appear (see Fig. 5) to run together in the brain for some distance before they separate to go into the two hemispheres. Isolated agraphia will therefore, under certain circumstances, appear as bilateral.

The theoretical types with which we have hitherto been engaged corresponded closely with well-known varieties of aphasia. There remain two, due to lesions of the commissures A B and A a, which must present themselves as cases of sensorial aphasia. Owing to the rarity of examples of the latter, it would have been but natural had I had no actual examples of it to adduce, though it would obviously have weakened my whole position, the full confirmation of which requires a filling up of every gap. I have, however, found the two missing types, and their entire correspondence with the theory of aphasia here developed is a warrant for the accuracy of the hypothesis.

6. Lesions of the path A B, would give rise to the following symptoms. Loss of:
(a) understanding of spoken language;

(b) understanding of written language.
    There are preserved:
(c) volitional speech.
    For the reasons stated above, there will be paraphasia. So far, the symptoms coincide with those of Wernicke's sensorial aphasia. Here, however, there subsist,
(d) volitional writing,
which will also have the characteristics of paragraphia;
(e) faculty of repeating words;
(f) of reading aloud;
(g) of writing to dictation.
    Owing to the interruption of communication between A and B, there must be a complete loss of intelligence for what is repeated, read aloud, written to dictation by the patient.
    There also subsists the
(h) power of copying words.

I shall now relate a case of my own which presents all these characteristics.

Case III.—Aortic Insufficiency. Cerebral Softening. Sensorial Aphasia.

J. U. Schwarz was admitted into the Inselspital on the 19th of May, 1884. Sixty years of age—nothing noteworthy in antecedents.

He was well up to the 15th of May. The next night his wife noticed that he became restless, spoke in his sleep, rose and returned to bed, &c. At 4 in the morning it became apparent that something had happened; what he said had no sense. He did not answer to questions; he tried very hard to make himself understood, and the same mutilated expressions were constantly repeated. His wife thought he had lost his reason. His apparent intention was to complain of severe pains in the forehead and nape of neck. This state of things went on, and as he was losing strength, he was taken to the hospital.

Patient is a rather fat, pale, man. Features flabby; expression dull. On admission, he gave the impression of a subject with psychical deficiencies. He talked a good deal, but repeated the same phrases. He points to his head and says, "Oh how stupid I am, I cannot," &c. It is difficult to make anything out of him, for he understands little that is said to him; but it is easy to ascertain that he is in possession of his intelligence, and that the apparent psychical deficiency consists only in his difficulty in understanding others, and in making himself understood. His actions leave no doubt on this point.

Spoken language.—The disturbance in his power to understand it is very evident (verbal deafness). If one stands behind him and talks to him, he turns round and asks: "Do you speak to me?" The simplest requests, to show his tongue, shut his eyes, are answered by: "I don't know what one wants."

Speech.—There is no deficiency in his vocabulary. He talks a good deal in a flowing manner: he seldom is short for a word; he occasionally uses a wrong or a mutilated one. But this is unfrequent, and in this respect he has greatly improved on what his wife described he was. He is in great difficulty when he has to name objects shown to him; he finds the names with the greatest difficulty, and assists himself with descriptions. Instead of "wine," he says "that is strong;" for "water," "that is weak," &c.

Repetition.—He obviously could repeat correctly all that was spoken before him; but he apparently did not understand what he did repeat, as for instance the words, "My name is Peter Schwarz, and I am already 4 years old," which did not draw any signs of denegation on his part.

Written Language.—He understands nothing printed, or handwritten. The simplest things placed before him he cannot read nor decipher. He knows the name of most letters, and gives it correctly; he only confounds the capital I.

Reading aloud.—He can make up letters into words, and he can read aloud by spelling; but it is evident that the sense of the word remains closed to him. Out of the sentence, "Will you have a glass of wine?" he goes correctly as far as "you" but has manifestly no idea of the meaning.

Writing.—His volitional writing is worse than his speaking—but he does write a few words correctly. In "Meine Frau" (my wife), he manages the first word, not the second.

Writing to dictation was not tested at the very beginning. Later it was found that he could do it well if each word was given singly; whole sentences are rendered inaccurately, words being missed.

Copying.—He copies perfectly, changing German into English characters, but does not understand anything of what he so writes.

Motility and Sensibility.—No difficulty in walking or standing. Movements of arms and legs quite normal; sensation likewise.

Reflexes.—Skin reflexes normal. Patellar and Achillis-tendon jerk absent.

Cerebral nerves.—1. Smell normal.—2. Nothing noteworthy.—3, 4, 6. Movements of the eye normal. Pupils small, react to light.—5. Normal.—7. No weakness of fascial muscles.—8. Hearing not very acute; but present on both sides; he hears the tick of the watch only when close to the ear.—9. Taste appears to be normal. He can recognise and name acid; seems to recognise sweet, but cannot name it. He calls bitter "strong." Deglutition normal. 10. Voice natural.—11. Movements of the tongue free.

In the further evolution of the case, the word deafness receded without disappearing altogether; on the 21st of May, the improvement was already very marked. On the 22nd the following conversation was held. "Shut your eyes."—He does it. "Take this glass of wine from the table."—He turns round and says: "Are you saying anything to me? I don't understand it." "Do you like red or white wine best?" "Here is some red wine." "Put your right leg out of the bed." "What shall I take?"—and he puts out the left. "Put your right forefinger to your nose."—"Some thing right? What must I do?" He puts the right leg out of bed. "Drink the Professor's health with this wine."—"As you wish . . ." The request is repeated. "Shall I take red wine for me or for you?" "Show your hand."—He does it. "Do you cough much?"—"Only to-day, as the weather is so bad." "What costs the cheapest wine you buy?"—"I don't know the words any more," &c.

His writing improves also. On the 21st he could write the alphabet easily. German and English characters are used promiscuously. On the 29th he made the first attempt, on being asked, to write a letter.

"*Ich soll*[17] Herrn Professor etwas wissen, *aber was soll ich etwas gheides wissen*. Ich weiss garnichts davon."

He still fails to make out written language; but this does not hold for numbers. He reads the multiplication table, and tells the results, though with a little uncertainty.

At the beginning of June he understands what is said to him much better; his speech is to a slight degree paraphasic. But one notices now that conversation is easier, that he has difficulty in finding the names of objects shown to him, and that he immediately forgets them when they are told. Thus, he was shown a knife and asked "What is this?"—"I have seen something like it, but I can't remember the name." "Is it a knife?"—"Yes, knife, knife!" "What is this?" showing him a cap. He mutters, but cannot find the word. "Is it a coat?"—"No," pointing to his own coat. "Is it a cap?"—"Yes, a cap." "Tell us what you have been eating."—"Eaten something, this morning at 8 o'clock drank something, and again at at 12 o'clock, but I can't tell more." "Take your pocket-handkerchief, and wipe your spectacles." Patient does it. "Take my purse, take five francs out of it, and give them to So-and-so." He takes the purse, and five francs out of it, but does not understand the rest.

His understanding of written language is very bad still, though when he reads aloud he makes out the meaning better, a fact which corresponds with his improvement as to spoken language. When he is not allowed to read aloud, he apparently spells inwardly.[18] Even what he copies to dictation is obscure to him. I dictated to him an I. O. U. for 20,000 francs, which he wrote down, and allowed me to put in my pocket without giving the least sign of emotion. Volitional writing is still accompanied with well-marked paragraphia, though there is improvement in this respect. He wrote the following letter to me on the 4th of June:—

"Juni Mittwoch d. 4ten.—Herr Professor Dr. Lichtheim. Ich möchte heute etwas schreiben. Ich weiss noch sehr wenig. Ich bin Arbergergasse No. 52, mit meiner meiner Lieben um 1 und ½ Stunde sehr gern gesehen. Ach wie tausend Mal so gern für seine liebes Herz. Ach gott wie gern sollte ich viel mehr wissen und mein liebes Herz müsste mal allte Tag, oft die weiss täglich hundert mal und ich weiss fasst noch nichts mehr was ich zu wissen sollte. O wie viel zu wenig daheim. Ich will am morgen Mittags daheim Arbergergasse zu meine Liebenfrau. Fünf mal heute noch. Ich will auch noch etwas schreiben.—Schwarz-Beer."

Patient left the hospital on the 6th of June, but came to see us once every week. Every time he showed further improvement. On the 23rd the following notes were taken:

1. *Volitional speech.*—Paraphasia is very slight; word-amnesia, on the other hand, is considerable, though not so apparent in current conversation. He remembers the names of objects a little better; still he is very deficient in this respect.
2. *Volitional writing* is improved. There is less paragraphia.
3. *Understanding of spoken language* is much better. Patient understands almost everything he is told, even the longer sentences. Complicated tasks are executed correctly. Still, beyond a certain point, he still manifests deficiency in this respect; and it is impossible to appeal to his self-observation.
4. He *repeats words* correctly, and in longer sentences. He does it more quickly and intelligibly.
5. *Reading aloud.*—More ready; but he still mainly does it by spelling. He understands better.
6. *Understanding of writing* more deficient than that of speech, though unquestionably improved. He understands short words at once. Longer ones take him an interval, during which he seems to put them together; he used to repeat them, but this being forbidden he appears to spell them inwardly.
7. *Copying and writing to dictation* are carried out properly. He understands much of what he writes. The experiment with the I. O. U. does not succeed any longer.

The last time the tests were applied was on the 25th of July. He still talks somewhat slowly, the arrangement of words is often peculiar, but it takes time to discover that words are wanting in his vocabulary. He is easily stopped by proper names, and finds them with difficulty. The word amnesia, however, is much less marked.

He seems to understand all that is said; one is occasionally obliged to repeat a question; and he himself repeats, as if with astonishment, proper names. Much paragraphia still present when he writes of his own accord, though a letter he wrote to me on that day shows a marked improvement. Progress is also noticed in the other respects.

On the 30th of July I was called to see him. About midnight his wife noticed that he suddenly became restless. He tried to get up, and fell. The left arm appeared to be paralysed; but he can give no account of the state of the sensorium. He has been restless since, and talked nonsense.

I found his consciousness slightly affected; he is continually babbling as a delirious fever-patient. He reacts a little when called, but does not recognise people about him.

The eyes are chiefly turned to the right; it is difficult to make him fix them; when called he answers "yes," but turns them more to the right, and does not follow the finger. Pupils rather contracted.

He appears to have headache on the right side, points to it with his hand, and applies a sponge to it. Left arm flaccid and paralysed; left leg apparently sound, yet on rising he bends towards the left side.

Left naso-labial fold somewhat effaced. Sensation and reflexes on the left apparently diminished. No paraphasia noticeable in what he talks. There was constant vomiting; and the patient was taken to another hospital, owing to my removal into other wards, and is still living.

A few remarks on this case, in which the symptoms agree with those postulated by an interruption

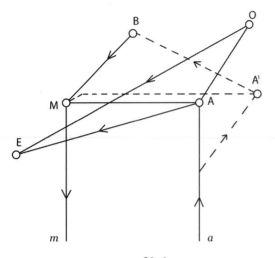

FIGURE 20–6.

in the commissure A B, may not be out of place. It may be asked why he spelt the words, though the path O A M *m* was intact. I think this is explained by the fact, that for fluent reading it is necessary to understand the words; we guess the words before we have actually read them through, and gain much time thereby. When we have to say long words in a foreign language, we also must spell to a certain extent. Our patient shows also a phenomenon which has been observed in other cases of the kind; he repeated the question of which he did not understand the meaning. This condition is closely allied to the *Echolalia* of Romberg; and Spamer,[19] who also deduced the possibility of this symptom from his schema, used this name. In our case it did not appear as if the repetition necessitated the understanding of the words heard, by means of a centripetal path[20] from M to B. The circumstance that the patient supplied his lost understanding of written language by reading aloud, must be explained differently. The case shows, with many others, that disturbances in the use of written language are much slower to disappear than those connected with speech. Paragraphia here persisted much longer than paraphasia, and the patient understood writing but very imperfectly, whilst verbal deafness had practically passed away.

This may be explained by assuming, that the recovery of the understanding of words is not effected by a new connection between A and B, but that the sound-representations are deposited at another point A which is connected with M, B, and *a*. We should thus obtain a state of things as represented in Dia-

gram 6, where the destroyed path A B is not shown, but where the vicarious connections are depicted by dotted lines (Fig. 20–6). With the assistance of the figure, one easily sees that the patient can easily understand by the ear what he reads aloud; whilst silent reading remains senseless. Silent spelling is already of assistance under these circumstances, because along with the innervation of the movement-representations the words are revived in A′ and make understanding possible; The commissure O A′ and A′ E, require to be used for a much longer time, before the disturbance in the writing can be overcome by their substitution.

The case I have just related is by no means an isolated one, but appears to be of the same category as that of Schmidt,[22] and that of Broadbent[23] mentioned by Skwortzoff as one of word-blindness. In other instances, the observations are not sufficiently full to allow us to decide whether the cases really belong to the same group.

7. The last interruption to be considered, that in the path A *a* does not really belong to the subject of aphasia, for the faculty of speech remains perfect. Still it is necessary to consider it here, because its symptoms cannot be properly understood except in connection with the present subject.

From the diagram we should conclude that there is a loss of:
(*a*) understanding of language;
(*b*) faculty of repeating;
(*c*) faculty of writing to dictation.
The following are preserved intact:
(*d*) volitional speech;
(*e*) volitional writing;
(*f*) understanding of writing;
(*g*) reading aloud;
(*h*) copying words.

There is no paraphasia nor paragraphia, because the path B M A B is whole; we could therefore designate such cases as "Isolated speech-deafness," as the incapacity for repetition and writing to dictation may be included under the term "speech deafness." But since there is a form of speech-deafness, in which, as we have seen, the faculty of repeating and writing to dictation is preserved, it is advisable to distinguish sharply these functions.

I have a personal observation to record of such a case which has already been published by Burckhardt.[24]

*Case IV. — Chronic Bronchitis. — Arterio-
sclerosis. — Two Apoplectic Seizures; After
the First, Paraphasia and Paragraphia
Gradually Receding; After the Second,
Persistent Word-deafness. — Incapacity of
Repeating and of Writing to Dictation. —
No Disturbance of Speech.*

Mr. L., aged 55, formerly a teacher and journalist, remained healthy till 1877. He then had an apoplectic fit, which was followed by troubles of language only, with the exception of a slight weakness in the muscles of the mouth on the left side of the face. These are fully described in Burckhardt's observation, to which the reader is referred for particulars. They consisted in paraphasia during volitional speech, repetition of words, and reading; paragraphia in writing to dictation. Volitional writing was very faulty, but not abolished. Nothing is said of the intelligence of language; but from the context and information given by his wife, it appears to have been intact. Evidence as to his understanding written language is wanting.

This association of symptoms may be identified with the one described under 3, as due to a break in M A, and the case is one I had in view when I said that the conditions of voluntary writing agree best with Diagram 2.

The state just described gradually improved, and a slight defect of speech only remained, consisting in the occasional misuse of a word.

In June 1882 he had a sudden attack; the symptoms seem to have been slight. A medical examination made immediately after showed an increase in the facial paralysis; and his wife said the defect of speech was more accentuated; he could not read nor write. We have here a discrepancy between the information given by the wife and that furnished by Burckhardt, who does not mention any disturbance of speech, and says he could read and write. I have mentioned the former statements because they do not agree so well with my views; but as they were made long after the event they do not deserve the same confidence as the notes taken at the time by Burckhardt. He was completely word-deaf.

The disturbances of language rapidly improved, even beyond the state in which he was before the attack. He recovered reading and writing completely; but the word-deafness remained the same. Intelligence free: patient felt weak, and did not like to leave his bed; he suffers from chronic catarrh and asthma.

I saw him first in July 1883; and again in June 1884; on both occasions his condition was the same.

[Passing over the general examination of the body, which presented no features of importance, we come to the functions of language.]

Understanding of speech. — Patient gives the impression of an absolutely deaf man, and differs in this respect from other cases of word-deafness. One cannot have the least communication with him except through writing; even his wife cannot make herself understood otherwise, as he can read from the lips but very few words, and these imperfectly.

I should probably have taken him for really deaf had I not been assured that he was acute of hearing, and could perceive all noises, which he said hurt him; and had I not tested the fact myself. Having written for him to raise his hand as soon as he heard the sound of a bell, he did so correctly, even when it was rung most gently behind him. It is the deficient attention he pays to sounds which gives one the impression that he is deaf. Then a few minutes later I rang again, but he did not react to the noise by raising his arm a little, until it was very loud. The same want of attention is manifest when one talks to him. He does not make the efforts to understand observed in patients with word-deafness, but remains indifferent; one has to push or shake him in order to make him attend. He hears when one whistles or sings, but does not recognize melodies. When his children sing in his room quartettes, of which he formerly was fond, he tells them to stop, and that they make too much noise. When I played the national anthem before him, he said, "Once more, I shall perhaps recognize it." But he cannot do so.

Speech. — He speaks with absolute accuracy, but with a slight drawl; very rarely, not oftener than would a healthy man, he stops for a word. He finds substantives, even complex ones, and proper names. I showed him a picture, and he said without the least hesitation, "Winterthur." On neither occasion could I detect the least trace of paraphasia.

Writing. — He writes fluently and correctly, and composes long articles for journals, of which I have seen several, and possess one.

Repeating is impossible to him, even when he is told by writing to do so. Thus when I said, "Ich heisse," he fixed his eyes upon my lips and finally brings out an "Ich," but nothing more.

Writing to dictation. — Asked to do so, he said: "But I can't hear." I nevertheless proceeded to dictate, upon which he remarked: "What a farce to dictate when one does not hear!"

Copying and reading aloud he carries out correctly and fluently.

Intelligence of written language is intact, as shown by what has already been said. He copies an I O U, written by myself, gives it to his wife, remarking, "You see you have got money."

Intelligence perfectly normal. The articles he writes are up to his usual standard and are often published in his newspaper. Advice from his medical attendant informs me that he has remained *in status quo* up to the present date.

There is in this case only one point which needs discussion here. It is whether the word-deafness produced by the second attack really caused no disturbance of speech. The patient had preserved from his first attack a difficulty with reference to language and writing. If we follow the description of Burckhardt, the second attack brought no change into this condition, and the slight alteration of speech which remained receded completely in the subsequent evolution of the case before I saw the patient. This is in contradiction with the wife's account, who, in answer to my questions, said that the speech had been temporarily worse after the second attack, when writing and reading disappeared for awhile. I have already said that these statements were not trustworthy, having been made three years after the event, whilst the observations of Burckhardt were noted at the time; but I deemed it necessary to mention them precisely, because they seemed to militate against my view. However, even if they were correct, I would adhere to my interpretation, and assume that, in the second attack, the centre A of the diagram had been transitorily affected also. Thus Wernicke's type of aphasia, which includes, besides word-deafness, paraphasia, agraphia and alexia, might have some to be observed for a short time. This state of things would have passed away quickly, and word-deafness only persisted, complicated with a gradually receding trace of the disturbance of speech left after the first attack. This interpretation is obviously more probable than the assumption, that the disturbance of speech was a direct symptom of the focal lesion of the second attack, and was transitory only, whilst the verbal deafness remained. The opposite course is indeed the usual one, verbal deafness disappearing very much more quickly than paraphasia.

In other respects also the case offers peculiarities. I have already adverted to the possibility of looking upon the patient as slightly deaf. The other cases of word-deafness I have seen were different in this respect; one was apt in them to overlook the symptom, the patients answering all questions, but not appositely, and the danger being then to diagnose confusion of ideas. Our patient, on the other hand, paid no attention to the questions, never returned any answer, and thus gave one the impression of being deaf.

Finally, the persistence of this symptom differentiates the present case from the others. Yet these peculiarities can lend only a high degree of probability to this differentiation; a single case does not warrant certainty, and further instances are required before we can decide. The case seems to be an isolated one; I have suspected from the description of others that they belonged to the same category, but the want of accuracy in the observations has not allowed me to reach a definite conclusion.

I think I have so far shown, that each of the seven forms of aphasia postulated by the diagram are found to exist; but there remains the question, as to whether all cases hitherto observed are reducible to these forms. If we examine a large number of the cases on record, it will be found that the majority present deficiencies of observation which allow the test to be applied to them only up to a certain point. In a large number of instances the probability is that they do really belong to one of the forms. But one readily obtains examples in which this is not the case; they seem to differ in one point or another from these morbid types. Do they constitute a serious objection to my theory? I do not think so; most of them can be shown to be reducible to the schema. I must first advert to the fact, that the seven forms hitherto discussed have their origin in *simple* interruptions; whilst there is no doubt that more than one of the paths may be affected simultaneously. A decisive proof of the reality of such combination types is to be found in "total aphasia," in which there is complete incapacity to speak (the "logoplegia" of the French), with word-deafness. Here there must be a break in the centripetal as well as the centrifugal portion of the arc. We possess several observations to this effect, in which the autopsies have confirmed this assumption. Under the definition of total aphasia just given, this type will include all cases where there is loss both of speech and of understanding of speech; a combination which will arise not only when M and A are injured, but also when other combined breaks in the two branches of the arc do occur: it will be evident from the diagram that six such combinations are possible, each giving rise to the symptom. It is very doubtful, however, if these theoretical possibilities are all embodied in actual cases; their respective degree of probability can be arrived at only when we know more clearly the anatomical disposition of the nervous paths. We must assume, however, that some other combined lesions occur besides that of A and M; certain observations point to this conclusion. Thus, for instance, the celebrated case of Lordat, which, though I know only through the fragmentary account of Kussmaul, may be explained on the assumption of a simultaneous break in M B and A B. It appears that, like our patient Schwarz, he could read spelling-wise, though without understanding what he did read. Aphasia due to lesion in M B and B A, would be differentiated from that due to lesion of M and A by the preservation of the faculty of reading aloud, of repeating words, and of writing to dictation; but there is no mention made of these functions in the account just referred to.

[. . .]

Notes

1. 'Der Aphasische Symptomencomplex;' Breslau, 1874.

2. 'Die Störungen der Sprache;' Ziemssen's 'Cyclopedia,' vol. xiii. Leipzig, 1877.

3. ['Wortklangsbilder;' or auditory word-impressions.]

4. ['Wortbewegungsbilder;' or kinaesthetic word-impressions.]

5. ['Klangbildercentrum;' and 'Bewegungsbildercentrum.']

6. ['Begriffe.']

7. 'Clinique Médicale,' vol. ii.

8. A rare species of aphasia, included by Kussmaul under the ataxic, and to which we shall allude presently, differs in this particular.

9. Loc. cit. p. 39.

10. Excepting a difference in the power of volitional writing. This point will be considered in detail further on.

11. Loc. cit. p. 39.

12. 'De la cécité et de la surdité des mots dans l'Aphasie,' Paris, 1881. On page 84 a Case of Broadbent is mentioned which could be opposed to that of Wernicke. It is one apparently of sensorial aphasia, for besides imperfect understanding of language, the speech consisted in a kind of unarticulated jargon. It is said that the writing was not involved. But apart from the fact, that it is doubtful whether this was really volitional writing, and not only that to dictation or to a copy, the whole description is given in such a fragmentary manner, that we cannot tell whether we have to do with true sensorial aphasia, or some variety of it. The case, therefore, cannot be brought as evidence on the subject before us. — Since this paper was in the press, I read a typical case of Wernicke's sensorial aphasia described by Grasset (Contribution clinique à Pétude des Aphasies. 'Montpellier médical,' Jan. 1884) and in which also there was complete agraphia. This case too, therefore, points to the correctness of Fig. 4.

13. 'Diseases of the Nervous System,' 7th ed., chap. vii.

14. See example given by Wernicke, loc. cit., p. 56.

15. We learn to write with the co-operation of auditory representations, hence, we cannot write without it. Every lesion of the path B M A (Fig.) 4 destroys the innervation of the auditory representation from the concept-centre, and must necessarily result in agraphia.

16. "Considérations sur l'agraphie à propos d'une observation nouvelle d'agraphie." — 'Revue de Médecine,' 1884, 11.

17. [The words in *italics* were written in English characters, the rest in German. The word "wissen" is apparently used for "schreiben." "Gheides" is meaningless.]

18. When questions were asked, he, at the beginning of his stay in the hospital, used to repeat them, it seemed to facilitate his comprehension; but occasionally did not understand them even after repeating them.

19. 'Ueber Aphasic und Asymbolie;' 'Archiv für Psychiatrie,' vi. 523.

20. I should not have mentioned this possibility, had not a case of Westphal's (cf. Spamer, p. 541) made such an interpretation probable.

21. The rapidity with which this occurs may seem an objection to the explanation. But the sensorial aphasia of Wernicke through lesions of A goes on diminishing likewise, a fact not susceptible of another interpretation.

22. 'Allg. Zeitschrift für Psychiatrie,' 1871, vol. 27, p. 304; quoted by Kussmaul, p. 176.

23. "Cerebral Mechanism of Thought and Speech" 'Med. Chir. Transactions, 1872,' vol. lv.; quoted after Skwortzoff, loc. cit., p. 38.

24. "Ein Fall von Worttaubheit." — 'Correspondenzblatt für Schweizer Aerzte,' 1882, No. 20.

21

Contributions to a Histological Localization of the Cerebral Cortex— VI. Communication: The Division of the Human Cortex

Korbinian Brodmann

The early beginnings of an attempt to reach a topographic parcellation of the cerebral cortex by using an anatomical-histological method, thereby gaining new guidelines for clinical and physiological localization, reach back only a few years. These first attempts start— when one disregards the, for the purpose of localization, inadequate myelinisation method—with the fact already recognized by Meynart (1868 and 1872) and Betz (1874), that regional differences exist in cell and fiber structures, i.e. in the laminar pattern (Schichtungstektonik) of the cross section of the cerebral cortex, and therefore base themselves on those histological structural relations existent in the cortex cerebri recently described on numerous occasions as cytoarchitectonical and myeloarchitectonical differences.

Excerpts from *Contributions to a histological localization of the cerebral cortex*, translated by Simran Karir and Katrin Amunts from Beiträge zur histologischen Lokalisation der Großhirnrinde. VI: Die Cortexgliederung des Menschen, in *Journal für Psychologie und Neurologie* X (6):231–246 (1908). (Neurobiological Laboratory of the University of Berlin)

It was to those individual cortex segments, marked by their particular clinical significance, to which the anatomical localizational research first turned its interest.

The first cortical region, which due to its specific laminar pattern has undergone an exact topical localization, is the region of the calcarine fissure, which is associated with vision. Bolton (1900) and after him—originally without knowledge of the preceding investigations by Bolton—I (1903) gave an exact spatial demarcation of the cortex type marked by the Stria Gennari of Vicq d'Azyr or of the "calcarina type"("Calcarinatypus") in the Lobus occipitalis in humans and discovered that the region in question— Bolton's *Visuo sensory area* or *Area striata*, as it was later more practically named by E. Smith—is limited to the actual cortex of the Fissura calcarina and its immediate vicinity.[1]

Elliot Smith and myself, localizational in comparison, dealt with this type of cortex. E. Smith (1904) described, based only on macroscopic sections however, the extent of the Stria Gennari—*Area striata*—in a large number of lower species of monkeys (and brains of Egyptians) and searched in particular to prove solid and legitimate relationships of the borders of the Area striata to particular sulci on the occipital lobe. I myself have in the same year proven the presence of the homologous field using series of microscopic serial sections at first on lower monkeys as well (1904) and shortly thereafter (1905) going through the whole row of mammals and in detail determined localizationally in each order except in the cetaceans and monotremes, of which material was missing, the location and size of the cortical area; I thereby came to findings that differed from those by E. Smith in that I discovered a vast variability in the behavior of the Area striata to individual sulci. Hermanides and

Köppen in 1903 sought to determine the location of "visual region" in lissencephalic brains (insectivores and Rodentia), but they (as by the way Watson as well) arrived at wrong homologues and, in addition, did not give an exact spatial boundary of their so-called "granular cortex." Köppen and Löwenstein describe in 1905 the location of the visual cortex in carnivores and ungulates. In the following year, Mott, obviously without prior knowledge of my older works on this subject, published findings on the development of the *"Visual Cortex"* in mammals, but he does not really give a topical localization of the field either.

The second gyrus, which was dealt with in regards to cortical topography, is marked by its close relationships to motility and is called the Regio Rolandica. We have Schlapp (1898), Cajal (1900), and Farrar

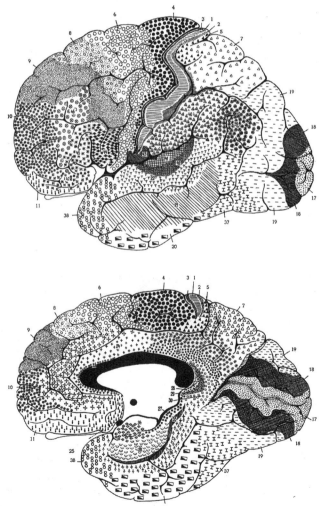

FIGURE 21–1. Lateral (*top*) and medial (*bottom*) views of the hemisphere of a human brain with cytoarchitectonic cortical areas.

(1903) to thank for the evidence that in the Sulcus centralis, a borderline is located between two sections of the cortex, which are cell—resp. fiberanatomically different; hence the important observation for clinicians and physiologists as well, that the frontal and back central gyri are constructed differently on their entire expansion. At the same time one should not forget, however, that already in 1874 Betz assumed that the lower 3/4 of both gyri had a different structure and only recognized a homogenous construction for the upper 1/6.

Localizational in a narrower sense, i.e., I dealt with the central gyri in humans (1903) for the purpose of spatially defining the different structure types on all sides. In the first of my contributions on histological localization, one finds that the topical demarcation of the "giant pyramidal type" ("Riesenpyramidentypus")—the *Area gigantopyramidalis*—is in the Gyrus centralis anterior, and at the same time it is already described there that in the Gyrus centralis posterior three areas, namely occupying the frontal bank, the crown of the gyrus and the ventral bank, may be separated and are different from one another as well as from the aforementioned one. The location of the homologous ("motor" ("motorischen")) type or the Area gigantopyramidalis has been defined in carnivores and ungulates by Köppen and Löwenstein (1905); Watson has done the same in insectivores (1907), as did I for all main orders of mammals (1905/06). O. Vogt in 1906 determined the relationship of the location of zones in the Area gigantopyramidalis, which can be electrically stimulated, using a number of different species of monkeys. The older work by Kolmer (1901), which also proceeds from the idea of a histotopography of the "motor" region of the cerebral cortex in humans, comes to findings that completely deviate from the ones mentioned above. He based his studies exclusively on the existence of one lone histological element, of the "motor cell type" (motorischen Zellart) in the same understanding as Nissl, and as such did not recognize the coarse regional differences in the tectonic structure of the entire cross section of the cortex in the area in question. He wrongly concluded that the biggest part of the parietal lobe together with both central gyri represent one uniform histological zone.

In the following years, localizational parcellations of the entire surface of the cortex were added to the above-mentioned specific studies, which focused on individual gyri marked by certain physiological features. To begin with, there exist two studies both stemming from 1905. One by Campbell, which by favoring myeloarchitectonics but also by considering the cellular structure provides a new histological parcellation of the cerebral cortex in humans (as an appendix in anthropoids, carnivores, and ungulates as well) and a second work by myself, which based on cytoarchitectonics offers a complete parcellation of the cortex in lower monkeys. Watson has recently (1907) published a complete parcellation of the cortex in insectivores. I myself could in the meantime finish the histotopography of the Cortex cerebri in prosimians, and I of late, after finishing this essential preliminary comparative anatomical work, was also able to finish the cytoarchitectonical localization of the human cerebral cortex, which I had begun years ago (Fig. 21–1, top and bottom).

[. . .]

Notes

1. It should be noted here that this anatomically defined demarcation is in complete agreement with the localization long since taught by Henschen, which is based on clinical observations of the human "visual sphere" ("Sehsphäre"). It remains an everlasting merit of Henschen's to have, by way of a clinical pathological method, more closely defined and spatially exactly determined a relatively undefined sensory region in the "occipital lobes" or in the "cuneus" or in the "vicinity of the calcarina." The histotopographical method seems to corroborate with his opinion.—Cf. Henschen, Clinical and anatomical contributions to the pathology of the brain. Vol. I-IV. 1890–1903.

22

The Agrammatical Language Disturbance: Studies on a Psychological Basis for the Teaching on Aphasia

Arnold Pick

I. TERM, HISTORY, DEFINITION AND CLASSIFICATION OF AGRAMMATISM

Kußmaul chooses the term agrammatism (Störung der Sprache, in *Handbuch der Pathologie und Therapie*, ed. by Ziemsen 1877, vol. 12, appendix, p. 193) to denote the various syntactical diction disturbances, which Steinthal (*Einleitung in die Psychologie und Sprachwissenschaft*. 1871. 2nd ed. 1881, cited here, p. 478) had earlier on already separated from the disturbance of the diction of words.

The beginning of the history of agrammatism dates back before Steinthal, since he too bases his grammatical disturbances, which he so painstakingly pared out of aphasia in general, on many Berlin dissertations, which he does not mention any further but which are partly considered here in casuistics.

Excerpts here are translated by Simran Karir and Katrin Amunts from Arnold Pick, *Die agrammatischen Sprachstörungen. Studien zur psychologischen Grundlegung der Aphasielehre* (1913), Reprint by Springer-Verlag, Berlin, Heidelberg, New York, Tokyo with an Introduction by Dorothea Weniger (1986), pp. 113–129.

Steinthal himself suggested, calling upon Aristotle's *On Interpretation*, the term "acataphasia" to designate the disturbance, but it did not prevail. Moreover, Kußmaul's term was most probably taken up in all languages because non-philologists easily understand it as well.

Linguistically [*sprachlich*] speaking, the term "asyntactism," chosen by individual authors (for example, in Bianchi's *Lehrbuch der Psychiatrie*, Engl. version, p. 341), may seem more appropriate than the others, if we define syntax, according to O. Dittrich (*Anz. F. indog. Sprach-und Altertk. XIX*, p. 13) "as a common teaching on inflection, as long as all the remaining means of inflection in words are treated as well and not only the case endings."[1]

Taking into consideration that the term syn- or rather asyntactism designates something completely different in linguistics, one hesitates to completely agree with Bianchi's term, which at first glance seems appropriate (cf. also V. Henry, *Et. sur l'analogie en générale etc.* 1883, p. 27); a further objection to this term will arise later on.

It is worth taking a plunge into the historical depths of this teaching for the following reason as well, namely because the same lack of clarity existed there, which resulted from the then exclusive theory that a very close relationship existed between thought and speech [*Sprache*] to the point where these two corresponded, and which we will still encounter in the latter phase of the teaching on aphasia. This may readily be seen in the statement by Steinthal, which is strongly influenced by the combination of both: "because the inability to form a sentence perhaps slightly touches the ability of logic" (p. 478). A suggestion, though, that Steinthal does in this case separate speech [*Sprechen*] in the third person, as a result of a lack of intelligence and agrammatism, which is determined somewhat differently, may be found therein, that he says in the description of a girl, who spoke of herself in the third person, and which Steinthal takes as sign of "low intelligence": "But she also spoke without *verba finita* and without conjunctions, exactly like a child, that is with the inability to really and fully formulate sentences though; she said, for example, 'Toni made, everything already made' ['Toni gemacht, alles schon gemacht'], or 'Toni flowers taken, keeper come, Toni hit' ['Toni Blumen genommen, Wärterin gekommen, Toni gehaut']."[2] But the same vacillation asserts itself in the basic account of that, which is hindered in acataphasia, when he describes the disturbance in the following way: "But the composition of sound [*Lautbild*] is associated with an idea, and it is a severer disturbance in language ability [*Sprachfähigkeit*] when the sick person is unable to reproduce, not the sound [*Lautbild*], but rather the idea. The real process of speaking, the function of transforming an opinion [*Anschauung*] into a concept [*Vorstellung*], i.e. the ability to formulate a sentence, is hindered."

A more precise, piece-by-piece account is needed to uncover all contradictions of the presently dominating opinions that arise in this interpretation; these shall only be touched upon here, as a further presentation of these opinions in the chapter about the path from thought to speech will bring about a self-explanatory clarity.

Still, in a later comment by Steinthal (l. c. p. 485), there clearly emerges a blurring of borders between speech [*Sprechen*] and thought, resulting in the definition of acataphasia becoming unclear, when he defines this latter as a "lack of strength to apperceive or to connect ideas according to grammatical rules."

It will be the task of further chapters to show the error in Steinthal's theory, presented here at the beginning, of a close parallelism between language and thought; but it has to be noted here, that modern authors as well, like Ziehen, who even in his latest article on aphasia in the *Eulenburgische Realenzyklopädie*, hold on to the opinion: "The arrangement of words into a sentence is not a feat of coordination of language, but rather depends on the associative connection of ideas."

Somewhat clearer are comments made by Kußmaul, who specifies the disturbance as one in the "ability to present one's train of thought"; the opinion of the connection between thought and speech, which he seems to not uphold, does lie hidden in the following though (l. c.): "To speech, the idea has to, as it moves logically through consciousness, be expressed in all its detail and twists and turns." (The emphasis not in Kußmaul.)

The error in the idea of such a parallelism between thought and linguistical presentation [*sprachliche Darstellung*] has already been pointed out in the introduction; one holds up in contrast the following statement by a philologist, taken from a small, recently rediscovered book from 1844: "As rich as a language might be in syntactical idioms, it is impossible that this language may offer similar idioms for every one of the innumerable changes that occur in a train of thought." (Weil, *De l'ordre des mots*, p. 38.)

This shall suffice for the moment, as we will take a closer look at this question later on; but it is suggested that the reader take note of how, as here with Kußmaul, a characteristic of logic clearly emerges in pathology and follows through to the psychology practiced in recent times.

A further fundamental deficit in Kußmaul's definition of agrammatism lies in the complete disregard of an important part of syntactically effective means of language [*syntaktisch wirksamen Sprachmittel*],[3] which is expressed in the sentence "The train of thought possesses two linguistical means [*sprachliche Mittel*] by which it presents itself: inflections and word order [*Wortstellung*], or, in a narrower sense, grammar and syntax. Syntax, in a broader sense, encompasses both."

That Kußmaul left out the musical elements of language, whose importance as a means of expression in a sentence we will soon briefly become preliminarily acquainted with, from the discussions on agrammatism, should be of no surprise; since he stood under the spell of contemporary opinions such as the ones voiced by H. Lotze (*Mikrokosmus*. Vol. 2, p. 229), he simply did not consider that a sentence is formed by an act of thought, which is cognitive opinionated, as well as emotional. This deficit goes back lastly to not having considered spoken language [*Sprechsprache*].

Broadbent dealt with the question in a more precise manner than Steinthal, especially in terms of pathology. Broadbent has to also be mentioned by name here, because he is the first person to have tried to determine the localization of agrammatism. He localizes those words that represent intellectual symbols in the "superadded convolution," which corresponds pretty exactly to what, many decades later, Flechsig calls centers of association [*Assoziationszentren*] in comparison to the centers of projection [*Projektionszentren*]; he localizes words, as motor processes, in the left third frontal convolution, which, as he supposes, serves in the choice of words that bring an idea to expression ("which is supposed to select the words for the expression of an idea"). Where thought and sentence formulation occurs cannot be precisely pinpointed, but the above-mentioned "superadded" convolutions of both hemispheres do play a part; the path that sentences, for the purpose of being expressed, take to the third left frontal convolution is not known.[4]

One should compare the latter belief by Broadbent with the newer opinion by v. Monakow, which is basically identical to the former's, in order to appreciate the historical significance of Broadbent's opinion; but with all the praise for the accomplishment, one cannot, on the other hand, overlook, as already Hughlings Jackson criticized at the time and as is still subject to frequent criticism now, in what gross fashion the procedures related to the mechanics of the brain and those that are psychological are blended. The opinion that Broadbent offers here on the formulation of thought is, besides the historical significance of this first attempt at the localization of agrammatism, of interest above all because the connection between the formulation of a sentence and choice of words is presented in such a manner that the former goes first; and it is this priority given to one process over the other that plays an important role in the following discussions dedicated to questions concerning language formulation [*Sprachformulierungen*]; the following will show that we, also now, come to the same results formulated here by Broadbent; this is therefore of such fundamental importance to the

question concerning localization, since it is now generally accepted that we normally speak by way of the temporal lobe, i.e. it helps us speak, because this is also where word selection takes place and therefore the first phase of formulating a sentence cannot be the function of the frontal lobe, which for speech comes into effect only later, nor of Broca's area.

Let's add to the historical overview just presented the fact that Broadbent, in the 1879 January issue of *Brain*, emerges correctly with the localization of agrammatism in the frontal brain and this then exhausts everything that can now still be considered historical in regards to this question; to continue this historical overview would only be a point for recapitulation of all those authors and their theories, who, because they are still current, will in the following presentation find enough opportunity to have their say. —

Hughlings Jackson is of the same narrow opinion, characterized above, concerning the extent of linguistic means [*Sprachmittel*] (*Brain. I* 1879, p.311), in that he separates the intellectual language [*intellektuelle Sprache*] from the emotional one, but what sets him apart is that one may clearly deduce from his statements on one-word sentences, which he differentiates according to an interjectional or propositional use of the word, that he, at least like this, judged, in an extraordinarily fine-tuned manner, musical elements as being the primary means by which emotions were expressed in language.

But what danger a sharp separation of "both these languages" poses—and not considering the emotional elements in the "intellectual" ones—may already be seen in the work of H. Jackson's successor, Roß (*On Aphasia* 1877, p. 2), who in a straightforward manner describes tone, melody, and rhythm as not belonging to intellectual language. When we later learn that in the teaching on word sequence [*Wortfolge*], one compares a grammatical one to an emotional one, then we clearly see therein the error of such a separation, as far as we, in this wide field, get to see how "both" languages come into effect in the same means of expression.

To further show that this theory has been neglected in contemporary language pathology will prove to be unnecessary here; it shall have to suffice, for the time being, to have pointed out that pathology has, up to the present time, been infected by this purely intellectual definition of linguistical means [*Sprachmittel*], which linguistics has long since mainly overcome, although Wundt as well, whose monograph serves as a main guide for pathologists, recognizes musical elements as a form of expression, and even in "pure logic"(cf. Husserl, *Logische Untersuchungen II*, p.14) the significance of these elements in comparison to the grammatical categories does find complete acknowledgement.

A radical quote by a modern linguist may show how this is perceived in current linguistics: "One falls under the illusion too quickly that language constitutes nothing more than that which one finds in black and white on paper. No, everything that happens while speaking and with the help of language tools [*Sprachwerkezeugen*] belongs to language: rhythm and intonation, singing, monotony, breadth or sharpness of that which is presented, but also the position [*Haltung*] of the mouth, if the lips are pulled wide or pointed, a protruding lower jaw, a limp, flu-ridden velum, etc." (From the *Gabelentz Die Sprachwissenschaft*. Vol. 2, p. 35).

How someone with a sense for the arts thinks may be inferred from the remark by C. Fiedler (*Schriften über Kunst*, ed. von Morbach 1896, p. 200), which states: "That all our sensual, emotional [*sinnlichseelischen*] abilities, our whole ability to sense, to feel, to perceive, to imagine participates in judging the worth of language, that it is the whole being that enters into the form of language." It may be pointed out here as well that the full weight of the meaning of the theories stressed here will emerge in the next chapter on sentence definition.

Of course, if even amongst language psychologists still too little attention has been paid to the fact that there also exist parts of sentences that are not words (e.g. sentence melody, which defines the question characteristic of a sentence), then it can be of no surprise if the correct point of view has not caught on amongst language pathologists yet. But slowly a change is coming about in the views of pathologists regarding the meaning of emotions also in the, to date, exclusively intellectually defined area of imagination [*Vorstellungsleben*]; in terms of the subject matter being discussed here, the since published work by Serog (*Zeitschr. f. d. ges. Neur. u. Psych.*, 1911, p. 107) should be pointed out, in which he agrees that emotions have a stronger influence on how words are organized [*Zusammenordnen*] than it merely being an arrangement of ideas by association, and which is a prerequisite for organized, goal-oriented thought [*Denken*]. We see here as well how pathology, which especially in this area could itself promote crucial, guiding facts, lags behind psychology.

Since the reasoning of Kußmaul's definition, a second issue has arisen, concerning the treatment of this problem, which poses some difficulty. Kußmaul's leanings towards the then-defining linguistical theory influenced him to give written language, as represented in the literature [*Dokumenten*], precedence in his observations, and nothing has changed in pathology since then, especially since Wundt does not use spoken language, colloquial language, as a basis for his language psychology either; if one can now, as was stressed in the introduction, infer the one-sidedness of Wundt's theory from this, then language pathology must look to lean more heavily on the living [*lebendige*] word; it will be shown that this psychology of colloquial language in its different, also social and dialect modifications, normally shows important relationships especially to agrammatism; an analysis of those means of expression, emerging in colloquial language, results in findings to be taken especial notice of here, as some of these means of expression, which are not at all detectable in written language or only become so in written language through the analysis of colloquial language, play an even greater role as their importance in how the sick person expresses himself increases through the demise of the rest, caused by the aphasic destructive process.

Kleist has very recently, to designate the processes coming into play here, coined the term "*Ausdrucksfindung*" [the search to express oneself], which in terms of the wider, encompassing meaning of the word "*Ausdruck*" [expression] is quite appropriate; but he also, on closer observation (as far as may be inferred from reports on his lecture), adheres to the articulated elements of language.

The theories that were taken into consideration, up until this point, regarding the definition of those disturbances collectively known as agrammatism identified a considerably richer amount of actual types of disturbances and not simply types whose characteristics varied by a few degrees, as do the older definitions, and they do so without incurring differences in regards to the means of expression taken into consideration. Contrary to this, though, a fact is now to be heeded by which such a difference is uncovered, and by further examining this fact (one of the desiderata of future pathological research), new insight into another area of psychological phenomena may be granted.

It was Rieß, the philologist, who in his 1894 epoch-marking work "Was ist Syntax?" pointed out that forms of inflection do not simply serve to express relationships among words, as one thought up until that point and as is still the case to date, in regards to the definition of agrammatism; since this—if correct—would be as important to the question concerning the breadth of the definition and psychological significance of the different kinds of agrammatisms as to linguistics and also as to the question concerning the localization of agrammatism and other related disturbances, then the essence of Rieß's proof shall be given here.

"The significance of forms of inflection is . . . varied. They serve to express relationships amongst words (e.g. most case forms, in their most frequent use), as well as to signal a further qualification that adds to the actual definition of the word (e.g. gender and number of the noun, the majority of tenses) and also to signal a modification in the meaning of a word (e.g. forms of comparison). The wrong theory, which simply ascribes a syntactical interest [*synktatisches Interesse*] to all forms of inflection and to all of their meanings, has led to a veiling and blurring of the essential varied nature of the inflection significances, which mostly remains unnoticed and is often completely overlooked.[5]

"In the same way as 'the father comes' ['der Vater kommt'] is syntactically the same as 'the brother comes' ['der Bruder kommt'], it is the same in regards to syntax if I say, 'the father comes' ['der Vater kommt'] or 'the fathers come' ['die Väter kommen']; if I say, 'the father comes' ['der Vater kommt'] or 'the father came' ['der Vater kam']. . . . And as Syntax does not take exception to '2 × 2 = 5,' which it does not at all know to differentiate from '2 × 2 = 4,' it, in the same way, does not take exception to 'my heads hurt' ['Meine Köpfe tun mir weh'], which similarly cannot be differentiated syntactically from 'my head hurts' ['Mein Kopf tut mir weh']. What was changed in these structures, which remained the same, is only the material content. This alone changes by changing comes [*kommt*] and came [*kam*], father [*Vater*] and fathers [*Väter*], head [*Kopf*] and heads [*Köpfe*], as it would change by replacing brother [*Bruder*] with father [*Vater*], 5 with 4. . . . That certain forms, similar for all words of the same kind [*Art*], serve to express certain terms or categories of thought, does not change the fact that we are exclusively dealing with the meaning of the individual word, by which a general term joins the specific word-term [*Wortbegriff*]. All this has nothing to do with syntax."

F. N. Finck later elaborates on this theory by Rieß, in that he contrasts one part of inflection suffixes, like the dual and plural endings, the designations signaling gender and elements of mood, as elements of qualification, with elements signaling relationships. The Latinist P. Morris (*On Princ. and Meth. in Latin Syntax*, 1902, p. 38) expresses Rieß's principle idea very well when he says that a clear separation of semantics (theory of meaning) and syntax, which for theoretical reasons is seldom done, could easily bring about the notion where the syntactical form could only represent the shell, which could be filled with any kind of content without changing its characteristic.

The validity of Rieß's argument leaves no doubt even for the layperson; it first of all has the following influence in the wake of the pathological [*Pathologische im Gefolge*], namely that those disturbances that Rieß specifies cannot exclusively be categorized as disturbances of syntax anymore, but rather fall into the category of semantics. (Cf. that which was said in the introduction following a program [*Programm*] by Meillet on an individual linguistics, regarding the rejection of a sharp separation of linguistical material to be used in teachings on aphasia.)

That a consideration of agrammatical disturbances in light of these theories will be an important task for future research; that important, at first purely theoretical results may come about for pathology, but also for the regular psychology of language, is reason to continue linguistic discussions that seem to be so far-reaching at the moment.

The next task for the study of agrammatical disturbances will be a separation of these according to Rieß's theories; if it turns out that those parts of syntax [*Formbildung*] that belong to semantics are, in those cases, not part of the disturbance, then this would mean for pathological agrammatism that we are essentially really dealing with a disturbance in the old sense. Realistically, this will not be the case though, since the grammatization of speech [Rede] may be seen as a uniform process. But such a conclusion then gains, in terms of questions concerning localization, more theoretical significance than that already at hand. Because if in such a case, with enough proof according to the whole clinical-anatomical position, localizations of lesions, postulated by the author, should confirm agrammatism, be they in the temporal lobe or elsewhere, then two theories of eminent importance may be abstracted from this. First of all, the main theory of a possible localization of a function, which lies closer to the intellectual functions than to those dealing with syntax, and whose acquisition in itself represents a valuable step in this direction. A second gain may be found therein, that, aside from the specific localization, to be further made use of, the close proximity of the brain processes, corresponding to both kinds of syntaxations as according to Rieß in the form of parallel processes, is given.

Following a suggestion by the French linguist Meillet, one designates, in contrast to the phonetical elements, called "phonämes," everything that in a word signals the grammatical form as "morphämes." The teachings on agrammatism would thereby in the broadest sense be a pathology of morphemes, and this entails more than simply the term agrammatism, as Meillet also includes syntax, which together with morphology represents both subdivisions of grammar. (Cf. the different works by Meillet and lastly his article on linguistics in "De la Méthode d. l. sciences". 2e série. 1911, p. 271 and 276 and especially his comments on p. 277, where he shows that the separation between morphology and syntax is artificial and cannot be actually performed.)

A.Dauzat (*Essai de Méthodol. Linguist.* 1906, p. 19) categorizes phonetics as the science of sound, next to semantics, the teaching of ideas in relation to sound. Semantics breaks down into three parts: morphology, lexicology, and syntax; morphology studies words in relation to their different definitions, syntax deals with words and the relationships amongst these. Here again is to be seen how the teachings on agrammatism reach out over the borders of syntax.

That such considerations, as presented above, are not unimportant to the question concerning pathology has been proven. An author who of late deals with agrammatism bases his definition of agrammatism, a term that cannot be too narrowly defined, on syntactical disturbances. Pelz (Zur Lehre von d. transkort. Aphasien. *Zeitschr. f. d. ges. Neur. u. Psychol.* XI, p. 129) speaks of a disturbance in the speech order or of a loosening of the organic compound sentence as being a form of agrammatism. If one disregards the term asyntactism, which would be most appropriate to describe the disturbance of speech order, then one cannot overlook, also if one were to exclude considerations influenced by Rieß, that next to this disturbance others are joined together under the common term agrammatism as well. That such a combination

is also clinically at least justified is proven by Pelz's case, in which he not only shows speech order, i.e. asyntactism, but also the other form, that is, speech using infinitives [*Sprechen in Infinitiven*] ("come, Hanchen come" ["Kommen, Hanchen kommen"], "today mama comes" ["heute Mama kommen"]).

Some words are to be assigned to another, recently established, area of agrammatism. Kleist (Über Störungen der Rede. Autorref. regarding the last-mentioned lecture) describes a more or less far-reaching simplification in expression [*Ausdrucksvereinfachung*] as being a kind of disturbance in expression [*Ausdrucksfindung*] that reaches its highest degree in agrammatism. One has to take note in regards to this, though, that this is not the only form of agrammatism that occurs in persons suffering from actual aphasia nor in those who are mentally ill.

It should be of no surprise that other general arguments made in previous linguistical studies might still be relevant as well. When Heilbronner states in his study on aphasia (in the *Handbuch der Neurol. I*, p. 987), that the separation of the two main types of agrammatism, the 'telegram style' [*Telegrammstil*] and the so-called *parler nägre*, is clinically hard to do, the following question, which expresses the stance justified by the preceding, is then to be pondered: The separation of both comes about either as a consequence of a different psychological or linguistic basis that makes the separation a clinical postulate then, or such a difference does not exist and neither does the clinical separation; but the clinical simultaneous occurrence of these types remains in both cases of importance in terms of localization and shall be assessed according to the answer in terms of the chosen alternative.

It should be noted, in addition to the preceding discussion on the definition of agrammatism, that some syntactical forms as well as some words serve to lend to expression that which later in the chapter will be said of the sentence, namely that it represents the speaker's point of view. We shall later come back to words expressing emotions and phrases with a similar effect; but only the following statement by a linguist shall be added here: "One understands that these forms of expression appear at any moment during conversation; a host of adverbs, adjectives, parts of sentences that we simply inject into sentences and that are the speaker's reflections or opinions. I will first of all present those forms of expression that relate a strong or weak feeling of security or trust, as for example *sans doute, peut-êàtre, probablement, surement,* etc. Every language has a group of such adverbs." (M. Bréal, *Essai de Sémantique* 1897, p. 255.)

Nothing would be simpler than to add to these linguistic facts, as far as they touch upon the question of agrammatism, similar discussions concerning pathology, as was done before with Rieß's conclusions. Seeing as the state of pathology offers even fewer actual points to latch onto than in Rieß's conclusion, it is simply noted here that the opinion derived from Meillet's comments is certainly worthy of the language pathologists' [*Sprachpathologen*] attention.

In this context, another fact is to be considered, which Marty (Unt. z. Grundleg. 1908, I, p. 532) brings up. He demonstrates how narrow the definition of syntax—that is, the teaching on sentences and sentence structure—is by showing that there exist word constructions that do have a complete meaning, yet are not sentences in the regular sense, but rather only names, and yet do show syntactical characteristics, as e.g. a father of five naughty children. Another objection in regards to defining the term too narrowly also arises from the fact that there exist expressions that do not consist of many parts [*Redegliedern*] (lego, wehe!), but are, according to the definition, real sentences. It remains to be seen if the facts that support the first objection are significant to pathology; in regards to the second, one should take a look at discussions on sentences, especially on one-word sentences.

Even if, in light of the linguistical facts just presented, the term agrammatism proves to be technically more adequate than the term "asyntactism" and is thereby further used without regarding such kinds of fundamental differences, one cannot, on the other hand, ignore that this broader agrammatism does also incorporate things that will have to be separated according to their pathological differences. In which way a separation will occur for pathology can hardly be foretold; one can at best think of a buffer from other disturbances also located in the temporal lobe (amnestical aphasia), that is, symptoms that for the moment are related to paraphasia; what significance this question concerning localization has for the author's localization of agrammatism, which he places in the temporal lobe, will have to be discussed in a chapter belonging to the section on pathology.

Only the following shall briefly be added: In accordance with Rieß's conclusions, just presented here, the effectiveness of grammatical elements affects the relations of words [*Wortbeziehungen*] as well as their meaning; these latter functions are most probably connected to the process of finding words [*Wortfindung*] and their localization may at least be near the temporal lobe, as the localization of the process of finding words is definitely in the temporal lobe.[6] Even now that we know everything on the general localization, the task at hand is not to separate the two simultaneously learned and carried out grammatical functions Rieß distinguished, but a further argument arises from the functions examined here, which supports the point of view that the localization of "grammatism" is in the temporal lobe.

In pathology, little attention has been paid to those questions, as were discussed above, and yet one cannot tell what advantages, and not only for pathology, would result from contemplating these, or even from simply heeding relevant facts that were not deemed important until now. At the time these lines were being written, Vix (Arch. f. Psych. 48, 3, p. 5 of the Sept. issue) reports on the recovery phase in a case of motor aphasia in addition to agrammatical disturbances: "Occasionally a word was, according to the proper language usage, not applied properly." One cannot very well, in light of these aphoristic descriptions, make any assumptions as to the peculiar symptoms described here, but this case, which still allows for the possibility that it may have something remotely in common with the subject matter at hand, shows how important it can be to not limit oneself only to theories readily accepted in pathology when it comes to the description as well as to assessing factual material.

What significance such cases, as just described, gain, how far-reaching this particular case could have been with a properly detailed report carried out in accordance to the opinions portrayed here, has been proven by the preceding statements. Nevertheless, to avoid any misunderstandings, the following comment is added. Earlier comments dedicated to progress in the teaching on localization and the author's position on the problem of localization of psychological functions, which have been stated elsewhere as well, cannot leave one doubting whether he thinks to have actually located the concerning function; it would be a regression back to Gall if one were now to localize the "grammatical function" or the "function concerning meaning" [*Bedeutungfunktion*]; but it may be considered to be an important development that we were able to find areas whose lesions regularly result in the disturbances of this function.

More facts will be presented in the following that help support the localization in the temporal lobe. It will be shown in the chapter on abstract thought that on a first, lowest level of abstract thought, the meaning of a word [*Obektwort*] is determined by how the object at hand uses it. Now cases of lesions in the temporal lobe (cf. the ones mentioned above by the author) prove through the simultaneous occurrence of amnestical aphasia (objects' lack of ability to designate [*Fehlen der Bezeichnung*]) and sensory apraxia (the object does not use [*Nichtauftauchen des Gebrauches des betreffenden Objektes*]) that both these phenomena are close to one another localizationally as well; from this follows that which further supports the aforementioned facts and explanations. The author will not go into the Vix case any further, which started off the last discussion, even though it would be very appropriate, considering the fact that it demonstrates apractical occurrences that support arguments made here; not only would the whole controversy around the localization of agrammatism have to be revisited, for which no occasion presents itself at the moment, but the rendering of the case would also have to be critically discussed, which would have to exceed the subject matter discussed in this chapter.

If our speech normally presents itself as an amalgamation, as a syntax of many signs, then the teaching on this amalgamation forms the basis for the explanation of the disturbances combined under the term agrammatism; and, accordingly, one has defined agrammatism in a wider sense as the pathology of syntax; but we will very soon see in great detail that means of expression in language far exceed this frame as well, which one has up until now considered tools of syntaxation and grammatization; one will nevertheless be able to accept the older definition, in this broader sense, if one keeps this in mind. One cannot further overlook that in forming sentences, certain language tools [*Sprachmittel*] are used that belong to the field of phonetics, where they are combined as its syntactical part. These theories are done justice, if one defines as follows: agrammatism is the form of pathologically changed speech in which processes related to the grammatical and syntactical structure of language are disturbed in different ways or occur only partly. This latter addition is important in order to determine those types of agrammatisms caused by deficient or lacking language development as well.

By defining the term in processes, the author shows that he leans towards functional psychology in contrast to structural psychology and expresses the rejection of pictures of memory [*Erinnerungsbilder*]. When the author recognizes specific functional mechanisms in these processes, which are coordinated, then his own opinion concerning the standing of the disturbance as well as its localizationability is thereby given; the definition should go beyond the realm of description and underline the author's opinion as to the kind of disturbance and its approximate location, which lie at the heart of the matter.

Mills (Journ. of Amer. Med. Assoc. 1904, II, p. 1945) characterizes the disturbance of agrammatism as a "difficulty in regaining those parts of speech which are concerned with qualifying and correlating. The grammar of language no longer exists for them." To further have to discuss the narrowness of this definition is, after the statements in this chapter, unnecessary.

Hacker (Arch. f. d. ges. Psychol. 21, p. 48) and lately, Köhler after him (ibid. Vol. 23, p. 427) separate acataphasia from agrammatism by determining the former disturbance as one where a whole or many sentences are wrongly used, so that they do not correspond to the content of the thought behind them, while agrammatism represents an incorrect linguistic [*sprachliche*] arrangement of the sentence structure. It's made obvious by what is outlined here—that a shift takes place regarding acataphasia compared to its original scope—but will not be further discussed at this place.

In addition to the definition given here, although not directly related to the subject matter at hand, but still of importance for specifying where agrammatism stands in terms of the relationships between speech [*Sprechen*] and thought, is an area touched upon in the introduction that deserves to be looked at. The fact brought up there is that, over time, a highly cultivated language, like the English language for example, will in the course of its evolution come to resemble Chinese, a language without inflections; many linguists came to a similar conclusion, namely that inflections are not unchanging characteristics clinging to Indo-Germanic languages, and one can rather prove that these languages were once without; this theory will, at least in evaluating the dissolution of languages into agrammatism, be an instructive test of Hughlings Jackson's belief of a regression to older stages of development. Also functional psychology, which the author supports in contrast to phenomenon psychology [*Erscheinungspsychologie*], will find support therein. A direct consequence of this, though, will be the afore-mentioned principle rejection of that theory, which states that agrammatism results from amnesia of words and thereby represents a special form of amnestical aphasia.

A subsequent consequence has to do with placing agrammatism in the context of paraphasia. v. Niessl, the last author to examine this question (*Die aphasische Symptome.* 1911, p. 137), categorized, in succession to Bonhöffer and Heilbronner, agrammatism as the fourth type of paraphasia, "when individual words are properly formed, but form grammatically incorrect sentences".[7] Even if we have already in the introduction rejected combining agrammatism and paraphasia as disturbances separated only by a small degree of difference, we must now further delve into this question, as Pelz lately describes (Zeitschr. f. d. ges. Neur. u. Psych. XI, p. 129) the severest degree of agrammatism as the "loosening of the speech order" ["Lockerung der Ordnung der Rede"], which results "in a complete confusion of words, void of any sense or order." He cites Pick's case of a transcortical sensorial aphasia as an example, in which "the individual, otherwise correct, words are senselessly lined up." We are of the opinion that by itself the senseless lining up of words does not at all have anything to do with agrammatism, and can state, based on W. James, that a senseless sequence of words can leave the impression of "making sense" if these simply possess the characteristic of being grammatical.[8]

We are further of the opinion that even the highest degree of paraphasia, that is the one in which not only are correct words senselessly lined up, but are spoken in complete jargon, does not necessarily constitute agrammatism, but that rather in those cases, where one actually speaks of agrammatism in the narrower sense of the definition, another disturbance is at play here, namely that described as agrammatism. This is proven in those cases that we do not consider to be agrammatical, especially by the whole tone and accent in which the sick person speaks; this is a disturbance of the executive in the advanced stages, while those higher processes, which we attribute to grammatisation, are completely undisturbed or may be so. This is also true of those statements by Pelz (l.c.) concerning these processes; this cannot be presented here in greater detail, but the reader is referred to discussions assigned to a later chapter ("The path from thought to speech").

The main task of this work will be to get to know those disturbances that present themselves as agrammatical as well as possible; one will very quickly see in the course of this presentation, but already with the teaching on means of expression occurring in sentences, and later in the discussion on those stages of the language process, in which the disturbance of grammatization takes place, that we are dealing with processes that precede word selection [*Wortwahl*]; that is, we are mainly concerned with psychological processes in no way connected to motor processes, which follow word selection; the immediate consequence to be drawn from this is that the processes resulting from paraphasia have nothing in common with those resulting from agrammatism, except that they are connected due to the sequence of linguistic processes [*Sprachvorgänge*]. This latter allows for the already mentioned combination of agrammatism and paraphasia, which in turn supports the localization of both in the temporal lobe.

It may of course not be overlooked that individual offences against grammar and syntax also occur, besides other disturbances of aphasic nature, and one can therefore only speak of agrammatism there, where these similar symptoms widely occur and may be observed more or less continuously. In the other cases, it remains to be seen what significance may be attributed to these disturbances; if they are not to be judged as disturbances that also occur in general, or if we are dealing with the manifestation of a disturbance where the sequence of individual processes that constitute the linguistic process are similar to the grammatical and syntactical ones, and thereby, as a weaker type of the latter disturbance, may be used to study it genetically and localizationally; it is to be particularly stressed that one cannot proceed any differently than when evaluating other phenomena, that thereby the point of views concerning the separation of direct and indirect signs, neighboring and distant effects, the diaschisis (v. Monakows) will be kept in mind.

In a later chapter we shall see that the disturbances collectively known as agrammatism partly manifest themselves in processes that the linguistic philosophers [*Sprachphilosophen*] since W. v. Humboldt designated as the "inner language form" ["innere Sprachform"], and that this term, or more precisely, the newly coined term by Marty, the so-called "constructive inner language form" ["konstruktive innere Sprachform"], describes these processes more precisely than do the old terms syntax and grammar. On the other hand, some disturbances will again seem to be subsumed under Marty's term that have nothing to do with agrammatism, the question here remaining quite controversial, despite its advanced age, and it shall thus have to suffice for the moment to have mentioned this area of research having proved to be a rich territory for pathology and by that alone therefore of significance to the definition. Differences of opinion, as the author cultivated with Ziehen for example, concerning if agrammatism may be seen as a psychological or a linguistic disturbance, can be now laid to rest; we are increasingly convinced that clear boundaries cannot be drawn between both, and that as with the process/occurrence of language comprehension, one cannot really tell where the psychological begins and, similarly here, cannot tell where the psychological ends. But if such boundaries are now still set up, then these are only practical points of view and considerations of the presentation, which are decisive for it. It has to be stated, though, that this controversy, seen from a higher standpoint, falls apart when the principle of parallelism is strongly taken into consideration; already H. Jackson, as we have already cited here, has rebuked as reprehensible the methodical combining of the psychological and physiological.

In conclusion to this introductory outline, let us mention a few words on the direction the following will take. Psychological and linguistic debates will take up a large part of our exposition; the whole has therefore, to bring an order into this wealth of material, been separated into a psychological and pathological part; the former will contain facts and interpretations taken also from the linguistic and the remaining medical sciences [Hilfswissenschaften], as these already serve as aids in linguistic psychology. The second, pathological part will not only comprise everything that has to do with the pathology of agrammatism, but will bring up for discussion all those general opinions in the teaching on aphasia, when the occasion arises for the author to take a stance. As far as the attempt will be made here to bring up all the material concerning linguistic psychology, this stance will then of course be more detailed.

In the first part, the psychological one, the processes on the path from thought to speech and the knowledge of the means of expression that serve this purpose, presented in the following chapters, will be decisive for systemizing the material; that is why a very detailed presentation will be included of all the aspects as well as all other moments that occur in those processes or influence these and will therefore be of importance for the understanding of the pathological aspect; it should of course already be implied that the author does not presume to be writing a work on linguistic psychology. One cannot of course do otherwise but to honor these facts, if but briefly, at the appropriate place, in their meaning to pathology, and thereby the psychological aspects, which at first do not seem to have a relation to the pathological ones, will close in on the pathologists' sphere of interest. The discussion will follow of those psychological occurrences that are important for the understanding of the pathology of these occurrences and whose psychology is to be made clear (psychology of grammar).

Next, children's language will form the basis for the understanding of hereditary [angeboren] agrammatism and be treated as the guide for the pathology of dissolution and re-evolution (of reformation of the occurrences); next will follow relevant facts from sign language and the remaining forms of expression relevant to the understanding of agrammatism. Such facts from philology and comparative linguistics [Sprachvergleichung] that show relationships or analogies to those deficient languages, just discussed, round up the end.

The pathological part shall first of all incorporate the symptomology and localization of agrammatism and a detailed discussion of all phases taken into consideration will follow this, in short all that shall be incorporated that from those conclusions drawn here seem of importance to the teaching on aphasia in general and especially for the relationship of agrammatism to the individual types of disturbances.

Notes

1. It should be noted here, with regards to the participation of what the author calls musical elements of language in the syntaxation of language, which, as we will soon see, is especially significant for agrammatism, that Dittrich also acknowledges, based on proof supporting comments made on the meaning of the word "Oh!", which follow the citation, the significance of these kinds of means of expression for the sentence's meaning. If the author keeps on using here, as in different places, the term musical [musisch], coined by him, even if we are dealing with a phenomenon that in linguistics is classified as being, to an extent, part of phonetics, it is to particularly underline the genetic as well as the localizational point of view by emphasizing the connection with the amusical [amusische] phenomenon, which is more familiar to the pathologist.

2. Let it be permitted to comment on this age-old interpretation. The fact that speaking of oneself in the third person exists other than as an agrammatical phe-

nomena, due to imbecility, suggests that one should, also for that phenomenon, consider the lack of intelligence as an explanation. But one may ask if this holds true in all cases. The author made an observation not long ago that cast doubt upon this. This regards a sick person with moderate 'word-deafness' [*Worttaubheit*], severe paraphasia, and paragraphia, word-amnesia affecting nouns and alexia; it was repeatedly observed that the 67-year-old man, who did not seem to be intellectually challenged, when speaking of himself constructed the whole sentence in the third person; the supposition arises, as he, besides this, occasionally also showed signs of agrammatism (weak conjugation, instead of hard ones), that speaking in the third person, based on the rarity of its occurrence, could simply be the result of a language disturbance. This phenomenon disappeared after a couple of weeks.

3. The historian will not overlook the welcome contrast that already the ideologues (S. Destut-Tracy: Élém. d'Idélogie 2. Part. Grammaire 2. Ed. 1817, p. 247) directly refer to the musical elements as "means of syntax."

4. "Where exactly the process of reasoning and propositioning or forming for the expression the product of intellectual action takes place cannot be stated; probably the whole area of superadded convolutions of both hemispheres is engaged in it; nor is the route known by which propositions pass to the third frontal gyrus for expression". (Med. Chir. Transact. 1872, Vol. 55, p. 191.)

5. That Rieß had a predecessor in the American anthropologist and linguist Powell (Evolut. of lang. in *I. An. Rep. Bureau of Ethnolog. Smithson. Inst.* 1881, p. 7), is proven by Örtel (Lect. on the study of lang. 1901, p. 275).

Powell says (l.c.), introducing his work, which shall not be expanded upon here: "It should be noted that paradigmatic inflections are used for two distinct purposes[:] qualifications and relation."

6. The author has access to two cases of lesions in the temporal lobe that simultaneously show a worsening of an already existing amnestical aphasia and a disturbance in word significance [*Wortbedeutung*].

7. When we put the weight of the counter-argument on the fact that it is not about having the group of words, known as sentence, resemble the assumed collection of letters, known as words, it then remains up to the proponents of the latter point of view to debate those people who argue against this as well (E. B. Huey, *The Psychol. and Paedag. of Reading*, 1910, p. 125, "we shall find that the word is not a mere collection of syllable and letters"). It should simply be mentioned here that it is by not taking into consideration the spoken language that one comes to the conclusion that a word is always made up of the same exact letters. It was argued elsewhere how such theories, which are described as misguided in light of modern linguistics, rest on a synthetic interpretation of the language process [*Sprachvorgang*] that would better be replaced by an analytical observation of the same.

8. "If the words stem from the same vocabulary and the grammatical structure is correct, then absolutely senseless sentences may be uttered . . . without it being obvious". (Prince. I, p. 263). Cf. ibid. the citation from a 784-page book full of the most unbelievable grammatically correct nonsense, as well as similar pieces of writing of cases on Dementia praecox.

[. . .]

23

The Cytoarchitectonics of the Fields Constituting Broca's Area

Ludwig Riegele

INTRODUCTION

The segment of the third frontal convolution in humans, named after its discoverer Broca, was determined in the last century using approximate morphological reference points provided by the gyral division. Broca let this region reach from the Sulcus subcentralis, located at the foot of the frontal central convolution, to about the Ramus horizontalis Fossae Sylvii, which, orbitalwards, it even exceeds by a little. Hervé later concluded, based on anthropological studies, that this convolution feature stretches much further onto the orbital surface of the front brain (Stinhirn) than Broca and the other authors believed. The gyrus lies in the caudal segment of the H-fissure and ends, according to Hervé, without a distinctively

Excerpts here are translated by Simran Karir and Katrin Amunts from *Die Cytoarchitektonik der Felder der Broca'schen Region*, in *Journal für Psychologie und Neurologie*, 42(5), 496–514 (1931). The author was at the Kaiser Wilhelm Institute in Berlin.

marked border, close to the Sulcus olfactorius. This demarcates a region that comprises the whole back part of the third frontal convolution. We will, in the following, call this region, as did Hervé, the Broca convolution or Broca's area, as opposed to Broca's spot (Brocasche Stelle). The demarcation of this cortex region, up until now, has only been possible using approximate morphological reference points, furrows, but architectonics, at the beginning of this century and based on inner structural characteristics, opened up the possibility of demarcating this region in the same exact way in every case. The myeloarchitectural division of the front brain by O. Vogt then showed that the cortex segment in question, which is different from neighboring regions because of its marrow fiber structure, being of the unitostriary (unitostriären) type (=the joining of both Baillarger's bands through thick individual fibers), encompasses the Regio unitostriata, the largest part of the lateral as well as the entire caudal orbital segment of the third frontal convolution. However, it does not, in most cases, reach up to the caudal border of the front central convolution, the Sulcus subcentralis, as Broca indicated, so that Vogt's fields **56** and **41** have to be counted as belonging to Broca's area.

Besides this, the Regio unitostriata in most cases exceeds the Sulcus transversus, which connects both Orbital-sulci towards the front and which, according to Hervé, makes up the front orbital border of Broca's area. The back orbital border of the Regio unitostriata is only partly created by the anatomically approximate caudal border of the orbital part of the Broca convolution, formed by the Sulcus marginalis superior, as by the Sulcus marginalis anterior. According to O.Vogt, the border (which at the same time represents the front brain's back boundary) runs through the Retzius's pars anterior Gyri olfactorii lateralis here.

Brodmann demarcated the Regio subfrontalis using a cytoarchitectural method. The borders of this region closely correspond, as the surface schema shows, with the borders O. Vogt defined in the Regio unitostriata. Campbell did not architecturally separate Broca's area from the third frontal convolution. According to v. Economo (who essentially follows the Brodmann division of the region into 3 fields), Broca's area basically has the same borders as Brodmann indicates, except on the orbital surface, where they only reach the Sulcus olfactorius.

O. Vogt, in 1910, divided his Regio unitostriata into 10 somewhat exact myeloarchitectural fields (**57-66**), while Brodmann could only divide the same region into 3 fields (**44**, **45** and **47**), by way of an architectural method. v. Economo, who also divides this region into 3 fields, does however, using a cytoarchitectural method, discover a row of modifications in these fields; e.g. in the area orbitalis: F_{FF}, F_F, F_{Fa}. These however, according to v. Economo, do not constitute sharply bordered fields, but continuous changes from one spot to another in the orbital field.

According to O. Vogt, the 10 myeloarchitectural fields of Broca's area, as the remaining fields on the cortex, do not continuously flow into each other, but represent sharply divided cortex regions, which Knauer could also confirm myeloarchitecturally in a few brains. C. and O. Vogt, based on many years of research, have concluded that every architectural field is characterized not only by definite myeloarchitectonics but also by special cytoarchitectonics.

O. Vogt described in 1910 the myeloarchitectonics of the 10 fields of his Regio unitostriata. The description of the cytoarchitectonics of these fields was as yet to be undertaken.

I have now, in a series of brains, examined these questions:

1. if and to what extent do cyto- and myeloarchitectural fields in Broca's area correspond to each other,
2. if individual fields show differences in all layers or only in single layers, and
3. if the discovered cytoarchitectural fields possess sharply defined borders, as do the myeloarchitectural fields, or continuously flow into each other.

Only gapless series were studied, as only these allow for an exact reconstruction of the fields. Using gapless series is especially essential for the region's orbital part, as the borders in most cases are located intrasulcally, and too much cortex substance would be lost, by cutting out small blocks, to be able to determine the size of the fields and the shape of their boundaries. The myeloarchitectonics of the fields of Broca's area were first examined in four series of myelin sheaths [*Markscheiden*], which were dyed using the Kultschitzky-Pal method. The cytoarchitectonics of these fields were determined by using gapless series of paraffin-incisions in many brains. The paraffin method has the advantage, besides being able to exactly reconstruct the fields, of being able to control the cytoarchitectural fields as well as their borders through the marrow fiber structure in the neighboring incision. If this latter is not as complete (*vollständig*) as with the Kultschitzky-Pal method, it nevertheless suffices for identifying the cyto- and myeloarchitectural fields.

By using these series, I was able to convince myself that every one of O. Vogt's myeloarchitectural fields corresponds to a cytoarchitectural one, and furthermore that not only do myeloarchitectural borders exist in Broca's area, but also cytoarchitectural ones. Fields, therefore, do not continuously flow into each other. The borders are easier to recognize in the marrow fiber structure than in the cell structure, as the field types are more clearly distinguishable here. If the borders, as is mostly the case in Broca's area, are located intrasulcally, they are more often less noticeable than in those parts where they lie extrasulcally. The oft-occurring different inclinations of the Sulcus' labia against the cutting plain on the frontal incisions make it hard to recognize these intrasulcally located borders. Further more, the architectonics of each field gradually changes going towards the Sulcus. This change is especially noticeable in the cell structure of the fields in Broca's area, where relatively weak laminary differences exist. Despite these circumstances, which are unfavorable for the recognition of borders, one discovers that borders, located in the fundus of steep furrows, are clearly recognizable, even if they are less noticeable in the cell structure than in the marrow fiber structure. The more obvious laminary differences in the cell structure in the fields of Broca's area are limited to a few layers, while the differences in the remaining fields are significantly slighter and therefore harder to recognize. The latter is mostly the case for the deeper located layers V and VI.

If my research, as well as Knauer's, determined the same number of fields as O. Vogt discovered, then these corresponding results, which many researchers have come to, mean that we are not dealing with accidental constructions, but rather with real and, in this region, constant differences. I was able, also in chimpanzees, to myeloarchitecturally locate on the orbital surface fields 60 to 66.

The fields have been photographically reproduced and enlarged 100 (or 50) times. In addition, only incisions from an A 43 r hemisphere were used. The majority of the sites chosen are from the peaks [Kuppe] in these fields, as these are easier to compare. Field 60 is the exception here, because it lies, for the most part, intrasulcally and is the most clearly marked in the cell—as in the marrow fiber structure inside of the Sulcus.

The following description of the cytoarchitectural fields is in large part based on direct observations of the incisions and less so of the photos, as some findings, which may be seen in the incisions, cannot be seen in the photos and, furthermore, a part of the finer differences, which can still be recognized in the original photo, is faded or entirely lost due to the printing. A description must therefore, in certain points, complement the graphic reproduction. I have not included a representation of the borders, as this would have considerably increased the parameters of this work.

[...]

The preceding description of the cytoarchitectural fields of the Regio unitostriata shows that all fields differ from one another through their structural differences. These do not refer to individual layers, but all layers of the cortex cross section. The differences do,

however, appear in varying degrees in the individual layers. The laminary differences are most pronounced in the outer layers. But they are sometimes also very noticeable in the inner layers, as for example in the V and VI of fields **64** and **65**, as well as **58** and **59**.

The individual layers vary in the different fields not only in their density, but also in the composition of elements, which change in form and size. So for example the *II*, which in the Regio unitostriata is made up of small and big corpuscles, as well as small pyramids, is, in the individual fields, a changing combination of these three elements. Namely, the pyramids dominate in the caudal lateral fields of the region, and the bigger corpuscles in the caudal orbital fields. The *II*, in the fields between these, has relatively few bigger corpuscles and small pyramids.

Cells of varying sizes appear in layers V and III_3 in the fields of the Regio unitostriata.

A varying ratio of big to small cells exists in these layers in different fields.

The boundaries of certain layers, as for example the *II* and *IV* with layers following inwards, are not very defined in the Regio unitostriata. The reason for this is the small difference in the cell density and cell size of neighboring layers [*II* and *III*] or a relatively similar composition of elements of differing sizes in neighboring layers [*IV* and *V*].

The *IV* in the Regio unitostriata is narrow and poor in granula. Smaller and bigger pyramids are embedded here.

The *Va* is distinguished by a larger number of mostly smaller pyramids, which are mixed in with some bigger ones. The number of pyramids increases going inwards, towards the *Vb*. In the *Vb*, where the elements are somewhat bigger than those in *Va*, transitions (Übergänge) from the bigger to the smaller elements can be found, as in *Va*. The big pyramids in V, in the caudal fields, adjacent to the Regio unitostriata, are significantly larger than the cells in *VI*. The *Vb* is embedded uniformly here. A three way division is thereby suggested in the V of the fields of the Regio unitostriata, in that a strip surfaces between *Vb* and *VI*, which has less and smaller cells, i.e. the bigger pyramids in V_b in this edge zone diminish or are absent. This zone on the edge is called *Vc* in those fields, where it is clearly distinguishable (**58, 59, 62**). It also changes its width in these fields.

The *VI* also shows, besides its varyingly sharp separation from V and the varyingly sharp division into *VIa* and *VIb*, differences in the size of its cells. Brodmann added the *VII* to the myelin [*Mark*], which is characterized ontogenetically by its very low amount of cells. O. Vogt realized that this was a special layer. It stands out in the Regio unitostriata, in that its cells are not spool-shaped but possess a that is mostly triangular to pyramid-form. Besides an irregular transition into the marrow, the cell size and –cell density of the individual fields in this layer do not vary greatly. The cells of *VII* are only somewhat smaller in the fields of the Regio unitostriata than the cells in $VI\beta$. They therefore contribute to the difference in cell size in the *VI* of the individual fields.

I already mentioned the discovery of distinct borders between the individual fields in the introduction.

From the description of the cytoarchitectonics of the fields of the Regio unitostriata at hand, it can be seen that cytoarchitectural structural differences do not only exist in individual layers, but in all layers, as well as in some sub-layers. And further more, the theory by C. and O. Vogt—that every field is not only characterized by distinct myeloarchitectonics, but also by distinct cytoarchitectonics—is proven true. If one sees a strong interdependency between the cytoarchitectonics and myeloarchitectonics of the fields of the Regio unitostriata, the question then arises whether the cytoarchitectural as well as the myeloarchitectural fields can, due to certain characteristics, be combined into subregions and divisions. O. Vogt divided the fields of his Regio unitostriata into two bigger subgroups, the Subregio subunitostriata and the Subregio unitostriata, which are each comprised of a certain number of fields, as can be seen below (Fig. 23–1).

The fact that cytoarchitectural differences are less noticeable than myeloarchitectural ones leads one to expect that the cytoarchitectural characteristics common to the subregions and divisions stand out less than the myeloarchitectural ones.

The Subregio subunitostriata differs in its cell structure from the Subregio unitostriata through the following distinguishable characteristics:

1. the vague separation of *II* from *III₁*, as well as the vague separation of *IV* from *Va*,
2. the pyramids of *III₂* are relatively smaller than those in *III₃*,
3. *IV* is relatively broader and possesses a higher content of bigger pyramids.

Of the divisions, it is especially the Divisio multostriata (field **60**) as well as the Divisio propebizonalis (field **66**) that are distinctly noticeable due to their cell structure, while the Divisio propebistriata (field **57**), also categorized as a field, is less distinguishable in its cell structure from its neighboring Divisio subunitostriata.

The Divisio multostriata (field **60**) differentiates itself cytoarchitecturally mainly through the *III*; it is namely especially the big pyramids in *III₃* as well as the width and the relatively small size of the remaining cells of this sublayer, and also the small cells in *III₂*, which separates the field in its cell structure from the neighboring divisions.

The Divisio propebizonalis (field **66**) is set apart by a rudimentary, very narrow *IV*, which has few cells, as well as by a relatively increased number of bigger elements in *II*.

The Divisio propebistriata (field **57**) has, compared to field **56**, a wider *IV*, which contains fewer mid-size pyramids and more granula, and also a *V*, which, in comparison with fields **56** and **58**, has smaller cells.

The Divisio subunitostriata, which comprises fields **58** and **59**, is characterized by a greater quantity of pyramids in *IV* than **57** and **60**, as well as a significant *Vc*, characterized by a lack of cells and small cells.

The Divisio propeunistriata of the Subregio subunitostriata, which comprises fields **61** and **62**, differentiates itself from the neighboring multostriata through *V*, which has large cells and also, compared

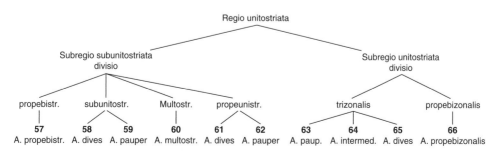

FIGURE 23–1.

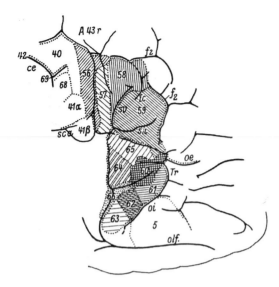

FIGURE 23–2. A 43. Right hemisphere. (A 43 refers to the case number.)

with the Divisio multostriata and subunitostriata, by smaller cells in III_3 and III_2.

The Divisio trizonalis of the Subregio unitostriata, which comprises fields **63**, **64** and **65**, distinguishes itself from neighboring divisions through its clearer separation of layers *II* and *IV* from the layers going inwards and also through a *V*, which has a high number of cells and large cells.

THE SYNTOPICAL VARIATION OF THE FIELDS CONSTITUTING BROCA'S AREA

As mentioned above, Broca's area divides into the same number of fields both cytoarchitecturally and myeloarchitecturally. These 11 fields were discovered in 16 hemispheres by three different researchers. They were reconstructed in every object; i.e. the borders discovered in the series were transcribed onto photographs of the brain's surface in the corresponding spots. The resulting surface projections provide a clear view of the mutual topical relationships of the fields in every object. The individual findings deviate from object to object, disregarding the intercerebral architectural differences, mainly in the varying size, in the changing large proportion of individual fields on the surface, as well as in the mutually changing position of the fields.

The sequence in which the individual fields appear, one after the other, is the same in all examined objects.

Fields **56-59** follow each other, going caudal to frontal, according to the numerical sequence established by O. Vogt. In contrast, the fields of the Regio unitostriata **60-66**, in the orbital part of Broca's area, do not succeed each other in a straight line, one after the other; rather, they are grouped around field **60**, forming a kind of circular arch, and these fields are located here in the same sequence in every hemisphere as well. A connecting line starts from field **60** and reaches, going medially to the Sulcus olfactorius, field **61**, then runs caudalwards to field **62**, then runs behind field **60** over fields **63** and **64** lateralwards to field **65**. Field **66** is located outside of this circular arch, at the medio-caudal end of the region.

Field **60**, which is cyto- and myeloarchitecturally different from the surrounding fields and compared to the remaining fields (**61-65** or rather **66**), has a central location, lying inside of the orbital surface of the front brain, always in a certain region called the Sulcus transversus.

It belongs to the so-called furrow-bound fields and can be located almost completely in the Sulcus transversus, but it can also stretch out quite a bit behind the Sulcus. This central field deviates relatively little in terms of its location—i.e. it often occupies the space between the Sulcus orbitalis internus and ex-

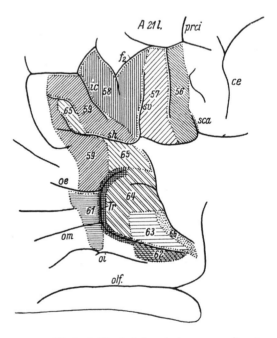

FIGURE 23–3. A 21. Left hemisphere according to Knauer (Die Myeloarchitektonik der Broca'schen Region. Neurol. Zentralblatt 28, 1909.) (A 21 refers to the case number.)

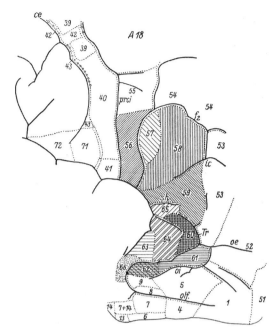

FIGURE 23–4. A18. Parcellation scheme by O. Vogt (Die myeloarchitektonische Felderung des menschlichen Stirnhirns. Journal für Psychologie und Neurologie 15, 221, 1910.) (A18 refers to the case number.)

ternus—but does, however, sometimes reach over to one or the other branch of both Sulci. In the context of the reoccuring same sequence, the relationships between the six fields surrounding field **60** change their location relative to field **60** and relative to each other, and these changes appear to depend both on how much surface area each actually occupies and how much surface area each proportionally occupies. The different extensions of the neighboring fields in the region in certain spots also influence the syntopy of the fields. These variations in the syntopy of the fields cannot be meaningless if closer relationships exist between some fields than in others. That such close relationships exist is made probable through the observation that the fibers of the Lamina tangentialis are located in the same direction in certain fields, while they lie differently in others. Also, some thick individual tangential fibers in some fields cross into neighboring fields. In contrast, this is not the case in others; that is, they abruptly end at the border.

A close connection between certain fields can manifest itself topically, in that these fields are located next to each other or rather share a particular border. Certain fields of the Pars. Orbitalis of the Regio – as far as may be judged at the moment – never lose con-

tact with each other this way. Field **64** is located at the caudal border of field **60**, and they thereby share the border that is almost longest, and in the same way field **62** stays in contact with field **63**.

Field **63** has more contact with field **60** than field **62** does. Fields **62** and **63**, because they are located more occipitalwards, may lose contact with field **60**.

It seems that those fields that border on each other (e.g. **60** and **64** as well as **61**), also share the longest boundary.

The fields of the lateral part of Broca's area also remain connected in the same way as the numerical sequence dictates. This is also the case when (as for example with A 22) a field that normally belongs to the orbital surface, such as field **65**, is pushed in between fields **58** and **59**.

Besides these relationships, which can be constantly observed in the field schema, one may also ob-

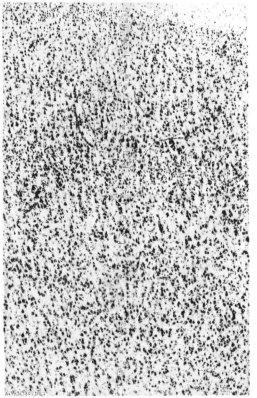

FIGURE 23–5. Plate 5, Figure 2, area 56 (shown in the right corner). Roman numbers indicate cortical layers. *Lower left corner*, identifier of the brain, section, region, hemisphere, and magnification. This area corresponds to area 44 of Brodmann (1909) and to FCBm of von Economo and Koskinas (1925). (Figure scanned from original article.)

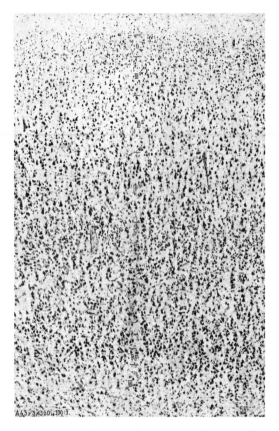

FIGURE 23–6. Plate 6, Figure 2, area 58. Areas (57–59) correspond to area 45 of Brodmann (1909) and to FDG of von Economo and Koskinas (1925). (Figure scanned from original article.)

serve a shift in the fields, due to a field being pushed in between two fields that normally share a border.

In this way, field **62** for example directly adjoins, occipitalwards, field **61**. But it can also be separated from field **61** by field **5**. Field **63** lies mostly between field **62** and **66**. It usually borders field **64** frontally and laterally. However, field **66** may push in between field **63** and **64**.

Field **65** may, on the one hand, be separated from field **60**, on which it usually borders, by field **59**; on the other hand, field **59** may be divided into two segments by field **65** (A 22 l and A 21 l, cf. Ill. 2). If field **65** is more strongly developed on the surface, then it may (as with A 22 r) border on fields **57** and **58** and **59**.

If field **65** is separated from field **60** by field **59**, then field **64** may reach frontalwards around field **60**.

Field **66**, which is normally located on the occipital side around fields **62** and **63** or between these, can also be inserted between field **63** and **64** in a

wedge shape (A 24 l) and can finally also reach field **60** (in doing so, field **62** and **63** are shifted frontalwards (A 43 r, cf. ill. 1). It frequently extends on the occipital side around fields **64, 63** and **62** (A 27 l and r, A 22 l and r).

Having been able to determine certain shifts in the location of fields by comparing data on fields (*Felderungsmaterial*) to date, it remains to be studied if, and how far, these shifts are connected with the furrowmolding (*Furchenausprägung*).

The question concerning the relationships of fields, or rather, their borders to furrows, has been posed by individual researchers since the existence of architectonics and has been answered in the same manner. O. Vogt, as well as a line of other authors, discovered that, on the one hand, fields did frequently end at furrows; however, on the other hand, there existed a whole row of borders that only partly had relationships to fields or not at all. There are furrows that, in every brain, stand in specific relation to certain fields. These, like the Sulcus transversus, contain the so-called furrow-bound fields. The position of some fields in regards to specific furrows is also almost constant. Field **61**, for example, lies almost in front and somewhat medially from the Sulcus transversus, or field **62** lies medially from the Sulcus orbitalis internus or between both its branches. The same holds true for the medial segment of field **61**.

Furthermore, some furrows exist that are frequently located at borders of certain fields, such as, for example, the Sulcus radiatus with the border of fields **58** and **59**. With the help of the surface projections, one may further discover that at every point where certain fields have, more than on average, strongly shifted in contrast to the neighboring fields, the furrowmolding deviates more strongly than the average. The furrows can finally, as C. and O. Vogt have shown with the opercular fields **56-58**, have shifted, when close similarity in the syntopy of the fields exist, by a whole furrow feature (*Zug*) in comparison to the fields.

From this it results that we are not in the position today, on the basis of observations made on the brain surface, to only specify the extension and boundaries of one single field. For furrow-bound fields, the possibility exists to specify an area that is the same in every brain, however not the exact location and boundary.

The latter might be possible for a region only after having mapped out the location for a very large number of fields.

[. . .]

24

The Phonological Development of Child Language and Aphasia as a Linguistic Problem

Roman Jakobson

I [. . .]

DISSOLUTION OF THE PHONOLOGICAL SYSTEM

The same considerations are valid *mutatis mutandis* for aphasic speech disturbances.

There are unfortunately only very few linguistically useful descriptions of aphasia, and these are based on only a small number of languages. The observations of linguists on infancy are for the most part all too superficial, but at least infants have been more often available to linguists than aphasics. We are indebted to psychiatrists and neurologists for a number of stimulating and fruitful ideas on particular linguistic functions, and especially on inner speech; but in the description and analysis of concrete linguistic, and especially phonological, facts they exhibit with few ex-

Excerpts from *Fundamentals of Language* (with Morris Halle), Mouton Hague, 1956.

ceptions an astonishing perplexity and lack of attentiveness. It is not to be denied that the detailed linguistic form of problematical disturbances is indispensable in determining their causes, just as a rigorous linguistic analysis is indispensable to their symptomatology. With complete justification Arnold Pick criticizes the poverty of the results that pathology has so far obtained in this respect, as well as the scantiness of the records and the usual "lack of word-by-word transcription of pathological speech forms" (α 50). This noted scholar, in fact, who endeavored to make extensive use of a linguistic point of view in aphasic theory, found it necessary, in a study that deals precisely with the phonological alterations of aphasic speech, to make the following apology: "Of course we were not able to indicate in the written reproduction of what was spoken those facts which would have required a phonetic transcription with which we are not familiar . . ." (δ 230). Karl Kleist, in the newest and most thorough survey of aphasia, also points out the seriousness of these deficiencies, concerning which he feels obliged to state: "The observations set forth in the literature regarding real linguistic deafness unfortunately very often do not provide any exact description of how much the patient was not able to grasp from linguistic impressions, or of how much he was still able to understand—in general, how he heard language." Most of the observations about "real linguistic dumbness" (sound-dumbness) are open to criticism for the same reasons.

The pathology of language makes a fundamental distinction between aphasic sound disturbances and the so-called arthritic lesions of the bulbar senso-motor apparatus (designated as dysarthria or anarthria according to their degree) and the direct mutilations of the articulatory organs (dyslalia, mechanical alalia), as well as the peripheral hearing defects. In aphasic sound disturbances neither the articulatory nor the auditory organs are themselves injured, nor is the bulbar apparatus, "on which sound formation depends"; rather, "something which we have learned—a possession of the memory—is lost."[1] But what then is the controlling factor of this mnemic possession? As was pointed out above, the important factor for children who are learning their language is not the ability to produce or to perceive a particular sound, but the distinctive linguistic value of the sounds in question. In the same way, the reduction in the ability to pronounce or to perceive sounds, therefore, is not essential to the unlearning of the aphasic; only the ability to distinguish functionally significant sounds is important. It is here that one finds the essential origin of aphasic disturbances of sound production and comprehension. In some cases the aphasic is occasionally able to produce the sounds in question and very often preserves them in sound gestures; but their distinctive (phonemic) value is lost in the "arbitrary linguistic signs." There develops in patients, then, on the one hand, sound coalescences and confusions, and on the other, an absolute non-recollection of these sounds—that is, the sound disappears without being replaced. In both cases a distinction ceases. For example, in the latter case, with the loss of the Czech phoneme r, the distinction between r and ϕ is lost. In the former case, the distinction between r and l is lost, so that either r falls together with l (*hrad* "city" > *hlad*), or r and l function as free variants (*hrad* "city" as well as *hlad* 'hunger' can be pronounced by patients with either r or l).

The notorious difficulties which commonly arise in the comprehensive description of the so-called "true aphasias" (*aphasies pures ou extrinsèques*), or in the establishment and classification of their different forms and stages, as well as in the examination and testing of individual patients, disappear automatically when one attempts, first of all, to answer the following question: what changes does the phonemic system—the system of sound values that distinguish meanings—undergo in aphasics?

If this question is considered, then indeed the succession of changes turns out to be absolutely fixed, whereas arthritic disturbances can be limited to any particular speech muscle or any sequence of sounds whatever (cf. § 8). Individual components of the phonemic system are eliminated in sound aphasia in a determined order of precedence.

As long as a part of the phonemic system continues to exist, it forms in its turn a system which is still ordered, although impoverished. And just as the child not only reduces his linguistic model but often attributes new values to the simplified system (cf. § 2), there is in the linguistic system of an aphasic as well not only a reduction of the former richer system, but sometimes also a remodeling. The curious change shown by the Czech aphasic examined by Pick (δ), who replaced the initial stress of the mother tongue with accentuation of the penultima, is to be connected with the simultaneous tendency toward the reduction of Czech vocalic quantitative oppositions. In the history of the West Slavic languages both phenomena—the loss of quantity and the transition from initial to penultimate stress—are more than once found linked together (Polish, some Czech and Slovak dialects). This connection has been explained by the fact that with the loss of quantity, the stress is naturally felt as more intense and that it is precisely the penultima in contrast to the initial syllable that gives greater prominence to the stress. The distinctions of stress are more emphatic in the rising-falling pattern of the word than in the simple falling, and more striking in the alternating stress of the next to the last and single syllable of the word than in the uniform initial stress.[2] A constructive adjustment is even manifested, therefore, in the destruction of the aphasic's phonological system, and it recalls the "reparatory substitute-function" which was repeatedly observed in new formations of agrammatism.

SOUND AND MEANING DISTURBANCES

The newest developments in aphasic theory suggest that an inquiry into the phonemic character of sound disturbances may be necessary. The effort of modern psychiatry, which goes back to Broca's clearsighted formulations (see esp. 91), to consider all phenomena of linguistic activity from the point of view of "their symbolic character, or sign nature" (cf. Thiele 949), is more and more consistently being applied to impairments of the "inner means of language," and it must naturally be extended to the "external means," that is, to the phonological form of the language, and accordingly to phonological disturbances. This programmatic reminder has, moreover, already been incorporated into the comprehensive interpretations of language pathology, and it has been explicitly pointed out that the study of aphasia cannot altogether dispense with phonology inasmuch as functions that are a part of phonology are also involved in establishing meaning (Pick ε 1419). A progression from the sphere of sound to that of meaning ought to be apparent in every theory. Yet even some of the newest investigations of aphasia "obscure this clear and unequivocal position," and therefore fail to analyze the comprehension of speech sounds in more detail. Isserlin has characterized this, with justified harshness, as "a grave and fatal error" (208).

"An abstracting and referential comprehension of the permanent or relatively permanent reality of things" (*ibid.*, 220), which fundamentally distinguishes our speech activity from the nonreferential acoustic-articulatory sensations of the babbling child, must be learned by the child in the acquisition of language. In true aphasia, on the other hand, this "imprinted fixation" (to use the term of the pathologists) of the mnemic phonological possession is lost.[3] Every attempt to restrict the speech sound to an external empiricism is unsuccessful, and another prominent scholar in modern speech pathology, K. Goldstein, teaches in agreement with contemporary linguistics that there is no distinction between sounds and words in this regard: "a sound is the same as a word . . . either a motor act or a linguistic entity" (β 765).

Phonemes and words are related in different ways to the sign function of language. While every word— *i.e.*, every grammatical form—has its own particular and constant meaning, the phoneme performs only the function of distinguishing meanings without possessing any positive meaning of its own. It distinguishes every word in which it occurs from all other words which *ceteris paribus* contain some other phoneme.[4] Accordingly, the disturbances of meaning and of phoneme comprehension are certainly to be distinguished; but at the same time one must not for-

get that they are two easily associated although independent aspects of an essentially uniform aphasia, and the sign value of language possession is impaired and diminished in both cases. The fundamental participation of the phoneme in meaning, namely its distinguishing function, is clearly demonstrated in the disturbance of sound comprehension as well as in the disturbance of meaning comprehension. A patient whose meaning comprehension is preserved but whose phoneme comprehension is damaged, and who has lost, *e.g.*, the distinction of liquids, surely knows the meanings of *Rippe* and *Lippe*. Both words are homonyms for him, however, and he cannot identify the meaning of either word in any given case so long as the context or the situation does not supply him with any more specific information.

On the other hand, patients with impaired meaning comprehension but uninjured sound comprehension can distinguish two words whose meanings they cannot understand but which are similar in sound by means of their non-significant phonological differences, and thereby perceive them as two different, although enigmatic, meaningful units (see *e.g.*, Isserlin 209).[5] Insofar as the aphasic loses the ability to separate closely related meanings in his use of language, words related in meaning are stripped of every functional distinction, and consequently the justification for preserving these distinctions is also lost. Word amnesia occurs, and one of the words related in meaning replaces the others and takes over their meanings. Thus a patient with meaning muteness characterized, *e.g.*, every useful activity with the verb "to build." Kleist refers to the similar word poverty of children learning to speak and to the equally large range of meaning of the small number of words which are available to them (γ 850).

Both meaning and sound disturbances result, therefore, in an expansion of homonymy. In the former, a phonological unit corresponds to a multiplicity of interlinked meanings, while in the latter such an interlinkage is never present, and a simple homophony occurs. Indeed, in both kinds of disturbances (just as in their exact correspondences in child language) an expanded ambiguity (polysemy) of the linguistic sign necessarily arises, and "the active use of the word as interpreter of the concept" is impaired. The more extensive the sound disturbance, the more the distinguishing of words, or of meanings, is hindered. With the decreasing number and frequency of phonemes and phoneme combinations, the number of homonyms (phonologically identical words), and especially the number of paronyms (phonologically similar words), which likewise obstruct the distinguishing of words, naturally increases. In homonymy the marks of distinction disappear, in paronymy they decrease in number. With whatever level of language aphasia is concerned, it is always the sign function of the linguistic units in question that is injured:[6] in phonemes, their distinctive value; in vocabulary, lexical meanings; and in morphological and syntactical forms, grammatical meanings. Often the lesions of the individual levels are connected with each other. If the distinction between two homogeneous units loses its linguistic value, one of these units is then supplanted by the other. We then speak of sound amnesia where sound disturbances are concerned, of word amnesia where disturbances of word meanings are concerned, and of agrammatism where disturbances of grammatical meanings are concerned. Or if both units, in spite of the loss of their different functions, are retained in a weaker stage of these disturbances but are confused and indiscriminately used for one another, then we speak of sound paraphasia,[7] of verbal paraphasia and of paragrammatism.

Jackson's warning of the year 1878 is still relevant: "We must not classify on a mixed method of anatomy, physiology and psychology, any more than we should classify plants on a mixed natural and empirical method, as exogens, kitchen-herbs, graminaceae, and shrubs" (115). A purely linguistic classification of aphasic disturbances is necessary, since it satisfies this call for a uniform criterion, and at the same time can be easily realized, since every aphasic disturbance is characterized by the loss of some linguistic value. The newest pathological works comply to an even greater extent with this formulation. In linguistics there are two aspects of the linguistic act that are distinguished—emissive and receptive—and correspondingly, in the study of aphasia, different kinds of linguistic muteness and deafness. On the other hand, linguistics distinguishes semantic and phonological units, i.e., primary signs, which are related to concrete entities, and secondary signs, which are related to signs. Similarly, aphasic disturbances, according to whether they impair semantic or phonological units (therefore signs for concrete entities or signs for signs), are classified in the newest pathological literature as meaning disturbances and sound disturbances. The fundamental linguistic classification of meanings as lexical and grammatical (or, according to Fortunatov's terminology, as real and formal) is also important for the study of aphasia and underlies the delimitation of agrammatism. Every linguistic unit functions in a sequence. Depending upon whether one treats (1A) the characteristics of the units in question, (1B) their characteristics in relation to the sequence, or finally (2) the characteristics of the sequence as such, one speaks, with regard to phonemes, (1A) of their qualities, (1B) of their prosodic features, (2) of combinations. Similarly the linguistic distinguishes, with regard to the word as a grammatical unit (1) morphology, namely (A) word formation and (B) word inflection, and (2) syntax, i.e., the form of word combinations. The consistent use of these distinctions could dispose of a number of misunderstandings in the study of aphasia.

LINGUISTIC CHARACTER OF APHASIC SOUND-DEAFNESS AND SOUND-MUTENESS

Complete or partial sound-deafness was often not only called "sensory aphasia," but was also interpreted as such. Indeed, the nature of the disturbance, as especially Pierre Marie convincingly showed, does not have its roots directly in the concrete acoustic, but rather in the conceptual, "semiotic" sphere ("an intellectual deficiency relating specifically to language," according to the formulation of this scholar). Not the perception as such, but rather its linguistic value is impaired. A patient who is unable to grasp certain elements of his language, but whose perception of all the remaining auditory sensations is normal (and, therefore, does not suffer from any auditory agnosia) cannot have any sensory defect.

It is impossible to explain the perception of speech sounds by a kind of elementary auditory perception independent of pitch differences and of noises. The perception of sounds is dependent on uniquely those laws which convert the acoustic-motor raw material into elements with semiotic (sign-functioning) value, and therefore on the structural laws of the phonemic system, and not on the acoustic characteristics of the sound in relation to pitch and noise. Every speech sound represents a complex of distinctive features, and each of these features functions as the member of a binary opposition which necessarily implies the opposite member. What the pathologist is confronted with is not the existence of three special delimited classes of sound perceptions, but primarily the essential distinction between three separate types of values that are performed by sound phenomena. Indeed, the same physical facts, *e.g.*, distinctions of pitch, can occur on the one hand as musical values, and on the other hand as a means of differentiating meaning. In the first case the absolute value of the pitch differences, or intervals and their scales, is important, whereas in language the contrast of a neutral (unmarked) and raised or lowered pitch is significant (cf. in the Yoruba language *tu*, in normal pitch "spear," in high register "untie," and in low register "rest").[8] Let us use the well-known and clear comparison of language with a board game. It is easily possible to use chessmen for checkers. "What constitutes them phenomenally and physically is completely inconsequential and can change arbitrarily. They become tokens of the game in question rather through game rules, which give them their fixed game meaning."[9] The interpretation and classification of sound phenomena is entirely different according to their function, and accordingly the following are distinguished: 1) differences of pitch as musically utilized sound phenomena, 2) sounds as linguistically utilized sound phenomena, and 3) sound phenomena which have neither musical nor linguistic value, but act rather as mere marks of different sounds ("noises" in normal usage).[10] In the every day life of the average person, language (or sound) plays a much more important role than music (or pitch), and in this connection it is completely understandable that in some people, especially those who are unmusical, simple tones can come to acquire linguistic values, and that thereby their similarities to vowel sounds easily emerge.[11]

It is customary to compare the agrammatic "telegraphic style" and the similar speech form of children in particular stages of development with imperfectly controlled foreign speech (see Isserlin 1022), but the analogy is also valid for phonemic disturbances. In the ordinary comprehension of the phonemes of a foreign language, there are striking correspondences which help to explain linguistically the pathological facts of sound-deafness. A speaker of Chinese who in listening to a European language does not perceive the difference between *r* and *l*, a Scandinavian who often does not distinguish the Russian or German *z* from *s*, a Russian or Bulgarian who commonly remains deaf not only to the quantitative but also to the pitch oppositions of the Serbocroatian syllabic phonemes are all thoroughly normal from a sensory point of view and suffer neither from impaired hearing nor from

any reduction in the ability to perceive. Since there is no distinctive difference in Chinese between the two liquids, in Russian or Bulgarian between long or short vowels, or vowels with rising and falling pitch, in the Scandinavian languages between voiced and voiceless sibilants, the non-native speaker is therefore not at all accustomed in the language in question to consider these, to him, irrelevant fine points, and his attention and memory must be thoroughly exercised and newly trained so that the otherwise equivalent words of the foreign language can be recognized and will no longer count as homonyms (*e.g.*, for a Swede, Russian *zlóva slóva* "of the bad word," or for a Bulgarian, Serbian *'sela* "of the village" with rising pitch on *e*, *'sela* "the villages" with falling pitch on *e*, and *'sēlā* "of the villages," a form which is distinguished only by means of the long vowels). The aphasic who has forgotten the common distinctive value between *r* and *l* or between *z* and *s*, or between rising and falling word pitch,[12] takes on the aspect of a foreigner in relation to his native language and therefore can no longer discriminate between such phonological differences.

But what is most difficult for a foreigner is not to grasp but to use, and especially to use correctly, a foreign phonemic distinction which is lacking in his own language. It is not just a question of the difficulty of the unfamiliar articulation. Even if a speaker of Chinese is successful in imitating the *r*-sound, which is not found in his language, he must still make a special effort to remember that it must actually be used in speech, and to be able to choose correctly between the two liquids in particular cases. Either he does not use the foreign phoneme, or *r* and *l* are confused (*Paris* can become *Palis* and at the same time *London*, *Rondon* and *reflector*, *lefrectol*). It is not difficult for a Bulgarian or Pole to lengthen a vowel at will, but it is a much more strenuous task for him actually to preserve these long vowels when he speaks Serbocroatian or Czech, and, what is more, in the correct places, since a phonemic opposition of long and short vowels does not occur in his native language.

The so-called aphemic disorders (sound-dumbness or, as it is sometimes called, partial motor aphasia) and in like manner the beginning stages of child language present a similar picture. Articulations whose autonomous phonemic value has been lost in patients and is not yet incorporated by the child are lacking or are used in place of each other. There are borderline cases: if the sound distinction in question or its use in words is indeed known but is felt as foreign or strange, it overstrains the attention; and while it is preserved in special situations, it is avoided in unaffected speech. Many Russians living in Czechoslovakia have learned the quantitative distribution of Czech vowels and can, if necessary, use them accurately, but in fluent speech they easily let this distinction go now and then. "A child," says Sully, "can often articulate better than he himself wants to." A one-and-a-half-year-old English girl, *e.g.*, who was teased because she constantly said *mudder*, laughingly quite accurately pronounced *mother*, with the interdental fricative, although she afterwards returned to her former pronunciation of this word (133). There are also less serious cases of sound-dumbness where the patient, under coercion, speaks more correctly for a while, only to slip back again into his usual sound poverty.

This aphasic mutilation of sounds resembles admittedly the so-called arthritic disturbances (*i.e.*, disturbances of the senso-motor apparatus), and this similarity has often misled observers. But as Liepmann (*β*) has clearly pointed out, a sharp fundamental distinction is necessary here. The lack of both masticating and swallowing disturbances and of other pseudobulbar symptoms, as well as very often the undisturbed state of the expressive elements of speech, proves that in aphemic disturbances "the conceptual design" rather than the articulation of speech or the kinaesthetic memory is impaired; or in other words, the knowledge of particular linguistic operations, rather than the innate instrument which is required for their performance, is lacking.

It has rightly been stressed that not only the mnemic connection of purely kinaesthetic elements, but also the mnemic connection of limb-kinetic complexes with the remaining possession of memory is a prerequisite for the completion of every action (cf. Isserlin 188). It must be added that as far as the speech sound is concerned there is a mnemic connection not only of the kinetic and superimposed acoustic components, but also, and more important, with that component of the speech sound concerned with content—*i.e.*, the sign-functioning element—to which the first two components are subordinated. Liepmann contrasts sound-deafness (and receptive aphasia in general) as "an agnosia for conventional signs, for linguistic symbols," with agnosis in the narrower sense, *i.e.*, "disturbances of sensory impressions which are not symbols" (*α* 484). Accordingly, one can separate sound-dumbness (and emissive aphasia in general) as

an apraxia for conventional linguistic signs, from true apraxis, *i.e.*, the inability to perform movements associated with objects, rather than symbolic movements.[13] With the failure of the sign-functioning value, the former can sometimes cease, while the latter can sometimes remain preserved.

The production of sounds is a goal-directed activity whose primary purposes lies in the distinctive value of the sound. To the extent that this activity is divested of its purpose, the inability arises, well-known to the pathologists, to accomplish a separate movement (in our case a self-sufficient articulation). Within the framework of another movement combined with it, however, (in our case an articulation which distinguishes words, *i.e.*, which is motivated by meaning) such a separate movement can be accomplished (see Pick *ε* 1441). Similarly, in apraxia, habitual movements toward an object succeed considerably better than the same movements without an object.

The autonomy of aphasic disturbances, in contrast to apraxia, finds its explanation in the sign function of speech elements, so that the mutually relative autonomy of aphasic phonemic and meaning disturbances corresponds to the entirely different sign function of the linguistic unit affected. Every morphological unit, from the smallest to the largest—*i.e.*, from the morpheme to the word—has a constant meaning, every phoneme a constant distinctive value. The morphological unit is related, as we have said, to something concrete, and this relation is for one and the same unit a manifold one: In the expressions *Bucephalus is a horse*, and *this cart-horse is a horse*, *e.g.*, the concrete relation of the expression *a horse*, but not its meaning, has changed, as Husserl specifies (*op cit.*, 46ff.). The phoneme is related to a morphological entity, and this relation is also, for one and the same phoneme, a manifold one. Thus the French nasal phoneme *ā*, *e.g.*, expresses simply that the different words and types of words in which it occurs (as *an*, *allant*, *enlever*, *vente*, *sang*, *lent*, etc.) contrast in their meaning with words containing a different phoneme in the same position (*e.g.*, *sang* with *saint*, *son*, *ça*, *sot* or *lent* with *lin*, *long*, *las*, *laid*, *loup*). The phoneme, therefore, has no direct relation to anything concrete and participates in the distinguishing of meanings without having any meaning itself. The relative frequency of cases of sound-dumbness in relation to the remaining forms of language-dumbness appears to be connected with this poverty of content, which opposes the phoneme to the meaningful units of language (see *e.g.*, Kleist 804). For the same reason, sentence into-nation (and the phonological elements characteristic of the sentence in general) often are preserved in aphasic sound disturbances. In contrast to the phoneme, they possess their own constant meaning, as, *e.g.*, the specific intonation at the end of the sentence, which marks the end of a meaningful unit.

Oddly enough, the same Pierre Marie who understood clearly the conceptual aspect of the speech sound, or of the loss of speech sounds in his analysis of sound-deafness, failed to appreciate the similar characteristics of sound-dumbness, although it is simply a question of recognizing the emissive counterpart to the corresponding receptive disturbance. Indeed, both types of disturbances, "in their nature and appearance," are connected very closely with each other. This same scholar even showed himself inclined to group sound-dumbness, not with the other forms of aphasia, in spite of its frequent connection with them, but with the arthritic disturbances, since the essential aphasic characteristic, the damage to "linguistic intelligence" (or in other words, the impairment of the intellectual functions of speech) is ostensibly absent in sound-dumbness.

According to Niessl von Mayendorf as well, there exists only a gradual distinction between aphasic sound-dumbness and dysarthria. It would be more correct, however, to speak of a gradual distinction between sound-deafness and sound-dumbness and, with Kleist and Fröschels (β 78), to consider the former, as opposed to the latter, as a lighter form, or retrogressive stage, of phonemic disturbance and to cite as analogous either the "hearing-dumbness" of the child (see §§ 5, 8) or the common inability to actively manipulate many foreign linguistic sound distinctions, when these are nevertheless controlled passively. Niessl believes that the boundary between aphasic and arthritic disturbances is "artificially and misleadingly drawn." An aphasic suffering from sound-dumbness as well as a child learning to talk or an adult attempting to speak a foreign language, speaks dysarthritically, and consequently suffers from an "ataxia of the speech muscles" (32f.). Nevertheless, the loss of babbling sounds by children is not to be explained by a suddenly appearing awkwardness of the speech muscles. Indeed, the nondistinction of rising and falling pitch or of long and short vowels in the Bulgarian pronunciation of Serbian words has nothing whatsoever to do with dysarthria, ataxia of the speech muscles or with the infrequent "tongue-lip

mechanism" (see Henschen VII, 129). These same sound features (distinctions of pitch and duration) are used by speakers of Bulgarian, although they have a different linguistic function, that is, they are used as features characteristic of the sentence (sentence intonation, tempo). The fact that, in polyglots suffering from sound-dumbness, one language can be affected while another remains undamaged proves that they cannot be suffering from an "ataxia of the speech muscles." And from the frequent cases of "single sound paraphasia," which one could interpret as an incomplete or partially restored sound aphasia (cf. § 10), it follows that phonemic distinctions can be lost without the loss of any articulation. Thus there are, *e.g.*, patients who produce both liquids, but nevertheless indiscriminately replace *r* with *l* and conversely *l* with *r* (cf. Stein γ 104).

Ombredane, the most distinguished observer of pathological sound change, understood well that partial sound-dumbness is fundamentally the reduction in the ability to differentiate (β 409). The system of distinguishable articulatory gestures ("gesticulation pneumo-laryngeal-buccal") is reduced, and since these are gestures which establish meanings ("gesticulation significative," see 363 ff.), the sign function is crucial for distinguishing them. Neither in the static description of such a gesture system nor in the analysis of its dissolution can one refrain from taking this point of view and get by on "purely physiological grounds."

II. STRATIFICATION OF THE PHONOLOGICAL SYSTEM

RELATIVE AND ABSOLUTE CHRONOLOGY OF PHONOLOGICAL DEVELOPMENT

Whether it is a question of French or Scandinavian children, of English or Slavic, of Indian or German, or of Estonian, Dutch or Japanese children,[14] every description based on careful observation repeatedly confirms the striking fact that the relative chronological order of phonological acquisitions remains everywhere and at all times the same.

While the succession of phonological acquisitions in child language appears to be stable in its fundamental characteristics, the speed of this succession, is, in contrast, exceedingly variable and individual, and two "newly added phenomena" which directly succeed each other in one child can in another child be separated by many months, and even by years. There are children who acquire the sound system of their native language especially quickly and who are in full possession of it by about the middle of their second year, while others still have not completely mastered their phonemic system at school age, as Gutzmann, e.g., established for German, or Helga Eng (58) for Norwegian, school children.[15]

At a particular stage of development, as Axel Kock has already observed, the Swedish child says *tata* for "kaka," the German child *topf* for "kopf," the English child *tut* for "cut," and the Japanese child also changes *k* to *t* (389).[16] The absolute chronology, in contrast to the relative chronology, however, is extremely vacillating. In many children, velar stops are acquired shortly after dentals at the beginning of the second year or sometimes even during the first year; in others, only about the third year. Often children replace all velars with corresponding dentals until their sixth year.[17] The lack of velars is not infrequently found even in school children of eight to nine years.[18] It is apparently a universal fact, then, that palatovelar sounds develop in child language only after dental sounds.

These cases of retarded language development, which are like a slow motion film, are especially instructive. Equally instructive, on the other hand, is the life-long preservation of one of the beginning stages of the language of imbeciles. In this case the infant sound system is preserved, and the fricatives continue to be replaced by stops (cf. Galant 430, Maupaté and the further bibliography in Nadoleczny α 149).

[. . .]

IDENTICAL LAWS OF SOLIDARITY IN THE PHONOLOGICAL DEVELOPMENT OF CHILD LANGUAGE AND IN THE SYNCHRONY OF THE LANGUAGES OF THE WORLD

If we consider now those acquisitions of the child's consonantal or vocalic system which exceed the minimum already discussed, a fact of great importance comes to light—the amazingly exact agreement between the chronological succession of these acquisitions and the general laws of irreversible solidarity (*solidarité irréversible*, cf. Jakobson 28) which govern the synchrony of all the languages of the world. Logically the solidarity, *i.e.* the necessary connexion of two elements, can, as is known, be "bilateral or unilateral, depending on whether the regularity in question is reversible or not" (cf. Husserl *op. cit.*, 265).

The acquisition of fricatives presupposes the acquisition of stops in child language; and in the linguistic systems of the world the former cannot exist unless the latter exist as well. Hence, there are no languages without stops, whereas P. Schmidt cites a number of Australian, Tasmanian, Melonesian, Polynesian, African and South American languages in which fricatives are completely unknown.[19] In Kara-Kalpak[20] and in Tamil,[21] to cite additional examples from another continent, there is no autonomous category of fricatives; stops and fricatives appear as combinatory variants of the same phoneme—the first as basic variants, the others as variants conditioned by the environment. In Tamil *e.g.*, stops become fricatives after a vowel.

The child first changes fricatives to the corresponding stops—*f* to *p*, *s* to *t*, and insofar as the palatovelar series is established before the appearance of fricatives, *x* and *ʃ* to *k*. For the change of *ʃ* > *k* (or ȝ > *g*) cf., *e.g.*, the formation *kam*, with which Edm. Grégoire at seventeen months repeatedly reproduced the name "Charles" (*β* 135),[22] or sound sequences such as *r'águ* "rezu," *mag'i* "muzik," which were frequently uttered by a two-year-old Russian boy (Blagoveščenskij 83). In the grouping of consonants into basic classes according to place of articulation, the traditional classification separates the alveo-palatals *ʃ*, ȝ from the palatals and classifies these consonant with the dentals. But this division is absolutely superficial and conventional. It is not based on any productive criterion and does not take into account the abundant linguistic evidence for the fundamental connection between the alveo-palatals and the true palatals. What characterizes the *ʃ*-sounds in contrast to the *s*-sounds is the greater retraction of the tongue and thereby the creation of a resonance chamber between the teeth on the one hand and the narrowing (or the closure) on the other. *ʃ*, ȝ and the corresponding affricates are thus distinguished from *s*, *z* and the corresponding affricates by the same characteristic feature as the palatal stops *c*, *ɟ* are from the dental stops *t*, *d*. In the former the place of articulation is located behind, and in the latter, before the dominant resonance chamber of the oral cavity.[23] This opposition corresponds to that of the velars and labials: the place of articulation is located, in the former, behind, and in the latter before, the undivided oral resonator. Thus, the velars and palatals (including the alveo-palatal consonants) can be opposed, as back or palato-velar sounds, to the labials and dentals, as front sounds.[24]

The acquisition of back consonants presupposes in the linguistic development of the child the acquisition of front consonants, i.e., labials and dentals; and, in particular, the acquisition of back oral and nasal stops presupposes the acquisition of front oral and nasal consonants. Similarly, the acquisition of back fricatives presupposes the acquisition of front fricatives, and, on the other hand, that of back consonants. The existence of back consonants in the languages of the world presupposes accordingly the existence of front consonants. That is, k as well as c (and η as well as n) require solidarity with p and t (or m and n), and x as well as $\int$ require solidarity with p and t (or m and η), and x as well as $\int$ require solidarity with f or s,[25] and in addition with k or c.

The solidarity is not reversible: the presence of front consonants (or individual classes of them) in no way requires the presence of back consonants (or individual classes of them). In other words, no language has back consonants without containing front consonants. On the other hand, there are some languages with labials and dentals, but without back consonants, as, e.g., the language of Tahiti in which both velars— k and η—have changed to '[26] and Kasimov-Tatar, in which all velars—both stops (voiceless and voiced, oral and nasal) and fricatives—were also replaced by the glottal stop.[27] In some languages the lack of palato-velar sounds is limited to oral consonants (e.g. in the language of Samoa, where k became the glottal stop, but where η was preserved),[28] and in many languages the system of nasal consonants is represented solely by m and n, whereas we know of no language which possesses back but not front nasal consonants. Accordingly, the velar nasal consonant appears in English, Scandinavian and German children, and, similarly, the palatal consonant in French, Czech and Serbocroatian children, only after m and n.

At first both of the back nasal consonants are replaced in the child by n, and, generally, the back consonants are replaced by the corresponding dentals. Thus, t is substituted both for k (cf. § 12) and for the palatal stop c (e.g., in Czech and, according to J. Lotz,

in Hungarian). When k finally appears, mistakes in the use of both phonemes (k, t) arise at first, especially those caused by a hypercorrect repression of the expected t in favor of k,[29] which is sometimes inaccurately interpreted as a sound change of $t > k$ (see Fröschels β 97). Consonant assimilations cannot be offered as evidence for a sound change of this kind either, as, e.g., in a Swedish child, gak "gata," geka, "Greta," gakk "god natt," guk "duk," gakka "docka" (Bolin 209). In the development of child language, k therefore merges with t, and only later does k emerge as a separate phoneme.[30] Occasionally, an intermediate stage is introduced between these two stages in which, although the velar series is not yet established, the two phonemes are already distinguished. In this case, a glottal stop corresponds to k (or velars, in general) of the mother tongue (cf. e.g., Ronjat 54). Exactly the same mutation occurs in the languages of the world, as we have mentioned above (cf. also § 18).

Just as the child (e.g., a Czech, Serbocroatian or Hungarian child) for a prolonged period possesses only one of the two series of back stops of his native language, a large number of the languages of the world contain only a single series of back stops, in contrast to the obligatory two series of front stops. With a few isolated and doubtful exceptions, the back oral stops are replaced only by velars, whereas the back nasal consonants are more frequently replaced by palatals. Both back as well as front fricatives can be replaced by a single series—the latter generally by dentals and the former often by palatals. If, in the languages of the world or in child language, the fricative consonants are limited to a single phoneme, this phoneme is as a rule represented by s.[31] Only the friction, and not the place of articulation, is relevant to this phoneme, when it is not opposed to any other fricative. One can accordingly characterize it as an "indefinite fricative phoneme." The same kind of phoneme possibly has back combinatory or expressive variants. Such was the case originally, e.g., with the Proto-Slavic s-phoneme, which was replaced by x after certain phonemes and, in addition, in some expressive formations. In cases where there is no opposition of front and back fricatives, however, this s-sound is not sharply differentiated from an $\int$-articulation either in the languages of the world or in child language.[32]

A so-called half-stop consonant (or affricate) which functions as an opposition to the corresponding stop consonant in phonemic systems, is acquired by the child only after the fricative of the same series. The son of Ronjat (54), *e.g.*, acquired the German initial *pf* only in his twenty-first month, whereas he had acquired initial *f* three months earlier. In the same chronological order, although later, the same phonemes appeared medially: *f* in his twenty-third month and *pf* in his thirtieth month. Similarly, the opposition of a stop and an affricate in the languages of the world implies the presence of a fricative of the same series (the pair *t-ts* implies the co-existence of the phoneme *s*, etc.). The number of such affricates in a phonemic system is therefore never greater, and is generally less, than the number of fricatives. Before the child acquires affricates, he substitutes either corresponding stops or fricatives for them, *e.g.*, *t* or *s* for *ts*, and *p* or *f* for *pf*.

An opposition of two vowels of the same degree of aperture is not acquired by the child as long as a corresponding vocalic opposition of a narrower degree of aperture is lacking. Only if y is opposed to *u* can *ϕ* arise, etc., as *e.g.*, in French, Scandinavian or German children. Correspondingly, in the vowel systems of child language the wider degrees of aperture are never represented by more phonemes than are the narrower degrees of aperture (cf. Trubetzkoy *op. cit.*, 88, 103). The phoneme *æ*, to which *a* as the palatal opposition of the same degree of aperture and *e* as the narrow opposition of the same series are opposed, appears relatively later in children, and is explained by the laws of solidarity already mentioned. Sully remarks that English *æ* "appears to be learned only after considerable practice" (126); similarly Saareste reports the difficulties which the same phoneme affords Estonian children, who usually replace it with *e* (20), and this is also the case with *æ* in Slovakian children.

A differentiation of rounded vowels according to degree of aperture cannot arise in child language as long as the same opposition is lacking for the unrounded vowels. The pair *u ~ o* cannot, therefore, precede the pair *i ~ e*, and there are no children who have an *o*-phoneme without having acquired an *e*-phoneme. On the contrary *o* is very often acquired considerably later than *e*.[33] Accordingly, a number of languages have an *e*-phoneme without any *o*-phoneme (cf. Trubetzkoy *op. cit.*, 98 on the Lezghian vowel system), but there is hardly any language with *o* and not *e*.

Rounded palatal vowels, which Rousselot characterized appropriately as "secondary," arise in child language only after the corresponding primary vowels,

i.e., after the rounded velar vowels and after the unrounded palatal vowels of the same degree of aperture. This is the case, *e.g.*, with Dutch and French children, and both sons of Grégoire "acquired them completely only after much practice that continued beyond the second year" (β 245). The existence of a secondary vowel in the languages of the world is dependent on the co-existence of the two corresponding primary vowels. Thus, *e.g.*, the vowel *ϕ* does not occur in a linguistic system as long as the vowels *o* and *e* are not present in the same system (cf. Trubetzkoy *op. cit.*, 102ff.).

LATE OR RARE PHONOLOGICAL ACQUISITIONS

Oppositions which occur in the languages of the world comparatively rarely are among the latest phonological acquisitions of the child. Thus, the geographical distribution of nasal vowels is relatively limited,[34] and, accordingly, these phonemes appear, in French and Polish children, *e.g.*, only after all of the remaining vowels have been acquired, generally not until about the third year.[35] On the other hand, nasal consonants, as we have stated, exist in all languages and are among the earliest linguistic acquisitions of the child.

The number of languages with a single liquid (whether *l* or *r*) is extraordinarily large, and in this connection Benveniste justly points out that the child has only a single liquid for a long time and acquires the other liquid only as one of his last speech sounds.[36]

The Czech *ř*, a sibilant opposition to *r*,[37] is one of the rarest phonemes that occur in language, and hardly any other phoneme of their native language presents such major and persistent difficulties to Czech children. It is also characteristic that Czech settlers in Russia easily loose this sound, as Prof. O. Hujer observed (the voiced combinatory variant becomes ʒ, the voiceless ʃ).

RELATIVE DEGREE OF SOUND UTILIZATION

The laws of irreversible solidarity determine the inventory of phonemic systems. In addition, the relative degree of utilization of particular phonemes in language (i.e., the relative frequency of their occurrence as well as their combinatorial capacity)[38] is also affected by these laws, provided that their validity is not restricted by specific structural principles. When, therefore, both phonemes—the implying as well as the implied—are introduced into child language, the implying element generally appears in speech more frequently than the other, takes part in a greater number of phoneme combinations, and possesses a more active assimilating force. Thus, in the sons of Grégoire, the predominance of the phomene *a* is still observable even after the development of the vowel system, "a predominance which still lasts and against which the other vowels must struggle" (β 171). As has been observed in Russian children, fricatives, even after they have become a part of the phonemic system, are still used less frequently than stops. In consonant clusters, the former are omitted more easily and for a longer period than the latter, and non-contiguous assimilation changes fricatives into stops rather than the reverse (see esp. Gvozdov, Rybnikov). Similarly, studies of regressive assimilation in the language of German children show that velars are commonly replaced by dentals (Meumann), and that "the labial quality stands out as the most important" (Röttger).

PANCHRONY OF THE LAWS
OF SOLIDARITY

One could easily increase the number of parallels between the phonological development of child language and the general laws which are brought to light by the synchrony of all of the languages of the world, and more extensive agreements will surely be uncovered as soon as more accurate information on child language from a great many different linguistic areas is obtained. Nevertheless, that such laws of irreversible solidarity exist in language can be considered as already established. Indeed, the domain of these laws is even considerably wider.

As we have said, the analysis of the most varied languages reveals general synchronic laws of solidarity. According to these laws, a secondary value cannot exist in a linguistic system without the corresponding primary value. From this fact two consequences necessarily emerge for the evolution of any given linguistic system as well: without the primary value, the corresponding secondary value cannot arise in a linguistic system, and without the secondary value, the corresponding primary value cannot be eliminated.

Thus, the laws of solidarity turn out to be panchronic. They retain their validity at every stage and in the course of every change of all of the languages of the world.

LAWS OF SOLIDARITY AND
SPEECH PATHOLOGY

The same laws determine, as we have seen (§ 14f.), the development of child language (*i.e.*, the building up of every individual linguistic competence): the acquisition of the secondary value presupposes the acquisition of the primary value. In addition, the dissolution of the individual linguistic competence is governed by the same regularity: the loss of the primary value presupposes the loss of the secondary-value. "Close analogies between immature child language and aphasia" (Fröschels β 49), or, more exactly, the infantilism or puelerism of aphasic speech, have repeatedly been pointed out.[39] The question of the parallels between the two areas, especially with reference to sound correspondences, requires a systematic survey.

The speech of dysarthritics suffers only to the extent that their speech apparatus suffers, and it does not reveal any constant sequence of mutilations: "if the lips are damaged the labials are affected, etc." (Liepmann α 489). Similarly, there is no permanent and uniform sequence of babbling sounds in the speech of the infant (cf. § 8). On the other hand, aphasic sound disturbances exhibit a strictly regular sequence of stages, and are therefore similar to those found in the actual linguistic progress of the child. Every attempt to make use of the principle of least effort already discussed (cf. § 5), or of any other mechanistic explanations, fails in this area.

The dissolution of the linguistic sound system in aphasics provides an exact mirror-image of the phonological development in child language. Thus, *e.g.*, the distinction of the liquids *r* and *l* is a very late acquisition of child language, and, as Fröschels observes, it is one of the earliest and most common losses in aphasic sound disturbances.[40] Also, in the restitution of language the "*r-l* symptom" often remains as the last distinct sign of an aphasic. Similarly, in those aphasics whose speech contained a uvular *r*, the confusions of the two liquids is characteristically almost a standard phenomenon (β 97f.), which once again confirms the insignificance of the place of articulation as far as the liquids are concerned.[41] The very late emergence of the sibilant ř in Czech child language is one of the most typical and well-known phenomena of Czech speech pathology (cf. Hlaváček, Kutvirtová). The nasal sounds, which in French children appear only after all of the other vowels, usually disappear earliest in French aphasics, as Ombredane states (α 955, β 468). English children acquire the interdental fricatives only after the corresponding *s*-sounds (cf. *e.g.*, Lewis 178), and, according to Head's statements, English aphasics loose the interdentals earlier than the *s*-sounds (*e.g.*, I 175, II 199f.). In the intervening period both children and aphasics replace the interdentals with *s*-sounds (*zis* "this," etc.).

In aphasics, secondary vowels are lost earlier than primary vowels; affricates are given up "in a childlike fashion";[42] fricatives then fall together, as in children, with the corresponding stops. Thus Bouman and Grünbaum report, concerning Dutch aphasics, that "an explosive sound is uttered in place of a spirant. The reverse confusion does not occur" (328).[43] According to the observations of Ombredane (α 947, β 408), *f* in French aphasics becomes *p* (*pu* "fou"), *s* becomes *t*, and *ʃ* becomes *k* (*ka* "chat," cf. § 14), if this latter change does not precede that of *ʃ* to *s* (see below).

Forward articulated consonants are more resistant than palatovelar sounds, and the latter become dentals for the most part, for which phenomenon there are again exact correspondences in child language. Nasal palato-velar sounds generally merge with *n* (velar *ŋ* in English as well as French and Czech *ɲ*),[44] and a parallel change occurs in fricatives and affricates, to the extent that these sounds are not yet eliminated. To this category belong the change of *ʃ*, *ʒ*, *tʃ* to *s*, *z*, *ts* in Czech aphasics, which was characterized by Haskovic as "infantile." And, finally, the back oral stops, as is well known, become *t* and *d*, or else the difference between *k*, *g* and *t*, *d* is preserved, but *k*, *g* are changed to the glottal stop, which, from the point of view of the phonemic system, subsumes only the distinctive feature of closure (or explosion) and consequently functions as an "indeterminate stop phoneme."[45]

A further impoverishment of the consonantal system results in the so-called "Paradeltazismus," *i.e.*, the merger of dentals and labials into a single series, which is represented for the most part by labial sounds. Labial consonants and the vowel *a* appear to

be the last sounds to resist the process of dissolution (cf. *e.g.*, Gutzmann ε 232), and this stage corresponds to the beginning stages of child language. Indeed, the agreement goes even further. For, even after the complete loss of the inventory of speech sounds, the interjectional language ("emotional language") of the aphasic can be spared, as Hughlings Jackson understood and stressed (cf. *e.g.*, Kussmaul 59ff.). In short, the higher strata are always abolished before the lower.

The order in which speech sounds are restored in the aphasic during the process of recovery corresponds directly to the development of child language. Prof. B. I. Jacobowsky, Director of the University Psychiatric Clinic in Uppsala, has drawn my attention to the rapid (approximately half an hour) course of development from speechlessness through aphasia to the complete recovery of language in the awakening process of mentally diseased patients who have been treated with insulin.[46] Thanks to the kind cooperation of Prof. Jacobowsky, I was able to observe that there are processes, similar to an accelerated film (cf. § 12), which are extraordinarily valuable for the study of the acquisition of speech sounds and which must be systematically observed and examined. A schizophrenic in the process of awakening at first omitted the liquids in the pronunciation of his name "Karlson," and for a while initial *k* could not be restored and was replaced by the glottal stop. For a considerable period the rounded palatal vowels, and in particular *r*, were omitted by Swedish insulin patients; the lack of aspiration in the unvoiced stops was also striking (cf. § 2), as was the strong palatalization of *t* (cf. § 25).

Notes

1. See Liepmann α 465, Kleist γ 928f.

2. Cf. my *O češskom stiche* (Berlin, 1923), 51 and 41.

3. The traditional concept of the "sound of the letter" in speech pathology shows, despite the naiveté of the term and of its motivation, that it is absolutely necessary to separate in the study of aphasia the linguistically relevant properties of the phoneme ("phonetic unity," in Kleist's terminology) from the simple combinatorial and optional variants. Froment (358) accordingly distinguishes between "fundamental sounds or phonemes" and "all the differences in pronunciation of the same sound."

4. If two words are distinguished by several phonemes (or by a sequence of them), the distinctive role is distributed among them.

5. The meaningfulness of the words is grasped, but there is no reaction to their individual meanings. One could cite similar examples of children who grasp certain phonological differences between words at the threshold of their language learning without having comprehended the meanings of these words.

6. Head's assertion, that every type of aphasia affects in some manner the "symbolic formulation," is thus correct. Moreover, de Saussure has penetratingly sketched this position: "In all cases of aphasia or agrapha, what is affected is less the faculty of producing a given sound or of writing a given sign than the ability to evoke by means of an instrument, regardless of what it is, the signs of a regular system of speech. . . . Beyond the functioning of the various organs, there exists a more general faculty which governs signs, and which would be the linguistic faculty proper" (*op. cit.*, 27).

7. More exactly, "single sound paraphasia," cf. Kleist γ 691.

8. See D. Westerman and J. Ward, *Practical phonetics for students of African languages* (Oxford, 1933), 169; cf. O. Gjerdman, "Critical remarks of intonation research," *Bull. of the School of Orient. Studies*, III, 495ff., and N. Trubetzkoy, *Grundzüge der Phonologie* (= *Trav. du Cercle Ling. de Prague*, VII), 182ff.

9. E. Husser, *Logische Untersuchungen*, II (Halle, 1913²), 69.

10. Cf. W. Köhler in *Zeitschr. f. Psychol.*, LXXII, 80ff.

11. Cf. esp. C. Stumpf, *Die Sprachlaute* (Berlin, 1926), 326ff.

12. Dr. Hjalmar Torp (Oslo) has drawn my attention to the frequent loss of the Norwegian pitch opposition in aphasics, and the pedologist Rutti Bjerknes (Presterod), to the lack of the same distinction in backward children. The falling "double pitch" (accent II) is thus replaced by the rising "single pitch" (accent I): '*lyse* "to shine" is pronounced like '*lyse* "the light"; on the Norwegian pitch opposition, see O. Broch in *Mélanges Pedersen*, 308ff., and C. Borgström in *Norsk Tidsskrift Sprogvidenskap*, IX, 260ff.

13. Pötzl correctly objects to the ranking of agnosia and apraxia above aphasic disturbances and advocates putting agnosia, language deafness, apraxia and language muteness together under a higher concept: "One may characterize these as disturbances of the selective comprehension, i.e. of a single integrated ability to perform" (45).

14. Data were available to us only from these languages (cf. below the bibliography employed). We were able to consider Swedish, Norwegian, and Danish of the Scandinavian languages; Russian, Polish, Czech, Serbocroatian and Bulgarian of the Slavic languages, and

the Zuñi language in New Mexico of the American Indian languages (see Kroeber).

15. According to Gutzmann's Berlin experience "almost half of the children just starting school, who were about six years old, did not have normal pronunciation" (α 19f.), whereas more recent statistical data indicate that only 1.21% of the school children of working and lower middle classes in Vienna still do not have normal pronunciation.

16. Cf. in French children *tā* "carte," *tata* "caca" (Bloch α 38), in Serbian children *tata* "kaka" (Pavlovič), in Estonian children *taal* "kukal" (Saareste 17)—in short, "children in all countries tend to substitute *t* for *k*" (Jespersen β 85).

17. See *e.g.*, Bloch α 42, Ronjat 58.

18. Cf. Gutzmann: "I have observed very intelligent children of eight and nine years who cannot pronounce *k*, although no reason whatever existed for it" (ε 111).

19. *Die Sprachfamilien und Sprachenkreise der Erde* (Heidelberg, 1926), 287. Cf. A: Sommerfelt: "These phonemes are unknown to all of the Australians and were unknown also to the Tasmanians. The *s* is found only at the northeast point of Cape York. In certain Melanesian languages as well, the *s* does not occur, as is also the case with the langauges of the Andaman Islands, where, in addition, spirants do not occur" (*La langue et la société*, Oslo, 1938, 51).

20. See E. Polivanov, *Nekotorye osobennosti karakalpakskogo jazyka* (Taschkent, 1933).

21. See J. R. Firth, *A short outline of Tamil pronunciation* (appendix to Arden's *Grammar of Common Tamil*, 1934²), and Trubetzkoy, *op. cit.*, 134f.

22. A backward girl (of four years) says *koko* "chaud" (Decroly).

23. Cf. A. Thomson, "Bemerkungen uber s-Laute," *Zeitschr. f. slav. Philol.*, XI (1934), 345ff., esp. 354f., also Rousselot, *Principes de phonétique expérimentale*, II (1925), 916f., J. Chlumsky[agu], *Les consonnes anglaises* (Prague, 1924), 23, and G. Panconelli-Calzia, *Die experimentelle Phonetik in ihrer Anwendung auf die Sprachweissenschaft* (Berlin, 1924), 79.

24. See my article in *Proceedings of the Third Int. Congress of Phonet. Sciences* (Ghent, 1939), 36. Brucke's assertion, that *s* was combined from both *s* and *x*, is correct from the standpoint of the systematic patterning of consonants; and Jan Hus, before the fifth century, showed his penetrating understanding of the problem when he separated the Czech *c*, *f*, *n*, *ʃ*, *ʒ*, from *t*, *d*, *n*, *s*, *z* by means of the same diacritic mark. Also, retroflex sounds, insofar as there are no palatals of the same manner of articulation which are opposed to them, rank with the palatal or back class of consonants. Characteristic in this

connection is the change of $t > k$, $n > \eta$ in Norwegian children: *ontli* "properly" $>$ *oŋkli* (G. Morgenstierne, *Indo-Iranian frontier languages*, II (1938), 49).

25. For stops (both nasal and oral, but not fricatives) the presence of the opposition dental $\sim$ labial is obligatory, insofar as there are no external obstacles (cf. §§ 13, 29).

26. See O. Dempwolff, *Vergleichende Lautlehre des austronesischen Wortschatzes*, I (1934), II (1937) = *Zeitschr. f. Eingeb. Spr.*, Supplements XV, XVII.

27. See E. Polivanov, *Vvedenie v jazsykoznanie* (Leningrad, 1928), 85f.

28. See Dempwolff, *o.c.*, II, 167ff.

29. Thus a child said *Duten Ta Herr Dotta*, but then for a while *Guken Gag Herr Goka* (Nadoleczny α 61).

30. The sounds *k* and *t* can appear at first only as two combinatorial variants. Thus the records of Grammont show that a child used the dental stop only intervocalically, but the velar initially and finally (e.g., *cateau* "gâteau," *cütine* "cuisine," *caté* "cassé," *pati* "partir," *peuteu* "monsieur," *pèti* "merci," *quépic* "qui pique"); the initial dental therefore becomes velar (*còtüc* "du sucre," *coupé* "souper"), the medial back sibilant becomes dental (*caté* "caché," *boudie* "bougie"), and the back stop is shifted by metathesis to initial position (*capet* "paquet," *cópou* "beaucoup," *coupé* "bouquet").

31. E.g., in Tungus (cf. A. Gorcevskij in *Sov. Sever*, I (1938),105ff.

32. Grégoire observes for children who are almost two years old: "The *s*'s were often lisped. These defective *s*'s cannot be considered as attempts at imitating ∫ of ʒ, since they were found in words where they replaced neither ∫ nor ʒ. The *s* must have sufficed to express both the hissing and hushing fricatives, since the incorrect articulation of *s* was close to that of ∫. It was necessary to wait until the articulation would be decided in favor of the two normal types" (β 205). Cf. the lisped character of the Danish *s*, to which no back sibilant phoneme is opposed.

33. See *e.g.*, Aleksandrov 92f., Pavlovič 48, Brenstiern 291, Ronjat 54.

34. See A. Isačenko, "A propos des voyelles nasales," *Bull. Soc. Ling.*, XXXVIII (1937).

35. See *e.g.* for French, Grégoire 246f., Ronjat 54 and for Polish, Oltuszewski 23ff., Brenstiern 292.

36. *Trav. du Cercle Ling. de Prague*, VIII (1939), 34f. Cf. similar observations in Egger 71 and Fröschels 105. Most descriptions report the very late adoption of the second liquid in child language. See *e.g.*, the characteristic example of a five-year-old in Barbelenet: "this child neither understands nor pronounces *r*; he always substitutes *l* for it" (34ff.).

37. Cf. J. Chlumský, "Une variété peu connue de l'R Linguale," *Rev. de Phonét.*, I (1911).

38. Cf. the pioneering programmatic paper of V. Mathesius, "Zum Problem der Belastungs-und Kombinationsfähigkeit der Phoneme," *Trav. du Cercle Ling. de Prague*, IV (1931).

39. In addition to Fröschels α, β, see *e.g.*, Feyeux 163, Head I, 221ff., Ombredane 409f., Pick γ, Torp 45f.

40. For examples, cf. Ombredane (α 947) for French, Torp (37) for Norwegian, V. Bogorodickij (*Fonetika russkogo jazyka v svete èksperimental'nyx dannyx*, Kazan, 1930, 337) for Russian, Pick (δ 237) for Czech.

41. Cf. esp. the paper of M. Dluska, "Quelques problèmes de phonétique en polonais etudiés expérimentalment," *Archivum Neophilologicum*, I (1934).

42. See *e.g.*, Kleist γ 805, 809, Ombredane 948.

43. Similarly Bogorodickij, *ibid.*, on Russian patients.

44. See Head I, 200, Ombredane α 948, Haškovec 595.

45. On the last change see Fröschels β 77; for the change of velar stops to dentals, Gutzmann gives German examples ε 170, 260, Head gives English examples II, 199f., and Pick gives Czech examples δ 337.

46. Cf. M. Sakel, *Neue Behandlungsmethode der Schizophrenie* (Vienna, 1935).

25

Grammatical Complexity and
Aphasic Speech

Harold Goodglass

J. Hunt

Linguistics challenges the student of aphasia to determine whether various levels of language are disturbed in brain-injured persons differentially according to their inherent "complexity" in the language. In the domain of phonology R. Jakobson (1942) has suggested in quite specific terms that in aphasia, phonemes are dissolved in an order of greater to lesser complexity. We would not expect a French aphasic, for example, to maintain the complex distinction between /i/ and /ü/ or /e/ and /ē/ if he had lost the more fundamental distinction of /a/ and /i/. This theory of Jakobson's has unfortunately not been followed by the required experimental investigation.

The present paper[1] deals with the related problem of differentially disturbed levels, not in phonology, but in grammar. The problem of grammatical disturbance

From *Word*, 14, 197–207 (1958). The authors are indebted to Professor Morris Halle of the Massachusetts Institute of Technology for suggesting the general design of the experiment described here. The assistance of Uriel Weinreich in formulating the linguistic issues is gratefully acknowledged.

in aphasia is significant not only for linguistics, but for neurophysiology and clinical diagnosis as well. Differential impairment of the grammatical structure of spoken language has been regularly described in cases of aphasia and most authorities have distinguished between an "agrammatic" form, marked by simplification and loss of grammatical detail, and a "paragrammatic" form, marked by confused and incomplete, but not necessarily simplified constructions. The similarities and differences between these two speech patterns have not been adequately accounted for theoretically, nor has an objective empirical means of distinguishing between them been developed.

For the purpose of the present experiment, we have chosen two English inflectional morphemes: the noun plural and the possessive. Apart from minor allomorphs of the plural these two morphemes have the same allomorphs, /-s, -z, and -əz/, in the same distribution. Thus, any differential treatment of the morphemes on the part of an aphasic cannot be due to a difference in phonemic form, but must be due to their different status in the grammatical system.

Our theory is that the possessive is more complex than the plural, and leads to the following specific hypotheses:

1. When they are given stimuli intended to elicit responses with plural nouns and responses with nouns in the possessive form, some aphasics should have more difficulty with the possessive form than with the plural, but none should have significantly more difficulty with the plural than with the possessive.
2. When required to discriminate incorrect usage of plural and of possessive word forms, some aphasics should make more errors with possessives, but none should make significantly more errors with plurals.

This prediction can be derived in several alternative ways and, for economy, the discussion of the theory has been combined with the discussion of the results in the final section of this paper.

The following secondary problems were also considered:

1. The final *s* indicating the third personal singular in verbs was included in the test for auditory discrimination of incorrect forms. It was predicted that this form, like the possessive -'*s*, should be more vulnerable than the plural -*s* to disturbance in aphasia.
2. It is important to determine whether the disturbance of grammatical discrimination in aphasia affects expressive and receptive language similarly in most patients, or whether it may appear in one modality without the other.
3. It is significant to determine whether difficulties with grammatical forms are only a reflection of the severity of aphasia, or whether there is evidence for specificity of this type of defect.

PROCEDURE

Two experimental tests were used in this study: an Expressive Final S test and a Receptive Final S test. (These terms relate, respectively, to the expressive and receptive use of language, i.e. to speaking and writing, on the one hand, and to understanding on the other.) In each item of the Expressive test, a simple declarative sentence of from five to seven words was read to the subject twice. The reading was followed immediately by two questions, the first of which required a one-word answer with a pluralized noun and the second an answer with a possessive form ending in -'*s*. Both responses were part of the original sentence. To illustrate:

Examiner reads:	My sister lost her gloves. *(Repeated.)*
Question 1.	What did she lose?
Question 2.	Whose gloves were they?
Examiner reads:	The baby dropped his toys. *(Repeated.)*
Question 1.	What did he drop?
Question 2.	Whose toys were they?

For the grading of an answer as "correct," it was necessary for the final *s* to be clearly heard, although a distorted pronunciation of the stem of the word was tolerated, and help with the initial sound of the word was given to patients with severe word-finding difficulty. The test consisted of twelve of these sets.

In the Receptive Final S test, 30 sentences of six to ten words each were divided into six categories, as follows:

A. Six sentences in which the final *s* is omitted from a possessive. E.g., *The ship anchor was lost in the storm.*
B. Six sentences in which the final *s* is omitted from a plural noun. E.g., *There were three book on the table.*
C. Six sentences in which the final *s* is omitted from a verb. E.g., *The soldier write home every week.*
X. Four correct sentences similar in structure to sentences of Type A.
Y. Four correct sentences similar in structure to sentences of Type B.
Z. Four correct sentences similar in structure to sentences of Type C.

These sentences were arranged in a random sequence and recorded on tape with each sentence repeated once, and a 15 second interval between the repetition and the first reading of the next sentence. The subject was instructed simply to listen carefully and to indicate whether each sentence sounded like correct English or not.

TABLE 25–1. Characteristics of Subjects Used in These Studies

Subject	Age	Type of Aphasia	Severity
Subjects Common to Both Experiments			
Sar.	46	Mixed, predom. Express.	Severe
Hig.	27	Mixed, predom. Express.	Severe
Ray.	38	Predominantely Expressive	Severe
Bar.	27	Expressive	Severe
Ton.	38	Expressive	Moderate
Hic.	70	Receptive	Mild
Mur.	62	Receptive	Mild-moderate
Chu.	26	Mixed, predom. Express.	Moderate
Cou.	38	Mixed, predom. Express.	Moderate
Cru.	32	Expressive	Moderate
Subjects Used in Receptive Experiment Only			
Com.	36	Mixed	Mild residual
Fie.	32	Expressive	Mild
Phi.	58	Expressive	Mild
Tay.	34	Expressive	Mild residual
Pei.	59	Expressive	Mild residual
Subjects Used in Expressive Experiment Only			
McC.	41	Mixed	Moderate-Severe
Pen.	38	Expressive	Moderate
Rol.	54	Expressive	Moderate
Del.	48	Mixed	Severe
Sla.		Mixed	Moderate-Severe
Murr.	62	Mixed	Moderate
Ren.	40	Expressive	Severe
Fei.	51	Expressive	Moderate-mild
Rya.	55	Expressive	Moderate

SELECTION OF SUBJECTS

Twenty of the 24 subjects used in this study were patients residing in the Aphasia Unit of the Boston Veterans Administration Hospital and four were patients at the Lemuel Shattuck Hospital.[1] They ranged in age from 25 to 70 years and included all types of aphasia, ranging in severity from mild to severe. Ten patients were subjects in both the expressive and the receptive experiments. Five subjects were retained only for the receptive experiment because they made no errors on the Expressive Final S test and had virtually normal speech patterns. It was felt that inclusion of their scores would distort the results of the study with spuriously high correlations. Nine patients who participated in the expressive experiment were no longer available for the receptive experiment. The characteristics of the subjects are summarized in Table 25–1.

RESULTS

Expressive Final S.   Examination of the first specific hypothesis requires comparison of the number of errors in the use of plural as compared to possessive final *s* in the Expressive Final S test. The patients were

TABLE 25–2. Number of Errors in Expressive Final S Experiment

Type of Error Subjects	Plural	Possessive	Total
High Error Group			
Ton.	0	8	8
Ray.	3	5	8
Bar.	7	9	16
McR.	5	8	13
Chu.	1	5	6
Hig.	1	4	5
Pen.	2	6	8
Rol.	8	11	19
Subtotal	27	56	83
Low Error Group			
Cou.	0	0	0
Hic.	1	2	3
Cru.	2	1	3
Mur.	1	0	1
Del.	1	2	3
Sla.	1	2	3
Murr.	0	1	1
Ren.	1	0	1
Fei.	2	1	3
Rya.	1	1	2
Subtotal	10	10	20
Total	37	66	103

easily dichotomized into those with high total errors (more than 4) and low total errors (less than 4). Table 25–2, summarizing the results on this test, is therefore presented with sub-totals for high- and low-error subjects. The difference in number of plural errors (37) and possessive errors (66), as tested by the Wilcoxon Signed Ranks method, is significant, with *p* less than .025.

By inspection, Table 25–2 reveals that the high total error group was consistently higher in possessive errors, while the low error group was equally divided in incidence of the two types of errors. The number of cases involved, however, is too small to rule out the effects of pure chance.

Receptive Final S. Examination of the second specific hypothesis requires comparison of the number of errors of types A, B, C, and XYZ (rejection of correct sentences). The data are summarized in Table 25–3. Application of the Wilcoxon Signed Ranks test to the comparison of errors yields the following:

A—B	Significant beyond .05 level
A—C	Not significant
C—B	Significant beyond .01 level.
A—XYZ/2	Just short of .05 level of significance.
B—XYZ/2	Not significant
C—XYZ/2	Significant beyond .01 level.

No useful dichotomy of high- and low-error subjects could be made for the Receptive Final S Test. In these data, the error score XYZ/2 (rejection of correct sentences) represents a measure of the subjects' tendency to make random errors due to confusability or to a fluctuating level of comprehension. It is apparent that Type B (plural) errors are no more frequent than the random error level, and that errors in detecting the omitted final *s* for possessive and verb forms occur significantly more often. Thus, the two specific hypotheses concerning the order of difficulty of grammatical forms for aphasics are supported.

ΣXYZ represents the number of rejections among the 12 grammatically correct sentences. This figure is divided by two to make it comparable to the error scores for types A, B, and C which are based on sets of six sentences.

Intercorrelations Among the Tests. Computation of rank-order intercorrelations among the several subscores of the tests permits examination of the secondary problems raised in connection with this study. These correlations are summarized in Table 25–4. In this table, the Functional Speech score, taken from the clinical aphasia examination, is used as a measure of the general severity of the aphasic speech handicap.

It is apparent, from the low correlations in the last section of the table, that difficulties with the *expressive* use of the *-s* are unrelated, in our subjects, to difficulties in *perceiving auditorily* the omission of the corresponding *-s* in the context of a sentence. Severity of aphasia is significantly predictive of difficulty with the possessive *-'s* on the expressive side, but only doubtfully related to difficulty with the plural *-s* (correlations of .53 and .38, respectively). On the receptive side, there is a sharp division in the clustering of the subscores. The XYZ, or random receptive error rank, is highly predictable from knowledge of the severity of

TABLE 25–3. Number of Errors in Receptive Final S Experiment

| | Type of Error | | | |
Subjects	Type A (Possessive)	Type B (Plural)	Type C (3rd Pers. Sing.)	ΣXYZ
McG.	2	4	4	2
Sar.	0	2	2	4
Hig.	2	0	1	.5
Ray.	0	0	1	1.5
Bar.	3	1	3	2
Com.	0	0	1	0
Tay.	1	0	1	0
Pei.	1	0	1	.5
Ton.	3	0	2	1.5
Fie.	1	0	3	0
Phi.	0	0	1	0
Hic.	3	0	1	0
Mur.	2	0	1	0
Chu.	1	1	4	.5
Cou.	5	1	1	.5
Cru.	2	1	3	1.5
Total	26	10	30	14.5

aphasia (rho = .82). Errors in the perception of the plural and third person singular -s are also strongly related to the severity and to each other. On the other hand, the non-perception of errors with possessive -'s is insignificantly correlated either with the severity of aphasia or with the other receptive subscores.

DISCUSSION

Jakobson's (1956) reformulation of agrammatism as "contiguity disorder" does not attempt a detailed prediction of the order of dissolution of grammatical processes in aphasia. However, his position does lead to the hypothesis that contiguity disorder first interferes with those obligatory grammatical forms which express syntactic relations and are not a matter of semantically determined choice. In the present experiment, the possessive and the third person verb suffixes are of this type, being highly determined by syntax, whereas the plural ending has a predominantly semantic function and is to a large degree independent of syntactic relationships. Thus, while this study is not a strong test of Jakobson's position, the results are in accord with his general formulation. In order to provide stronger support for an interpretation of the data in these terms, it would be necessary to produce parallel findings with other pairs of endings which may have either a semantic or an automatized, syntactic function in different settings. In English, these include the noun ending /iŋ/ (as in *clipping, beginning*) vs. the /iŋ/ of the verb in the progressive present; the /ər/ of agency (*seller, buyer*) vs. the comparative /ər/. The results should also discriminate patients who have the clinical speech pattern of agrammatism from the non-agrammatic.

Chomsky's theory of syntax (1957) provides specific predictions about the order of complexity of grammatical structures. According to this theory, some sentences in a language belong to a basic level ("kernel sentences"), whereas others are formed from kernel sentences by transformations. Elaborations or substi-

TABLE 25–4. Intercorrelations Among the Subscores of the Final S Tests

Correlations between:	N	rho	Significance
Expressive Final S			
Functional speech vs. possessive errors	14	.53	.05
Functional speech vs. plural errors	14	.38	n.s.
Possessive vs. plural errors	17	.48	.05
Receptive Final S			
Functional speech vs. Type A (poss.) err.	16	.32	n.s.
Functional speech vs. Type B (pl.) errors	16	.73	.01
Functional speech vs. Type C (3rd pers) err.	16	.68	.01
Functional speech vs. XYZ (random) errors	16	.82	.01
Type A vs. Type B	16	.32	n.s.
− A − C	16	.24	n.s.
− B − C	16	.75	.01
− A − XYZ	16	.25	n.s.
− B − XYZ	16	.75	.01
− C − YXZ	16	.60	.01
Expressive and Receptive			
Possessive vs. Type A.	10	.08	n.s.
Plural vs. Type B	10	.32	n.s.
Possessive vs. XYZ	10	.78	.01
Plural vs. XYZ	10	.57	.05

tutions on the phrase structure level, which remain on the basic kernel level, are regarded as grammatical processes of a lower order than transformations.

Now, sentences containing possessives in English are not kernel sentences, but transforms of kernels. For example, *John's hat* . . . is a transform of the kernel sentence *John has a hat* and, in general, *X's Y*, wherever it occurs, is a transform of *X has Y*. The formation of the plural form a singular noun, on the other hand, is a process within the phrase structure level and is thus less complex. The results in the present study are consistent with Chomsky's position insofar as the noun plural was less disturbed than the grammatically more complex possessive. Perhaps a stricter test of Chomsky's theory would compare the

use of a transform with the particular kernel from which it was derived. The experimental advantage of making the responses phonetically identical could be retained, as in the following type of completion item:

> *The soldier mails a letter home every night. He did the same last night. What did he do with the letter? He ___ ___ it.* (Kernel sentence)
> *And what happened to the letter? It was ___ ___.* (Passive transformation)

This line of investigation is now being followed intensively.

Chomsky's theory does not account for the patients' difficulties with the -s of the third person singular verb form. The addition of this suffix is a change at the phrase structure level, yet it was found more subject to disturbance than the possessive transformation. At the risk of introducing an additional principle for the explanation of a further fact, we may conjecture that another factor at work in determining the survival value of a grammatical structure is its redundancy. The -s of the verb form is completely determined by the subject of the verb, and its omission does not appreciably increase the ambiguity of the sentence in which it appears.

Our limited sample gives no support to the hypothesis that a common factor explains disturbances both in grammatical expression and in auditory discrimination of grammatical forms. It is true that the receptive task used here was not directly analogous to the expressive: it required only a recognition of the correct or incorrect-sounding sentence, without demonstration of response to the meaning. However, our finding is in line with Pick's observation (1931) that expressive and receptive agrammatism occurred independently of each other. It is interesting to note that the disturbance in *recognizing* the missing -'s is particularly poorly related to the other -s difficulties. However, in view of our small sample, it would be premature to offer explanations before the finding is verified in further research.

The present study demonstrates the need for more detailed investigations of agrammatism based on sound linguistic theory regarding the hierarchical structure of grammar. This approach has proved fruitful in the present experiment and promises to add both to the understanding of aphasic symptoms and to the refinement of linguistic theory.

Note

1. The authors are indebted to Miss Mary Hyde, Speech Therapist at the Lemuel Shattuck Hospital, for her assistance in testing patients.

References

Chomsky, N., *Syntactic Structures.* The Hague: Mouton & Co., 1957.

Jakobson, R., "Kindersprache, Aphasie, und allgemeine Lautgesetze," *Uppsale Universiteis Årsskrift,* 1942:9.

Jakobson, R., "Two Aspects of Language and Two Types of Aphasic Disturbances," in R. Jakobson and M. Halle, *Fundamentals of Language,* The Hague, Mouton & Co., 1956.

Pick, A. (edited by R. Thiele), "Aphasie," in A. Bethe, (ed.), *Handbuch der normalen und pathologischen Physiologie,* Berlin, J. Springer, 1931.

26

The Organization of Language and the Brain

Norman Geschwind

Language disorders after brain damage help in elucidating the neural basis of verbal behavior.

Many problems relating to the functions of the nervous system can effectively be studied by investigation in animals, which permits controlled and repeatable experiments on large groups of subjects. When we come, however, to consider the relationship of the brain to language, we must recognize that our knowledge is based entirely on findings in man. Some authors would even argue that language is exclusively a human attribute, so that no experiments on animals could ever be relevant. Although I believe that forerunners of language do exist in lower forms (1), the

Reprinted with permission from *Science* 170:940–944. Copyright 1970 American Association for the Advancement of Science.

The author was James Jackson Putnam Professor of Neurology at the Harvard Medical School and director of the Neurological Unit, Boston City Hospital, Boston, Massachusetts 02118. This article is based on a paper presented 28 December 1969 at the Boston meeting of the AAAS.

direct contributions to this area of experimentation on the brains of animals still lie in the future.

BRAIN LESIONS IN MAN

Information in this area has come from several sources. Cases of brain tumor are of limited value, since tumors distort the brain and produce effects at a distance. Cases of penetrating brain wounds (2) have been of considerable use but are not the best source of anatomical data, since postmortem information is usually lacking. Analysis of the sites at which the skull was penetrated is of use statistically, but, because of variations in the paths taken by missiles, cannot provide precise data concerning the location of lesions producing language disorders. Stimulation during surgery (3) has been another most important source of information but, because of limitation of time at operation and the accessibility of only certain structures, has not covered the full range of phenomena observed clinically.

The elegant studies of Milner and her co-workers on patients undergoing excision of cortical regions for epilepsy represent the largest corpus of truly experimental studies of the higher brain functions in man (4). They are limited, however, with respect to the range of phenomena observed. Furthermore, since most of these patients were undergoing removal of areas of brain which had been the site of epileptic discharges since childhood, there is reason to believe that the effects seen after surgery may not represent the full range of phenomena seen after damage to the adult brain. The Wada test (5), in which sodium amytal is injected into one carotid artery, has been a major source of knowledge concerning the lateralization of language functions in the brain.

Although important information has been obtained by the above methods, it is still true that the bulk of our knowledge concerning the relationship of the brain to language has been derived from the study of adults in whom delimited areas of brain have been damaged as the result of occlusion of blood vessels, who have been studied carefully over long periods, and whose brains have been subjected to careful postmortem examination. Although fully suitable cases of this type are not common, the experience of nearly 100 years of study has built up a large body of reliable knowledge.

APHASIC DISORDERS

The generic term *aphasia* is used to describe the disorders of language resulting from damage to the brain. Early in the history of the study of aphasia the distinction between language and speech was stressed. In disorders of speech the verbal output was impaired because of weakness or incoordination of the muscles of articulation. The criterion of a disorder of language was that the verbal output be *linguistically* incorrect. The muscles of articulation might be used normally in nonlinguistic activities. Similarly, in aphasic disorders of comprehension the patient might lose the ability to comprehend spoken or written language and yet show normal hearing or vision when tested nonverbally. Furthermore, these disorders could occur without impairment of other intellectual abilities. The

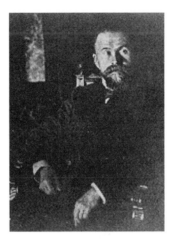

FIGURE 26–1. Carl Wernicke (1848–1904), who, at the age of 26, published the monograph *Der aphasische Symptomencomplex*, which was to be the major influence on the anatomical study of aphasia in the period preceding World War I. During his tenure as professor at Breslau, his assistants and students included many of the later leaders of German neurology, such as Otfrid Foerster, Hugo Liepmann, Karl Bonhoeffer, and Kurt Goldstein. (Figure scanned from original article.)

aphasias were thus the first demonstrations of the fact that selective damage to the brain could affect one class of learned behavior while sparing other classes, and thus gave origin to the field of study of brain-behavior relationships. The discovery of these phenomena was one of the greatest achievements of the last half of the 19th century.

Some cases of aphasia had been described before the mid-1800's, but it was Paul Broca who in 1861 began the study of the relationship of aphasia to the brain, with two major contributions (6). He was the first to prove that aphasia was linked to specific lesions, and to show that these lesions were predominantly in the left half of the brain. The man who was, however, most responsible for initiating the modern study of this field was Carl Wernicke (Fig. 26–1), who in 1874, at the age of 26, published his classic work, *The Symptom Complex of Aphasia*, which carried the appropriate subtitle, "A Psychological Study on an Anatomical Basis" (7). Wernicke established clearly the fact that there were linguistic differences between the aphasias produced by damage in the left temporal lobe, in what is now called Wernicke's area, and those produced by lesions in the frontal lobe in Broca's area (Fig. 26–2) (8).

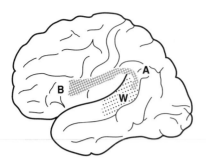

FIGURE 26–2. Lateral surface of the left hemisphere of the human brain. *B*, Broca's area, which lies anterior to the lower end of the motor cortex; *W* (*open circles*), arcuate fasciculus, which connects Wernicke's to Broca's area. (See text.)

LINGUISTIC CHANGES IN APHASIA

The aphasic of the Broca's type characteristically produces little speech, which is emitted slowly, with great effort, and with poor articulation. It is not, however, only at the phonemic level that the speech of these patients is abnormal, since the patient clearly fails to produce correct English sentences. Characteristically the small grammatical words and endings are omitted. This failure persists despite urging by the examiner, and even when the patient attempts to repeat the correct sentence as produced by the examiner. These patients may show a surprising capacity to find single words. Thus, asked about the weather, the patient might say, "Overcast." Urged to produce a sentence he may say, "Weather . . . overcast." These patients invariably show a comparable disorder in their written output, but they may comprehend spoken and written language normally. In striking contrast to these performances, the patient may retain his musical capacities. It is a common but most dramatic finding to observe a patient who produces single substantive words with great effort and poor articulation and yet sings a melody correctly and even elegantly. Because Broca's area lies so close to the motor cortex (Fig. 26–2), this latter region is often damaged simultaneously, so that these patients frequently suffer from paralysis of the right side of the body.

The Wernicke's aphasic contrasts sharply with the Broca's type. The patient usually has no paralysis of the opposite side, a fact which reflects the difference in the anatomical localization of his lesion. The speech output can be rapid and effortless, and in many cases the rate of production of words exceeds the nor-

mal. The output has the rhythm and melody of normal speech, but it is remarkably empty and conveys little or no information. The patient uses many filler words, and the speech is filled with circumlocutions. There may be many errors in word usage, which are called paraphasias. These may take the form of the well-articulated replacement of single sounds (so-called literal or phonemic paraphasias), such as "spoot" for "spoon," or the replacement of one word for another (verbal paraphasias), such as "fork" for "spoon." A typical production might be, "I was over in the other one, and then after they had been in the department, I was in this one." The grammatical skeleton appears to be preserved, but there is a remarkable lack of words with specific denotation.

The Wernicke's aphasic may, in writing, produce well-formed letters, but the output exhibits the same linguistic defects which are observed in the patient's speech. He shows a profound failure to understand both spoken and written language, although he suffers from no elementary impairment of hearing or sight.

The localization of these forms of aphasia has been confirmed repeatedly. It is important to stress this point, since there is a common misconception that the classical localizations were rejected because powerful arguments were raised against their validity. The two authors whose names are most frequently quoted as critics are Kurt Goldstein and Henry Head. As I have pointed out in greater detail elsewhere (9), Goldstein, who had been a student under Wernicke at the University of Breslau, despite the holistic views which he expressed in his philosophical discussions, actually explicitly stated his support of the classical localizations throughout his career. Head did indeed violently attack these views early in the first volume of his famous work on aphasia (10). His argument was, however, vitiated by the fact that, later in the same volume, the localizations which he himself supported turned out to be essentially identical to the ones he had previously dismissed as invalid.

WERNICKE'S THEORY

Wernicke's contribution lay not only in establishing the syndrome patterns and their localizations but also in providing a theoretical analysis of the mechanisms of aphasia (Fig. 26–2). He pointed out that Broca's area was located just in front of the cortical region in which lay the motor representation for the face, tongue, lips, palate, and vocal cords—that is, the organs of speech. It seemed reasonable to assume that Broca's area contained the rules by which heard language could be coded into articulatory form. This formulation still appears reasonable. There is no need to assume that this coding need be a simple one. By contrast, Wernicke's area lies next to the cortical representation of hearing, and it was reasonable to assume that this area was somehow involved in the recognition of the patterns of spoken language. There is also no need to assume that this coding is a simple one.

Wernicke then added the natural assumption that these two areas must be connected. The general pattern was now clear. Destruction of Wernicke's area would lead to failure to comprehend spoken language. Wernicke pointed out that, for most people, written language was learned by reference to the spoken form and that therefore a lesion of this region would abolish comprehension of printed and written language. The act of speaking would consist in arousing in some way the auditory form of words, which would then be relayed forward to Broca's area to be transduced into the complex programming of the speech organs, and therefore, with damage to Wernicke's area, language output would also be disordered.

The model could readily be complicated further. Wernicke himself and those who followed him filled in further details. The comprehension of written language would require connections from the visual to the speech regions, and destruction of these connections should be able to cause isolated difficulties in reading comprehension. Since the language abilities were localized in the left hemisphere, language performances by the right hemisphere would depend on information transmission over the corpus callosum.

Clearly the validation of a theory is not a function of its surface plausibility but is dependent on other factors. It is important to remember that Wernicke's theory has been the only one in the history of aphasia which could in a real sense be put to experimental test. It was possible, on the basis of the theory, to predict that certain lesions should produce symptoms not previously described. Furthermore, it was possible, on being confronted with previously undescribed syndromes, to predict the site of the anatomical lesion. The most dramatic examples of this appear in the writings of Hugo Liepmann (11) on the syndromes of the corpus callosum. On the basis of his clinical examination he predicted the presence of callosal lesions, which were later confirmed at postmortem examination.

Several remarkable disorders of language have been described which fit readily into the Wernicke theory. In pure word deafness, the patient, with intact hearing as measured by ordinary nonverbal tests, fails to comprehend spoken language although he has essentially normal ability to express himself verbally and in writing and to comprehend written language. In this syndrome the area of damage generally lies deep in the left temporal lobe, sparing Wernicke's area but destroying both the direct auditory pathway to the left hemisphere and the callosal connections from the opposite auditory region. Although elementary hearing is intact because the right auditory region is spared, there is no means for auditory stimulation to reach Wernicke's area, and therefore the patient does not understand spoken language, although his ability to express himself in spoken and written language and his comprehension of the written language are essentially intact (12).

In conduction aphasia, there is fluent paraphasic speech, and writing, while comprehension of spoken and written language remains intact. Despite the good comprehension of spoken language there is a gross defect in repetition. The lesion for this disorder typically lies in the lower parietal lobe (Fig. 26–2), and is so placed as to disconnect Wernicke's area from Broca's area. Because Broca's area is preserved, speech is fluent, but abnormal. The preservation of Wernicke's area insures normal comprehension, but the gross defect in repetition is the result of disruption of the connection between this region and Broca's area. The disorder in repetition exhibits some remarkable linguistic features which are not yet explained. The disorder is greatest for the small grammatical words such as *the*, *if*, and *is*; thus, a patient who may successfully repeat "big dog" or even "presidential succession" may fail totally on "He is here." The most difficult phrase for these patients to repeat is "No ifs, ands, or buts." In many of these patients the ability to repeat numbers may be preserved best of all, so that, given a phrase such as "seventy-five percent," the patient may repeat the "seventy-five" rapidly and effortlessly but may fail on "percent" (12).

PURE ALEXIA WITHOUT AGRAPHIA

Many examples of pure alexia without agraphia were described in the 1880's, but the first postmortem study of this syndrome was described in 1892, by Dejerine (13). His patient suddenly developed a right visual

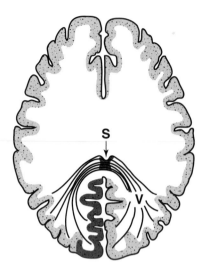

FIGURE 26–3. Horizontal section of the human brain, illustrating the mechanism of pure alexia without agraphia. V, visual region. The visual cortex on the left is destroyed (*thick black line*). As a result, the patient can perceive written material only in the intact right visual region. For this material to be appreciated as language, it must be related to the speech areas on the left side through the splenium, which is the posterior portion of the corpus callosum. As a result of damage to the splenium (S), this transfer cannot take place, and therefore the patient cannot comprehend the written words whose form he perceives clearly.

field defect and lost the ability to read. He could, however, copy the words that he could not understand. He was able, moreover, to write spontaneously, although he could not read later the sentences he had written. All other aspects of his use and comprehension of language were normal. At postmortem Dejerine found that the left visual cortex had been destroyed. In addition, the posterior portion of the corpus callosum was destroyed, the part of this structure which connects the visual regions of the two hemispheres (Fig. 26–3). Dejerine advanced a simple explanation. Because of the destruction of the left visual cortex, written language could reach only the right hemisphere. In order to be dealt with as language it had to be transmitted to the speech regions in the left hemisphere, but the portion of the corpus callosum necessary for this was destroyed. Thus, written language, although seen clearly, was without meaning. This was the first demonstration of the effects of a lesion of the corpus callosum in preventing transfer of information between the hemispheres.

Dejerine's thesis has received striking confirmation. In 1925 Foix and Hillemand (*14*) showed that destruction of the left visual cortex in the absence of a callosal lesion does not produce this syndrome. In 1937 Trescher and Ford (*15*) described the first case in which a surgical lesion of the corpus callosum was shown to have a definite effect. Their patient had sustained section of the posterior end of the corpus callosum for removal of a tumor from the third ventricle. The patient could not read in the left visual field, but could read normally on the right side. This result is implied by the Dejerine theory and was confirmed by Maspes in 1948 (*16*) and more recently by Gazzaniga, Bogen, and Sperry (*17*). Many authors have confirmed Dejerine's anatomical findings. Michael Fusillo and I studied a patient with alexia without agraphia who demonstrated another intriguing disorder (*18*, *19*). For approximately 3 months after his stroke he suffered from a disorder of verbal memory, which then cleared, leaving him with the reading difficulty, which remained unchanged until his death several months later. At postmortem, in addition to the anatomical findings of destruction of the left visual cortex and of the posterior end of the corpus callosum, the brain showed destruction of the left hippocampal region. It is now generally accepted that bilateral destruction of the hippocampal region leads to a permanent memory disorder. The transient memory disorder in our patient appeared to be the result of the destruction of the left hippocampal region — that is, the one located in the same hemisphere as the speech areas. Presumably it is the left hippocampal region which is necessary for the memory functions of speech cortex. After a period, the brain manages to compensate, presumably by making use of the opposite hippocampal region. Since publication of our paper (*18*), I have seen several other cases of this syndrome in which memory disorder was present at the onset. It is well known that the posterior cerebral artery supplies not only the visual cortex and the posterior end of the corpus callosum but also the hippocampal region. In a certain number of cases of occlusion of the left posterior cerebral artery, all of these structures are damaged. In other cases, however, the hippocampal region is spared. Meyer and Yates (*20*) and Milner (*4*) have demonstrated that, after removal of the left anterior temporal region for epilepsy, a verbal memory disorder is observed, which is, however, generally much milder than that found in the case Fusillo and I reported, and which is not present after right anterior temporal ablation. The mildness of the disorder after left temporal ablation is probably the result of the fact that these patients had suffered from left temporal epilepsy for years and had therefore already begun to use the right hippocampal region to a considerable degree.

ISOLATION OF THE SPEECH AREA

Another syndrome, called "isolation of the speech area," is explained readily by the Wernicke theory. This syndrome was described first by Kurt Goldstein (21) and has been described more recently by Geschwind, Quadfasel, and Segarra (22). We studied our patient for nearly 9 years after an episode of carbon monoxide poisoning. During this period she showed no evidence of language comprehension in the ordinary sense, and never uttered a sentence of propositional speech. She was totally helpless and required complete nursing care. In striking contrast to this state were her language performances in certain special areas. She would repeat perfectly, with normal articulation, sentences said to her by the examiner. She would, however, go beyond mere repetition, since she would complete phrases spoken by the examiner. For example, if he said, "Roses are red," she would say, "violets are blue, sugar is sweet, and so are you." Even more surprising, it was found that she was still capable of verbal learning. Songs which did not exist before her illness were played to her several times. Eventually, when the record player was started she would begin to sing. If the record player was then turned off she would continue singing the words and music correctly to the end, despite the lack of a model. Postmortem examination by Segarra showed a remarkable lesion, which was essentially symmetrical. The classical speech area, including Wernicke's area, Broca's area, and the connections between them, was intact, as were the auditory inflow pathways and the motor outflow pathways for the speech organs. In the regions surrounding the speech area either the cortex or the underlying white matter was destroyed. The speech area was indeed isolated. The patient's failure to comprehend presumably resulted from the fact that the language inputs could arouse no associations elsewhere in the brain, and since information from other portions of the brain could not reach the speech areas, there was no propositional speech. On the other hand the intactness of the speech region and its internal connections insured correct repetition. The preservation of verbal learning is particularly interesting. In addition to the speech area, the hippocampal region, which is involved in learning, was also preserved, and this probably accounts for her remarkable ability to carry on the memorizing of verbal material.

CALLOSAL SYNDROMES

Although pure alexia without agraphia (13) was the first syndrome in which damage to the corpus callosum was shown to play a role by interrupting transfer of information between the hemispheres, it was a group of Wernicke's students, including Hugo Liepmann, Kurt Goldstein, and Karl Bonhoeffer, who elucidated the full syndrome of callosal disconnection in cases in which eventually there was careful postmortem confirmation of the predicted sites of the lesions (11, 12). While the callosal syndromes continued to be recognized by German authors (23), their existence was either forgotten or indeed totally denied in the English-language literature. In November 1961, Edith Kaplan and I presented a patient to the Boston Society of Psychiatry and Neurology who was, we believed, suffering from a callosal disconnection syndrome—a diagnosis which was later confirmed at postmortem examination by Segarra. [Since that time several cases of confirmed callosal disconnection have been described (24).] I will mention here briefly only a few of the aspects of our patient's condition which fit into the Wernicke theory. When writing with the right hand the patient produced linguistically correct words and sentences and carried out calculations correctly. When writing with the left hand he produced incorrect words (for example, "run" for "go") and performed calculations incorrectly. The theory outlined above implies that, for writing to be carried out correctly with the left hand, the information must be transmitted from the speech areas across the corpus callosum, whose interruption in our patient explained his failures. Similarly, the patient could correctly name objects (concealed from vision) which he palpated with the right hand. On the other hand he would misname objects palpated with the left hand, although it could be shown by nonverbal means that his right hemisphere recognized the object. Thus, if a pencil was placed in his left hand the patient could draw the object previously held in that hand. Again, the Wernicke theory implies that, for an individual to correctly name an object held in the left hand, the information must be transmitted from the sensory regions in the right hemisphere to the speech regions via the corpus callosum, which had been destroyed in this patient. On the other hand, the patient could read in the left as well as the right visual field. This led us to conclude that the destruction of the corpus callosum had spared the posterior end, a prediction also confirmed at postmortem.

CEREBRAL DOMINANCE

Let me turn to another bit of knowledge which fits very well into the scheme presented above. One of the most remarkable features of man is cerebral dominance—that is, the fact that in the adult the capacities for speech are overwhelmingly controlled by the left hemisphere. Out of 100 adult aphasics, at least 96 percent have damage to the left side of the brain (25). We do not know of any example in any other mammal of a class of learning which is predominantly controlled by one half of the brain (26). What underlies human speech dominance? It is widely stated in the literature that the human brain is symmetrical, and this had led either to the assumption that speech dominance must reflect some subtle physiological difference between the hemispheres, or indeed even to the assumption that speech dominance is somehow acquired as the result of postnatal experience. My colleague Walter Levitsky and I (27) decided to reinvestigate this problem, particularly since we found that some earlier authors had claimed that there were in fact anatomical differences between the hemispheres. We demonstrated that such differences exist and are indeed readily visible to the naked eye. The area that lies behind the primary auditory cortex in the upper surface of the temporal lobe is larger on the left side in 65 percent of brains, and larger on the right in only 11 percent. This region on the left side is, on the average, nearly a centimeter longer than its fellow on the opposite side—that is, larger by one-third than the corresponding area on the right. More recently Wada (28) has confirmed our results. He has, in addition, studied this region in the brains of infants and has found that these differences are present at birth. This region which is larger in the left hemisphere is, in fact, a portion of Wernicke's area, whose major importance for speech was first shown nearly 100 years ago. It is reasonable to assume that there are other anatomical asymmetries in the hemispheres of the human brain, reflecting other aspects of dominance.

The study of the organization of the brain for language has been based of necessity on investigations in man. The bulk of our information in this area has come from careful studies of patients suffering from isolated damage as a result of vascular disease, whose brains have, after death, been subjected to careful anatomical examination. Disorders of language resulting from brain damage, almost always on the left side, are called aphasias. Carl Wernicke, nearly 100 years ago, described the linguistic differences between aphasias resulting from damage in different anatomical locations and outlined a theory of the organization of language in the brain. Not only have Wernicke's localizations stood up under repeated examination but his theory has been the only one which as permitted the prediction of new phenomena, or has been able to account for new observations. Several remarkable disorders, such as isolated disturbances of reading and the symptomatology of the corpus callosum, are examples of the explanatory power of this theory.

The phenomenon of cerebral dominance—that is, the predominant importance of one side of the brain for a class of learned behavior—occurs, as far as we know, in no mammal other than man. The dominance of the left side of the brain for speech is the most striking example of this phenomenon. Contrary to generally accepted views, there is a striking anatomical asymmetry between the temporal speech region on the left side and the corresponding region of the right hemisphere.

References and Notes

1. I have argued elsewhere that language is based on the striking development of the angular gyrus region in man, a region which receives inputs from all cortical sensory areas [see N. Geschwind, in *Monograph Series on Languages and Linguistics, No. 17* (Georgetown Univ. Press, Washington, D.C., 1964), pp. 155–169; *Brain* 88, 237 (1965); *ibid.*, p. 585]. D. Pandya and H. Kuypers [*Brain Res.* 13, 13 (1969)] have shown that a forerunner of this region exists in the macaque. R. A. Gardner and B. T. Gardner [*Science* 165, 664 (1969)] and D. Premack (in a paper presented at the Symposium on Cognitive Processes of Nonhuman Primates, Pittsburgh, March 1970) have described what appears to be a definite degree of linguistic behavior in chimpanzees.

2. A. R. Luria, *Traumatic Aphasia* (Mouton, The Hague, 1969).

3. O. Foerster, in *Handbuch der Neurologie*, O. Bumke and O. Foerster, Eds. (Springer, Berlin, 1936), vol. 6, pp. 1–448; W. Penfield and L. Roberts, *Speech and Brain-Mechanisms* (Princeton Univ. Press, Princeton, N.J., 1959).

4. See for example, B. Milner, in *Interhemispheric Relations and Cerebral Dominance*, V. B. Mountcastle, Ed. (Johns Hopkins Press, Baltimore, 1962), pp. 177–195.

5. J. Wada and T. Rasmussen, *J. Neurosurg.* **17**, 266 (1960); C. Branch, B. Milner, T. Rasmussen, *ibid.* **21**, 399 (1964).

6. A. L. Benton [*Cortex* **1**, 314 (1964)] summarizes the earlier literature; R. J. Joynt (*ibid.*, p. 206) gives an account of Broca's contributions.

7. C. Wernicke, *Der aphasische Symptomen-complex* (Franck and Weigert, Breslau, 1874). An English translation has recently appeared in *Boston Studies in the Philosophy of Science*, R. S. Cohen and M. W. Wartofsky, Eds. (Reidel, Dordrecht, 1969), vol. 4, pp. 34–97. For a more complete evaluation of Wernicke's work, see N. Geschwind, *ibid.*, pp. 1–33.

8. R. Jakobson [in *Brain Function*, E. C. Carterette, Ed. (Univ. of California Press, Berkeley, 1966), vol. 3, pp. 67–92] has given a vivid description of these linguistic differences.

9. N. Geschwind, *Cortex* **1**, 214 (1964).

10. H. Head, *Aphasia and Kindred Disorders of Speech* (Cambridge Univ. Press, London, 1926).

11. H. Liepmann, *Drei Aufsatze aus dem Apraxiegebiet* (Karger, Berlin, 1908).

12. N. Geschwind, *Brain* **88**, 237 (1965); *ibid.*, p. 585. There is another, less readily understood, lesion in some cases of pure word deafness which is discussed in these two communications.

13. J. Dejerine, *Mem. Soc. Biol.* **4**, 61 (1892).

14. C. Foix and P. Hillemand, *Bull. Mem. Soc. Med. Hop. Paris* **49**, 393 (1925).

15. J. H. Trescher and F. R. Ford, *Arch. Neurol. Psychiat.* **37**, 959 (1937).

16. P. E. Maspes, *Rev. Neurol.* **80**, 100 (1948).

17. M. S. Gazzaniga, J. E. Bogen, R. W. Sperry, *Brain* **88**, 221 (1965).

18. N. Geschwind and M. Fusillo, *Arch. Neurol.* **15**, 137 (1966).

19. For a review of the different varieties of alexia, see D. F. Benson and N. Geschwind, in *Handbook of Clinical Neurology*, P. J. Vinken and G. W. Bruyn, Eds. (North-Holland, Amsterdam, 1969), vol. 4, pp. 112–140.

20. V. Meyer and H. J. Yates, *J. Neurol. Neurosurg. Psychiat.* **18**, 44 (1955).

21. K. Goldstein, *Die transkortikalen Aphasien* (Fischer, Jena, 1917).

22. N. Geschwind, F. A. Quadfasel, J. M. Segarra, *Neuropsychologia* **4**, 327 (1968).

23. J. Lange, in *Handbuch der Neurologie*, O. Bumke and O. Foerster, Eds. (Springer, Berlin, 1936), vol. 6, pp. 885–960; O. Sittig, *Über Apraxie* (Karger, Berlin, 1931).

24. N. Geschwind and E. Kaplan, *Neurology* **12**, 675 (1962); M. S. Gazzaniga, J. E. Bogen, R. W. Sperry, *Proc. Nat. Acad. Sci. U.S.* **48**, 1765 (1962).

25. For a review, see O. Zangwill, *Cerebral Dominance and Its Relation to Psychological Function* (Thomas, Springfield, Ill., 1960).

26. In *submammalian* forms there are examples of behaviors whose neural control appears to be predominantly unilateral—for example, bird song [see F. Nottebohm, *Science* **167**, 950 (1970)]. these may represent, not an earlier stage of dominance, but rather a separate development.

27. N. Geschwind and W. Levitsky, *Science* **161**, 186 (1968).

28. J. Wada, paper presented at the 9th International Congress of Neurology, New York, 1969.

29. The work discussed has been supported in part by grant NS 06209 from the National Institutes of Health to the Boston University School of Medicine.

27

Broca's Area and Broca's Aphasia

Jay P. Mohr

[. . .]

THE CLINICAL SYNDROME OF BROCA'S APHASIA AND ITS ANATOMIC FOUNDATION

The literature contains a long list of articles concerning a syndrome referred to as Broca's aphasia. In most of these articles, primary emphasis has been placed on the description of the clinical features, with much less effort devoted to autopsy correlation of the clinical syndrome with the lesion topography.

The clinical features of the syndrome that have evolved in the literature over the past 110 years are more complex, involve more evidence of deficit in

Excerpts reprinted from *Studies in Neurolinguistics*, Haiganoosh Whitaker & Harry A. Whitaker, eds.; J. P. Mohr, "Broca's Area and Broca's Aphasia," 1979, with permission from Elsevier. This paper was supported by grants HL 14888-02, NS 10828-01A1, and HS 00188.

The author was at the Massachusetts General Hospital and Harvard Medical School, Boston, Massachusetts.

language usage, including easily documented deficits in "comprehension," appear more severe, and are much more thoroughly described than those met in the older literature, which presents autopsy data showing infarction limited to LF3 and its immediate surroundings. However, the uncomfortable possibility suggested by the more complex clinical syndrome is that the underlying lesion far exceeds that of LF3 and adjacent structures.

Despite the impressive list of authors who have written on Broca's aphasia, many have not cited personal cases that document their views, and few have provided autopsy or other laboratory evidence corroborating the lesion topography. In some, even the etiology of the case material has been unclear. Vascular material appears to have been the source material for Broca, Wernicke, Déjerine, Marie, Liepmann, Alajouanine, Nielsen, Kreindler and Fradis, and Goodglass, Quadfasel, and Timberlake. War material was used by Head, Kleist, Goldstein, Conrad, Russell and Espir, and Luria. Weisenburg and McBridge, and deAjuriaguerra and Hécaen, used a wide etiologic spectrum of cases. Brown presented an abscess case. Textbook authors usually have not specified their material. Included in this group are Brain, Critchley, Lhermitte and Gautier, Benson and Geschwind, and Adams and Mohr.

Perhaps as troublesome has been the frequently unstated time course over which the syndrome changed from or to the state described as Broca's aphasia. In the few cases reported, the late description of a deficit referred to as Broca's aphasia is better correlated with a lesion far larger than Broca's area, as illustrated in Tables 27–1 and 27–2. The two notable exceptions were Broca's own cases, further described at the end of this review.

Traditional Formulations of Broca's Aphasia

Wernicke (1874) might be credited with the first textbook characterization of Broca's aphasia. In 1874, he confined his remarks to a few simple features without citing actual cases: following "destruction of the speech movement images . . . the patient understands everything but has either suddenly become mute or has at most a few simple words at his disposal" (p. 57).

By 1908 (Wernicke, 1908, pp. 272–273) his description had enlarged considerably under the term *motor aphasia*, which he equated with *Broca's aphemia*, due to involvement of Broca's convolution. Still without cited cases, Wernicke described three main features:

1. "The power of articulate speech is wanting. The patients have forgotten the process, the mechanism, which they formerly called into action to produce its sounds." He considered the patients mute or at best minimally able to speak, using "senseless syllables," short words or phrases, profane expressions. Dyspraxia of bulbar musculature for other movements, right lower facial and tongue weakness, but no elementary weakness of the bulbar musculature were also described.

2. "In the main, the power of understanding speech is retained at least this appears to be the case on ordinary tests. . . . There is almost invariably a certain inability to understand complicated constructions and the finer differentiations of speech. . . . I no longer am of the opinion that in pure motor aphasia the ability to understand speech always remains unim-

paired." Here Wernicke considerably modified his earlier views, but did not indicate whether he considered this wider deficit to reflect a lesion larger than Broca's area.

3. "Written language . . . is lost simultaneously with articulate speech." This statement is the first of along series of opinions concerning the intimate relationship between written and spoken speech stemming from Broca's original cases.

Wernicke considered the prognosis "generally unfavorable" for restoration of speech function.

This complex, severe, and persisting syndrome, together with the inference that Broca's area is the site of the responsible lesion, has persisted largely unchanged over the years under the label motor or Broca's aphasia (Adams & Mohr, 1974; Bastian, 1897; Benson & Geschwind, 1971; Brain, 1962; Brown, 1972; Déjerine & Mirallié, 1896; Hécaen, 1972; Heilbronner, 1910; Kreindler & Fradis, 1968; Lhermitte & Gautier, 1969; Lichtheim, 1885; Liepmann, 1915; Nielsen, 1962; Weisenburg & McBride, 1964; Wyllie, 1894). This description has also found application in war-injury studies where efforts have been made to correlate the clinical deficit with the skull defect or operative findings (Conrad, 1954; Goldstein, 1948; Head, 1926; Russell & Espir, 1961).

Several earlier authors took the trouble to present exemplary personal case reports and/or excerpted cases from the literature (Lichtheim, Wyllie, Bastian, Weisenburg and McBride, Nielsen), but only Dejerine appears to have published autopsied case reports.

Remarkably, despite the paucity of autopsy material for this larger syndrome, most of the differences of opinion revolve around individual features of the syndrome, in particular the explanations for deficits in behavior apart from disordered speaking. Disturbance in silent reading "comprehension" has been noted since the earliest reviews (Bastian, 1897; Wyllie, 1894). The explanations of dyslexia are typified by Bastian (1897):

In reading, a proper comprehension of the meaning of the text requires a conjoint revival of the words in the visual and the auditory word-centres, but that for this mere comprehension it is not necessary for the stimulus to pass on also to the glossokinesthetic (Broca's) centre, as it must do in reading aloud. It may, however, be freely admitted that if the way is open, and this latter centre is in a

TABLE 27–1. Autopsy Documented Cases of Broca's or Total Aphasia Found in the Literature[a]

*F3 B 51 Broca (case Leborgne)

SYL T 23 Dejerine (Moutier 70)

SYL T . . Moutier (case Maillard)

SYL B . . Bastian (Moutier 98)

OI T . . Mills (Henschen 1069)

FOI B 45 Bernard (Moutier 84)

SYL B 59 Moutier (case Chissadon)

FOI B 55 Preston (Moutier 96)

FOI B . . Broadbent (Moutier 51)

SYL T . . Vulpian & Mongie (Moutier 40)

SYL T 80 Bernard (Moutier 86)

SYL T 54 Bernheim (Moutier 90)

SYL T . . Comte

*F3 B . . Broca (case Lelong)

SYL T 39 Giraud (Moutier 64)

SYL B . . Archambault (Moutier 31)

FOI T 43 Pitres (Moutier 74)

FOI B 25 Lange (Moutier 52)

SYL T . . Bleuler (Moutier 92)

EN B . . Ballet (Moutier 132)

FOI T 80 Moutier (case Fauchier)

SYL B 56 Skwotzoff (Moutier 78)

F3 B 25 Baldisseri (Henschen 719)

SYL T 39 Rosenthal (Moutier 78)

F3 B 25 Böe (Henschen 779)

F3 B 43 Ballet & Boix (Moutier 130)

F3 B . . Rosenstein (Wyllie 3)

F3 B 45 Atkins

F3 B . . Magnan

F3 B 61 Chauffard & Rathery (Henschen 849)

F3 B . . Malicherg (Henschen 1052)

FOI T 69 Demange (Moutier 80)

F3 B . . Ogle

F3 B . . Sheinker & Kuhr

F3 B . . Magnan

F3 B 55 Nielsen (case Lulu)

F3 B 50 Hervey (Moutier 127)

F3 B . . Banti (Bastian 7)

F3 B 68 Nielsen (case Ingols)

| 10 | 20 | 30 | 10 | 20 | 30 | 10 | 20 | 30 | 10 | 20 | 30 |
| Days | | | Weeks | | | Months | | | Years | | |

(Time after onset when the last or only examination was described in the Case Report)

[a]Key: F3 Broca's area (3rd Frontal), FOI frontal operculum and anterior insula, OI operculum and insula, SYL Sylvian region, EN encephalitis, B Broca's aphasia, T total aphasia, . . age not stated, PH putaminal hemorrhage.

TABLE 27–2. Autosopy Documental Cases of Broca's Aphasia Considerd Ameliorated Found in Literature

OI B 32 Monakow (Henschen 1113)

OI T 57 Improved Monakow (Henschen 1114)

OI T 45 Improved Dejerine (Henschen 866)

F3 B 20 Disappeared Luys (Henschen 1031)

F3 B . . Recovered Wadham

F3 B 20 Recovered Dejerine (Henschen 865)

FOI B 61 Ameliorated Leva (Moutier 95)

OI T 25 Recovered Lange (Henschen 986)

F3 B 25 Improved DeFont (Henschen 905)

F3 B . . None Bourneville

PH B 61 Improved Nielsen

OI B 62 Improved . . . Cured DuFour (Henschen 885)

F3 B 20 Rapid Foulis (Henschen 908)

OI B 38 Later DuFour (Henschen 883)

F3 B 32 Rapidly Dejerine (Henschen 871)

F3 B 70 Cleared Bramwell

F3 B Transient Tuke

F3 B 65 Improving . . . . Normal Simon (Henschen 1240)

F3 B . . 10 Days Barlow

F3 B 49 Cleared Monokow (Henschen 1116)

10	20	30	10	20	30	12	15	25	35	5	10	15	20
Days			Weeks			Months				Years			

(Time after onset when initial examination was described, followed by repeat examination or comment regarding outcome)

[a]Key: F3 Broca's area (3rd Frontal), FOI frontal operculum and anterior insula, OI operculum and insula, SYL Sylvian region, EN encephalitis, B Broca's aphasia, T total aphasia, . . age not stated, PH putaminal hemorrhage.

healthy condition, it does commonly receive in reading to one's self a slight stimulus from the auditory word-centre, a fact which is often enough shown by the occurrence of involuntary half-whispered mutterings when reading. It may also be admitted that the rousing of all three centres does give assistance in the comprehension of anything difficult, as is shown by the common practice of reading aloud any passage the meaning of which may be at all obscure [p. 1009].

This principle has remained the explanation offered into modern times (Luria, 1966, p. 190).

Auditory comprehension and other disturbances in language formulations have been less easily explained. Opinion has been divided as to whether or not such disturbances even occur. Lichtheim (1885, p. 471), Wyllie (1894, pp. 318–319), Bastian (1897,

p. 1005), and Liepmann (1915, pp. 526–527) considered motor aphasia to be free of such deficits. Others concurred with Wernicke's views (Déjerine & Mirallié, 1896, pp. 102–105; Heilbronner, 1910, pp. 1021–1028). Marie (1906b) took the extreme position that Broca's aphasia represents Wernicke's aphasia plus anarthria. Modern authors' views on this point are less clearly stated, partially because the current, revised syndrome lays stress on different features of the deficit (as will be explained further).

Writing disturbances have been explained by citing two separate mechanisms. Bastian (1897), almost alone in his opinion, maintained that any dysgraphia is secondary to involvement outside Broca's area, usually affecting the second frontal gyrus, so-called "Exner's writing center." A few subsequent authors (Brain, 1962; Henschen, 1925) have entertained these views, while others (Mohr et al., 1973) have been content to indicate a certain degree of independence between writing and speaking performances without making anatomic inferences. The overwhelming weight of opinion has favored a coexisting deficit in writing and speaking. Where anatomic comments are included, the lesion is considered to involve Broca's area and need be no larger. The opinions of Jackson (1932) typify most authors: "speaking is propositionizing . . . that the speechless patient cannot propositionize *aloud* is obvious—he never does. But this is only the superficial part of the truth. He cannot propositionize internally . . . the proof that he does not speak internally is that he cannot express himself in writing. . . . He can say nothing to himself, and therefore has nothing to write." Given such reasoning, little additional explanation was required to account for the easily observed deficits in auditory comprehension noted by all authors, including Liepmann (1915), Pick (1973), Isserlin (1936), Lhermitte and Gautier (1969), Brown (1972), and others. None—as best can be determined by the present reviewer—based their views on personal cases with pathoanatomic correlation of the clinical deficits. Yet none expressed disagreement that the lesion lay in Broca's area.

Of the many features of this larger syndrome referred to as Broca's aphasia, the deficit in spoken speech has received the greatest attention. Broca (1861) has described the recurrent utterances and partial syllables that characterized the limited speaking behavior of his two patients. Jackson (1932), Wernicke (1908), Liepmann (1915), Pick (1973), Kleist (1934), Alajouanine, Ombrédane, and Durand (1939), Goodglass *et al.* (1964), and Brown (1972) have written and rewritten the basic features of verbal stereotypes, recurrent utterances, and condensed grammatical sentence structure that characterize speaking in cases of Broca's aphasia. Save for Kleist (1934), none have described clinical cases with individual pathologic correlation, although all authors have stated or implied that the lesion lies in Broca's area or immediately surrounding regions or needs to involve no additional areas for this characteristic speaking performance. In modern times, the work of Goodglass *et al.* (1964) provides an exemplary documentation of the clinical and linguistic features in clinical cases referred to as Broca's aphasia. Twenty-two of 53 patients studied with the Boston Veterans Administration Diagnostic Aphasia Test were characterized as cases of Broca's aphasia. They showed poor scores on melodic line, length of uninterrupted word groups, verbal agility in articulation, and correct grammatical form. Virtually no jargon in connected speech, impaired auditory comprehension, or problems in naming objects were found. The cases studied were all allowed at least two months after stroke onset before they were studied. Of particular interest to the present reviewer was the remark that "It appeared that most Broca's aphasics either remained grossly impaired or quickly attained a level of residual aphasia in which the classical features of agrammatism, telegraphic speech, and laborious articulation were no longer apparent." (Goodglass *et al.*, 1964). These observations corroborate those of the present review (Mohr *et al.*, 1975) that rapid amelioration of speech deficit occurs (in the local Broca's-area infarct), or when persisting, severe deficit is found in which disturbed language function is easily demonstrated (in the larger syndrome of Sylvian operculum infarction). Like most other authors, Goodglass *et al.* (1964) had no autopsy correlation in their clinical cases, but they appeared to consider that the presumed infarction involved Broca's area, since they speculated that "Broca's area contains critical structures which are so concentrated that a direct injury is likely to be permanently and severely damaging to speech." This speculation, based as it was on the litany, and not on the personal autopsy experience of the authors, is representative of the degrees to which this larger syndrome has been considered to reflect Broca's-area infarction by most authors.

Several authors have been impressed with the deficits in language behavior other than speaking to a degree that serious doubts were raised as to whether the term *motor aphasia* is appropriate for such cases. The painstaking work of Weisenburg and McBride (1964) represents some of the most detailed documentation of this larger deficit. Their criticisms of the concept of motor aphasia were based on a thorough literature review and 42 personal cases of "expressive" or "expressive–receptive" aphasia. Their efforts clearly documented the larger deficit and their reasons for objecting to motor aphasia as an inappropriate concept, but their case material could scarcely be considered an appropriate source for criticisms of the anatomic basis of the syndrome: Their 42 cases encompassed a broad etiologic spectrum including ischemic stroke, hemorrhage, tumor, cyst, gunshot wound, and subdural hematoma. None of the cases were autopsied, and in the early 1930s, save for the rare operated case, the topography of the lesion in each case was inferred on clinical criteria alone. The opportunity to relate the larger syndrome to a brain lesion far exceeding the confines of Broca's area and immediately adjacent brain tissue was not taken up by Weisenburg and McBride nor by a large number of other authors who also pointed out that the syndrome involved a deficit in language functions apart from that evident in speaking aloud. With few exceptions, Broca's-area lesion has been considered sufficient to cause this large deficit.

Kleist (1934, p. 930) considered the persisting and severe deficit to require infarction deep into the hemisphere, so as to disrupt the white matter fibers that served as projection and association pathways for Broca's area. By inference, these deeper lesions would mean a larger infarct, although Kleist did not specify the upper division of the left middle-cerebral artery as such. Foix (1928) earlier had made a similar inference by referring to deeper branches of the middle-cerebral artery. Goldstein (1948, pp. 204–205) made suggestions similar to those of Kleist, but also failed to specify the vascular territory involved in the larger lesion. Remarkably few cases of this larger syndrome have been autopsied and described in the literature (see Tables 27–1 and 27–2); those reported have proven difficult to classify simply as Broca's aphasia because they were examined only in the late stages, raising the possibility that they represented improved total aphasia.

The theoretic problems raised by the notions of total aphasia reflect sufficiently on those of Broca's aphasia to warrant further consideration of total aphasia. The term emerged in the late 19th century in the works of most textbook authors (Déjerine & Mirallié, 1896; Heilbronner, 1910; Liepmann, 1915; Wernicke, 1908). Liepmann's (1915) account is typical:

> More frequently than a lesion confined to the *frontal* or *temporal* speech region, we find, as a result of the arterial distribution bringing all the blood in the whole region of speech, through the *Art. foss. sylvii*, lesions, that affect both regions, and therefore causing *total* or almost total (motor and sensory) aphasia. Following the retrogression of the word-deafness, one sees, years later, a clinical picture, in which the symptoms of *motor* aphasia predominate. Word-dumbness conceals the paraphasia; the disturbance of speech understanding is no longer very serious. Writing and reading . . . are very poor. Hence it happens, that old cases, in which the lesions occur in both speech regions, are often classed clinically only as motor aphasia.

> In these cases, disturbances in speaking, writing and reading, are particularly stable [pp. 529–530]. (emphasis Liepmann)

This description by Liepmann bears a close resemblance to that currently referred to as Broca's aphasia in the later stages.

The existence of this syndrome prompts a detailed examination of the timecourse data for published cases labeled as Broca's aphasia. Protocols for most of the wholly clinically described cases of Broca's aphasia usually show that the authors dealt with chronic cases, at least two months (Goodglass *et al.*, 1964), as long as six years (Alajouanine *et al.*, 1939), and ten years (Goldstein, 1948, case 6, pp. 208–245) after onset. The autopsy material (Tables 27–1 and 27–2) further reveals that the later a case labeled as Broca's aphasia is documented clinically, the greater the likelihood that a large lesion is found at autopsy. This material also documents the frequency with which cases quite similar in detailed clinical features are given the label total aphasia (Tables 27–1 and 27–2).

Personal Observations

Mohr *et al.* (1975) have succeeded in acquiring autopsy or other laboratory corroboration of lesion topography for ten cases suffering cerebral infarction, all of whom broadly satisfied the criteria currently used for Broca's aphasia months after their stroke. Seven were studied by computerized axial tomogram (CT scan), two by arteriogram, and one by autopsy. The lesion topography in each case far exceeded Broca's area. In most, the lesion was best explained by total or near-total infarction of the area of supply of the upper division of the left middle-cerebral artery, encompassing the operculum from anterior frontal through Broca's area (LF3) to anterior parietal regions, the insula, both banks of the central (Rolandic) fissure, the entire infarct usually extending deep into the hemisphere (Fig. 27–1).

The initial deficit in these cases was uniformly severe, closely approximating Liepmann's (1915) descriptions of total aphasia. They later evolved, as described by Liepmann (1915), toward a state more or less conforming to current descriptions of Broca's aphasia. In all cases the later syndrome emerged from one more severe. Weeks, but usually months and occasionally years were required before this later state was fully established.

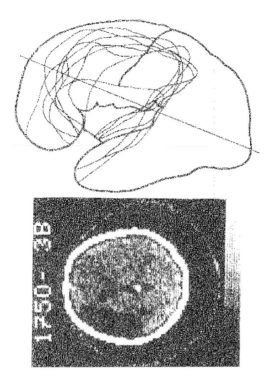

FIGURE 27–1. (*Top*) Syndrome of infarction in the upper division of the middle cerebral artery, projected on a lateral view of the left hemisphere. (*Bottom*) An example of a computed tomography scan with the large lesion evident. The plane of section for the scan is indicated by the line drawn through the top diagram. (Figure scanned from original article.)

All cases experienced hemiplegia at onset. None were able to stand for over a week; all walked with a heavy circumducted gait, the arm essentially useless, the right lower face densely paretic. The six seen the day of onset experienced head and conjugate eye deviation to the side of the lesion, all six improving to full head and eye control within a week. Hemianopia was present for several days. After several months, a syndrome of spastic hemiparesis still disabled all patients although they achieved independence with a cane after prolonged physiotherapy.

Initially, all cases were mute and unable to write legibly with either hand; most graphic efforts were hopeless loops or marks without communicative value. Evidence of disturbed comprehension, for many complete, was present in auditory and visual language tasks. Two cases followed for years (Mohr *et al.*, 1973) underwent steady evolution toward much improved auditory comprehension, but began to speak only after ten months in one case, three years

in the other. The most successful improvements occurred in two other cases, who performed Marie's three-paper test correctly at three months in the case of a 25-year-old left-handed man, and seven months in a 44-year-old right-handed man. Save for these two cases, deficits in language tasks were easily demonstrated months and even years after onset, if testing was carried beyond ordinary social conversation into more formal years, particularly in spelling. All patients emerged from mutism into stereotype utterances, which soon became agrammatic laconic efforts at spontaneous speech; this difficulty was similarly reflected in misspelled dysgrammatic efforts at writing. Considerable variation in dyspraxia of the upper extremities, oral, and respiratory apparatus was observed.

Corroborative cases were culled from the retrospective autopsy series from the Massachusetts General Hospital for a 10-year period (mentioned previously). Fifteen of the 39 cases of left-cerebral infarction affecting the territory of supply of the upper division of the left middle-cerebral artery were described as having deficits in speaking and in language use persisting months and years, conforming (where data was available) to features broadly classifiable as Broca's aphasia. In all such cases, the lesion far exceeded Broca's area, usually involving the bulk of the territory of supply of the upper division.

Formulation of the Syndrome of Upper Division Infarction

These personal and retrospective autopsy cases, compared with the few described and the fewer autopsied cases in the literature, prompt a formulation of this syndrome that differs from the traditional and current notions of Broca's aphasia.

Broca's aphasia, as currently defined, is not a result of infarction of Broca's area and immediate surrounds. It reflects a major infarction involving most of the territory of supply of the upper division of the left middle-cerebral artery. As a clinical entity, the evidence to date suggests that the deficit profile known as Broca's aphasia is observed only later after the infarction. The initial syndrome is more severe, described traditionally as total aphasia. After weeks or months, the gradual emergence of stereotypes, agrammatism, and protracted dyspraxia in speaking evolves slowly toward the long-standing deficit profile of Broca's aphasia, which remains little changed after months and years.

Subsequent studies may reveal that the complex syndrome of Broca's aphasia can occur acutely, without evolving from the more obvious syndrome of total aphasia. But in such case, the prediction is made that a large lesion will be found, far exceeding Broca's area.

This formulation of the upper-division syndrome makes the terms *Broca's aphasia* and *total aphasia* seem inexact, even inappropriate in principle. Neither convey the anatomic or functional implications implicit in this new formulation. The upper-division syndrome is a complex, wide-ranging deficit profile, involving formulation and production of spoken and written communication, including "central" language functions as well as the more elemental organization of sensory, motor, and praxic skills for execution of such spoken and written efforts. The major disorganization of these systems is more easily understood when the great extent and depth of the lesion are appreciated. Less fanciful explanations are required to account for the deficit, and the long periods of time required for improvement are more easily accounted for than by traditional implications that all this complex behavior depended upon the herculean homuncular functions of Broca's area. Although much of the mystique of aphasiology might be lost by these formulations of the upper-division syndrome, a close alignment with views of cerebral functions based on other physiologic studies might be the result.

BROCA'S CASES

In retrospect, had Broca emphasized the extent of the lesion topography in his two cases, he might have prevented over a century of controversy. When account is taken of lesion topography, Broca's cases appear relatively straightforward examples of the upper-division syndrome now referred to as Broca's aphasia: two chronic cases, seen 18 months and 10 years, respectively, after infarction, having severe speaking deficit confined to limited verbal stereotypes, conversationally satisfactory "comprehension," and, in the one case with autopsy findings, major infarction affecting the territory of supply of the upper division of the left middle-cerebral artery (Fig. 27–2).

Broca saw neither case acutely. He used only conversational and not more formal grammatical tasks such as spelling, which might have shown a deficient performance sharply contrasting with the conversa-

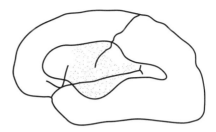

FIGURE 27–2. Topography of the infarct found in Broca's case Lebornge (drawing traced from Moutier).

tional evidence of good comprehension. In accordance with then-current ideas that stroke disease affected the brain in a slowly expanding fashion (Marie, 1906b), Broca understandably sought the site of "origin" of the stroke; he deliberately ignored the larger zone of infarction (which he considered the later spreading effect of the stroke) in favor of the portion involving the inferior frontal region, where he envisaged the stroke "began." By faithfully adhering to then-current notions of the pathophysiology of stroke, Broca missed the opportunity to formulate for all time the clinical, temporal, and pathologic features of the upper-division middle cerebral artery syndrome that should justifiably bear his name. Instead, his name came to be associated with a syndrome improperly correlated with brain infarct topography and with an area of the brain whose infarction produces only a modest long-term clinical deficit.

To avoid future ambiguities, the terms *Broca's aphasia, total aphasia,* and even *Broca's area* might preferably fall into disuse, in favor of other terms, such as the opercular syndromes, that better describe the spectrum observed, including that end of the spectrum that Broca observed but did not interpret as such. Considering that Boulliaud gave Broca his original inspirations, the eclipse of Broca's epomyn seems a less than historic tragedy, since Boulliaud's own efforts have already largely passed into oblivion.

References

Adams, R. D., Mohr, J. P. 1974. Affections of speech. In M. M. Wintrobe *et al.* (Eds.), *Harrison's principles of internal medicine.* (7th ed.) New York: McGraw-Hill, Pp. 137–148.

Alajouanine, T., Ombrédane, A., & Durand, M. 1939. *Le syndrome de désintégration phonétique dans l'aphasie.* Paris: Masson.

Atkins, R. 1876. Case of sudden and complete aphasia and partial right hemiplegia, lesion of Broca's convolution, with a small haemorrhage in substance of corpus callosum &c. *Journal of Mental Science*, 22, 406–416.

Bailey, P., & von Bonin, G. 1951. *The isocortex of man.* Urbana: University of Illinois.

Bastian, H. C. 1897. Some problems in connexion with aphasia and other speech defects. *Lancet*, 1, 1005–1017, 1132–1137, 1187–1194.

Benson, D. F., & Geschwind, N. 1971. The aphasias and related disturbances. In A. B. Baker (Ed.), *Clinical neurology.* Vol. 1. New York: Harper. Pp. 1–25.

Bourneville. 1874b. Athérome généralisé: oblitérations multiples (aphasie; sphacèle du pied, etc.). *Progrès Médical*, 2(20), 278–280.

Bourneville. 1874b. Athérome généralisé: oblitérations multiples (aphasie; sphacèle du pied, etc.). *Progrès Médical*, 2(21), 296–298.

Brain, W. R. 1962. *Speech disorders.* London: Butterworths.

Bramwell, B. 1898. A remarkable case of aphasia. *Brain: A Journal of Neurology*, 21, 343–373.

Broca, P. 1861. Remarques sur le siége de la faculté du langage articulé, suivies d'une observation d'aphémie (perte de la parole). *Bulletins de la Société Anatomique de Paris*, 6, 330–357.

Brodmann, K. 1909. *Vergleichende Lokalisationslehre der Grosshirnrinde in ihren Prinzipien dargestellt auf Grund des Zellenbaues.* Leipzig: Barth.

Brown, J. W. 1972. *Aphasia, apraxia and agnosia.* Springfield, Ill.: Charles C Thomas.

Bruandet (Interne des hopitaux). 1900. Un cas d'hemispasme facial. *Revue Neurologique*, 8, 658–660.

Bruyn, G. W., and Gathier, J-C. 1970. The operculum syndrome. In P. J. Vinken & G. W. Bruyn (Eds.), *Handbook of clinical neurology.* Vol. 2. Amsterdam: North-Holland Publ. Pp. 776–783.

Chouppe. 1870. Ramollissement superficiel du cerveau intéressant surtout la troisième circonvolution frontale gauche, sans aphasie. *Bulletins de la Société Anatomique de Paris*, 45, 365–366.

Cole, M. F., & Cole, M. 1971. *Pierre Marie's papers on speech disorders.* New York: Hafner.

Comte, A. 1900. *Des paralysies pseudo-bulbaires.* (Thesis) 8°, No. 436. Paris: Steinheil.

Conrad, K. 1954. New problems of aphasia. *Brain: A Journal of Neurology*, 77(4), 491–509.

Critchley, MacD. 1970. *Aphasiology and other aspects of language.* London: Arnold.

DeAjuriaguerra, J., and Hécaen, H. 1964. *Le cortex cérébral.* Paris: Masson.

deBoyer, H. C. 1879. *Études topographiques sur les lésions corticales des hémisphères cérébraux.* (Thesis) Paris: Delahaye.

Déjerine, J. 1885. Étude sur l'aphasie dans lésions de l'insula de Reil. *Revue de Médecine (Paris)*, 5, 174–191.

Déjerine, J. 1891. Contribution à l'étude de l'aphasie motrice sous corticale et de la localisation cérébrale des centres laryngés (muscles phonateures). *Comptes Rendus Hebdomadaires des Séances et Mémoires de la Socièté de Biologie*, 3, 155–162.

Déjerine, J. 1906. L'aphasie motrice. Sa localisation et sa physiologie pathologique. *Presse Medicale*, 14(57), 453–457.

Déjerine, J., & Mirallié, C. 1896. *L'aphasie sensorielle.* Paris: Steinheil.

Flechsig, P. 1901. Developmental (myelogenetic) Localisation of the cerebral cortex in the human subject. *Lancet*, ii, 1027–1029.

Foix, C. 1928. Aphasies. In G. H. Roger, F. Widal, & P. J. Teissier (Eds.), *Nouveau traité de médecine.* Vol. 18. P. 135. Paris: Masson et Cie.

Foulis, D. 1879. A case in which there was destruction of the third left frontal convolution without aphasia. *British Medical Journal*, 1, 383–384.

Friedlich, A. L., Castleman, B., & Mohr, J. P. 1968. Sudden stroke in a woman with dyspnea and anemia. *New England Journal of Medicine*, 278, 1109–1118.

Geschwind, N. 1965a. Disconnexion syndromes in animals and man: I. *Brain: A Journal of Neurology*, 88, 237–294.

Geschwind, N. 1965b. Disconnexion syndromes in animals and man: II. *Brain: A Journal of Neurology*, 88, 585–644.

Goldstein, K. 1948. *Language and language disturbances.* New York: Grune & Stratton.

Goodglass, H., & Kaplan, E. 1972. *The assessment of aphasia and related disorders.* Philadelphia: Lea & Febiger.

Goodglass, H., Quadfasel, F. A., & Timberlake, W. T. 1964. Phase length and type and severity of aphasia. *Cortex*, 1, 133–153.

Head, H. 1926. *Aphasia and kindred disorders of speech.* New York: Macmillan.

Hécaen, H. 1972. *Introduction à la neuropsychologie.* Paris: Larousse (Librairie).

Heilbronner, K. 1910. Die aphasischen, apraktischen und agnostischen Störungen. In M. Lewandowsky (Ed.), *Handbuch der Neurologie.* Vol. 1. Berlin: Springer-Verlag. Pp. 982–1093.

Henschen, S. E. 1922. *Klinische und pathologische Beiträge zur Pathologie des Gehirns.* Vol. VII. Stockholm: Nordiske Bokhandeln.

Henschen, S. E. 1925. Clinical and anatomical contributions on brain pathology; (Abstracts and comments by Walter F. Schaller); Fifth Part: Aphasia, amusia and akalkulia. *Archives of Neurology and Psychiatry*, 13, 226–249.

Isserlin, M. 1936. Aphasie. In O. Bumke and O. Foerster (Eds.), *Handbuch der Neurologie*. Vol. 6. Berlin: Springer-Verlag. Pp. 627–806.

Jackson, J. H. 1932. *Selected writings*. London: Hodder & Stoughton.

Jefferson, G. 1950. Localization of function in the cerebral cortex. *British Medical Bulletin*, 6, 333–340.

Kleist, K. 1934. *Gehirnpathologie*. Leipzig: Barth.

Kreindler, A., & Fradis, A. 1968. *Performances in aphasia*. Paris: Gauthier-Villars.

Kugler, J. 1964. *Electroencephalography in hospital and general consulting practice*. Amsterdam: Elsevier.

Lhermitte, F., & Gautier, J.-C. 1969. Aphasia. In R. J. Vinken & G. W. Bruyn (Eds.), *Handbook of clinical neurology*. Vol. 4. Amsterdam: North-Holland Publ. Pp. 84–104.

Lichtheim, L. 1885. On aphasia. *Brain: A Journal of Neurology*, 7, 433–484.

Liepmann, H. 1915. Diseases of the brain. In C. W. Barr (Ed.), *Curschmann's textbook on nervous diseases*. Vol. 1. Philadelphia: Blakiston. Pp. 467–551.

Luria, A. R. 1966. *Higher cortical functions in man*. New York: Basic Books.

McAdam, D. W., & Whitaker, H. A. 1971. Language production: Electroencephalographic localization in the normal human brain. *Science*, 172, 499–502.

Magnan. 1879. On simple aphasia, and aphasia with incoherence. *Brain: A Journal of Neurology*, 2, 112–123.

Marie, P. 1906a. Revision de la question de l'aphasie: L'aphasie de 1861 à 1866; essai de critique historique sur la genèse de la doctrine de Broca. *Semaine Médicale*, 26, 565–571.

Marie, P. 1906b. Revision de la question de l'aphasie: La troislème circonvolution frontale gauche ne joue aucun rôle spécial dans la fonction du langage. *Semaine Médicale*, 26, 241–247.

Marie, P. 1906c. Revision de la question de l'aphasie: Que faut-il penser des aphasies sous-corticales (aphasies pures)? *Semaine Médicale*, 26, 493–500.

Marie, P. 1907. Rectifications à propos de la question de L'aphasie. *Presse Medicale*, 15(4), 25–26.

Marie, P., & Moutier, F. 1906a. Examen du cerveau d'un cas d'aphasie de Broca. *Bulletins et Mémoires de la Société Médicale des Hopitaux de Paris*, 23, 743–744.

Marie, P., & Moutier, F. 1906b. Nouveau cas d'aphasie de Broca sans lésion de la troisième frontale gauche. *Bulletins et Mémoires de la Société Médicales des Hopitaux de Paris*, 23, 1180–1183.

Marie, P., & Moutier, F. 1906c. Nouveau cas de lésion corticale du pied de la 3e frontale gauche chez un droitier sans trouble du langage. *Bulletins et Mémoires de la Société Médicale des Hopitaux de Paris*, 23, 1295–1298.

Marie, P., & Moutier, F. 1906d. Sur un cas de ramollissement du pied de la 3e circonvolution frontale gauche chez un droitier, sans aphasie de Broca. *Bulletins et Mémoires de la Société Médicale des Hopitaux de Paris*, 23, 1152–1155.

Mettler, F. A. 1949. *Selective partial ablation of the frontal cortex: A correlative study of the effects on human psychotic subjects*. New York: Haeber.

Mohr, J. P. 1968. Cerebral control of speech. Letters to the Editor. *New England Journal of Medicine*, 279, 107.

Mohr, J. P. 1973. Rapid amelioration of motor aphasia. *Archives of Neurology*, 28, 77–82.

Mohr, J. P., Funkenstein, H., Finkelstein, S., Pessin, M., Duncan, G. W., & Davis, K. 1975. Broca's area infarction versus Broca's aphasia. *Neurology*, 25, 349.

Mohr, J. P., Leicester, J., Stoddard, L. T., & Sidman, M. 1971. Right hemianopia with memory and color deficits in circumscribed left posterior cerebral artery territory infarction. *Neurology*, 21, 1104–1113.

Mohr, J. P., Sidman, M., Stoddard, L. T., Leicester, J., & Rosenberger, P. B. 1973. Evolution of the deficit in total aphasia. *Neurology*, 23, 1302–1312.

Moutier, F. 1908. *L'aphasia de Broca*. (Thesis) Paris: Steinheil.

New, P. F. J., Scott, W. R., Schnur, J. A., Davis, K. R., & Taveras, J. M. 1974. Computerized axial tomography with the EMI scanner. *Radiology*, 110, 109–123.

Nielsen, J. M. 1962. *Agnosia, apraxia, aphasia*. New York: Hafner.

Ogle, W. 1867. Aphasia and agraphia. *St. George's Hospital Reports*, 2, 83–122.

Ojemann, R. G., Aronow, S., & Sweet, W. H. 1966. Scanning with positron-emitting isotopes in cerebrovascular diseases. *Acta Radiologica*, 5, 894–905.

Penfield, W. 1958. *The excitable cortex in conscious man*. Springfield, Ill.: Charles S Thomas.

Penfield, W., & Rasmussen, T. 1968. *The cerebral cortex of man*. New York: Hafner.

Penfield, W., & Roberts, L. 1959. *Speech and brain mechanisms*. Princeton, N.J.: Princeton University Press.

Pick, A. 1973. *Aphasia*. (Translated and edited by J. W. Brown) Springfield, Ill.: Charles C Thomas.

Robb, J. P. 1948. Effects of cortical excision and stimulation of the frontal lobe on speech. *Research Publications, Association for Research in Nervous and Mental Disease*, 27, 587–609.

Russell, W. R., & Espir, M. L. E. 1961. *Traumatic aphasia*. London: Oxford University Press.

Scheinker, I., & Kuhr, B. M. 1948. Motor aphasia and agraphia caused by small vascular lesion confined to third and second convolutions of left frontal lobe. *Research Publications, Association for Research in Nervous and Mental Disease*, 27, 582–586.

Simpson, J. H. 1867. On a case of extensive lesion of the left posterior frontal convolution of the cerebrum, without aphasia. *Medical Times and Gazette, 2,* 670.

Singer, M., & Yakovlev, P. I. 1954. *The human brain in sagittal section.* Springfield, Ill.: Charles C Thomas.

Taveras, J. M., & Wood, E. H. 1964. *Diagnostic neuroradiology.* Baltimore: Williams & Wilkins. Pp. 1.691–1.718.

Tuke, J. B., & Fraser, J. 1872. Case with a lesion involving Broca's convolution without Broca's aphasia. *Journal of Mental Science, 18,* 46–56.

Wadham, W. 1869. On aphasia. *St. George's Hospital Reports, 4,* 245–250.

Weisenburg, T., & McBride, K. E. 1964. *Aphasia.* New York: Hafner.

Wernicke, C. 1874. *Der Aphasische Symptomencomplex.* Breslau: Cohn & Weigert.

Wernicke, C. 1908. The symptomcomplex of aphasia. In A. Church (Ed.), *Modern clinical medicine. New York: Appleton. Pp.* 265–324.

Wyllie, J. 1894. *The disorders of speech.* Edinburgh: Oliver.

Yakovlev, P. I. 1970. Whole brain serial histological sections. In C. G. Tedeschi (Ed). *Neuropathology: Methods and diagnosis.* Boston: Little, Brown. Pp. 371–378.

Author Index

Note: Page numbers followed by f and t refer to figures and tables, respectively.

Subject Index

Note: Page numbers followed by f and t refer to figures and tables, respectively.